Body Image, Eating, and Weight

Massimo Cuzzolaro · Secondo Fassino
Editors

Body Image, Eating, and Weight

A Guide to Assessment, Treatment, and Prevention

Springer

Editors
Massimo Cuzzolaro
Formerly University Sapienza of Rome
Editor-in-Chief of Eating and Weight Disorders
Campiglia Marittima (LI)
Italy

Secondo Fassino
Department of Neuroscience
University of Turin
Torino
Italy

ISBN 978-3-319-90816-8 ISBN 978-3-319-90817-5 (eBook)
https://doi.org/10.1007/978-3-319-90817-5

Library of Congress Control Number: 2018955861

This Springer imprint is published by the registered company Springer Nature Switzerland AG
The registered company address is: Gewerbestrasse 11, 6330 Cham, Switzerland

Preface

The living human body feels, conceives, imagines, represents, evaluates, loves, hates, and manipulates itself. The relationship between a human being and his/her own body is a borderland, an area of study and practice open to philosophers, historians, sociologists, artists, anthropologists, anatomists, aesthetic physicians, plastic surgeons, neuroscientists, neurosurgeons, neurologists, psychiatrists, psychologists, and bioethicists.

Disturbances of the so-called body image are crucial issues in eating and weight disorders.

The book deals with the interface between body image and eating and weight disorders (anorexia nervosa, bulimia nervosa, binge eating disorder, orthorexia nervosa, overweight, obesity, etc.) to offer a comprehensive and up-to-date review of research findings and theoretical assumptions.

Disorders of body experience may be associated with identified lesions and diseases affecting the nervous system or be part of some psychiatric syndromes without established neurobiological alterations. They challenge the descriptive classifications of mental disorders. In fact, body image disturbances are also linked to intrapsychic mechanisms as well as different cultural inputs across the lifespan.

The first chapter of the book explores the umbrella concepts of body image and body schema from different viewpoints.

The knotty problems of definition and classification of eating disorders, body image disorders, and obesities are discussed to shed light on the current debate (Chaps. 2, 4, and 13).

Chapter 3 is devoted to the body image assessment methods in children, adolescents, and adults.

Chapter 5 reviews the syndrome that in the last three decades has been called body dysmorphic disorder, while the historical roots of the invention of dysmorphophobia at the end of the nineteenth century are analyzed in Chap. 6.

Neuroscientific and brain imaging studies on body image in eating and weight disorders are examined in Chap. 7.

Five chapters (Chaps. 8–12) discuss body image disturbances in different eating disorders, according to the current classifications, while four chapters (Chaps. 14–17) examine body image problems in higher-weight children, adolescents, adults, and after weight loss.

Chapters 18 and 19 consider specific issues associated with native gender, gender identity, and sexual orientation.

The effects of sexual abuse on body image and eating and weight-control behaviors are explored in Chap. 20. Feminist perspectives on the etiology and treatment of body image disturbance in eating disorders are the subject of Chap. 24.

Two chapters review studies on body shame (Chap. 27) and the consequences of social weight stigma (Chap. 28), while Chap. 31 investigates some cultural differences.

Chapter 29 reviews the studies on body image, eating, and weight disorders in models, dancers, and aesthetic athletes.

Treatment of body image disturbances associated with eating and weight disorders is the topic of five chapters devoted to pharmacotherapy (Chap. 26), psychodynamic psychotherapies (Chap. 21), family functioning (Chap. 22), transdiagnostic cognitive behavioral therapy (Chap. 23), and virtual reality, a new promising research field described in Chap. 25.

Chapter 30 discusses the experiments of integrated prevention of eating and weight disorders and the role of body image in those programs.

All the authors tried to offer a clear even if problematic overview of the above-mentioned topical questions.

Health professionals who work in the fields of eating disorders, obesity, body image, adolescence, public health, and prevention should be interested.

Rome, Italy Massimo Cuzzolaro
Turin, Italy Secondo Fassino

Contents

Contributors

Giovanni Abbate-Daga Eating Disorders Center, Department of Neuroscience, University of Turin, Turin, Italy

Federico Amianto Eating Disorders Center for Treatment and Research, Department of Neuroscience, University of Turin, Turin, Italy

Matteo Balestrieri University of Udine, Udine, Italy

Ottavio Bosello Department of Medicine, University of Verona, Verona, Italy

Anna Brytek-Matera SWPS University of Social Sciences and Humanities, Katowice, Poland

Federica Buongiorno Department of Medicine, University of Padova, Padova, Italy

Luca Busetto Department of Medicine, University of Padova, Padova, Italy

Rachel M. Calogero Department of Psychology, Western University, London, ON, Canada

Simona Calugi Department of Eating and Weight Disorders, Villa Garda Hospital, Garda (VR), Italy

Giovanni Castellini Psychiatric Unit, Department of Health Sciences, Florence University School of Medicine, Florence, Italy

Gianluca Castelnuovo Istituto Auxologico Italiano IRCCS, Psychology Research Laboratory, Ospedale San Giuseppe, Verbania, Italy

Department of Psychology, Catholic University of Milan, Milan, Italy

Roberto Cattivelli Istituto Auxologico Italiano IRCCS, Psychology Research Laboratory, Ospedale San Giuseppe, Verbania, Italy

Department of Psychology, Catholic University of Milan, Milan, Italy

Cesare Cavalera Department of Psychology, Catholic University of Milan, Milan, Italy

Massimo Cuzzolaro Formerly Medical Pathophysiology Department, Eating Disorders and Obesity Unit, Sapienza University of Rome, Rome, Italy

Antonios Dakanalis Department of Medicine and Surgery, University of Milano Bicocca, Milan, Italy

Department of Brain and Behavioral Sciences, University of Pavia, Pavia, Italy

Department of Clinical Psychology and Psychobiology, University of Barcelona, Barcelona, Spain

Applied Technology for Neuro-Psychology Lab, Istituto Auxologico Italiano, Milan, Italy

Riccardo Dalle Grave Department of Eating and Weight Disorders, Villa Garda Hospital, Garda (VR), Italy

Daniela Degortes Department of Neurosciences, University of Padova, Padua, Italy

Claudia Delicato Department of Translational Medicine, Institute of Psychiatry, University of Eastern Piedmont, Novara, Italy

Maria Pia Donataccio Department of Medicine, University of Verona, Verona, Italy

Lorenzo M. Donini Sapienza University of Rome, Rome, Italy

Giuseppe Fariello Department of Diagnostic Imaging, Ospedale San Pietro Fatebenefratelli, Rome, Italy

Secondo Fassino Eating Disorders Center for Treatment and Research, Department of Neuroscience, University of Turin, Turin, Italy

Angela Favaro Department of Neurosciences, University of Padova, Padua, Italy

Marta Ferrer-García Department of Clinical Psychology and Psychobiology, University of Barcelona, Barcelona, Spain

Rita Francisco School of Human Sciences, Universidade Católica Portuguesa, Lisboa, Portugal

Santino Gaudio Department of Neuroscience, Functional Pharmacology, Uppsala University, Uppsala, Sweden

Centre for Integrated Research (CIR), Area of Diagnostic Imaging, Departmental Faculty of Medicine and Surgery, Università "Campus Bio-Medico di Roma", Rome, Italy

Carla Gramaglia Department of Translational Medicine, Psychiatry Institute, Università del Piemonte Orientale, Novara, Italy

SC Psichiatria—AOU Maggiore della Carità di Novara, Novara, Italy

Giovanni Gravina Hospital San Rossore, Pisa, Italy

Melinda A. Green Body Dissatisfaction and Eating Disorder Research Laboratory, Department of Psychology, Cornell College, Mt Vernon, IA, USA

José Gutiérrez-Maldonado Department of Clinical Psychology and Psychobiology, University of Barcelona, Barcelona, Spain

Caterina Lombardo Department of Psychology, Sapienza University of Rome, Rome, Italy

Emilia Manzato University of Ferrara, Ferrara, Italy

Gian Mauro Manzoni Istituto Auxologico Italiano IRCCS, Psychology Research Laboratory, Ospedale San Giuseppe, Verbania, Italy

Faculty of Psychology, eCampus University, Novedrate (Como), Italy

Enrica Marzola Eating Disorders Center, Department of Neuroscience, University of Turin, Turin, Italy

Angela Meadows School of Psychology, University of Exeter, Exeter, UK

Walter Milano ASL Napoli 1, Napoli, Italy

Mental Disorders Department, Eating Disorders Unit, Napoli, Italy

Enrico Molinari Istituto Auxologico Italiano IRCCS, Psychology Research Laboratory, Ospedale San Giuseppe, Verbania, Italy

Department of Psychology, Catholic University of Milan, Milan, Italy

Alessio Maria Monteleone Department of Psychiatry, University of Campania "L. Vanvitelli", Naples, Italy

Palmiero Monteleone Department of Psychiatry, University of Campania "L. Vanvitelli", Naples, Italy

Department of Medicine, Surgery and Dentistry "Scuola Medica Salernitana", University of Salerno, Salerno, Italy

Umberto Nizzoli Eating Disorders and Addictions Services of Reggio Emilia, Reggio Emilia, Italy

Italian Society for the Study of Eating Disorders (SISDCA), Reggio Emilia, Italy

Margherita Novelli Istituto Auxologico Italiano IRCCS, Psychology Research Laboratory, Ospedale San Giuseppe, Verbania, Italy

Giada Pietrabissa Istituto Auxologico Italiano IRCCS, Psychology Research Laboratory, Ospedale San Giuseppe, Verbania, Italy

Department of Psychology, Catholic University of Milan, Milan, Italy

Alessandra Pokrajac-Bulian University of Rijeka, Faculty of Humanities and Social Sciences, Department of Psychology, Rijeka, Croatia

Valdo Ricca Psychiatric Unit, Department of Health Sciences, Florence University School of Medicine, Florence, Italy

Giuseppe Riva Centro Studi e Ricerche di Psicologia della Comunicazione, Università Cattolica del Sacro Cuore, Milan, Italy

Applied Technology for Neuro-Psychology Lab, Istituto Auxologico Italiano, Milan, Italy

Alessandro Rossi Istituto Auxologico Italiano IRCCS, Psychology Research Laboratory, Ospedale San Giuseppe, Verbania, Italy

Paolo Santonastaso Department of Neurosciences, University of Padova, Padua, Italy

Federica Scarpina Istituto Auxologico Italiano IRCCS, Psychology Research Laboratory, Ospedale San Giuseppe, Verbania, Italy

"Rita Levi Montalcini" Department of Neuroscience, University of Turin, Turin, Italy

Sami Schiff Department of Medicine, University of Padova, Padova, Italy

Silvia Serino Centro Studi e Ricerche di Psicologia della Comunicazione, Università Cattolica del Sacro Cuore, Milan, Italy

Applied Technology for Neuro-Psychology Lab, Istituto Auxologico Italiano, Milan, Italy

Patrizia Todisco Eating Disorders Unit, Villa Margherita, Vicenza, Italy

Angiola Vanzo Department of Food Hygiene and Nutrition, ULSS 8 Berica, Vicenza, Italy

Giorgia Varallo Istituto Auxologico Italiano IRCCS, Psychology Research Laboratory, Ospedale San Giuseppe, Verbania, Italy

Valentina Villa Istituto Auxologico Italiano IRCCS, Psychology Research Laboratory, Ospedale San Giuseppe, Verbania, Italy

Umberto Volpe Department of Psychiatry, University of Campania "L. Vanvitelli", Naples, Italy

Patrizia Zeppegno Department of Translational Medicine, Psychiatry Institute, Università del Piemonte Orientale, Novara, Italy

SC Psichiatria—AOU Maggiore della Carità di Novara, Novara, Italy

Body Schema and Body Image: History and Controversies

1

Massimo Cuzzolaro

1.1 Introduction

The language is a primary clinical and research tool. The expressions *body schema* and *body image* have been increasingly used in the scientific literature of the twentieth century, especially the second one (Fig. 1.1). They appear in neurological, psychiatric, psychological, psychoanalytical, sociological, and phenomenological studies of body experience, sometimes as distinct concepts, at other times as synonyms.

In 1986, Shaun Gallagher put the accent on the "conceptual confusion and the terminological ambiguity" connected with the use of these expressions and proposed "a phenomenological clarification" [1] (p. 541). He suggested that *body image* should indicate "a conscious awareness of one's own body", perceptual, cognitive, emotional, and differentiated from the environment (p. 544). In contrast, he defined the *body schema* as a non-conscious system of sensory-motor capacities, a pre-personal, holistic "performance of the body" that functions in communion with its environment (p. 549 and 552). In 2005, Gallagher confirmed and developed his distinction in a book that was a relevant contribution to the recent theory of *embodied cognition* [2].

Recurrently, scientists and philosophers have tried to more clearly define these possible two types of body representation and the interactions between *the body we perceive* and *the body we act with* [3, 4]. However, a shared and consistent definition of these two concepts, with a clear distinction between them, does not exist yet.

Some old and recent books and articles may offer a powerful lens through which to inspect the remote antecedents of these two metaphorical terms and their still uncertain boundaries. Table 1.1 is an arbitrary choice of some significant stages in

M. Cuzzolaro
Formerly Medical Pathophysiology Department, Eating Disorders and Obesity Unit, Sapienza University of Rome, Rome, Italy

M. Cuzzolaro, S. Fassino (eds.), *Body Image, Eating, and Weight*,
https://doi.org/10.1007/978-3-319-90817-5_1

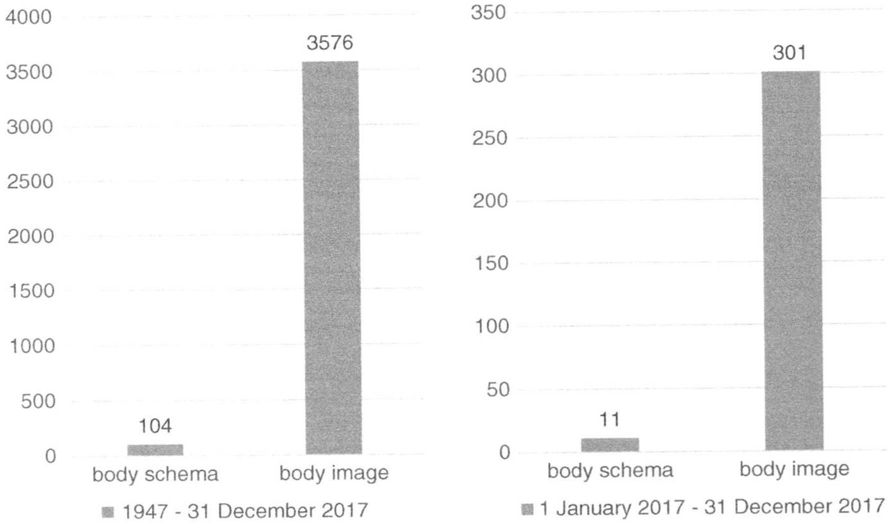

Fig. 1.1 Number of PubMed articles with a title that contains *body schema* or *body image*

Table 1.1 A list of some historical steps in the study of mental body representations

Year	First author	Concepts and words
1545	A. Paré	Paré first described a phenomenon that was later called 'phantom limb'
1794	C.F. Hübner	*Caenesthesis* (coenaesthesia, or coenaesthesis, or coenesthesia, or cenesthesia)
1882	J. Cotard	*délire des négations* (delusion of negation)
1891	E. Morselli	*dismorfofobia* (dysmorphophobia)
1898	L. Dugas	*dépersonnalisation* (depersonalization)
1900	C. Wernicke	*Somatopsyche* (self-consciousness of the body)
1903	P.M.F. Janet	*obsession de la honte du corps* (the obsession of body shame)
1905	P. Bonnier	*schéma corporel* (body schema)
1908	A. Pick	*Autotopagnosie* (autotopagnosia, somatotopagnosia)
1914	J. Babinski	*anosognosie* (anosognosia), *anosodiaphorie* (anosodiaphoria)
1923	P.F. Schilder	*Körperschema*
1935	P.F. Schilder	body image
1937	W. Penfield	cortical *homunculus sensorius* and *homunculus motorius*
1939	J.J. Lhermitte	*l'image de notre corps* (the image of our own body)
1967	A. Stunkard	obesity and the body image
1984	J. Rodin	normative discontent
2000	T. Cash	body image and human appearance
2001	C. Semenza	towards a neuropsychological-based theory of body representation

the history of the studies on mental body representations, which are mentioned in detail in this chapter (italics for German, French, Latin, and Italian original words).

1.2 From the Concept of *Caenesthesis* to the DSM-5

For a long time, body awareness was regarded as an assemblage of sensations. In 1794, the word *Caenesthesis* appeared for the first time in the doctoral thesis of Christian Friedrich Hübner, inspired by the German physiologist and physician Johann Christian Reil (1759–1813) [5].

The term comes from the Greek κοινός (general) and αἴσθησις (sensation). The equivalent words are in German *Gemeingefühl* (general sensibility) or *Coenesthesie*, in French *sensibilité générale* or *cénesthésie* or *coenesthésie*, and in English *coenaesthesia*, or *cenesthesia*, or *coenesthesia*, or *coenaesthesis*.

Reil observed that some changes in cenesthesia were primary and not due to other disorders. He included in this class of his psychiatric taxonomy cases of hypochondria, melancholia, and dysfunction of appetites (e.g. polydipsia, bulimia, pica, nymphomania) [6]. About 100 years later a related word appeared in France, *cénestopathies* [7], to indicate the idiopathic disturbances of bodily sensations.

By the way, few years after Hübner's thesis, in a 118-page article [8], Reil coined another successful neologism, from the Greek ψυχή (soul) and ιάτρευσις (medical care): *Psychiaterie* (psychiatry) that he subsequently changed to *Psychiatrie*. Reil's paper documents that the word was created to highlight the need for a new primary medical discipline, the others being pharmacy (general or internal medicine) and surgery [9]. According to the author, human diseases are produced by the interaction of physicochemical and mental causes and the so-called *psychic therapy* is an essential treatment for both somatic and mental disorders, together with drugs and surgery.

From Reil and the so-called romantic medicine up to the first decades of the twentieth century, the expressions *cenesthesia* and *cenestopathy* became common in medicine to indicate the general sense of bodily existence and, in particular, the general feeling of well-being or malaise [10, 11]. Then, they were replaced by the expressions *body schema* and *body image*, apparently more specific, and the phenomenon of painful and disabling bodily sensations—often *sine materia* or medically unexplained—received many different names.

The DSM-IV classification included under the label of *somatoform disorders* seven clinical pictures: somatization disorder, undifferentiated somatoform disorder, somatoform disorder not otherwise specified, conversion disorder, pain disorder, body dysmorphic disorder (BDD), and hypochondriasis.

In DSM-5, BDD was set among the *obsessive-compulsive and related disorders* while hypochondriasis and related conditions were replaced by two only diagnostic

Table 1.2 Somatic symptoms and illness anxiety disorders in DSM-5

Somatic symptom disorder	Illness anxiety disorder
The person reports one or more chronic somatic symptoms about which he/she is excessively preoccupied or fearful	The person has heightened bodily sensations and is intensely anxious about the possibility of an undiagnosed illness
Distress and abnormal thoughts, feelings, and behaviours	
In both cases, the person may or may not have a known medical condition	

categories: *somatic symptom disorder* and *illness anxiety disorder* (Table 1.2). The presence of somatic symptoms is only required for the first disorder, while high health anxiety is a shared diagnostic criterion.

This sweeping change has been criticized. In particular, by eliminating the concept of *medically unexplained symptoms*, the new classification appears too broad and could lead to more psychiatric diagnoses among persons with medical diseases.

1.3 To Feel One's Own Body in a Right or Distorted Way

More scientific studies on the mental representation of the body began in the second half of the nineteenth century. The conceptual boundaries between neurology and psychiatry were (and continue to be) uncertain, and some classic and recent case studies about disturbances of the self-representation of the body are still hard to understand and classify as neurological or mental disorders [12].

In the late nineteenth century, the German physiologist Hermann Munk (1839–1912) made small experimental lesions on the brain of dogs to prove that representations of the body were stored in definite cortical regions. In particular, he found that specific areas of the parietal cortex received sensory inputs from distinct parts of the body and presumed that these cortical areas saved the corresponding images [13].

In the wake of Munk, another eminent neurologist, Carl Wernicke (1848–1905), assumed that the cortex of the brain merged together the sensory signals sent by various body portions and built a sort of picture of each body segment in the space.

As a result, he accounted for the awareness of one's body in the space as a bottom-up phenomenon produced by the cortical integration of many different, external (tactile, visual, auditory), and internal (muscular, visceral) sensory inputs. To define the integrating self-consciousness of the body, Wernicke coined the neologism *Somatopsyche* [14].

A lot of clinical observations have proved that the experience of one's own body may be distorted in very many ways.

The medical history of an unexpected possible consequence of an amputation was initiated by Ambroise Paré (1510–1590), a notable French barber-surgeon of the Renaissance, who is considered the father of modern surgery. Paré operated on wounded soldiers and wrote that some of them complained of pain in amputated limbs [15]. Three centuries after, during the American Civil War, the surgeon Silas Weir Mitchell (1829–1914), observed the same phenomenon, characterized by both painful and non-painful sensations, and coined the expression *phantom limb* [16].

The majority of the individuals born with underdeveloped or absent limbs (phocomelia, amelia) do not report this syndrome. However, some persons with these malformations testify the existence of phantom sensations. If the cortical representation of the body is developed with experience or innate is still an open question [17].

Parenthetically, it may happen that a person who has lost a lot of weight still perceives his/her body as much heavier. This phenomenon is sometimes called *phantom fat* or, more accurately, *vestigial effects of overweight* [18].

Some persons feel a body part that does no longer exist. Other individuals do not feel a body part that is present. In 1882, Jules Cotard created the expression *délire des négations* (*delusion of negation*) and described 11 clinical cases (three men and eight women) with this symptom [19]. The affected persons denied the existence of their body or some body parts, rejected the need to eat, believed that the internal organs were displaced, or were putrefying.

A recent clinical and neuroimaging study of 12 patients with Cotard's syndrome found that these symptoms occur in the context of a broad spectrum of medical, neurological, and psychiatric disorders with various brain changes and lesions, in particular in the non-dominant hemisphere [20].

In 1891, the alienist Enrico Morselli described a morbid condition in which a person is afflicted by the preoccupation with some unreal or negligible imperfections in his/her physical appearance and coined the Italian neologism *dismorfofobia* (dysmorphophobia) (see Chap. 6 of the present volume).

In DSM-III-R, the word *dysmorphophobia* was officially replaced by the expression *body dysmorphic disorder* (BDD) (see Chap. 5 of the present volume).

In 1898, Ludovic Dugas (1857–1942) coined the term *depersonalization* to label a singular experience: the individual becomes a stranger to himself, he does not feel his body as his own, his voice sounds unfamiliar, etc. [21].

In 1903, the neurologist and neurosurgeon Otfrid Foerster (1873–1941) described a 50-year-old woman who suffered from a similar enigmatic disorder: she did not feel her head, eyes, hands anymore. Furthermore, well-known persons and objects did not look familiar to her. Following Wernicke, Foerster called that disordered representation of the body parts *Afunktion der Somatopsyche* [22].

Two years later, Gaston Deny and Paul Camus published an article about comparable symptoms: a woman who did not feel her head, hair, limbs anymore [23]. She felt her body changed and had to touch herself unceasingly.

DSM-5 classified these clinical pictures as *depersonalization-derealization disorders* [24].

1.4 Unawareness of Deficits and Illnesses

Lucius Annaeus Seneca (4 BC–AD 65) was likely the first to describe a phenomenon of non-awareness of cortical blindness in the *Epistula L ad Lucilium* [25]. Many centuries after, other cases of non-awareness of illness (in particular, cortical blindness and left hemiplegia) were reported by Constantin von Monakow (1853–1930) [26], Gabriel Anton (1858–1933) [27, 28], and Arnold Pick (1851–1924) [29].

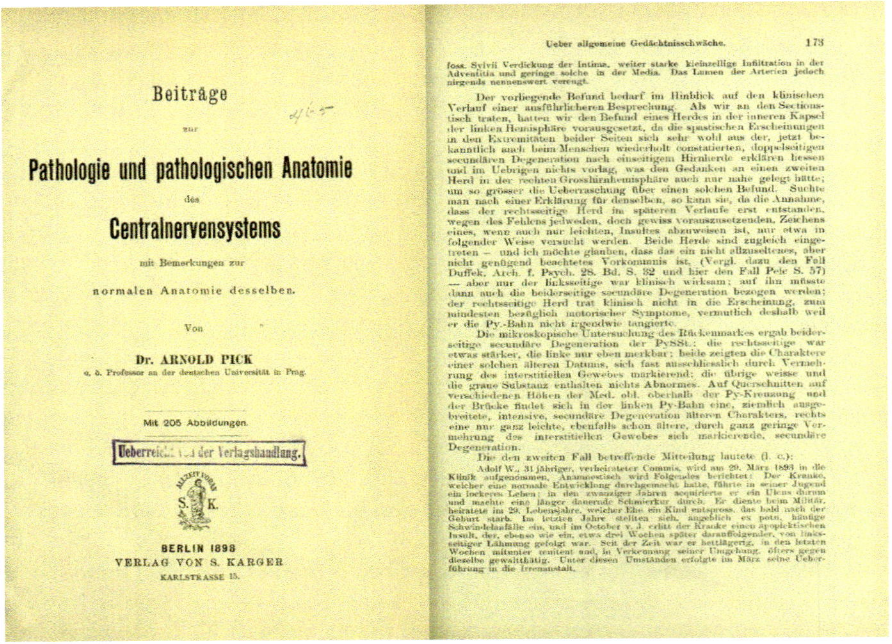
Beiträge

zur

Pathologie und pathologischen Anatomie

des

Centralnervensystems

mit Bemerkungen zur

normalen Anatomie desselben.

Von

Dr. ARNOLD PICK

o. ö. Professor an der deutschen Universität in Prag.

Mit 205 Abbildungen.

Ueberreicht von der Verlagshandlung.

S. K.

BERLIN 1898

VERLAG VON S. KARGER

KARLSTRASSE 15.

Ueber allgemeine Gedächtnisschwäche. 173

foss. Sylvii Verdickung der Intima, weiter starke kleinzellige Infiltration in der Adventitia und geringe solche in der Media. Das Lumen der Arterien jedoch nirgends nennenswert verengt.

Der vorliegende Befund bedarf im Hinblick auf den klinischen Verlauf einer ausführlicheren Besprechung. Als wir an den Sectionstisch traten, hatten wir den Befund eines Herdes in der inneren Kapsel der linken Hemisphäre vorausgesetzt, da die spastischen Erscheinungen in den Extremitäten beider Seiten sich sehr wohl aus der, jetzt bekanntlich auch beim Menschen wiederholt constatierten, doppelseitigen secundären Degeneration nach einseitigem Hirnherde erklären liessen und im Uebrigen nichts vorlag, was den Gedanken an einen zweiten Herd in der rechten Grosshirnhemisphäre auch nur nahe gelegt hätte; um so grösser die Ueberraschung über einen solchen Befund. Suchte man nach einer Erklärung für denselben, so kann sie, da die Annahme, dass der rechtsseitige Herd im späteren Verlaufe erst entstanden, wegen des Fehlens jedweden, doch gewiss vorauszusetzenden, Zeichens eines, wenn auch nur leichten, Insultes abzuweisen ist, nur etwa in folgender Weise versucht werden. Beide Herde sind zugleich eingetreten – und ich möchte glauben, dass das ein nicht allzuseltenes, aber nicht genügend beachtetes Vorkommnis ist. (Vergl. dazu den Fall Duffek, Arch. f. Psych. 28. Bd. S. 32 und hier den Fall Pelc S. 57) — aber nur der linksseitige war klinisch wirksam; auf ihn müsste dann auch die beiderseitige secundäre Degeneration bezogen werden; der rechtsseitige Herd trat klinisch nicht in die Erscheinung, zum mindesten bezüglich motorischer Symptome, vermutlich deshalb weil er die Py.-Bahn nicht irgendwie tangierte.

Die mikroskopische Untersuchung des Rückenmarkes ergab beiderseitige secundäre Degeneration der PySSt.: die rechtsseitige war etwas stärker, die linke nur eben merkbar; beide zeigten die Charaktere einer solchen älteren Datums, sich fast ausschliesslich durch Vermehrung des interstitiellen Gewebes markierend; die übrige weisse und die graue Substanz enthalten nichts Abnormes. Auf Querschnitten auf verschiedenen Höhen der Med. obl. oberhalb der Py-Kreuzung und der Brücke findet sich in der linken Py-Bahn eine, ziemlich ausgebreitete, intensive, secundäre Degeneration älteren Charakters, rechts eine nur ganz leichte, ebenfalls schon ältere, durch ganz geringe Vermehrung des interstitiellen Gewebes sich markierende, secundäre Degeneration.

Die den zweiten Fall betreffende Mitteilung lautete (l. c.):

Adolf W., 31 jähriger, verheirateter Commis, wird am 29. März 1893 in die Klinik aufgenommen. Anamnestisch wird Folgendes berichtet: Der Kranke, welcher eine normale Entwicklung durchgemacht hatte, führte in seiner Jugend ein lockeres Leben; in den zwanziger Jahren acquirierte er ein Ulcus durum und machte eine länger dauernde Schmierkur durch. Er diente beim Militär, heiratete im 29. Lebensjahre, welcher Ehe ein Kind entspross, das bald nach der Geburt starb. Im letzten Jahre stellten sich, angeblich ex potu, häufige Schwindelanfälle ein, und im October v. J. erlitt der Kranke einen apoplektischen Insult, der, ebenso wie ein, etwa drei Wochen später darauffolgender, von linksseitiger Lähmung gefolgt war. Seit der Zeit war er bettlägerig, in den letzten Wochen mitunter renitent und, in Verkennung seiner Umgebung, öfters gegen dieselbe gewaltthätig. Unter diesen Umständen erfolgte im März seine Ueberführung in die Irrenanstalt.

Fig. 1.2 Adolf W, a case of non-awareness of left hemiplegia (Arnold Pick, 1898)

For example, Pick reported that Adolf W, a 31-year-old patient with a severe left hemiplegia without somato-sensory deficits in the paralysed limbs, was not aware of his handicap. He wanted to show that he could walk as before and wondered about the fact that he had been dismissed from the army. The post-mortem neuropathological diagnosis was neurosyphilis with encephalomalacia of the left temporal lobe and the right thalamus [29] (p. 173–180) (Fig. 1.2).

In 1914, Joseph Babinski (1857–1932) coined the word *anosognosie* (anosognosia, from the Greek alpha privative + νόσος, illness + γνῶσις, knowledge) to denote the condition of a person who is unaware of his/her disability due to a brain injury (e.g. hemiplegia) [30]. Besides, he created the term *anosodiaphorie* (anosodiaphoria, from the Greek διαφορά, difference) for a person who verbally acknowledges a deficit but appears indifferent to it.

It is worth mentioning that in his article Babinski spoke of *hémiplegie organique cérébrale* (organic brain hemiplegia) and *troubles mentaux* (mental disorders): he considered hemiplegia as a brain disease but anosognosia and anosodiaphoria as mental disorders. Babinski aimed to mark the bounds of neurology by the evidence of definite alterations of the nervous system associated with specific symptoms.

The loss of motor awareness follows, in particular, right-hemisphere damage and represents an opportunity to study the neurocognitive basis of body awareness. Some authors suggested that right-hemisphere spatial capacities may underlie our ability to take third-person perspectives (more *objective*) about our body. They found that patients with anosognosia performed worse than controls in 'third-person perspective taking abilities' [31].

What, if anything, links up Babinski's anosognosia with *lack of insight* observed in many psychiatric disorders, including anorexia nervosa (AN) and BDD?

Insight is a multidimensional concept with inconsistent definitions.

In the psychoanalytic literature, the concept of *insight* has a more comprehensive meaning, and its cornerstone is the experiential recognition of unconscious mental processes and conflicts, emotional states, defence mechanisms, transference, resistance to change, advantages by illness. The expression *insight-oriented therapy* is often used in this sense.

In the psychiatric mental status evaluation, the concept of *insight* involves two main components: (a) the patient's knowledge that his/her symptoms are morbid phenomena, and (b) the recognition of the need for treatment.

There are three main interpretations of *lack of insight*:

- It is an intrinsic component of the psychiatric disorder itself (e.g. during a severe manic episode).
- It is a psychological defence mechanism (denial) that protects the patient from the disturbing awareness of a disease.
- It is a neuropsychological deficit resulting from a brain lesion or dysfunction.

Intellectual insight usually indicates the objective knowledge of a problematic situation without the drive to change.

DSM-5 introduced a *dimensional insight specifier* among the diagnostic criteria for BDD to indicate the *degree of delusionality* (see Chap. 5 of the present volume). However, expressions such as *good, fair, poor, limited, absent*, or *improving insight* are sketchy and superficial evaluations.

Several standardized scales of insight have been published and may be helpful [32]. They are primarily used in the research setting but rarely in everyday clinical practice.

To clarify the relationship of the terms—*anosognosia* and *insight*—to the referent phenomena, Marková and Berrios suggested that *awareness* and *insight* are "the narrower and wider form of self-knowledge patients have concerning their conditions" [33] (p. 421). Self-knowledge is narrow (*awareness*) when it refers to the impairment of a specific function, as in the neurosciences, and is wide (*insight*) when it relates to the mental symptoms, as in psychopathology.

However, the distinction is not indisputable, and it is not proven that the underlying mechanisms are entirely different.

1.5 The Emergence of Fat Phobia and Drive for Thinness as Symptoms

Physicians and neurologists such as Richard Morton (1637–1698) [34], Robert Whytt (1714–1766) [35], William Gull (1816–1890) [36, 37], Ernest-Charles Lasègue (1816–1883) [38], Jean-Martin Charcot (1825–1893) [39], and Georges Gilles de la Tourette (1857–1904) described patients with symptoms very similar to those of contemporary AN except for fear of fatness and weight and shape worries. By the way, Gilles de la Tourette wrote that Charcot observed at least four cases of persons with *anorexie hystérique* (hysterical anorexia) who died [40] (p. 531). Therefore, they were not less seriously ill than patients of our days.

Before Gull and Lasègue, in 1860, a rarely mentioned French alienist, Louis-Victor Marcé (1828–1864), used the term *anorexie* to designate the chief symptom of two girls (14 and 19 years old), *le refus d'aliments* (the refusal of food). Marcé made it clear that the nature of the illness was psychopathological. He brought to light that body experience was deeply troubled in these cases, but considered the clinical picture as a form of hypochondria and spoke of *délire hypochondriaque* (hypochondriacal delusion) [41, 42].

Pierre Marie Félix Janet (1859–1947) was the first scientist to report in detail the case of an unmarried woman of 27 years, called Nadia, whose core symptom was the food refusal "*pour la crainte d'engraisser*" (for fear of becoming fat) [43] (p. 33–40). Her daily diet included one cup of tea with the juice of one lemon, two cups of consommé, one egg yolk, and one teaspoon of vinegar.

Nadia—a pseudonym that was chosen by herself—was described as thin but her weight was never mentioned. Would she meet DSM-5 diagnostic criteria for AN [24]? It is an impossible question to answer because we don't know if Nadia's body weight was significantly low, that is less than minimally normal (DSM-5 Criterion A, see Chap. 4 of the present volume).

The girl told Janet that her intense body uneasiness started from a very early age—even from her fourth year—because she was told she was too tall for her age. Then she found her arms too fat and her hands too long and ridiculous. Moreover, she felt ashamed of feet, hips, and legs, at which she thought everyone was looking.

From puberty, Nadia rejected her usual food, in spite of intense hunger because she wanted to be thin, without sex, indeed without a body. Until her twentieth year, she removed her pubic hair that she considered "*monstruosité … ornement de sauvage*" (monstrosity … savage ornament) [43] (p. 39).

She refused maturity: "Je ne voulais, dit-elle, ni grossir, ni grandir, ni ressembler à une femme parce que j'aurais voulu rester toujours petite fille … j'avais peur d'être moins aimée ... si on me voyait bien en pleine lumière on serait dégoûté et on ne m'aimerait plus" (I did not wish, she said, to gain weight, or to grow tall, or to resemble a woman because I always wanted to remain a little girl … I was afraid of not being loved as before … a person who saw me in a good light, would be disgusted and would not love me anymore) [43] (p. 40).

Nadia was referred to Janet at the age of 22 as a case of *anorexie hystérique*, but he challenged this diagnosis, which he considered, moreover, uncertain and in need of elucidation. The French alienist judged that his patient did not present two essential symptoms, required to identify a hysterical anorexia: loss of appetite (due to a supposed hysterical anaesthesia of gastric nerves) and psycho-motor paroxysms. He concluded that Nadia suffered primarily from an obsessional contempt and shame of her entire body that he classified as a form of "obsession de la honte du corps" (obsessional body shame) [43] (p. 36) (Fig. 1.3).

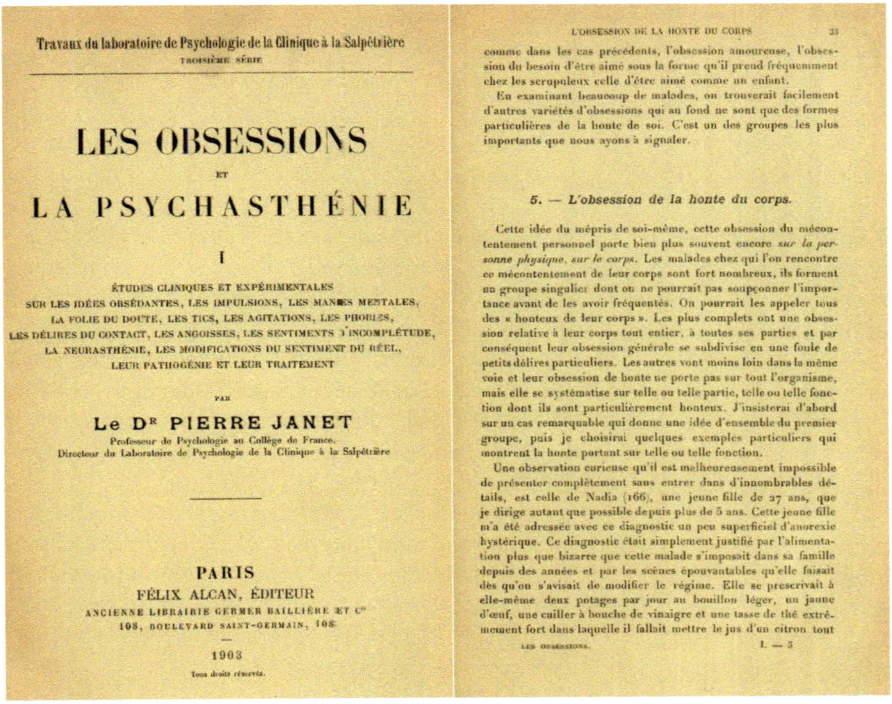

Travaux du laboratoire de Psychologie de la Clinique à la Salpêtrière
TROISIÈME SÉRIE

LES OBSESSIONS
ET
LA PSYCHASTHÉNIE

I

ÉTUDES CLINIQUES ET EXPÉRIMENTALES
SUR LES IDÉES OBSÉDANTES, LES IMPULSIONS, LES MANIES MENTALES,
LA FOLIE DU DOUTE, LES TICS, LES AGITATIONS, LES PHOBIES,
LES DÉLIRES DU CONTACT, LES ANGOISSES, LES SENTIMENTS D'INCOMPLÉTUDE,
LA NEURASTHÉNIE, LES MODIFICATIONS DU SENTIMENT DU RÉEL,
LEUR PATHOGÉNIE ET LEUR TRAITEMENT

PAR

Le DR PIERRE JANET
Professeur de Psychologie au Collège de France,
Directeur du Laboratoire de Psychologie de la Clinique à la Salpêtrière

PARIS
FÉLIX ALCAN, ÉDITEUR
ANCIENNE LIBRAIRIE GERMER BAILLIÈRE ET Cie
108, BOULEVARD SAINT-GERMAIN, 108

1903
Tous droits réservés.

L'OBSESSION DE LA HONTE DU CORPS 33

comme dans les cas précédents, l'obsession amoureuse, l'obsession du besoin d'être aimé sous la forme qu'il prend fréquemment chez les scrupuleux celle d'être aimé comme un enfant.

En examinant beaucoup de malades, on trouverait facilement d'autres variétés d'obsessions qui au fond ne sont que des formes particulières de la honte de soi. C'est un des groupes les plus importants que nous ayons à signaler.

5. — L'obsession de la honte du corps.

Cette idée du mépris de soi-même, cette obsession du mécontentement personnel porte bien plus souvent encore *sur la personne physique, sur le corps*. Les malades chez qui l'on rencontre ce mécontentement de leur corps sont fort nombreux, ils forment un groupe singulier dont on ne pourrait pas soupçonner l'importance avant de les avoir fréquentés. On pourrait les appeler tous des « honteux de leur corps ». Les plus complets ont une obsession relative à leur corps tout entier, à toutes ses parties et par conséquent leur obsession générale se subdivise en une foule de petits délires particuliers. Les autres vont moins loin dans la même voie et leur obsession de honte ne porte pas sur tout l'organisme, mais elle se systématise sur telle ou telle partie, telle ou telle fonction dont ils sont particulièrement honteux. J'insisterai d'abord sur un cas remarquable qui donne une idée d'ensemble du premier groupe, puis je choisirai quelques exemples particuliers qui montrent la honte portant sur telle ou telle fonction.

Une observation curieuse qu'il est malheureusement impossible de présenter complètement sans entrer dans d'innombrables détails, est celle de Nadia (166), une jeune fille de 27 ans, que je dirige autant que possible depuis plus de 5 ans. Cette jeune fille m'a été adressée avec ce diagnostic un peu superficiel d'anorexie hystérique. Ce diagnostic était simplement justifié par l'alimentation plus que bizarre que cette malade s'imposait dans sa famille depuis des années et par les scènes épouvantables qu'elle faisait dès qu'on s'avisait de modifier le régime. Elle se prescrivait à elle-même deux potages par jour au bouillon léger, un jaune d'œuf, une cuiller à bouche de vinaigre et une tasse de thé extrêmement fort dans laquelle il fallait mettre le jus d'un citron tout

LES OBSESSIONS. I. — 3

Fig. 1.3 Pierre Janet: anorexia nervosa as obsession of body shame

In the first volume of his treatise, Janet indicated Nadia as the "*Observation 166*" among 325 patients (230 women and 95 men) with obsessive thoughts [43] (p. XII).

Nadia was proud of imposing on herself a strict regimen and resisting to her great hunger. From time to time she capitulated and ate greedily everything she could with subsequent guilt and shame, but no mention of vomiting [43] (p. 36). Some authors considered Nadia an early example of *bulimia* [44].

As to bulimia, almost three decades after Janet, the physician and psychoanalyst Mosche Wulff (1878–1971), published an account on four women with overwhelming cravings for food [45]. He put the accent on the relationship of this syndrome to craving (in German: *Sucht*) and anticipated recent studies on addictive eating and food addiction [46]. Wulff's patients appear similar to the clinical pictures currently named *bulimia nervosa* (BN) or *binge eating disorder* (BED) [47, 48]. It is worth noting that shame and disgust (in German: *Ekel*) with the body were present in all cases (Table 1.3).

In the same years, also Ellen West—another classical case history—suffered from an intense body disparagement [49, 50].

Eating symptoms started with a bulimic phase when Ellen was 20 years old. For a tormenting dread of becoming fat, she used high doses of laxatives, thyroid tablets, and self-induced vomiting. Her weight varied again and again. During the last

Table 1.3 Wulff's four cases of binge eating

Case	Binge eating	Purging behaviours	Overweight/obesity	Disgust with the body
A	Yes	–	Yes	Yes
B	Yes	Vomiting	–	Yes
C	Yes	–	Yes	Yes
D	Yes	Vomiting	–	Yes

18 months of her life, she was underweight and amenorrhoeic, until her suicide, at the age of 33. Emil Kraepelin (1856–1926) made a diagnosis of manic-depressive psychosis. Ludwig Binswanger (1881–1966)—who treated Ellen West at the end of her life and, at least two decades after her death, published a detailed biographical account—discussed some diagnostic hypotheses: obsessive-compulsive neurosis, personality disorder, phobia, overvalued idea, delusional idea, manic-depressive psychosis, schizophrenia. He concluded that Ellen suffered from a progressive schizophrenic psychosis. This diagnosis had been supported by another famous psychiatrist, Eugen Bleuler (1857–1939).

As from Janet's case of Nadia, during the last century, eating patterns and body appearance concerns have become more and more intertwined. The rising interest in eating disorders (ED) has dragged a growing attention to the study of the so-called *body image*. However, for the same reason, research mainly focused on teen girls and young women and for a long time overlooked older people, men, higher weight individuals, disfiguring conditions, gender dysphoria, etc.

1.6 Bonnier and the Concept of Body Schema

Two years after Janet's description of the body appearance obsessions that afflicted Nadia, another French scientist, the otologist Pierre Bonnier (1861–1918), used for the first time the word *schéma* (English: *schema*). It indicated an internal, spatial, and topographic representation of one's own body [51].

He distinguished this new concept from the classical and more vague notions of *cenesthesia* and *cenestopathy*.

Bonnier—who had already published a book entitled *Le vertige* (vertigo)—was especially interested in the notion of *spatial sense*, the perception of our postures and gestures in the space and as to other persons and objects in the environment. He postulated the existence of a *body schema* to explain the human ability to locate a perceived stimulus accurately: inside the body, on its periphery, or at some distance from it.

A defective account of the space occupied by the body and its parts and of the localization of sensory inputs was the main feature of the disorders Bonnier collected under the labels *hyperschématie* (overestimation of body parts or the whole body), *hyposchématie* (underestimation), and *paraschématie* (displacement of body parts).

Besides he called *aschématie* the loss of body consciousness with a global disorientation and defined it with these words: "an anaesthesia confined to the topographic notion, to the spatial representation" of the body [52] (p. 605).

In his article, Bonnier reported some brief clinical observations, based only on the subjective complaints of some patients, in the absence of objective findings, such as a neurological assessment. In his opinion, all the patients suffered from a vestibulopathy. In fact, some of them showed psychiatric symptoms without evidence of neurological lesions: hysteria (patient h), depersonalization (patients b, d, h and perhaps i), and autoscopy (patient f).

In the following years, the expression *body schema* was increasingly used in the scientific literature, but Bonnier was rarely cited [53].

Henry Head (1861–1940) and Gordon Morgan Holmes (1876–1965) hypothesized the existence of two different schemata: a *postural schema* or *model* (recognitions of postures and gestures) and a *superficial schema* or *model* (localization of a stimulus applied to one point of the body surface). The schemata are plastic and continuously updated. Lesions of the cortex (in particular of the left parietal cortex) can damage them separately. Furthermore, Head and Holmes used the word *schema* to indicate the preconscious processes and reserved the term *image* to the conscious body representations [54, 55].

In the same years, also Arnold Pick (1851–1924) suggested that there is not one body schema but multiple body representations, based on different sensations, that contribute to the consciousness of one's own body (*Bewusstseins vom eigenen Körper*) [56]. Pick coined the word *Autotopagnosie* (autotopagnosia) to indicate a specific impairment of body recognition, the inability to locate body parts on command, e.g. the person cannot touch the part of his/her body that the examiner indicates verbally.

Autotopagnosia may affect localization only of one's body parts, only of other people's body parts, or both. It can be understood as a visuo-spatial deficit, as a semantic deficit, or both. In fact, *autotopagnosia*—or, better, *somatotopagnosia*—is an elusive and multifaceted phenomenon and in Pick's observations, the impaired representation in the brain of the lexicons was probably more relevant than the damaged body representation [57]. These phenomena have been more recently named *selective impairment of semantic memory* and *category and modality-specific aphasias*, in particular, *body-specific aphasias* [58, 59].

The expression *body schema* is still used, although rarely (Fig. 1.1), also in the studies on eating and weight disorders [60].

1.7 Schilder and the Concept of Body Image

The expression *body image* appeared in 1935, when the Viennese neuropathologist and psychoanalyst Paul Ferdinand Schilder (1886–1940) published, in English, *The image and appearance of the human body* [61].

Schilder called *body image* the multifaceted human experience of embodiment. From his point of view, it encompasses perceptions, emotions, feelings, thoughts, beliefs, actions, and interactions. His exact words are these:

> "The image of the human body means the picture of our own body which we form in our mind, that is to say the way in which the body appears to ourselves. There are sensations which are given to us. We see parts of the body surface. We have tactile, thermal, pain

impressions. There are sensations which come from the muscles and their sheaths, indicating the deformation of the muscle; sensations coming from the innervation of the muscles (energy sense, von Frey); and sensations coming from the viscera. Beyond that there is the immediate experience that there is a unity of the body. This unity is perceived, yet is more than a perception. We call it a schema of our body or bodily schema, or, following Head, who emphasizes the importance of the knowledge of the position of the body, postural model of the body. The body schema is the tri-dimensional image everybody has about himself. We may call it 'body image'. The term indicates that we are not dealing with a mere sensation or imagination. There is a self-appearance of the body. It indicates also that, although it has come through the senses, it is not a mere perception. There are mental pictures and representations involved in it, but it is not mere representation" [61] (Loc. 207–215).

This definition is anything but clear. Schilder speaks of a "picture of our own body which we form in our mind … tri-dimensional image everybody has about himself" and defines it negatively as "not mere perception … not mere representation".

Schilder's name is primarily connected to the expression *body image* or *bodily image* that has been translated into many languages (French *image du corps*, German *Körperbild*, Spanish *imagen corporal*). However, in the 1935 book, the words *schema* and *image* coexisted in the introduction and many chapters, without a clear distinction.

In 1923, Schilder had published a German book entitled *Das Körperschema* [62], focused on "those mechanisms of the central nervous system which are of importance for the building up of the spatial image which everybody has about himself" [61] (Loc. 146). Ever since then, it was clear to the scientist that:

"It would be erroneous to suppose that phenomenology and psychoanalysis should or could be separated from brain pathology … such a study must be based not only on physiology and neuropathology, but also on psychology" [61] (Loc. 150–154).

Schilder's solution encompassed empirical investigations and an eclectic approach. The primary sources were neurological studies, psychoanalytic theory, *Gestaltpsychologie*, and the bio-psycho-social model supported, in those years, in the United States, by the psychiatrist Adolf Meyer (1866–1950).

So, the 1935 book was explicitly addressed to neurologists, psychologists, and philosophers and divided into three parts: (1) *The physiological basis of the body image*, (2) *The libidinous structure of the body image*, and (3) *The sociology of the body image*. At the end of the book, two appendices were reserved for: (1) *Case histories of organic brain lesions*; (2) *Some remarks on the anatomy and physiology of the nervous system*.

In his book, Schilder first described in detail some phenomena such as finger agnosia, alloaesthesia, autotopagnosia, phantom limb, and anosognosia. Then, from a psychoanalytic point of view, he examined the role of narcissism and erogenous zones in the libidinal development of body image, and some clinical pictures such as hysteria, hypochondria, and depersonalization. Finally, he contemplated the social space and tackled topics such as bodily expression of emotions, erythrophobia (fear of blushing as an instance of social neurosis), and cultural norms for appearance and beauty. Especially in the third part of his book, Schilder highlighted the variability of the body image and the crucial influence of interpersonal relationships.

Only 4 years after Schilder's book, Jean Jacques Lhermitte (1877–1959), a French neurologist, published *L'image de notre corps* [63]. He declared that Bonnier's *body schema*, Wernicke's *Somatopsyche*, Head's *postural and superficial models*, and Schilder's *body image* were different names of the same thing, the *image of our own body*.

Like Schilder, Lhermitte considered *body image* and *body schema* as interchangeable terms. However, his viewpoint was different from Schilder's multidisciplinary statement of the problem. Lhermitte favoured the neurological outlooks and gave more space to the body image alterations due to a specific brain or peripheral lesion—for example, *les membres phantômes* (phantom limb)—than to some psychiatric syndromes.

After Schilder, neurological and psycho-sociological studies of body self-representations often followed separate roads.

As a consequence, many psychologists have not taken into account the neurological research on the self-representation of the body. On the other hand, most neurophysiological studies have not considered, for example, the role of the narcissism, i.e. "the fact that the 'self' and particularly the body is loved by its owner" [64] (p. 302). Some psychoanalysts observed that the concept of body image should collect both the imaginary and symbolic aspects of identity. The self-representation of the body "has a prominent role in building the necessary narcissistic illusion of the unity of the self" [64] (p. 302) and underlies a *first-person perspective*: '*I* am in this environment'.

In the last decades, Thomas Cash was a scientist who specially developed and supported a multidimensional approach to the study and treatment of the *inside* and the *outside* view of human appearance, the self- and social-perception of physical attractiveness, etc. [65–68]. In 2000, he founded the journal *Body image: an international journal of research*. In 2012, he was the editor-in-chief of the *Encyclopedia of body image and human appearance* that takes up the same two words present in Schilder's title: image and appearance [68].

In the last 70 years, the term *body image* has been more and more used (Fig. 1.1), also in the area of eating and weight disorders.

1.8 Penfield's *Homunculus* and Cerebral Cartography

In the middle between Schilder and Lhermitte, in 1937, Wilder Penfield and Edwin Boldrey published, in a seminal paper, the results of the electrical stimulation of the human cerebral cortex [69]. The observations were made during 163 neurosurgical operations executed by Penfield since 1928. The stimuli were carried out as an aid in searching an epileptogenic focus that needed to be eradicated, or to define the areas that, in case of infiltrating tumour, could be removed without producing paralysis. So the authors were able to relate the stimulation of a particular point of the cortex with sensory and motor phenomena concerning a specific body part.

The results showed that, in each cerebral hemisphere, the somato-motor cortex is primarily located in the frontal lobe, in the precentral gyrus, just anterior to the central sulcus (sulcus of Rolando), and extends down to the Sylvian fissure. Conversely, the somato-sensory cortex is principally located in the parietal lobe of the brain, in the postcentral gyrus, just posterior to the central sulcus.

Both areas are organized in a somato-topic way and represent the contralateral side of the body. Furthermore, Penfield and Boldrey found that the amount of the cortex dedicated to each body part is not proportionate to the surface area of that body part. For example, the extent of cortex devoted to the thumb and lips is vast.

It is worth noting that, in a figure of their article, the researchers sketched a bizarre creature—that they named *homunculus*—to give a visual image of the size and the sequence of the cortical areas corresponding to the different body parts. So, the trunk, the legs, and the head of the figurine are exceedingly small compared with the tongue, the lips, and the hands. The authors observed:

> "The homunculus may be said to be both motor and sensory as the sequence pattern is roughly the same, although there are differences" [69] (p. 432).

The brain was not included in this first illustration.

In 1950, Penfield and another neurosurgeon, Theodore Rasmussen, published a book where the *homunculus* was drawn differently [70] (p. 214–215), in relation with the brain, "draped along the cortical surface and interhemispheric fissure" [71] (p. 330).

Four years later, in a book by Penfield and Jasper [72], three sets of *homunculi* appeared: the first was near to the central sulcus, the second near to the Sylvian fissure and the insula, and the third in the supplementary motor cortex. One more homunculus was placed in the thalamus.

As Schott noticed, Penfield's *homunculus* was a curious method of illustration which gives rise to some unexpected problems. "It was a deceptively simple and yet naïve concept … of doubtful scientific value, since facts and fancy have been confused" [71] (p. 329).

In those same years, the concept of *body image* was added to the older notion of *body schema*, and both terms were used in neurology, psychology, and psychiatry in an often confused and sometimes reified way, as if a *homunculus* were placed in some part of the brain to represent the body.

1.9 Higher Weight Persons: Normative Discontent

The first systematic studies on body image in subjects with obesity date back to the 1960s when Albert J Stunkard and collaborators published two pioneering articles [73, 74]. Five results deserve attention, given that they have been later repeatedly confirmed [75]:

- Not all higher weight individuals present a body image disturbance, but body dissatisfaction is a frequent psychological correlate of obesity, particularly in women
- The disturbances, if present, resemble those reported among persons suffering from objective deformities, for example, of the face
- The main feature is that body weight is an overriding concern
- The disturbance is not proportionate to the excess body weight and is not necessarily affected by weight reduction
- Adolescence is a critical period for the development of body weight and shape concerns.

The obesity galaxy is vast and heterogeneous. It is well known that many factors show modulating effects on body uneasiness, e.g. gender, age, ethnicity, cultural anti-fat bias, social class, onset age of overweight, degree of obesity, history of weight cycling, presence of binge eating, history of childhood teasing and parental criticism about weight, and negative body talk among peers [76] (see Chaps. 10, 13–17, 28, and 30 of the present volume).

Apart from obesity, a great many people experience body dissatisfaction.

In particular, in 1984, Rodin, Silberstein, and Striegel-Moore found that most women—also those in their healthy weight range—were dissatisfied with their body weight and coined the expression *normative discontent* [77]. The term means that it is normal, or even better it is prescribed to be ceaselessly dissatisfied with something. In this case, normative discontent involves body weight and shape, but it can be observed in any realm in present-day societies, and an extreme consequence is the so-called plastic surgery and cosmetic procedures addiction [78].

Normative discontent stereotypes associated with body appearance are pervasive also for men [79], children [80], and in non-Western cultures [81]. Body dissatisfaction is often associated with disordered eating behaviours, in particular through the subscription to inflexible eating rules [82].

1.10 Eating Disorders, Body Dysmorphic Disorder, and Hypochondriasis

Many shared transnosographic factors underpin the current, purely descriptive, diagnostic categories of ED, BDD, obsessive-compulsive disorders (OCD), and hypochondriasis.

Psychiatry as a distinct discipline is about two centuries old and psychiatric labelling has continuously changed over that time. The American Psychiatric Association's *Diagnostic and Statistical Manual of Mental Disorders* is now in its fifth edition (DSM-5) [24]. It remains a descriptive, prototypical classification, based on consensus more than pathophysiology and, for the most part, categories are not defined by natural boundaries [83, 84]. Therefore, diagnostic uncertainties are not surprising.

In 1860, Louis-Victor Marcé linked up anorexia symptoms of two girls to hypochondriasis [41]. In 1891, Enrico Morselli stressed the obsessional features of a new syndrome he called *dysmorphophobia* (see Chap. 6 of the present volume). In 1903, Janet considered the eating disorder of Nadia as an obsessive-compulsive disorder focused on body shame and implicitly related it to Morselli's dysmorphophobia, without citing it [43]. Janet's patient Nadia showed not only weight phobia but also other appearance concerns that today would justify a DSM-5 double diagnosis of comorbidity, ED and BDD. According to the French alienist, Nadia was thin and pretty enough, but she felt her face very ugly, red, and pimply. She was ashamed to be seen in the street and, at home, preferred the dark corners [43] (p. 38–39).

The relationships among ED, BDD, and hypochondriasis—all conditions that deeply involve the body experience—are still debated.

In the DSM-5, the diagnosis of hypochondriasis was replaced by two new categories, *illness anxiety disorder* and *somatic symptom disorder*, kept separate from ED and BDD. However, also recently some authors supported a transdiagnostic perspective and stressed the functional links of hypochondriac, obsessive, dysmorphic, and ED-related *unwanted mental intrusions*. They suggested that these intrusions (sensations, thoughts, images, impulses) are a transnosographic variable and might contribute to identifying common elements and phenomenological resemblances among the four diagnostic classes [85].

DSM-5 included BDD among the obsessive-compulsive and related disorders but differentiated them from ED and emphasized the distinction (see Chaps. 4 and 5 of the present volume).

However, many studies have identified phenotypic and endophenotypic similarities between BDD and ED (particularly AN). Traumatic experiences of neglect, abuse, and being teased and bullied at school are shared risk factors for both BDD and ED [86, 87]. Patients with AN and BDD show poorer *self-esteem* and higher *perfectionism* than healthy controls. The levels of self-esteem and perfectionism are comparable [88].

As to neurocognitive aspects, recent studies found that persons with BDD, compared to healthy controls, show differences in *visual processing* [89], in particular, *gestalt processing* with a dominance of detailed processing over global processing. Persons with BDD and those with ED both present a *selective visual attention* and overfocus on perceived flaws in their body appearance [90]. Functional magnetic resonance imaging (fMRI) demonstrated similar abnormalities in AN and BDD in processing visual information [91].

Do individuals with AN and BDD differently evaluate others' faces and bodies? A study found similar behavioural phenotypes. Compared to healthy control subjects, both participants with BDD and AN (weight-restored) evaluated more negatively others' faces and bodies and rated them as more overweight. Furthermore, they were more triggered to think of their physical features, even for images distant from their primary concerns [92].

Body checking is a variant of compulsive checking very common in BDD and ED [93]. It includes reassurance repeatedly seeking, frequently weighing, and mirror gazing for long periods of time. Experimental and self-report studies suggest that low cognitive confidence plays an essential role in OCD, BDD, and ED. *Cognitive confidence* is a form of metacognition. It refers to the level of faith one has regarding one's own cognitive abilities: perception, attention, reality monitoring, memory, etc. The relationship between compulsive checking and cognitive confidence appears paradoxical: repetitive checking behaviours decrease confidence and certainty [94], and creates a vicious circle.

As to comorbidity, Dingemans et al. found that BDD is a distinct comorbid disorder in almost half of the patients with ED [95]. An Australian study in a community sample of adolescents confirmed the associations of BDD with ED [96]. Appearance concerns other than body weight and shape are common in individuals with ED and comorbidity of BDD with an ED is presumably underdiagnosed in many clinical centres for ED [97].

However, does a person with a diagnosis of ED and BDD suffer from two distinct morbid entities? How useful for treatment can be such dual diagnosis? Is the so-called *body image disturbance* substantially different in ED and BDD?

1.11 To Classify Body Schema/Image Disorders

How many body representations should we postulate to account for the complexity of bodily experience and its countless alterations [3, 12, 98]? See Table 1.4 for an only partial list.

Table 1.4 Some disorders of body experience and misidentification syndromes

Name	Definition
Allochiria	Mislocation of sensory stimuli
Anorexia nervosa	Intense fear of gaining weight, disturbance in the way one's body weight and shape are experienced
Anosodiaphoria	Indifference to the existence of a serious handicap
Anosognosia	Unawareness of a deficit (e.g. cortical blindness, hemiplegia)
Apraxia	Skilled movements are impaired in the absence of peripheral deficits
Asomatognosia	Unawareness, loss of recognition of part of the body (e.g. the hemiplegic side of the body), expressed verbally or through neglect
Autotopagnosia (somatotopagnosia)	Inability to locate different body parts on command
Autoscopy (heautoscopy, out of the body experience)	Seeing a double of oneself, seeing one's own body at a distance, seeing it from a viewpoint outside the physical body
Body dysmorphic disorder (dysmorphophobia)	Perception of and torturing preoccupation with an imaginary or insignificant defect in one's physical appearance
Body integrity identity disorder	Urge to be amputated without a necessity
Body-specific aphasia	Loss of lexical knowledge of body parts, disruption of body semantics
Body weight and shape dissatisfaction	It is often measured as the difference between current and idealized body weight and shape
Bulimia nervosa	Excessive concerns about one's body weight and shape

(continued)

Table 1.4 (continued)

Name	Definition
Conversion disorder	Impairment of a body function *sine materia*
Capgras syndrome (delusion of doubles)	Delusional belief that others have been replaced by doubles, identical or near identical imposters
Capgras syndrome, reverse (reverse subjective double)	Delusional belief that the person is a double, the mind has been replaced, but the appearance is the same
Clonal pluralization	Delusional belief that some other persons look like the individual both physically and psychologically
Cotard's syndrome (delusion of negation)	Various delusional beliefs that one's own body no longer exists, is putrefying, is enormous, has lost organs or blood
Depersonalization	The individual becomes a stranger to himself, he feels his body, his voice as unfamiliar
Fregoli syndrome	The individual believes that persons, usually unknown, are other persons, well known, in disguise
Fregoli syndrome, reverse	The individual believes that others completely misidentify him/her
Gerstmann's syndrome	Finger agnosia, left-right confusion, acalculia, agraphia
Hypochondriasis	Heightened bodily sensations and tormenting anxiety about the possibility of an undiagnosed illness
Intermetamorphosis	Delusional belief that others temporarily change into someone else (appearance and personality)
Koro	Severe anxiety related to the belief that one's genitalia are shrinking or receding, with possible death
Macrosomatognosia	To feel the whole body or body parts bigger
Microsomatognosia	To feel the whole body or body parts smaller
Mirror sign (Capgras syndrome with one's own image)	Inability to recognize one's image in a mirror
Misoplegia	Hatred for paralysed limbs
Personal (unilateral) neglect	Lack of exploration of half of the body contralateral to the damaged brain hemisphere (usually the right hemisphere)
Phantom limb	Awareness of an amputated limb: an individual who has lost a part of his/her body still perceives it with or without pain
Polyopic heautoscopy	Seeing a number of doubles of oneself, sometimes of the opposite sex (heterosexual heautoscopy)
Prosopagnosia	Face blindness, a deficit of the ability to recognize familiar faces, including one's own face
Somatoparaphrenia	Denial of ownership of one's body part—e.g. a paralysed limb—that is attributed to another person
Subjective doubles syndrome	Delusional belief that other persons look like the individual but have different minds and live different lives
Taijin-kiofu-sho	Extreme self-consciousness regarding one's appearance. Four subtypes: Phobia of blushing, phobia of one's own foul body odour, phobia of a deformed body or face, phobia of one's own glance or eye-to-eye contact. (see Chap. 5 of the present volume)

Table 1.5 Some possible taxonomies for body experience and misidentification syndromes

Taxonomies based on clinical pictures	Abnormal body experiences with abnormal beliefs (absent insight)
	Abnormal body experiences without abnormal beliefs (good insight)
	Abnormal beliefs without abnormal body experiences (e.g. mistake the index finger for the thumb)
	Body unawareness vs. extreme self-consciousness regarding one's appearance
	Deficits (e.g. emisomatognosia) vs. distortions (e.g. macrosomatognosia)
	My body vs. your body
	Perceptual vs. mnestic body images
	Short-term vs. long-term body representations
A dyadic taxonomy	*Body schema disorders*: alterations of sensorimotor representations that are used for actions (e.g. emisomatognosia)
	Body image disorders: perceptual, conceptual, and emotional body representations that are not used for action (e.g. dysmorphophobia)
A triadic taxonomy	*Body schema disorders*: alterations of sensorimotor representations that guide actions (e.g. emisomatoagnosia)
	Body structural description disorders: visuo-spatial body map disorders (e.g. autotopoagnosia)
	Body semantics disorders (e.g. body-specific aphasia)

One may try to classify the very different syndromes described by neurologists and psychiatrists using several criteria [3]. Following Frédérique de Vignemont, Table 1.5 lists some possible taxonomies of body representation disorders.

The principle of double dissociation is often used in neuropsychological research and inspires the dyadic and triadic taxonomies:

> "A double dissociation is observed if a patient or group of patients is impaired on A, but not on B, and if another patient or group of patients is impaired on B, but not on A. If A and B are two body-related tasks, then there must be two independent processing systems of body information which can be functionally dissociated by lesions" [3] (p. 67).

1.12 Conclusive Remarks

A human being relates to his/her own body through interoception, proprioception, movement, vision, touch, taste, olfaction, emotions, feelings, social interactions, language, and semantic understanding. Furthermore, the concept of body image can be applied both to one's own body and to the appearance of someone else.

Disorders of body experience may be the result of noticeable lesions and diseases affecting the nervous system or be associated with several psychiatric syndromes without established neurobiological alterations. They challenge the current descriptive classifications of mental disorders.

The concepts of *body schema* and *body image* date back to the first decades of the twentieth century [51, 62, 63, 99]. Like the old word *coenaesthesia*, these more recent expressions merge various components of bodily experience (psychological, socio-cultural, neurological, and psychopathological) in the frontier between soma and psyche.

Sometimes *body schema* and *body image* are used to indicate two different types of body representation, respectively, unconscious and conscious, related to the body we act with and the body we perceive, connected to the unconscious sensorimotor and postural control of one's own body and the conscious appraisal of one's physical appearance. However, the distinction is still unclear, and these terms have been and continue to be used in a confused way. They appear as muddled metaphors that cover a variety of meanings and may apply to very different disorders such as anosognosia, Cotard's syndrome, AN, ideomotor apraxia, finger agnosia, BDD, body-specific aphasia, body weight and shape dissatisfaction, and so forth.

Both constructs originated from the observation of particular pathological phenomena that were interpreted as disorders involving an abstract and no well-defined construct called *body schema* or *body image*. From that time forth, a growing number of symptoms were classified as *body schema disorders* or *body image disorders* and used to confirm the validity of those theoretical concepts. This process is an obvious logical fallacy (*petitio principii*): a hypothesis, which in the beginning was proposed to be proved, is assumed to explain another hypothesis and, then, the second to confirm the first [100].

In the last decades, a growing number of neuropsychological and neuroimaging studies have made use of *domain-specific* (distinct cortical systems) and *domain-general* (a single general network) approaches aimed to investigate various dimensions of body awareness and body representation. The observation of the rare clinical cases in which only one type of body representation is impaired, while other types are preserved (neuropsychological dissociation) is always enlightening [4, 101]. Apposite testing instruments, designed to identify "the content and the format of the representation(s) and the processes that such representations would undergo in relevant tasks" [57] (p. 235) have been built, and scientists are now trying to develop cognitive, neuropsychology-based, theories of body representations.

As to treatment, at present, a pragmatic, eclectic, multidisciplinary approach is often the only available resource to take care of body experience disturbances.

References

1. Gallagher S. Body image and body schema: a conceptual clarification. J Mind Behav. 1986;7(4):541–54.
2. Gallagher S. How the body shapes the mind. Oxford: Oxford University Press; 2005.
3. de Vignemont F. Body schema and body image. Pros and cons. Neuropsychologia. 2010;48(3):669–80.
4. Pitron V, de Vignemont F. Beyond differences between the body schema and the body image: insights from body hallucinations. Conscious Cogn. 2017;53:115–21.
5. Hübner CF. Caenesthesis. Dissertatio inauguralis medica. Halae: Typis Bathianis; 1794.

6. Starobinski J. A short history of bodily sensation. Psychol Med. 1990;20:22–33.
7. Dupré E, Camus P. Les cénestopathies. L'Encéphale. 1907;2(2):606–31.
8. Reil JC. Über den Begriff der Medicin und ihre Verzweigungen, besonders in Beziehung auf die Berichtigung der Topik der Psychiaterie (On the term of medicine and its branches, especially with regard to the rectification of the topic in psychiatry). Beyträge zur Beförderung einer Kurmethode auf psychischem Wege (Contributions to the Advancement of a Treatment Method by Psychic Ways) 1808;1(2):161–279.
9. Marneros A. Psychiatry's 200th birthday. Br J Psychiatry. 2008;193(1):1–3.
10. Hinsie L, Campbell R, Cuzzolaro M, Zanda G, editors. Dizionario di psichiatria. Roma: Astrolabio-Ubaldini; 1979.
11. Fuchs T. [Coenesthesia. On the history of general sensibility]. Z Klin Psychol Psychopathol Psychother 1995;43(2):103–12.
12. Code C, Wallesch C-W, Joanette Y, Lecours AR, editors. Classic cases in neuropsychology. New York: Psychology Press; 1996.
13. Munk H. Über die Functionen der Grosshirnrinde. 2nd ed. Berlin: Hirshwald; 1890.
14. Wernicke C. Grundriss der Psychiatrie in klinischen Vorlesungen. Leipzig: Thieme; 1900.
15. Paré A. La Méthode de traicter les playes faites par les arquebuses et aultres bastons à feu. Paris: V. Gaulterot; 1545. http://catalogue.bnf.fr/ark:/12148/cb31058163n.
16. Mitchell SW. Phantom limbs. Lippincott's magazine of popular literature and science, 1871;8:563–9.
17. Reilly KT, Sirigu A. Motor cortex representation of the upper-limb in individuals born without a hand. PLoS One. 2011;6(4):e18100.
18. Cash T, Counts B, Huffine C. Current and vestigial effects of overweight among women: fear of fat, attitudinal body image, and eating behaviors. J Psychopathol Behav Assess. 1990;12:157–67.
19. Cotard J. Du délire des négations. Arch Neurol. 1882;4:152–70; 282–96.
20. Sahoo A, Josephs KA. A neuropsychiatric analysis of the cotard delusion. J Neuropsychiatry Clin Neurosci. 2017;30(1):58–65. https://doi.org/10.1176/appi.neuropsych.17010018.
21. Dugas L. Un cas de dépersonnalisation. Rev Philos France Let. 1898;45(1):500–7.
22. Foerster O. Ein Fall von elementärer allgemeiner Somatopsychose (Afunktion der Somatopsyche). Mschr Psychiat Neurol. 1903;14(3):189–205.
23. Deny G, Camus P. Sur une forme d'hypochondrie aberrante due à la perte de la conscience du corps. Rev Neurol. 1905;9:461–8.
24. American Psychiatric Association. Diagnostic and statistical manual of mental disorders, DSM-5. 5th ed. Arlington: American Psychiatric Publishing; 2013.
25. Seneca LA. Lettere a Lucilio (Epistulae morales ad Lucilium). Milano: Garzanti; 2008. p. 62–5.
26. von Monakow C. Experimentelle und pathologisch-anatomische Untersuchungen über die Beziehungen der sogenannten Sehsphäre zu den infracorticalen Opticuscentren und zum N. opticus. Arch Psychiatr Nervenkr. 1885;16(2):151–99.
27. Anton G. Beiträge zur klinischen Beurtheilung und zur Localisation der Muskelsinnstörungen im Grosshirne. Zeitschrift für Heilkunde. 1893;14:313–48.
28. Anton G. Über die Selbstwahrnehmung der Herderkrankungen durch den Kranken bei Rindenblindheit und Rindentaubheit. Arch Psychiatr Nervenkr. 1899;32(1):86–127.
29. Pick A. Beiträge zur Pathologie und pathologischen Anatomie des Centralnervensystems: mit Bemerkungen zur normalen Anatomie desselben. Berlin: Springer; 1898.
30. Babinski J. Contribution à l'étude des troubles mentaux dans l'hémiplégie organique cérébrale. Rev Neurol. 1914;27:845–8.
31. Besharati S, Forkel SJ, Kopelman M, Solms M, Jenkinson PM, Fotopoulou A. Mentalizing the body: spatial and social cognition in anosognosia for hemiplegia. Brain. 2016;139(Pt 3):971–85.
32. Marková IS. Insight in psychiatry. Cambridge: Cambridge University Press; 2005.
33. Marková IS, Berrios GE. Awareness and insight in psychopathology: an essential distinction? Theory Psychol. 2011;21(4):421–37.

34. Morton R. Phthisiologia, seu exercitationes de phthisi (London, S. Smith, 1689). Venetia: Typis Hieronymi Albrizzi; 1696.
35. Silverman JA. Robert Whytt, 1714-1766, eighteenth century limner of anorexia nervosa and bulimia, an essay. Int J Eat Disord. 1987;6(1):143–6.
36. Gull WW. Anorexia nervosa (apepsia hysterica, anorexia hysterica). Trans Clin Soc Lond. 1874;7:22–8.
37. Gull WW. Anorexia nervosa. Lancet. 1888;i:516–7.
38. Lasègue C. De l'anorexie hystérique. Arch Gen Med. 1873;21:385–403.
39. Mistura S. Professor J.M. Charcot on anorexia. Eat Weight Disord. 1997;2(2):105–8.
40. Gilles de la Tourette GAÉB. Traité clinique et thérapeutique de l'hystérie. Paris: E. Plon, Nourrit et Cie; 1895.
41. Marcé LV. Note sur une forme de délire hypocondriaque consécutive aux dyspepsies et caractérisée principalement par le refus d'aliments. Ann Med Psychol. 1860;16(3éme série):15–28.
42. Silverman JA. Louis-Victor Marcé, 1828–1864: anorexia nervosa's forgotten man. Psychol Med. 1989;19(4):833–5.
43. Janet P. Les obsessions et la psychasthénie (1903). Tome I. Paris: Félix Alcan Éditeur; 1903.
44. Pope HG Jr, Hudson JI, Mialet JP. Bulimia in the late nineteenth century: the observations of Pierre Janet. Psychol Med. 1985;15(4):739–43.
45. Wulff M. Su un interessante complesso sintomatico orale e sui suoi nessi con la tossicomania (versione italiana a cura di G. Binni e M. Cuzzolaro di: Über einen interessanten oralen Symptomen-Komplex und seine Beziehung zur Sucht, Internationale Zeitschrift für Psychoanalyse, 18, 281-302, 1932). Psicobiettivo. 2001;21:73–88.
46. Cuzzolaro M. Eating Disorders. In: Sbraccia P, Finer N, editors. Obesity: pathogenesis, diagnosis, and treatment. Cham: Springer; 2017. p. 1–24.
47. Stunkard A. A description of eating disorders in 1932. Am J Psychiatry. 1990;147:263–8.
48. Russell G. The history of bulimia nervosa. In: Garner DM, Garfinkel PE, editors. Handbook of treatment for eating disorders. New York: Guilford; 1997. p. 11–24.
49. Der BL. Fall Ellen West (II). Schweiz Arch Neurol Psychiatr. 1944;54:69–117.
50. Der BL. Fall Ellen West (III). Schweiz Arch Neurol Psychiatr. 1945;55:16–40.
51. Bonnier P. L'aschématie. Rev Neurol. 1905;54:605–9.
52. Bonnier P. Le vertige (deuxième édition). Paris: Masson; 1904.
53. Vallar G, Rode G. Commentary on bonnier P. L'aschematie. Rev Neurol (Paris) 1905;13:605-9. Epilepsy Behav. 2009;16(3):397–400.
54. Head H, Holmes G. Sensory disturbances from cerebral lesions. Brain. 1911;34(2–3):102–254.
55. Head H. Studies in neurology. London: Oxford University Press; 1920.
56. Pick A. Zur Pathologie des Bewusstseins vom eigenen Körper. Neurologishes Centralblatt. 1915;34:257–65.
57. Semenza C, Delazer M. Pick's cases on body representation. In: Code C, Wallesch C-W, Joanette Y, Lecours AR, editors. Classic cases in neuropsychology, vol. 2. New York: Psychology Press; 2003. p. 223–40.
58. McCarthy RA, Warrington EK. Past, present, and prospects: reflections 40 years on from the selective impairment of semantic memory (Warrington, 1975). Q J Exp Psychol (Hove). 2016;69(10):1941–68.
59. Chen L, Lambon Ralph MA, Rogers TT. A unified model of human semantic knowledge and its disorders. Nat Hum Behav. 2017;1(3):pii: 0039.
60. Wignall SJ, Thomas NA, Nicholls MER. Fat or fiction? Effects of body size, eating pathology, and sex upon the body schema of an undergraduate population. Body Image. 2017;23:135–45.
61. Schilder P. The image and appearance of the human body: studies in the constructive energies of the psyche. London: K. Paul, Trench, Trubner (reprinted by Routledge and transferred to digital printing in 2007: ISBN 978-1-136-33835-9, Kindle); 1935.
62. Schilder P. Das Körperschema. Ein Beitrag zur Lehre vom Bewusstsein des eigenen Körpers. Berlin: Springer; 1923.
63. Lhermitte JJ. L'image de notre corps (1939, Éditions de la Nouvelle Revue Critique). Paris: L'Harmattan; 1998.

64. Morin C, Thibierge S. Body image in neurology and psychoanalysis: history and new developments. J Mind Behav. 2006;27(3/4):301–18.
65. Cash T, Pruzinsky T, editors. Body images: development, deviance and change. New York: Guilford; 1990.
66. Cash T, Pruzinsky T. Body image. A handbook of theory, research and clinical practice. New York: Guilford; 2002.
67. Cash T, Smolak L. Body image. A handbook of science, practice and prevention. 2nd ed. New York: Guilford; 2011.
68. Cash TF, editor. Encyclopedia of body image and human appearance. Amsterdam: Elsevier Academic Press; 2012.
69. Penfield W, Boldrey E. Somatic motor and sensory representation in the cerebral cortex of man as studied by electrical stimulation. Brain. 1937;60(4):389–443.
70. Penfield W, Rasmussen T. The cerebral cortex of man. New York: Macmillan; 1950.
71. Schott GD. Penfield's homunculus: a note on cerebral cartography. J Neurol Neurosurg Psychiatry. 1993;56(4):329–33.
72. Penfield W, Jasper H. Epilepsy and the functional anatomy of the human brain. Boston: Little, Brown & Company; 1954.
73. Stunkard A, Mendelson M. Obesity and the body image. I. Characteristics of disturbances in the body image of some obese persons. Am J Psychiatry. 1967;123(10):1296–300.
74. Stunkard A, Burt V. Obesity and the body image: II. Age of onset of disturbances in the body image. Am J Psychiatry. 1967;123:1443–7.
75. Weinberger NA, Kersting A, Riedel-Heller SG, Luck-Sikorski C. Body dissatisfaction in individuals with obesity compared to normal-weight individuals: a systematic review and meta-analysis. Obes Facts. 2016;9(6):424–41.
76. Cuzzolaro M. Obesity. Psychiatric aspects. In: Capodaglio P, Faintuch J, Liuzzi A, editors. Disabling obesity from determinants to health care models. New York: Springer; 2013. p. 183–97.
77. Rodin J, Silberstein L, Striegel-Moore R. Women and weight: a normative discontent. Neb Symp Motiv. 1984;32:267–307.
78. Kuczynski A. Beauty junkies. New York: Doubleday; 2006.
79. Tantleff-Dunn S, Barnes RD, Larose JG. It's not just a "woman thing:" the current state of normative discontent. Eat Disord. 2011;19(5):392–402.
80. Costa Lda C, Silva DA, Alvarenga Mdos S, de Vasconcelos Fde A. Association between body image dissatisfaction and obesity among schoolchildren aged 7-10years. Physiol Behav. 2016;160:6–11.
81. Alipour B, Abbasalizad Farhangi M, Dehghan P, Alipour M. Body image perception and its association with body mass index and nutrient intakes among female college students aged 18-35 years from Tabriz, Iran. Eat Weight Disord. 2015;20(4):465–71.
82. Duarte C, Ferreira C, Trindade IA, Pinto-Gouveia J. Normative body dissatisfaction and eating psychopathology in teenage girls: the impact of inflexible eating rules. Eat Weight Disord. 2016;21(1):41–8.
83. Shorter E. What psychiatry left out of the DSM-5. Historical mental disorders today. New York: Routledge; 2015.
84. Kendell R, Jablensky A. Distinguishing between the validity and utility of psychiatric diagnoses. Am J Psychiatry. 2003;160(1):4–12.
85. Pascual-Vera B, Roncero-Sanchis M, Belloch FA. Are unwanted mental intrusions a transdiagnostic variable? Psicothema. 2017;29(2):166–71.
86. Buhlmann U, Marques LM, Wilhelm S. Traumatic experiences in individuals with body dysmorphic disorder. J Nerv Ment Dis. 2012;200(1):95–8.
87. Palmisano GL, Innamorati M, Susca G, Traetta D, Sarracino D, Vanderlinden J. Childhood traumatic experiences and dissociative phenomena in eating disorders: level and association with the severity of binge eating symptoms. J Trauma Dissociation. 2017;19(1):88–107.

88. Hartmann AS, Thomas JJ, Greenberg JL, Matheny NL, Wilhelm S. A comparison of self-esteem and perfectionism in anorexia nervosa and body dysmorphic disorder. J Nerv Ment Dis. 2014;202(12):883–8.
89. Beilharz F, Castle DJ, Grace S, Rossell SL. A systematic review of visual processing and associated treatments in body dysmorphic disorder. Acta Psychiatr Scand. 2017;136(1):16–36.
90. Kollei I, Horndasch S, Erim Y, Martin A. Visual selective attention in body dysmorphic disorder, bulimia nervosa and healthy controls. J Psychosom Res. 2017;92:26–33.
91. Li W, Lai TM, Bohon C, Loo SK, McCurdy D, Strober M, et al. Anorexia nervosa and body dysmorphic disorder are associated with abnormalities in processing visual information. Psychol Med. 2015;45(10):2111–22.
92. Moody TD, Shen VW, Hutcheson NL, Henretty JR, Sheen CL, Strober M, et al. Appearance evaluation of others' faces and bodies in anorexia nervosa and body dysmorphic disorder. Int J Eat Disord. 2017;50(2):127–38.
93. Kachani AT, Barroso LP, Brasiliano S, Hochgraf PB, Cordas TA. Body checking and obsessive-compulsive symptoms in Brazilian outpatients with eating disorders. Eat Weight Disord. 2014;19(2):177–82.
94. Hermans D, Engelen U, Grouwels L, Joos E, Lemmens J, Pieters G. Cognitive confidence in obsessive-compulsive disorder: distrusting perception, attention and memory. Behav Res Ther. 2008;46(1):98–113.
95. Dingemans AE, van Rood YR, de Groot I, van Furth EF. Body dysmorphic disorder in patients with an eating disorder: prevalence and characteristics. Int J Eat Disord. 2012;45(4):562–9.
96. Schneider SC, Baillie AJ, Mond J, Turner CM, Hudson JL. The classification of body dysmorphic disorder symptoms in male and female adolescents. J Affect Disord. 2017;225:429–37.
97. Kollei I, Schieber K, de Zwaan M, Svitak M, Martin A. Body dysmorphic disorder and nonweight-related body image concerns in individuals with eating disorders. Int J Eat Disord. 2013;46(1):52–9.
98. de Vignemont F. Cerveau. In: Marzano M, editor. Dictionnaire du corps. Paris: Presses Universitaires de France; 2007. p. 173–7.
99. Schilder P. Immagine di sé e schema corporeo (The image and appearance of the human body: studies in the constructive energies of the psyche, London, K. Paul, Trench, Trubner, 1935; also New York, International Universities Press, 1950). Milano: Franco Angeli; 1973.
100. Poeck K, Orgass B. The concept of the body schema: a critical review and some experimental results. Cortex. 1971;7(3):254–77.
101. Ogden JA. Autotopagnosia. Occurrence in a patient without nominal aphasia and with an intact ability to point to parts of animals and objects. Brain. 1985;108(Pt 4):1009–22.

2 Diagnostic Classification of Body Image Disturbances

Secondo Fassino and Enrica Marzola

2.1 Introduction

Body image disturbances characterize multiple clinical conditions as described in the Diagnostic and Statistical Manual of Mental Disorders [1]. In fact, body image is a "multifaceted psychological experience of embodiment" including thoughts, feelings, and behaviors related to the subjective perception of one's own body [2]. Body image is strictly related to one's own identity and self-esteem, essential components of mental health. The development of body image takes place along the life span also depending on significant others and peers' influences.

Major body image disturbances affect the field of eating disorders (EDs) but can also be found in patients affected by body dysmorphic disorder (BDD) and delusional conditions like those of the psychotic spectrum. Moreover, body image is also strictly connected to personality. Individuals' self-schemas related to appearance underpin the subjective investment in one's own appearance [3, 4]. The psychopathology of anorexia nervosa (AN), bulimia nervosa (BN), and BDD has as a hallmark a core emotional and cognitive disturbance of body image [5–7]. This chapter will provide the reader with an overlook of the main findings on body image across these clinical conditions.

Weight, body image dissatisfaction, clinical conditions, and psychosocial functioning are greatly connected although imperfectly understood. Although body image dissatisfaction is common at all sizes, in the general population high body mass index (BMI) is typically linked to increased body image dissatisfaction [8]. Overweight and obesity as well as severe emaciation are frequently highly stigmatized resulting in negative social and economic consequences [9]. Relatedly, body dissatisfaction is associated to depression and poor self-esteem [8] potentially playing a role in a whole variety of psychiatric conditions.

S. Fassino (✉) · E. Marzola
Eating Disorders Center for Treatment and Research, Department of Neuroscience, University of Turin, Turin, Italy
e-mail: secondo.fassino@unito.it

M. Cuzzolaro, S. Fassino (eds.), *Body Image, Eating, and Weight*,
https://doi.org/10.1007/978-3-319-90817-5_2

2.2 Eating Disorders

Feeding and eating disorders (EDs) is a DSM-5 category which includes: anorexia nervosa (AN), bulimia nervosa (BN), binge eating disorder, avoidant/restrictive food intake disorder, rumination disorder, PICA, other specified feeding or eating disorder, unspecified feeding, or eating disorder. Such disorders are characterized by persistent disturbances of eating behaviors entailing an altered consumption or absorption of food in turn significantly impairing sufferers' physical health and/or psychosocial functioning. Body image disturbance is particularly common in EDs, especially AN.

With more detail, patients with AN restrict their caloric intake often becoming severely underweight show a persistent fear of gaining weight and see themselves as "fat" even when emaciated to death. Two subtypes of AN exist: individuals with restricting type AN (R-AN) lose weight by restricting their diet and eventually over-exercising while those affected by binge-purging type AN (BP-AN) also starve but also show binge episodes followed by purging behaviors including vomiting, using laxatives or diuretics in addition to over-exercise. Bulimic patients engage in recurrent episodes of binge eating followed by purging behaviors including vomiting and/or using diuretics or laxatives and/or over-exercising. For both AN and BN diagnoses, weight and body shape impact strongly on individuals' self-esteem. It is noteworthy that body image disturbances and body dissatisfaction frequently occur even before the development of a full-blown ED [10]. See Chaps. 4, 8–12 of the present book.

2.2.1 Body Image Is a Multidimensional Construct

Many components can be called into question when dealing with body image, a multidimensional construct, in EDs. In fact, Hilde Bruch in her seminal publications [11] had already described the perceptual deficit in AN and since decades research acknowledged that AN people tend to overestimate their body size [12]. More recently, body image concerns have also been linked to certain temperamental profiles and other ED core features like interoceptive awareness and feelings of ineffectiveness [13]. Relatedly, studies from our group showed that in both AN and BN need for approval, as measured by the Attachment Style Questionnaire [14] and depressive symptomatology as measured by the Beck Depression Inventory [15], was found to be the best predictor of body dissatisfaction [16]. Moreover, body dissatisfaction plays a role in maintaining EDs, especially AN, further reinforcing treatment resistance [17]. Furthermore, our group found also that individuals with early-onset AN are characterized by greater body dissatisfaction and pursuit of thinness than those with a late-onset disorder [18]. See Chap. 1 of the present book.

2.2.2 The Predictive and Therapeutic Value of Body Image

Body image can predict the development of an ED. In fact, body dissatisfaction is known to be an important risk factor of restrictive dieting which can predict and maintain EDs. Also, body dissatisfaction predicts relapse in both AN and BN with recovered individuals reporting how body image concerns can hinder recovery and the maintenance of a healthy weight over the long run. Body image disturbances have been linked to poor interoceptive awareness and ineffectiveness in addition to other temperamental characteristics [19].

Body dissatisfaction, body image disturbances and distorted body size estimation in EDs have been the target of therapeutic attempts as well. Therapeutic strategies have the overarching goal to enhance AN patients' accuracy through providing objective feedback. Standardized measures of body size estimation have been used as well as patients' body exposure to a mirror, helping patients to develop a more objective perception of their own body shape. Nevertheless, such treatment approaches are not fully manualized so evidence is lacking on their effectiveness. Working on body image in treatment means to address, for example, also interpersonal relationships [20]. In fact, AN has been described as "valuable and visible" [20], and it has been found how body dissatisfaction can be a way to communicate for patients [21]. Relatedly, research from our group showed that day hospital interventions can be effective in improving body dissatisfaction, working on interpersonal relationships in a psychodynamic framework [22]. This is consistent with previous observations of a relationship between attachment style and body dissatisfaction [16].

That said, body image cannot be addressed as a stand-alone therapeutic treatment for EDs although manualized interventions on body dissatisfaction in EDs, especially AN, are currently lacking. Cognitive approaches to AN rely mainly on Cash's work [23] and try to help patients develop a more positive relationship with their own body, avoiding excessive looking in the mirror, repeated weighing, and body checking. Patients report such behaviors as having an anxiolytic effect on the short run but over the medium run represent maintaining factors. Patients are indeed encouraged to start using other strategies (yoga, listening to music, talking with a friend, etc.) in order to fight anxiety and dysphoric mood without creating dangerous vicious cycles. It is usually helpful in treatment to focus on the functional aspects of patients' body and the possibilities connected to a healthy body (i.e., restarting sport activities). Also, body image usually does not improve early in treatment in AN, and it can also be a target for patients' anxiety during weight restoration.

2.2.3 Body Image Across Feeding and Eating Disorders

Lines of research aiming to directly compare AN and BN with respect to body image have yielded mixed results. For example, it has been found that adult patients with AN and BN did not differ in their assessment of their ideal body size, using silhouettes, even when controlling for perceived current body size [24]. Other studies failed to find any differences between AN and BN patients on perceived weight and overall appearance [25]. Ideal body image has been assessed also with a software image warping system based on biometric data derived by real body shapes [26]; as a result, BN sufferers did not differ from healthy controls in their ideal body shape while those with AN reported a significantly thinner ideal body shape than both groups. Other studies assessed body image dissatisfaction using the body dissatisfaction subscale of the Eating Disorder Inventory (EDI) [27]; reporting more severe scores among patients with BN when compared to those with AN [28, 29]. In contrast, using the same assessing method, another study found patients with AN and BN as reporting similar body dissatisfaction scores [30]. A meta-analysis, putting together all the available studies on this topic, concluded that BN patients reported substantially greater body dissatisfaction than AN individuals on both weight-related and overall measurements when compared to clinical and non-clinical groups [5].

A few studies analyzed the comparison between AN and BN individuals reporting few statistically significant differences in body image. Patients of both clinical conditions reported comparable body image dissatisfaction, investment, and disturbance coupled with quality of life, preoccupation with weight, and overall distress [24, 25]. However, this is a debated topic since other studies found differences between AN and BN groups with respect to body image dissatisfaction, as measured with self-report [28, 29] or schematic figural measures [26, 30]. Moreover, a meta-analysis performed by Cash and Deagle [5] found BN patients as more body dissatisfaction than AN patients. Methodological issues could be responsible for these differences.

AN and BN individuals were found to have different coping with body image threats or challenges. Appearance fixing, experiential avoidance, and positive rational acceptance were found as comparable between diagnostic groups but those with BN resulted more prone to cope with body image-related stress by eating (or over-eating) than AN individuals [6]. Independently from eating, difficulties in coping with body image threats or challenges could mirror the subjective overevaluation of body image and appearance [31] which is a hallmark of AN and BN. Such an impairment in coping strategies is also thought to act as a maintaining factor for both conditions since it reinforces aberrant eating patterns [32]. See Chaps. 4, 8–12 of the present book.

2.3 Body Dysmorphic Disorder

Body dysmorphic disorder (BDD) is characterized by excessive concern and preoccupation with an imagined or a slight defect in bodily appearance that is not better accounted for by another mental disorder. The DSM-5 [1] classifies BDD in the obsessive–compulsive and related disorders category. BDD becomes a chronic disorder in a substantial proportion of cases impairing sufferers' quality of life and psychosocial functioning [33–35]. Furthermore, it is frequently accompanied by other psychiatric comorbidities [36]. The preoccupations caused by the appearance are intrusive, unwanted, time-consuming, and difficult to resist or control. BDD sufferers perceive themselves as unattractive and in turn are prone to evaluate themselves negatively. Time-consuming rituals are performed as a response to anxiety and shame which are generated by the aforementioned preoccupations; mirror gazing and constant comparing of their perceived physical defects with others are commonly reported. Although on the one hand these rituals tend to be reassuring, research showed that sufferers of BDD feel more anxious and distressed after mirror gazing when compared to the general population [37]. Nose, skin, and hair are common body areas that frequently trigger patients' concern. Affected individuals often seek unnecessary dermatologic treatment and cosmetic surgery without reporting any treatment-related relief.

Data in literature show that individuals with BDD evaluate their appearance more negatively than both healthy controls and other psychiatric patients [38, 39]. Recent research showed that BDD individuals reported greater negative body-related cognitions than depressed patients and the general population [40] providing support to a sort of specificity of their preoccupation with appearance and body image although studies comparing also patients with EDs are needed. In this light, research in the field of EDs demonstrated that salience, namely a strong focus on body-related cognitions including negative cognitions, is a proxy for body image-related cognitive disturbance [41, 42]. Relatedly, Kollei and coworkers [40] found that salience and negativity characterized BDD as well thus suggesting a similar cognitive pattern across disorders.

Body dissatisfaction also impacts on quality of life, with BDD individuals reporting the poorest quality of life scores when compared to healthy controls, patients with eating disorders, depression, diabetes, or a recent myocardial infarction [34, 39, 43].

Data on body exposure [40] found BDD patients as reporting more negative body-related cognitions than depressed patients and healthy controls providing support to earlier descriptions of BDD patients [44]. With respect to body image dissatisfaction, those affected by BDD were as body dissatisfied as individuals with an ED but overall more dissatisfied than healthy controls [39]. Relatedly, it has been consistently found that those with BDD tend to focus their body dissatisfaction on their face and hair when compared to gender-matched healthy controls [36, 39]. However, differently from the ED group, BDD individuals reported the higher facial dissatisfaction confirming earlier studies [45] reporting body weight/shape concerns as less marked for patients with BDD in comparison to those with an eating disorder. In fact, no differences between ED and BDD groups emerged in body dissatisfaction, preoccupation, and body checking. Nevertheless, participants with BDD reported more avoidant behaviors and more negative overall self-evaluation due to physical appearance although measured on a single item [45].

Another difference between BDD and ED groups is that self-evaluative and appearance-managing investment is higher in BDD as well as appearance fixing behaviors, including mirror checking and thinking on how to change their perceived imperfections engaging in repetitive behaviors to improve, being reassured or disguise them [39, 46, 47]. This is in line with everyday clinical practice since BDD patients frequently seek cosmetic and dermatological treatments rather than psychiatric therapies, as shown also in literature [48, 49].

BDD is characterized by strong psychological underpinnings, with strategies as mirror checking and camouflaging aiming to decrease inner distress and anxiety [50]. As earlier studies demonstrated, individuals with BDD do not report strong efforts to contrast their obsessions [51] with eventual attempts at avoiding or fighting intrusive thoughts about subjective physical defects being frequently unsuccessful in turn maintaining and enhancing the vicious cycle between intrusive thoughts and pathological behaviors [44]. In this light, rumination, worry, and appearance comparisons tend to maintain patients' preoccupation and distress [50]. See Chaps. 5 and 6 of the present book.

2.4 Psychosis

Findings on body image disturbances in the psychotic spectrum are sparse. The clinical relevance of the different multifaceted disturbances of body image and experience in schizophrenia was introduced and highlighted since 1911 when Bleuler published his original concept of schizophrenia and introduced the term into the psychiatric literature. Furthermore, he emphasized body image disturbances as frequent ancillary symptoms of schizophrenia. Also Kraepelin [52] described various body sensations as interesting symptoms in schizophrenia. Successively body image-related issues in schizophrenia have been addressed by clinical reports and phenomenological considerations [53–56].

Body image disturbances in schizophrenia are often represented by symptoms of disembodiment, that is a sensation of lacking a physical form, and being disintegrated. Different classifications have been proposed in order to capture such a phenomenological variety of body-related psychopathology [54, 57–60]. Also in schizophrenia as in other mental conditions, body image represents an umbrella term for different aspects of such a multidimensional construct. Nevertheless, it could be of importance to discriminate (a) body size perception; (b) the perceptual body schema; (c) the attitudinal and cognitive body concept which encompasses individuals' thoughts, beliefs, and knowledge of their body; and (d) the affective component which is mainly represented by body satisfaction and dissatisfaction [55, 61–65].

Notwithstanding, there is little in the way to garner empirical data on this topic with the existing studies providing mixed results. For example, some earlier studies found patients underestimate or overestimate their body size as well as being overall inaccurate about their body size perception. Also, desomatization, lack of boundaries, and disintegration emerged. Schizophrenic patients have a prevalence rate of body image disturbances and configural processing deficits potentially influencing their perception of actual and ideal body size ranging between 15 and 31% [57, 66–68] which is even higher, even up to 74%, when somatic hallucinations are considered [69].

Those with acute paranoid schizophrenia reported great body image distortions and perceptions; such body image distortions tend to fluctuate according to the major psychotic delusional symptomatology [64, 69] and tend to persist in chronic states even when acute symptoms are reduced. With more detail, anxiety symptoms have been reported to be associated with patients' underestimation of the lower extremities while grandiosity was deemed to correlate with an overestimation of the lower extremities [69].

A prospective study on body image pathology in acutely ill schizophrenic patients assessing body image in a multidimensional way with a longitudinal design showed that some body image distortions are specific for those with a paranoid and schizoaffective disorder. It is well known in literature that the size of certain body is frequently overestimated by healthy individuals as well as those affected by anxiety or depressive disorders. Paranoid and schizoaffective patients were reported to underestimate the size of their legs and such an underestimation was not due to a general distorted perception of their body. Moreover, this distortion of body image persisted even after normalization of acute psychotic symptoms. This is of interest because disturbances of body concept changed after treatment while disturbances of body size perception were unmodified after stabilization of psychotic symptoms.

Also, body image phenomena and medication dosage and side effects were not associated so medications should not be deemed responsible for the specific body image distortions found in patients with paranoid schizophrenia and schizoaffective disorder.

The distorted body perception found in schizophrenia could have some neurological correlates. In fact, Cumming [70] acknowledged that body schema is "a fact of perception" in which the parietal lobe is highly implicated, mostly in conjunction with the somatoaesthetic afferent system and the thalamus. For example, the phenomenon of underestimation of lower extremities could mime a neglect syndrome with an impairment of sensory and association cortex in turn altering the processing of the central nervous system. In this light, other perceptual disturbances have also been described in schizophrenia, including visual spatial perception [71], proprioception, [72] and pain perception [73, 74]. Relatedly, psychodynamic interpretations have been proposed as well, suggesting a sort of "scotomising of the body existence" [75] in order to avoid a body disintegration.

Earlier observational studies found that psychotic patients experience body disturbances [66] although research. With more detail, individuals affected by psychosis report body disintegration, disembodiment, and abnormal body sensations also due to multi-sensory processing dysfunction [76]. It has been reported by scientific literature that psychotic patients tend to underestimate or overestimate certain body parts [76, 77]. In this light, the role of psychiatric comorbidity should also be taken into account when evaluating the extent to which patients perceive their body image as distorted. Although data are mixed, depressed patients have been described as experiencing higher body dissatisfaction than psychotic patients [76]. In fact, patients diagnosed with schizophrenia, schizoaffective disorder, and depression reported comparable head and trunk size perceptions; nevertheless, psychotic patients underestimated the size of their lower extremities [76].

Lines of research also examined current self and ideal self body perceptions coupled with attitudes toward obesity in psychotic versus depressed and non-psychotic patients upon admission to an acute psychiatric unit. It has been found that psychotic and non-psychotic patients with a mood disorder had similar body perceptions after controlling the findings for BMI. With more detail, the mean actual self body image in non-psychotic and psychotic patients corresponded to an overweight BMI. Also body image discrepancy was reported as similar between groups, with both non-psychotic and psychotic patients desiring an ideal body image corresponding to a BMI in the normal range. Patients' perception on body image perception and discrepancies should be addressed in treatment, mostly when counselling psychotic patients on weight loss in order to favor a healthy weight management [78]. Importantly, research assessing body image upon hospital admission to an acute psychiatric unit highlighted that the psychotic episode did not distort body perceptions [79]. This finding could be biased by the effectiveness of the psychopharmacological treatment delivered for baseline acute agitation, the structured setting of the acute psychiatric unit, the severity of the psychotic illness, potentially not distorting body image perception. Interestingly, after controlling for BMI, female patients reported their perceived body image as overweight and heavier than that reported by males, and this is in line with the data in the general population [80]. Therefore, female patients experienced greater discrepancy between actual and ideal body image than males, independently from other confounding factors.

This is consistent with studies in the general population finding women as reporting more body dissatisfaction than males in turn being more prone to exercise to lose weight [81]. It should also be borne in mind that body dissatisfaction tends to decrease self-esteem potentially contributing to the maintenance of a mood or psychotic disorder. Research showed that psychotic and non-psychotic patients had comparably neutral attitudes toward obese individuals—although depressed patients reported more stigma toward obesity than non-depressed individuals—[79].

2.5 Personality

It is well known how body image perceptions can be influenced by sociocultural factors, also including the thin ideals proposed by the media [82, 83]. In this light, personality traits might also be a relevant underpinning of body image concerns [84]. In fact, personality is the characteristic manner in which people feel, think, and behave. Several dimensions can be acknowledged; with more detail, according to the big five model [85] neuroticism, extraversion, openness, agreeableness, and conscientiousness can be recognized as major dimensions [86, 87]. Such personality dimensions impact on a number of individuals' areas including: depressive symptoms, well-being, quality of life, cardiovascular disease, and mortality risk [88, 89].

For example, those with high neuroticism, that is susceptibility to emotional instability, are prone to be markedly self-conscious [85], to place much importance on their appearance [90], and to have high ideals of attractiveness [91]. Still, individuals who are high on neuroticism are more likely to be report negative body image concerns because are more sensitive to rejection [92]. In contrast, people scoring higher on extraversion, namely a dimension synthetizing quantity and intensity of interpersonal interactions, experience more positive emotions [93]; as a result, these individuals might be at a lower risk of negative body image because overall less vulnerable to sociocultural factors that trigger negative body image. A recent review confirmed that negative body image was associated with higher levels of neuroticism and lower levels of extraversion [94]. Relatedly, agreeableness—another personality dimension describing individuals' tendency to cooperate and live in social harmony—was unrelated to body image. After considering also study quality, negative body image was demonstrated as associated with higher neuroticism, lower extraversion, and lower conscientiousness, namely organization and goal-directed behaviors. With respect to body image, neuroticism was important in male and female samples while agreeableness was unimportant for both males and females. Altogether, these results demonstrate how personality can be a relevant correlate of negative body image.

References

1. American Psychiatric Association. Diagnostic and statistical manual of mental disorders. 5th ed. Arlington, VA: American Psychiatric Association; 2013.
2. Cash TF. Body image: past, present, and future. Body Image. 2004;1(1):1–5.
3. Cash TF, Melnyk SE, Hrabosky JI. The assessment of body image investment: an extensive revision of the appearance schemas inventory. Int J Eat Disord. 2004;35(3):305–16.
4. Markus H. Self-schemata and processing information about the self. J Pers Soc Psychol. 1977;35:63–78.
5. Cash TF, Deagle EA 3rd. The nature and extent of body-image disturbances in anorexia nervosa and bulimia nervosa: a meta-analysis. Int J Eat Disord. 1997;22(2):107–25.
6. Fairburn CG, Harrison PJ. Eating disorders. Lancet. 2003;361(9355):407–16.
7. Phillips KA. Body dysmorphic disorder: the distress of imagined ugliness. Am J Psychiatry. 1991;148(9):1138–49.
8. Sarwer DB, Thompson JK, Cash TF. Body image and obesity in adulthood. Psychiatr Clin North Am. 2005;28(1):69–87.
9. Puhl RM, Heuer CA. The stigma of obesity: a review and update. Obesity (Silver Spring). 2009;17(5):941–64. https://doi.org/10.1038/oby.2008.636. Epub 2009 Jan 22.
10. Stice E, Shaw HE. Role of body dissatisfaction in the onset and maintenance of eating pathology: a synthesis of research findings. J Psychosom Res. 2002;53(5):985–93.
11. Bruch H. Perceptual and conceptual disturbances in anorexia nervosa. Psychosom Med. 1962;24:187–94.
12. Garner DM, Garfinkel PE, Stancer HC, Moldofsky H. Body image disturbances in anorexia nervosa and obesity. Psychosom Med. 1976;38(5):327–36.
13. Zanetti T, Santonastaso P, Sgaravatti E, Degortes D, Favaro A. Clinical and temperamental correlates of body image disturbance in eating disorders. Eur Eat Disord Rev. 2013;21(1):32–7. https://doi.org/10.1002/erv.2190. Epub 2012 Jul 17.
14. Feeney JA, Noller P, Hanrahan M. Assessing adult attachment. In: Sperling MB, Berman WH, editors. Attachment in adults: clinical and developmental perspectives. New York, NY: Guilford Press; 1994. p. 128–52.
15. Beck AT, Ward CH, Mendelson M. An inventory for measuring depression. Arch Gen Psychiatry. 1961;4:561–71.
16. Abbate-Daga G, Gramaglia C, Amianto F, Marzola E, Fassino S. Attachment insecurity, personality, and body dissatisfaction in eating disorders. J Nerv Ment Dis. 2010;198(7):520–4. https://doi.org/10.1097/NMD.0b013e3181e4c6f7.
17. Fassino S, Abbate-Daga G. Resistance to treatment in eating disorders: a critical challenge. BMC Psychiatry. 2013;13:282.
18. Abbate-Daga G, Pierò A, Rigardetto R, Gandione M, Gramaglia C, Fassino S. Clinical, psychological and personality features related to age of onset of anorexia nervosa. Psychopathology. 2007;40(4):261–8. Epub 2007 Apr 17.
19. Garner DM. Eating disorder inventory-3. Professional manual. Lutz, FL: Psychological Assessment Resources, Inc; 2004.

20. Schmidt U, Treasure J. Anorexia nervosa: valued and visible. A cognitive-interpersonal maintenance model and its implications for research and practice. Br J Clin Psychol. 2006 Sep;45(Pt 3):343–66.
21. Marzola E, Abbate-Daga G, Gramaglia C, Amianto F, Fassino S. A qualitative investigation into anorexia nervosa: the inner perspective. Cogent Psychol. 2015;2:1032493.
22. Abbate-Daga G, Marzola E, De-Bacco C, Buzzichelli S, Brustolin A, Campisi S, Amianto F, Migliaretti G, Fassino S. Day hospital treatment for anorexia nervosa: A 12-month follow-up study. Eur Eat Disord Rev. 2015;23(5):390–8. Epub 2015. PubMed PMID:25974364
23. Cash TF. The body image workbook. New Harbinger: Oakland, CA; 1997.
24. Williamson DA, Cubic BA, Gleaves DH. Equivalence of body image disturbances in anorexia and bulimia nervosa. J Abnorm Psychol. 1993;102(1):177–80.
25. Ben-Tovim DI, Walker MK. A quantitative study of body-related attitudes in patients with anorexia and bulimia nervosa. Psychol Med. 1992;22(4):961–9.
26. Tovée MJ, Benson PJ, Emery JL, Mason SM, Cohen-Tovée EM. Measurement of body size and shape perception in eating-disordered and control observers using body-shape software. Br J Psychol. 2003;94(Pt 4):501–16.
27. Garner DM, Olmsted MP, Polivy J. Development and validation of a multidimensional eating inventory for anorexia nervosa and bulimia. Int J Eat Disord. 1983;2:15–34.
28. Garner DM, Garfinkel PE, O'Shaughnessy M. The validity of the distinction between bulimia with and without anorexia nervosa. Am J Psychiatry. 1985;142(5):581–7.
29. Ruuska J, Kaltiala-Heino R, Rantanen P, Koivisto AM. Are there differences in the attitudinal body image between adolescent anorexia nervosa and bulimia nervosa? Eat Weight Disord. 2005;10(2):98–106.
30. Benninghoven D, Raykowski L, Solzbacher S, Kunzendorf S, Jantschek G. Body images of patients with anorexia nervosa, bulimia nervosa and female control subjects: a comparison with male ideals of female attractiveness. Body Image. 2007;4(1):51–9. Epub 2007 Jan 18.
31. Shafran R, Fairburn CG, Robinson P, Lask B. Body checking and its avoidance in eating disorders. Int J Eat Disord. 2004;35(1):93–101.
32. Engel SG, Robinson MD, Wonderlich SJ, Meier BP, Wonderlich SA, Crosby RD, Steffen KJ, Mitchell JE. Does the avoidance of body and shape concerns reinforce eating disordered attitudes? Evidence from a manipulation study. Eat Behav. 2006;7(4):368–74. Epub 2006 Jan 23.
33. Grant JE, Kim SW, Eckert ED. Body dysmorphic disorder in patients with anorexia nervosa: prevalence, clinical features, and delusionality of body image. Int J Eat Disord. 2002;32(3):291–300.
34. Phillips KA, Menard W, Fay C, Pagano ME. Psychosocial functioning and quality of life in body dysmorphic disorder. Compr Psychiatry. 2005;46(4):254–60.
35. Phillips KA, Pagano ME, Menard W, Stout RL. A 12-month follow-up study of the course of body dysmorphic disorder. Am J Psychiatry. 2006;163(5):907–12.
36. Phillips KA, McElroy SL, Keck PE Jr, Pope HG Jr, Hudson JI. Body dysmorphic disorder: 30 cases of imagined ugliness. Am J Psychiatry. 1993;150(2):302–8.
37. Buhlmann U, Teachman BA, Naumann E, Fehlinger T, Rief W. The meaning of beauty: implicit and explicit self-esteem and attractiveness beliefs in body dysmorphic disorder. J Anxiety Disord. 2009;23(5):694–702. https://doi.org/10.1016/j.janxdis.2009.02.008. Epub 2009 Feb 14.
38. Didie ER, Kuniega-Pietrzak T, Phillips KA. Body image in patients with body dysmorphic disorder: evaluations of and investment in appearance, health/illness, and fitness. Body Image. 2010;7(1):66–9. https://doi.org/10.1016/j.bodyim.2009.09.007. Epub 2009 Nov 25.
39. Hrabosky JI, Cash TF, Veale D, Neziroglu F, Soll EA, Garner DM, Strachan-Kinser M, Bakke B, Clauss LJ, Phillips KA. Multidimensional body image comparisons among patients with eating disorders, body dysmorphic disorder, and clinical controls: a multisite study. Body Image. 2009;6(3):155–63. https://doi.org/10.1016/j.bodyim.2009.03.001. Epub 2009 May 1.
40. Kollei I, Martin A. Body-related cognitions, affect and post-event processing in body dysmorphic disorder. J Behav Ther Exp Psychiatry. 2014;45(1):144–51. https://doi.org/10.1016/j.jbtep.2013.09.005. Epub 2013 Oct 7.

41. Cooper MJ, Fairburn CG. Thoughts about eating, weight and shape in anorexia nervosa and bulimia nervosa. Behav Res Ther. 1992;30(5):501–11.
42. Hilbert A, Tuschen-Caffier B. Body-related cognitions in binge-eating disorder and bulimia nervosa. J Soc Clin Psychol. 2005;24(4):561–79.
43. Phillips KA. Quality of life for patients with body dysmorphic disorder. J Nerv Ment Dis. 2000;188(3):170–5.
44. Veale D. Advances in a cognitive behavioural model of body dysmorphic disorder. Body Image. 2004;1(1):113–25.
45. Rosen JC, Ramirez E. A comparison of eating disorders and body dysmorphic disorder on body image and psychological adjustment. J Psychosom Res. 1998;44(3–4):441–9.
46. Phillips KA, McElroy SL, Keck PE Jr, Hudson JI, Pope HG Jr. A comparison of delusional and nondelusional body dysmorphic disorder in 100 cases. Psychopharmacol Bull. 1994;30(2):179–86.
47. Veale D, Riley S. Mirror, mirror on the wall, who is the ugliest of them all? The psychopathology of mirror gazing in body dysmorphic disorder. Behav Res Ther. 2001;39(12):1381–93.
48. Crerand CE, Phillips KA, Menard W, Fay C. Nonpsychiatric medical treatment of body dysmorphic disorder. Psychosomatics. 2005;46(6):549–55.
49. Sarwer DB, Crerand CE. Body dysmorphic disorder and appearance enhancing medical treatments. Body Image. 2008;5(1):50–8. https://doi.org/10.1016/j.bodyim.2007.08.003. Epub 2008 Feb 5.
50. Neziroglu F, Khemlani-Patel S, Veale D. Social learning theory and cognitive behavioral models of body dysmorphic disorder. Body Image. 2008;5(1):28–38. https://doi.org/10.1016/j.bodyim.2008.01.002. Epub 2008 Mar 11.
51. Phillips KA, Gunderson CG, Mallya G, McElroy SL, Carter W. A comparison study of body dysmorphic disorder and obsessive-compulsive disorder. J Clin Psychiatry. 1998;59(11):568–75.
52. Kraepelin E. Psychiatrie. Ein lehrbuch fur studierende und arzte. 7. Auflage ed. Leipzig: Barth; 1913.
53. Fisher S. Body experience in fantasy and behaviour. New York: Appleton Century; 1970.
54. Fisher S. Development and structure of the body image, vol. 1&2. Hillsdale, NJ: Lawrence Erlbaum Associates Publishers; 1986.
55. Kolb LC. Disturbances of the body image. In: Reiser MF, editor. American handbook of psychiatry, vol. 4. 2nd ed. New York: Basic Books; 1975. p. 810–37.
56. Rohricht F, Priebe S. Storungen des korpererlebens bei schizophrenen patienten (disturbances of body experience in schizophrenia patients). Fortschritte fur Neurologie und Psychiatrie. 1997;65:323–36.
57. Lukianowicz N. "body image" disturbances in psychiatric disorders. Br J Psychiatry. 1967;113(494):31–47.
58. Lipowsky ZJ. The importance of body experience for psychiatry. Compr Psychiatry. 1977;18:473–9.
59. Sims A. Symptoms in the mind. An introduction to descriptive psychopathology. London, Philadelphia, Toronto, Sydney, Tokyo: W.B. Saunders Company LTD; 1995.
60. Cutting J. Principles of psychopathology: twoworlds-two minds-two-hemispheres. Oxford, New York, Tokyo: Oxford University Press; 1997.
61. Shontz FC. Body image and its disorders. Int J Psychiatry Med. 1974;5:461–72.
62. Shontz FC. Body image and physical disability. In: Cash TF, Pruzinsky T, editors. Body images - development, deviance and change. NewYork, London: The Guilford Press; 1990. p. 149–69.
63. Joraschky P. Das korperschema und das korper-selbst (the body schema and the body self). In: Brahler E, editor. Korpererleben in der Schizophrenie (Body Experience in Schizophrenia). Berlin, Heidelberg, New York, Tokyo: Springer; 1986. p. 34–49.
64. Rohricht F. Korperschema, korperbild und korperkathexis in der akuten Schizophrenie (body schema, body concept and body cathexis in acute schizophrenia). In: Rohricht F, Priebe S, editors. Korpererleben in der schizophrenie (Body experience in schizophrenia). Gottingen, Bern, Toronto, Seattle: Hogrefe; 1998. p. 91–104.

65. Thompson JK, Penner LA, Altabe MN. Procedures, problems, and progress in the assessment of body images. In: Cash TF, Pruzinsky T, editors. Body images - development, deviance and change. New York, London: The Guilford Press; 1990. p. 21–48.
66. Chapman LJ, Chapman JP, Raulin ML. Body-image aberration in schizophrenia. J Abnorm Psychol. 1978;87(4):399–407.
67. Soria Bauser D, Thoma P, Aizenberg V, Brüne M, Juckel G, Daum I. Face and body perception in schizophrenia: a configural processing deficit? Psychiatry Res. 2012;195(1–2):9–17. https://doi.org/10.1016/j.psychres.2011.07.017. Epub 2011 Jul 30.
68. Weiner IB. Psychodiagnosis in schizophrenia. Abingdon: Routledge; 2013.
69. Kato S, Ishiguro T. Clinical courses of hypochondriac-cenesthopathic symptoms in schizophrenia. Psychopathology. 1997;30(2):76–82.
70. Cumming WCK. The neurobiology of the body schema. Br J Psychiatry. 1988;153(Suppl. 2):7–11.
71. O'Donnell BF, Swearer JM, Smith LT, Nestor PG, Shenton ME, McCarley RW. Selective deficits in visual perception and recognition in schizophrenia. Am J Psychiatry. 1996;153(5):687–92.
72. Ritzler B, Rosenbaum G. Proprioception in schizophrenics and normals: effects of stimulus intensity and interstimulus interval. J Abnorm Psychol. 1974;83(2):106–11.
73. Guieu R, Samuélian JC, Coulouvrat H. Objective evaluation of pain perception in patients with schizophrenia. Br J Psychiatry. 1994;164(2):253–5.
74. Dworkin RH. Pain insensitivity in schizophrenia: a neglected phenomenon and some implications. Schizophr Bull. 1994;20(2):235–48.
75. Benedetti G. Todeslandschaften der seele (death landscapes of the soul). Gottingen: Vandenhoeck & Ruprecht; 1983.
76. Priebe S, Röhricht F. Specific body image pathology in acute schizophrenia. Psychiatry Res. 2001;101(3):289–301.
77. Cleveland SE. Judgments of body size in a schizophrenic and a control group. Psychol Rep. 1960;7:304.
78. Pulvers KM, Kaur H, Nollen NL, Greiner KA, Befort CA, Hall S, Born W, Fitzgibbon ML, Ahluwalia JS. Comparison of body perceptions between obese primary care patients and physicians: implications for practice. Patient Educ Couns. 2008;73(1):73–81. https://doi.org/10.1016/j.pec.2008.04.002. Epub 2008 Jun 25.
79. Hassamal S, Trutia A, Dalkilic A, Pandurangi AK. A pilot study of body image perceptions, and attitudes toward obesity in hospitalized psychotic and non-psychotic patients. Asian J Psychiatr. 2017;26:8–12. https://doi.org/10.1016/j.ajp.2016.12.014. Epub 2016 Dec 30.
80. Betz N, Mintz L, Speakmon G. Gender differences in the accuracy of self-reported weight. Sex Roles. 1994;30(7–8):543–52.
81. Davis C, Cowles M. Body image and exercise: a study of relationships and comparisons between physically active men and women. Sex Roles. 1991;25(1–2):33–44.
82. Grabe S, Ward LM, Hyde JS. The role of the media in body image concerns among women: a meta-analysis of experimental and correlational studies. Psychol Bull. 2008;134(3):460–76. https://doi.org/10.1037/0033-2909.134.3.460.
83. Groesz LM, Levine MP, Murnen SK. The effect of experimental presentation of thin media images on body satisfaction: a meta-analytic review. Int J Eat Disord. 2002;31(1):1–16.
84. Dionne MM, Davis C. Body image and personality. In: Cash TF, editor. Encyclopedia of body image and human appearance. London, UK: Elsevier; 2012. p. 136–40.
85. Costa PT, McCrae RR. Revised NEO personality inventory and NEO five-factor inventory: professional manual. Odessa, FL: Psychological Assessment Resources; 1992.
86. John OP, Naumann LP, Soto CJ. Paradigm shift to the integrative big five trait taxonomy: history, measurement, and conceptual issues. In: John OP, Robins RW, Pervin LA, editors. Handbook of personality: theory and research. 3rd ed. Guilford: New York, NY; 2008. p. 114–58.
87. McCrae RR, Costa PT. The five-factor theory of personality. In: John OP, Robins RW, Pervin LA, editors. Handbook of personality: theory and research. 3rd ed. Guilford: New York, NY; 2008. p. 159–81.

88. Friedman HS, Kern ML. Personality, Well-being, and health. Annu Rev Psychol. 2014;65:719–42. https://doi.org/10.1146/annurev-psych-010213-115123.
89. Ozer DJ, Benet-Martínez V. Personality and the prediction of consequential outcomes. Annu Rev Psychol. 2006;57:401–21.
90. Davis C, Dionne M, Shuster B. Physical and psychological correlates of appearance orientation. Personal Individ Differ. 2001;30:21–30. https://doi.org/10.1016/S0191-8869(00)00006-4.
91. Roberts A, Good E. Media images and female body dissatisfaction: the moderating effects of the five-factor traits. Eat Behav. 2010;11(4):211–6. https://doi.org/10.1016/j.eatbeh.2010.04.002. Epub 2010 May 21.
92. Benford K, Swami V. Body image and personality among British men: associations between the big five personality domains, drive for muscularity, and body appreciation. Body Image. 2014;11(4):454–7. https://doi.org/10.1016/j.bodyim.2014.07.004. Epub 2014 Aug 12.
93. Steel P, Schmidt J, Shultz J. Refining the relationship between personality and subjective Well-being. Psychol Bull. 2008;134(1):138–61. https://doi.org/10.1037/0033-2909.134.1.138.
94. Allen MS, Walter EE. Personality and body image: a systematic review. Body Image. 2016;19:79–88. https://doi.org/10.1016/j.bodyim.2016.08.012. Epub 2016 Sep 14.

3 Body Image: Methods of Assessment in Children, Adolescents, and Adults

Enrica Marzola, Massimo Cuzzolaro,
and Giovanni Abbate-Daga

3.1 Introduction

Body image is a broad and multifaceted construct that describes subjective perceptions of and attitudes toward the body, mostly its appearance. A whole variety of assessments are available to capture the different components of this construct. Relatedly, body dissatisfaction has been defined as displeasure with one's appearance [1]; this is likely to occur in case of body image discrepancies, namely those situations when the subjective perceptions of one's physical appearance do not mirror the characteristics one would like to possess.

Several factors contribute to making the evaluation of body image difficult. For example, although the majority of works on this topic report on body image as a stable trait, body image experiences vary over time and depending on different situations. This element increases the complexity of such an assessment; in fact, the scientific investigation of body image could require the assessment of evaluative/affective body image states in different experimental conditions. Still, another variable aspect is represented by age. Many instruments have been developed over time to measure various aspects of body image across different stages of life. Finally, gender and ethnicity are other factors which should be taken into account when assessing body image.

Hereunder a look at some largely used methods of assessment of body image across ages and stages of life will be provided.

E. Marzola · G. Abbate-Daga (✉)
Eating Disorders Center, Department of Neuroscience, University of Turin, Turin, Italy
e-mail: giovanni.abbatedaga@unito.it

M. Cuzzolaro
Formerly Medical Pathophysiology Department, Eating Disorders and Obesity Unit, Sapienza University of Rome, Rome, Italy

M. Cuzzolaro, S. Fassino (eds.), *Body Image, Eating, and Weight*,
https://doi.org/10.1007/978-3-319-90817-5_3

3.2 Assessment of Body Image in Adults

3.2.1 Body Shape Questionnaire (BSQ)

The BSQ [2] is a 34-item tool developed to assess body shape-related concerns about among young women. The BSQ is based on the notion that disturbance of body image is a central feature of both anorexia nervosa and bulimia. Although many assessment procedures have been developed that deal with various aspects of body image, the BSQ is one of the few measures that focus on concerns about body shape. This point is especially important because worries about body shape are a key feature of anorexia. In particular, the BSQ focuses on the phenomenological experience of "feeling fat." The BSQ can be used for both assessment purposes and to evaluate response to treatment.

3.2.2 Assessment of Body-Image Cognitive Distortions (ABCD)

Cognitive biases or distortions related to body image are not frequently assessed and measured. Cash, Muth, Williams, and Rieves [3] pioneered a 63-item self-report questionnaire called the Body-Image Cognitive Distortions Questionnaire (BCDQ) to fill this gap. In such a work, the BCDQ was positively related to poorer evaluations of appearance, more dysfunctional appearance schemas, heightened overweight preoccupation, and greater body-image dysphoria. Using this unpublished measure Cash [4] identified eight types of cognitive distortions related to body-image cognitions: (1) the Beauty-or-Beast distortion, referring to polarized thinking; (2) Unfair-to-Compare, namely those biased comparisons with one's own ideal and actual people. (3) The Magnifying Glass, with selective attention paid to a disliked feature of one's appearance. (4) The Blame Game, entailing that some aspect of one's appearance caused injustices in life. (5) Mind Misreading, occurring when one's negative body-image ideas are projected to somebody else's presumed thoughts. (6) Misfortune Telling relates to predictions that one's appearance could adversely affect one's future. (7) Beauty Bound poses that one cannot do certain things because of one's looks. (8) Moody Mirror entails a negative mood state that generalizes to feelings about one's appearance.

The ABCD [5] is a 37-item measure which represents eight distortions derived by the BCDQ [3] with five items each. It can be used to assess body image-related cognitive errors or distortions in different situations. Items are rated on a 5-point scale ranging from 0 (not at all like me) to 4 (exactly like me). Items read like the following: "Imagine that you leave for work or school one morning feeling that you don't look quite as good as you usually do. Would you think, "I really look terrible today?", "Imagine someone comments favorably on your appearance. Would you then have thoughts about aspects of your appearance that you think would never be complimented?"; "Imagine that you're invited to a party on the beach. Would you think that because of something about your appearance you probably won't fit in or enjoy participating?"; "Imagine that you're single and go out on a blind date. You both seem to have a pretty good time. Your date says, "I'll call you in a couple of days", but never does. Would you think, "My looks probably messed things up?"

3.2.3 Multidimensional Body-Self Relations Questionnaire (MBSRQ)

The MBSRQ [6] is a 69-item self-report inventory focused on the assessment of self-attitudinal aspects of body-image, including evaluative, cognitive, and behavioral components. The MBSRQ can be used with adults and adolescents (15 years or older) but is not appropriate for children. It is composed by seven-factor subscales: appearance evaluation, appearance orientation, fitness evaluation, fitness orientation, health evaluation, health orientation, illness orientation and additional three subscales: body areas satisfaction scale, overweight preoccupation, self-classified weight.

When mainly interested in the appearance-related subscales of the MBSRQ, the 34-item MBSRQ-AS (MBSRQ-Appearance Scales), a shorter version of questionnaire excluding both fitness and health items. The 34-item MBSRQ-AS includes the following subscales:

- Appearance Evaluation (AE) a 7-item scale of one's appraisals of one's physical appearance. Internal consistency was 0.90. Higher scores indicate a more positive body image evaluation.
- Appearance Orientation (AO): it describes the investment in physical appearance.
- Overweight Preoccupation (OPS): a 4-item scale with responses anchored at a 5-point response scale. It captures the anxiety of becoming fat, attention to weight, eating restraint, and dieting. Higher scores indicate greater preoccupation. Internal consistency was 0.74 for men and 0.80 for women.
- Self-Classified Weight (SCW): this scale describes one's weight perception, ranging from very underweight to very overweight.
- Body Areas Satisfaction Scale (BASS): a 9-item scale with responses anchored at a 5-point response scale. The higher the score on the BASS the greater the satisfaction with specific physical areas including face, weight, lower torso. Internal consistency was 0.80 for men and 0.82 for women.

3.2.4 Body-Image Ideals Questionnaire (BIQ)

The BIQ is a 22-item scale [7–9] which evaluates individuals' body-image taking into account the eventual congruence or discrepancy between idealized physical qualities and self-perception, coupled with the subjective relevance of such ideals. It showed internal consistency of 0.79 for men and 0.75 for women. Participants are asked to rate perceived incongruities from their ideals on 11 physical characteristics including weight, body proportions, overall appearance, etc. A 4-point scale is used to report individuals' evaluations; responses range from 0 = Exactly As I Am to 3 = Very Unlike Me. Importance is rated on a 4-point scale as well, ranging from 0 = Not Important to 3 = Very Important. Scores are the mean of the Discrepancy/ Importance cross-products.

3.2.5 Situational Inventory of Body-Image Dysphoria (SIBID)

When completing the SIBID [10, 11], individuals are asked to rate the frequency of negative body image emotions in 48 distinct situations including eating, exercising, looking in the mirror, being with attractive people, and trying on clothes. The 20-item brief version of the original SIBID, the SIBID-short form (SIBID-S) [12], measures negative body-image emotions in 20 situational contexts including body exposure and interpersonal situations. A 5-point scale ranging from 0 = Never to 4 = Always or Almost Always is used to rate such negative body image emotions. Internal consistency was strong for both men (0.94) and women (0.96). Higher SIBID-S scores indicate more marked situational body image dysphoria.

3.2.6 Body-Image Quality of Life Inventory (BIQLI)

The BIQLI [13–15] is a 19-item measure of negative versus positive impact of body image on a variety of facets of individuals' life, psychosocial functioning, and well-being, including mood, sex life, and relationships. BIQLI internal consistency has been showed to be 0.96. A 19-item mean is generated by the 7-point response bipolar scale ranging from −3 to +3. The higher the score, the better the body-image quality of life.

3.2.7 Body-Image States Scale (BISS)

The BISS [16] is a 6-item assessment of momentary evaluative/affective experiences of one's body-image states with an internal consistency ranging from 0.87 to 0.89 for each context. It can be reliably used by both genders. Participants are presented with five situational contexts that could trigger body image concerns or challenges [16]. Such triggers include: being on a beach in a bathing suit, weighing oneself and realizing to have gained weight, looking at fashion models, being dressed nicely but receiving no compliments. Participants are required to imagine themselves currently in each situation and rate how they would feel "right now, at this very moment" on each BISS item. The higher the BISS score, the more positive the body-image reactions to the contextual challenges. The BISS is anchored at a 9-item Likert-type scale, and the six items tap dissatisfaction versus satisfaction concerning the following six domains: overall appearance, body size/shape, weight, feelings of physical attractiveness/unattractiveness, current feelings about one's look and appearance. The instructions state: "For each of the items below, check the box beside the one statement that best describes how you feel right now, at this very moment. Read the items carefully to be sure the statement you choose accurately and honestly describes how you feel right now" [16]. The BISS has been applied to several contexts given its brevity (i.e., six items) and bipolarity (i.e., both positive and negative experiences).

3.2.8 Appearance Schemas Inventory-Revised (ASI-R)

The 20-item ASI-R [11, 17] is a measure of dysfunctional investment in appearance including the importance, influence, and meaning of appearance on one's life. Two scales are investigated: (a) self-evaluative salience, a 12-item measure assessing the extent to which individuals' appearance is deemed relevant to self-worth. Examples are: "When I see good-looking people, I wonder about how my own looks measure up"; "My physical appearance has had little influence on my life (reverse-scored)"; (b) motivational salience, an 8-item measure of subjective motivation to maintain or improve individuals' appearance. Examples are: "I try to be as physically attractive as I can be"; "I spend little time on my physical appearance (reverse-scored)". Internal consistency for the self-evaluative salience was 0.86 and for the motivational salience 0.83. Respondents are asked to rate their responses on a 5-point bipolar scale ranging from strongly disagree to agree strongly. A final score is obtained by the mean of the items. Higher scores indicate more psychological investment in individuals' appearance.

3.2.9 Body Image Coping Strategies Inventory (BICSI)

The 29-item BICSI [18] evaluates three different coping strategies applied to body image: (a) appearance fixing, namely the individuals' efforts to change their appearance by modifying a physical feature perceived as flawed; (b) avoidance, that is the attempt to elude potential challenges to body-image -related thoughts and feelings; (c) positive rational acceptance which describes those mental and behavioral activities that enhance the acceptance of one's experiences via positive self-care or rational self-talk. Individuals are required to think about situations that might challenge their body image and to rate how appropriate each statement is about their coping, ranging from 0 = definitely not like me to 3 = definitely like me. Cash and collaborators [18] found significant associations between the BICSI and other measures of body image and psychosocial functioning. For example, those who reported higher levels of avoidant coping showed also greater body-image dissatisfaction potentially also impacting on their personal worth and sense of self. Regarding psychosocial functioning, those who showed avoidant coping reported lower levels of self-esteem, less social support, and more marked eating concerns.

3.2.10 Body Exposure during Sexual Activities Questionnaire (BESAQ)

The BESAQ [19] is a 28-item measure which quantifies one's anxious attentional focus on and avoidance of body exposure while having sexual relations. As an example, respondents are asked the following: "I don't like my partner to see me completely naked during sexual activity." "During sexual activity, I try to hide certain areas of my body." "I am self-conscious about my body during sexual activity." Responses are rated on a 5-point frequency scale (0 = "Never" to 4 = "Almost Always"). The higher the score, the greater the self-conscious focus and avoidance. BESAQ's internal consistency (Cronbach's alpha) resulted in 0.95 for men and 0.96 for women. In fact, body-image evaluations can have an impact on individuals' sexual interest and experiences during sexual activities. Consistently, body dissatisfaction has been found to inhibit sexual behaviors and interfere with the quality of sexual experiences [19, 20] reported higher BESAQ scores as associated with poorer sexual functioning. Those reporting greater anxious/avoidant appearance self-focus during sex reported less positive experiences in the majority of aspects of their current sexual functioning including enjoyment of their sex life, desire for sex, and sexual arousal. This datum held true for women and men.

3.2.11 Virtual Reality

Virtual reality (VR) has also been applied to the assessment of body image in both clinical and non-clinical samples. VR allowed the development of three—dimensional figures able to reproduce their own body and each body component. Additionally, VR makes it possible to modify such elements allowing clinicians and researchers to obtain ideal and perceived body image. The application of VR for the assessment of body image has been pioneered by the Italian group of Riva and coworkers developing the Body Image Virtual Reality Scale (BIVRS) [21, 22], a software package for the assessment of body image disturbances. The BIVRS is a non-immersive, three-dimensional graphical interface; participants are asked to select one figure out of nine, both female and male, encompassing underweight and overweight. Participants are required to specify what figure represents their self-perceived and their desired body size. The discrepancy between the measures mentioned above is used as an indicator of body image dissatisfaction. Concerning the methods with silhouettes, the BIVRS is way more realistic making participants' choice easier. Another application has been developed in Spain [23], with a specific focus on eating disorders. This software allows participants to modify the size of their body parts. It is an immersive application so participants can change their figure in the virtual environment and it is possible to measure several dimensions of body image (e.g., perceived versus desired body) and body weight (actual versus desired weight).

3.2.12 Body Image Disturbance Questionnaire (BIDQ)

The BIDQ [24] is a 7-item measure of negative body image which asks participants to quantify their concerns about physical appearance. Assessing these preoccupations (ranging from not at all preoccupied to extremely preoccupied on a 5-point scale), the BIDQ investigates unattractive body parts, distress caused by physical defects, impact of body image on relationships, schoolwork, and work activities, avoidant behaviors body-image related.

3.2.13 Body Uneasiness Test (BUT)[1]

The BUT is a 71-item self-report questionnaire developed in Italy [25, 26] to evaluate concerns about the one's body image. It was normed and validated on large samples of patients with eating disorders, obesity (class I, II, and III), and controls. It is easy to use and requires no more than 20 min. The test consists of two parts: BUT-A (34 items) which measures feelings and behaviors toward one's own body and physical appearance; and BUT-B (37 items) which looks at worries about specific body parts or functions (see Appendix 1). A preliminary validation study of the questionnaire was presented at the 5th International Conference on Eating Disorders (New York, 24–26 April 1998) and published in Italian [25, 26]. A new validation study of the test was published in 2006. The test was submitted to 531 subjects (491 females) suffering from eating disorders (ED) and a general population sample of 3273 persons (2016 women) with Body Mass Index (BMI) < 25 kg/m^2 and Eating Attitudes Test-26 (EAT-26) scores under the cut-off 20 (scores ≥20 indicate possible cases of eating disorders) [27]. One year after, a multicenter study validated the instrument again using a clinical sample of 1812 patients with class I, II, and III obesity (women 1411; age range 18–65 years; BMI ≥ 30 kg/m^2). The non-clinical group, of 457 adult normal-weight subjects (women 248; BMI between 18.5 and 25 kg/m^2; EAT-26 score < 20), was matched for age class and educational qualification [28]. Both 2006 and 2007 analyses confirmed a structural five-factor model for BUT-A. The factors were defined as follows:

- WP: Weight Phobia (fear of being or becoming fat)
- BIC: Body Image Concerns (over-concern with physical appearance)
- A: Avoidance (avoidance behavior related to body image)
- CSM: Compulsive Self-monitoring (compulsive checking of physical appearance)
- D: Depersonalization (detachment and estrangement feelings toward the body)

All the BUT-A subscales showed Cronbach's alpha coefficients higher than 0.7. The test–retest reliability was satisfactory [27, 28]. Normative values for BUT scores

[1] This subchapter is an abstract of the BUT validation studies [27 and 28], with permission. Copyright Clearance Center's RightsLink, order numbers 4243170986838 and 4243170744101.

in non-clinical samples of normal-weight non-eating disordered subjects, from adolescence to old age, males and females, were calculated. Women obtained significantly higher scores (higher levels of body image concerns) than men in the Global Severity Index (GSI, see Appendix 2) and in all the five subscales. The females under 40 years had significantly higher scores compared to the others. Conversely, in men, there were non-significant differences between the different age groups [27, 28].

As for the comparison between women with ED and controls, the results demonstrated excellent predictive validity for anorexia nervosa (AN) and bulimia nervosa (BN). The BUT subscale D (depersonalization) had the best predictive validity for ED. It is interesting to note that this important psychopathological dimension is often neglected in the psychometric assessment of body image disturbances [27]. As regards obesity, females obtained significantly higher scores than males [28]. About the different age groups, both men and women with obesity aged 18–49 displayed significantly higher scores than older subjects. The result is in keeping with a decrease in body uneasiness with increased age. According to some researchers, the more or less satisfying feelings with the image of one's body are the result of two different factors: the aesthetic judgment of one's physical appearance and the importance or salience that is attributed to it. From this point of view, older people could be aware of their physical defects—both from early in life and those due to aging—but they would regard these as less critical than younger people do. As to BMI, persons with obesity had higher BUT scores than normal-weight individuals. In males of all age groups, the significant differences were mainly due to the BMI values. Conversely, in females, there were no statistically significant effects of the BMI values on the scores of most of the BUT subscales. We could think that in women the intensity of body uneasiness is not correlated to the actual degree of obesity [28]. The BUT takes its place in the range of instruments employed to study body image with good psychometric characteristics and remarkable possibilities of use as a diagnostic and prognostic test [27, 28]. As a screening tool in prevention programs, it might allow us to single out subjects at risk in whom body uneasiness and disordered eating are associated. In clinical practice, it might be of use in the study of the clinical course and outcomes of illnesses like AN and BN and other ED in which the improvement of body image disturbance not always goes with the improvement of body weight and unhealthy eating and weight-control behaviors. The study of negative body image associated with obesity and the inquiry of the effects on body image of medical or surgical therapies aimed at reducing weight might be another noteworthy field of application.

In the last years the BUT has been used in several different clinical and research areas such as eating disorders [29, 30], obesity [31–34], body dysmorphic disorder and muscle dysmorphia [35, 36], gender incongruence/dysphoria [37–39], neuropsychology [40], obstetrics and gynecology [41, 42], oncology [43], sexology [44, 45], dermatology [46], bariatric surgery and body contouring [47–51], plastic and reconstructive surgery [52–54].

3.3 Assessment of Body Image in Children and Adolescents

Scientific literature has increasingly investigated the development of body image dissatisfaction in young children, also because it may represent a risk factor for the onset of unhealthy eating behaviors and full-blown eating disorders in life (e.g., eating disorders, obesity; [55]).

In fact, young children tend to be dissatisfied with their bodies as well: evidence reported that kids as young as 8 years try diets, would like to be thinner than their current body sizes and to weigh less [56, 57]. This fact is of keen interest for families, teachers, pediatricians, and health educators because body image dissatisfaction in children predicts poor psychological well-being thus potentially triggering the onset of unhealthy eating behaviors later in life [58]. In contrast, the identification of kids with body image concerns could improve early prevention of psychological suffering and eating disorders.

Also, gender can influence body image dissatisfaction in children aged 8 years or older; in fact, girls reported greater body image dissatisfaction, more marked preoccupation with their weight, and more concerns about dieting than boys [59–62]. Over time, body dissatisfaction tend to increase [59, 60, 63].

Although a debated topic, race has also been found to impact on body image satisfaction in childhood. Some lines of research showed that Caucasian children have more body image discrepancies than other ethnic groups [64, 65] while some studies suggested that children from various ethnic groups (e.g., Caucasians, Hispanics, African Americans, Asians) report similar body image concerns [57, 66–68].

With young people, several methods to assess body image are available.

3.3.1 Figure Rating Scale

This assessment consists of seven gender-specific line drawings of increasing size, ranging from 1 (thinnest figure) to 7 (thickest/heaviest figure; [66]). According to participants' gender, boys and girls require separate sets of silhouettes. Respondents are required to choose those figures that most accurately represent their current body size and variations of ideal body type. Body dissatisfaction is measured by the difference between current and ideal body types [69]. It has been shown that children of different backgrounds can reliably complete this measure without requiring extensive interviews with a test–retest reliability of $r = 0.71$ [66]. Also, concurrent validity has been investigated in children for the Figure Rating Scale, with larger discrepancies correlating with lower self-esteem [70] and greater dieting [71]. Previous studies found that children can provide valid ratings of their current body figure [66, 72, 73] even if as young as 5 years [74].

3.3.2 Test for Body Image Distortion in Children and Adolescents (BID-CA).

According to the BID-CA [75], a string with standardized measures (length: 180 cm, approx. 71 in.; diameter: 0.6 cm, approx. ¼ in.) is used to ask participants to estimate the following: (a) size of their upper arm at the level of their armpit; (b) their waist at the level of their belly button; and (c) their thigh at the level of their crotch. Participants are asked in a non-specific way to use the string to form a cycle describing the aforementioned body circumferences as they perceive them. Such circumferences are then measured. Three Body Image Distortion Indices (BID-I) are calculated for tea upper arm, waist and thigh, as follows: BID-I arm/waist/thigh = (circumference perceived/circumference actual) × 100. A mean BID-I can be calculated as well.

3.3.3 Children Body Image Scale (CBIS)

The CBIS [76] is a pictorial measure which asks children to choose a figure of a child from seven photographic figures of children encompassing thin and obese sizes. Participants are asked to select two pictures: (a) what that they find most similar to their perceived body, and (b) what they deem their ideal body. The discrepancy between these two figures represents body dissatisfaction. This perceived–ideal discrepancy has been reported as a sound measure of construct validity in 8–12-year-old children [77]. Interestingly, the size of each figure of the CBIS is based on a measured body mass index (BMI), as a proxy for body fatness as assessed by population BMI norms. As a result, this makes it possible to determine a child's accuracy of perception of their body size when the CBIS is coupled with the child's measured BMI.

Conclusions

In closing, body image can be assessed in multiple ways across the life span, and many variables should be accounted for when investigating such a construct. In fact, body image describes subjective perceptions of and attitudes toward the body, mostly its appearance. Relatedly, body image varies over time, and it also depends on different situations. Also, healthy individuals, as well as people with several psychiatric disorders, are characterized by body image concerns. Still, age, gender and ethnicity make the assessment of body image even more complicated. Notwithstanding, different instruments have been proposed in the literature to capture this construct as reliably as possible, across different study settings. The relevance of the measurement of body image concerns—even in kids—is represented by the fact that body image dissatisfaction could be a risk factor for the onset of unhealthy eating behaviors and full-blown eating and weight disorders in life.

Appendix 1: Body Uneasiness Test, English Version

	BUT	Never	Seldom	Sometimes	Often	Very often	Always
	Mark with an X the answer which best expresses your experience at the moment						
1	I spend a lot of time in front of the mirror	0	1	2	3	4	5
2	I don't trust my appearance: I'm afraid it will change suddenly	0	1	2	3	4	5
3	I like those clothes which hide my body	0	1	2	3	4	5
4	I spend a lot of time flunking about some defects of my physical appearance	0	1	2	3	4	5
5	When I undress. I avoid looking at myself	0	1	2	3	4	5
6	I think my life would change significantly if I could correct some of my aesthetic defects	0	1	2	3	4	5
7	Eating with others causes me anxiety	0	1	2	3	4	5
8	The thought of some defects of my body torments me so much that it prevents me being with others	0	1	2	3	4	5
9	I'm terrified of putting on weight	0	1	2	3	4	5
10	I make detailed comparisons between my appearance and that of others	0	1	2	3	4	5
11	If I begin to look at myself. I find it difficult to stop	0	1	2	3	4	5
12	I would do anything to change some parts of my body	0	1	2	3	4	5
13	I stay at home and avoid others seeing me	0	1	2	3	4	5
14	I am ashamed of the physical needs of my body	0	1	2	3	4	5
15	I feel I am laughed at because of my appearance	0	1	2	3	4	5
16	The thought of some defects of my body torments me so much that it prevents me studying or working	0	1	2	3	4	5
17	I look in the mirror for an image of myself which satisfies me and I continue to search until I am sure I have found it	0	1	2	3	4	5

	BUT	Never	Seldom	Sometimes	Often	Very often	Always
	Mark with an X the answer which best expresses your experience at the moment						
18	I feel I am fatter than others tell me	0	1	2	3	4	5
19	I avoid mirrors	0	1	2	3	4	5
20	I have the impression that my image is always different	0	1	2	3	4	5
21	I would like to have a thin and bony body	0	1	2	3	4	5
22	I am dissatisfied with my appearance	0	1	2	3	4	5
23	My physical appearance is dissappointing compared to my ideal image	0	1	2	3	4	5
24	I would like to undergo plastic surgery	0	1	2	3	4	5
25	I can’t stand the idea of living with the appearance I have	0	1	2	3	4	5
26	I look at myself in the mirror and have a sensation of uneasiness and strangeness	0	1	2	3	4	5
27	I am afraid that my body will change against my will, in a way I don’t like	0	1	2	3	4	5
28	I feel detached from my body	0	1	2	3	4	5
29	I have the sensation that my body does not belong to me	0	1	2	3	4	5
30	The thought of some defects of my body torments me so much that it prevents me having a sexual life	0	1	2	3	4	5
31	I observe myself in what I do and ask myself how I seem to others	0	1	2	3	4	5
32	I would like to decide what appearance to have	0	1	2	3	4	5
33	I feel different to how· others see me	0	1	2	3	4	5
34	I am ashamed of my body	0	1	2	3	4	5

	BUT	Never	Seldom	Sometimes	Often	Very often	Always
	Mark with an X the answer which best expresses your experience at the moment *Of my body, in particular, I hate*						
1	Height		1	2	3	4	5
2	The shape of my head		1	2	3	4	5
3	The shape of my face		1	2	3	4	5
4	Skill		1	2	3	4	5
5	Hair		1	2	3	4	5
6	Forehead		1	2	3	4	5
7	Eyebrows		1	2	3	4	5
8	Eyes		1	2	3	4	5
9	Nose		1	2	3	4	5
10	Lips		1	2	3	4	5
11	Mouth		1	2	3	4	5
12	Teeth		1	2	3	4	5
13	Ears		1	2	3	4	5
14	Neck		1	2	3	4	5
15	Chin		1	2	3	4	5
16	Moustache		1	2	3	4	5
17	Beard		1	2	3	4	5
18	Hairs		1	2	3	4	5
19	Shoulders		1	2	3	4	5
20	Arms		1	2	3	4	5
21	Hands		1	2	3	4	5
22	Chest		1	2	3	4	5
23	Breasts		1	2	3	4	5
24	Stomach		1	2	3	4	5
25	Abdomen		1	2	3	4	5
26	Genitals		1	2	3	4	5
27	Buttocks		1	2	3	4	5
28	Hips		1	2	3	4	5
29	Thighs		1	2	3	4	5
30	Knee i		1	2	3	4	5
31	Legs		1	2	3	4	5
32	Ankles		1	2	3	4	5
33	Feet		1	2	3	4	5
34	Odour		1	2	3	4	5
35	Noises		1	2	3	4	5
36	Sweat		1	2	3	4	5
37	Blushing		1	2	3	4	5

Appendix 2: BUT Scoring Instructions

BUT•A (items 1–34)
Global measure
GSI (Global Severity Index): the average rating of all 34 items
Subscales
WP (Weight Phobia): average (9 + 10 + 18 + 21 + 24 + 31 + 32 + 33)
BIC (Body image concerns): average (3 + 4 + 6 + 12 + 15 + 22 + 23 + 25 + 34)
A (Avoidance): average (5 + 8 + 13 + 16 + 19 + 30)
CSM (Compulsive self-monitoring) average (1 + 11 + 17 + 20 + 27)
D (Depersonalization): average (2 + 7 + 14 + 26 + 28 + 29)
BUT•B (items 1–37)
Global measures
PST (Positive symptom total): the number of body parts or functions rated higher than zero.
PSDI (Positive symptom distress index): the average rating of those items constituting the PST

References

1. Rosen JC. Body-image disorder: definition, development, and contribution to eating disorders. In: Crowther JH, Tennenbaum DL, Hobfoll SE, MAP S, editors. The etiology of bulimia nervosa: the individual and familial context. Washington, DC: Hemisphere Publishing Corp; 1992. p. 157–77.
2. Cooper PJ, Taylor MJ, Cooper Z, Fairburn CG. Development and validation of the body shape questionnaire. Int J Eat Disord. 1987;6:485–94.
3. Cash TF, Muth J, Williams P, Rieves L. New assessments of body image: measuring cognitive and behavioral components. Poster presented at the annual meeting of the Association for Advancement of Behavior Therapy. New York; 1996.
4. Cash TF. The body image workbook: an 8-step program for learning to like your looks. Oakland, CA: New Harbinger Publications; 1997.
5. Jakatdar TA, Cash TF, Engle EK. Body-image thought processes: the development and initial validation of the assessment of body-image cognitive distortions. Body Image. 2006;3(4):325–33. Epub 2006 Nov 2.
6. Brown TA, Cash TF, Mikulka PJ. Attitudinal body-image assessment: factor analysis of the body-self relations questionnaire. J Pers Assess. 1990;55(1–2):135–44.
7. Cash TF. Body-image assessments: manuals and questionnaires. Available from the author's web site at http://www.body-images.com. 2004.
8. Cash TF, Szymanski ML. The development and validation of the body-image ideals questionnaire. J Pers Assess. 1995;64:466–77.
9. Szymanski ML, Cash TF. Body-image disturbances and self-discrepancy theory: expansion of the body-image ideals questionnaire. J Soc Clin Psychol. 1995;14:134–46.
10. Cash TF. The situational inventory of body-image dysphoria: contextual assessment of a negative body image. Behav Ther. 1994;17:133–4.
11. Cash TF. Manuals for the appearance schemas inventory, body image ideals questionnaire, multi- dimensional body-self relations questionnaire, and situational inventory of body-image dysphoria. Available from the author at http://www.body-images.com. 2000.
12. Cash TF. The situational inventory of body-image dysphoria: psychometric evidence and development of a short form. Int J Eat Disord. 2002;32(3):362–6.
13. Cash TF, Fleming EC. The impact of body image experiences: development of the body image quality of life inventory. Int J Eat Disord. 2002;31(4):455–60.

14. Cash TF, Grasso K. The norms and stability of new measures of the multidimensional body image construct. Body Image. 2005;2(2):199–203. Epub 2005 May 31.
15. Cash TF, Jakatdar TA, Williams EF. The body image quality of life inventory: further validation with college men and women. Body Image. 2004;1(3):279–87.
16. Cash TF, Fleming EC, Alindogan J, Steadman L, Whitehead A. Beyond body image as a trait: the development and validation of the body image states scale. Eat Disord. 2002;10(2):103–13.
17. Cash TF, Melnyk SE, Hrabosky JI. The assessment of body image investment: an extensive revision of the appearance schemas inventory. Int J Eat Disord. 2004;35:305–16.
18. Cash TF, Santos MT, Williams EF. Coping with body-image threats and challenges: validation of the body image coping strategies inventory. J Psychosom Res. 2005;58(2):190–9.
19. Cash TF, Maikkula CL, Yamamiya Y. "Baring the body in the bedroom": body image, sexual self-schemas, and sexual functioning among college women and men. Electron J Hum Sex. 2004;7 www.ejhs.org
20. Wiederman MW. Body image and sexual functioning. In: Cash TF, Pruzinsky T, editors. Body image: a handbook of theory, research, and clinical practice. New York: Guilford Press; 2002. p. 287–94.
21. Riva G. Virtual reality in psychological assessment: the body image virtual reality scale. Cyber Psychol Behav. 1998;1(1):37–4.
22. Riva G, Melis L. Virtual reality for the treatment of body image disturbances. Stud Health Technol Inform. 1997;44:95–111.
23. Perpiñá C, Botella C, Baños RM. Virtual reality in eating disorders. Eur Eat Disord Rev. 2003;11(3):261–78.
24. Cash TF, Phillipsb KA, Santos MT, Hrabosky JI. Measuring "negative body image": validation of the body image disturbance questionnaire in a nonclinical population. Body Image. 2004;1(4):363–72.
25. Cuzzolaro M, Vetrone G, Marano G, Battacchi MW. BUT: una nuova scala per la valutazione del disagio relativo all'immagine del corpo. Psichiatria dell'Infanzia e dell'Adolescenza. 1999;66:417–28.
26. Cuzzolaro M, Vetrone G, Marano G, Battacchi M. Body Uneasiness Test (BUT) [Codice di identificazione: #768]. In: Conti L, editor. Repertorio delle scale di valutazione in psichiatria, vol. 3. Firenze: SEE; 2000. p. 1759–61.
27. Cuzzolaro M, Vetrone G, Marano G, Garfinkel PE. The body uneasiness test (BUT): development and validation of a new body image assessment scale. Eat Weight Disord. 2006;11(1):1–13.
28. Marano G, Cuzzolaro M, Vetrone G, Garfinkel PE, Temperilli F, Spera G, et al. Validating the body uneasiness test (BUT) in obese patients. Eat Weight Disord. 2007;12(2):70–82.
29. Ravaldi C, Vannacci A, Bolognesi E, Mancini S, Faravelli C, Ricca V. Gender role, eating disorder symptoms, and body image concern in ballet dancers. J Psychosom Res. 2006;61(4):529–35.
30. Brytek-Matera A, Fonte ML, Poggiogalle E, Donini LM, Cena H. Orthorexia nervosa: relationship with obsessive-compulsive symptoms, disordered eating patterns and body uneasiness among Italian university students. Eat Weight Disord. 2017;22(4):609–17.
31. Dalle Grave R, Calugi S, Magri F, Cuzzolaro M, Dall'aglio E, Lucchin L, et al. Weight loss expectations in obese patients seeking treatment at medical centers. Obes Res. 2004;12(12):2005–12.
32. Dalle Grave R, Cuzzolaro M, Calugi S, Tomasi F, Temperilli F, Marchesini G, et al. The effect of obesity management on body image in patients seeking treatment at medical centers. Obesity (Silver Spring). 2007;15(9):2320–7.
33. Corica F, Corsonello A, Apolone G, Mannucci E, Lucchetti M, Bonfiglio C, et al. Metabolic syndrome, psychological status and quality of life in obesity: the QUOVADIS study. Int J Obes. 2008;32(1):185–91.
34. Pokrajac-Bulian A, Toncic M, Anic P. Assessing the factor structure of the body uneasiness test (BUT) in an overweight and obese croatian non-clinical sample. Eat Weight Disord. 2015;20(2):215–22.

35. Pollice R, Bianchini V, Giuliani M, Zoccali G, Tomassini A, Mazza M, et al. Early diagnosis of dysmorphophobia and others dysmorphic disorders: a possible operative model. Clin Ter. 2009;160(1):5–10.
36. Segura-Garcia C, Ammendolia A, Procopio L, Papaianni MC, Sinopoli F, Bianco C, et al. Body uneasiness, eating disorders, and muscle dysmorphia in individuals who overexercise. J Strength Cond Res. 2010;24(11):3098–104.
37. Bandini E, Fisher AD, Castellini G, Lo Sauro C, Lelli L, Meriggiola MC, et al. Gender identity disorder and eating disorders: similarities and differences in terms of body uneasiness. J Sex Med. 2013;10(4):1012–23.
38. Castellini G, Lo Sauro C, Ricca V, Rellini AH. Body esteem as a common factor of a tendency toward binge eating and sexual dissatisfaction among women: the role of dissociation and stress response during sex. J Sex Med. 2017;14(8):1036–45.
39. Fisher AD, Ristori J, Castellini G, Sensi C, Cassioli E, Prunas A, et al. Psychological characteristics of Italian gender dysphoric adolescents: a case-control study. J Endocrinol Investig. 2017;40(9):953–65.
40. Padulo C, Delli Pizzi S, Bonanni L, Edden RA, Ferretti A, Marzoli D, et al. GABA levels in the ventromedial prefrontal cortex during the viewing of appetitive and disgusting food images. Neuroscience. 2016;333:114–22.
41. Mento C, Le Donne M, Crisafulli S, Rizzo A, Settineri S. BMI at early puerperium: body image, eating attitudes and mood states. J Obstet Gynaecol. 2017;37(4):428–34.
42. Gueli Alletti S, Vizzielli G, Lafuenti L, Costantini B, Fagotti A, Fedele C, et al. Single-institution propensity-matched study to evaluate the psychological effect of minimally invasive interval debulking surgery vs standard laparotomic treatment: from body to mind and back. J Minim Invasive Gynecol. 2017. 10.1016/j.jmig.2017.12.007
43. Zucchetti G, Bellini S, Bertolotti M, Bona F, Biasin E, Bertorello N, et al. Body image discomfort of adolescent and young adult hematologic cancer survivors. J Adolesc Young Adult Oncol. 2017;6(2):377–80.
44. Maseroli E, Fanni E, Cipriani S, Scavello I, Pampaloni F, Battaglia C, et al. Cardiometabolic risk and female sexuality: focus on clitoral vascular resistance. J Sex Med. 2016;13(11):1651–61.
45. Maseroli E, Scavello I, Cipriani S, Palma M, Fambrini M, Corona G, et al. Psychobiological correlates of vaginismus: an exploratory analysis. J Sex Med. 2017;14(11):1392–402.
46. Granstrom S, Langenbruch A, Augustin M, Mautner VF. Psychological burden in adult neurofibromatosis type 1 patients: impact of disease visibility on body image. Dermatology. 2012;224(2):160–7.
47. Pecori L, Serra Cervetti GG, Marinari GM, Migliori F, Adami GF. Attitudes of morbidly obese patients to weight loss and body image following bariatric surgery and body contouring. Obes Surg. 2007;17(1):68–73.
48. De Panfilis C, Cero S, Torre M, Salvatore P, Dall'Aglio E, Adorni A, et al. Changes in body image disturbance in morbidly obese patients 1 year after laparoscopic adjustable gastric banding. Obes Surg. 2007;17(6):792–9.
49. Migliori FC, Gabrielli A, Rizzo R, Serra Cervetti GG. Breast contouring in postbariatric patients: a technique selection algorithm. Obes Surg. 2010;20(5):651–6.
50. Capoccia D, Monaco V, Coccia F, Leonetti F, Cavaggioni G. Axis II disorders, body image and childhood abuse in bariatric surgery candidates. Clin Ter. 2015;166(4):e248–53.
51. Pavan C, Marini M, De Antoni E, Scarpa C, Brambullo T, Bassetto F, et al. Psychological and psychiatric traits in post-bariatric patients asking for body-contouring surgery. Aesthet Plast Surg. 2017;41(1):90–7.
52. Migliori F. "upside-down" augmentation mastopexy. Aesthet Plast Surg. 2011;35(4):593–600.
53. Nicoletti G, Sasso A, Malovini A, Ponchio L, Scevola S, Faga A, et al. The role of rehabilitative camouflage after cervicofacial reconstructive surgery: a preliminary study. Clin Cosmet Investig Dermatol. 2014;7:43–9.
54. Baldelli I, Santi P, Dova L, Cardoni G, Ciliberti R, Franchelli S, et al. Body image disorders and surgical timing in patients affected by Poland syndrome: data analysis of 58 case studies. Plast Reconstr Surg. 2016;137(4):1273–82.

55. Levine MP, Smolak L. The prevention of eating problems and eating disorders. Mahwah, NJ: Lawrence Erlbaum; 2005.
56. Jung J, Peterson M. Body dissatisfaction and patterns of media use among preadolescent children. Fam Consum Sci Res J. 2007;36:40–54.
57. Robinson TN, Chang JY, Haydel KF, Killen JD. Overweight concerns and body dissatisfaction among third-grade children: the impacts of ethnicity and socioeconomic status. J Pediatr. 2001;138(2):181–7.
58. Stice E. Risk and maintenance factors for eating pathology: a meta-analytic review. Psychol Bull. 2002;128(5):825–48.
59. Gardner RM, Sorter RG, Friedman BN. Developmental changes in children's body images. J Soc Behav Personal. 1997;12:1019–36.
60. Lowes J, Tiggemann M. Body dissatisfaction, dieting awareness and the impact of parental influence in young children. Br J Health Psychol. 2003;8(Pt 2):135–47.
61. Phares V, Steinberg AR, Thompson JK. Gender differences in peer and parental influences. J Youth Adolesc. 2004;33:421–9.
62. Wood KC, Becker JA, Thompson JK. Body image dissatisfaction in preadolescent children. J Appl Dev Psychol. 1996;17:85–100.
63. Hendy HM, Gustitus C, Leitzel-Schwalm J. Social cognitive predictors of body image in preschool children. Sex Roles. 2001;44:557–97.
64. Lawrence CM, Thelen MH. Body image, dieting, and self-concept. J Child Clin Psychol. 1995;24:41–8.
65. Thompson SH, Corwin SJ, Sargent RG. Ideal body size beliefs and weight concerns of fourth-grade children. Int J Eat Disord. 1997;21(3):279–84.
66. Collins E. Body figure perceptions and preferences among preadolescent children. Int J Eat Disord. 1991;10:199–208.
67. Kelly NR, Bulik CM, Mazzeo SE. An exploration of body dissatisfaction and perceptions of black and white girls enrolled in an intervention for overweight children. Body Image. 2011;8(4):379–84. https://doi.org/10.1016/j.bodyim.2011.05.003. Epub 2011 Jun 22.
68. Xanthopoulos MS, Borradaile KE, Hayes S, Sherman S, Vander Veur S, Grundy KM, Nachmani J, Foster GD. The impact of weight, sex, and race/ethnicity on body dissatisfaction among urban children. Body Image. 2011;8(4):385–9. https://doi.org/10.1016/j.bodyim.2011.04.011. Epub 2011 Jun 12.
69. Fallon AE, Rozin P. Sex differences in perceptions of desirable body shape. J Abnorm Psychol. 1985;94(1):102–5.
70. Tiggemann M, Wilson-Barrett E. Children's figure ratings: relationship to self-esteem and negative stereotyping. Int J Eat Disord. 1998;23(1):83–8.
71. Kostanski M, Gullone E. Dieting and body image in the child's world: conceptualization and behavior. J Genet Psychol. 1999;160(4):488–99.
72. Poudevigne MS, O'Connor PJ, Laing EM, R Wilson AM, Modlesky CM, Lewis RD. Body images of 4-8-year-old girls at the outset of their first artistic gymnastics class. Int J Eat Disord. 2003;34(2):244–50.
73. Rolland K, Farnill D, Griffiths RA. Children's perceptions of their current and ideal body sizes and body mass index. Percept Mot Skills. 1996;82(2):651–6.
74. Williamson S, Delin C. Young children's figural selections: accuracy of reporting and body size dissatisfaction. Int J Eat Disord. 2001;29(1):80–4.
75. Schneider N, Martus P, Ehrlich S, Pfeiffer E, Lehmkuhl U, Salbach-Andrae H. The assessment of body image distortion in female adolescents with anorexia nervosa: the development of a test for body image distortion in children and adolescents (BID-CA). Eat Weight Disord. 2009;14(2–3):e128–36.
76. Truby H, Paxton SJ. The children's body image scale: reliability and use with international standards for body mass index. Br J Clin Psychol. 2008;47(Pt 1):119–24.
77. Truby H, Paxton SJ. Development of the children's body image scale. Br J Clin Psychol. 2002;41(Pt 2):185–203.

4 Diagnostic Classification of Eating Disorders: The Role of Body Image

Umberto Volpe, Alessio Maria Monteleone, and Palmiero Monteleone

4.1 Introduction

A disordered body image is retained a hallmark feature of eating disorders (ED), and it is included as a diagnostic criterion for the two main phenomenological ED entities, namely anorexia (AN) and bulimia nervosa (BN), in all major contemporary psychiatric diagnostic systems. However, in the first diagnostic formulations of AN, the most well-known and long-studied ED, this aspect was almost completely neglected. William Whitney Gull, who coined the term "anorexia nervosa" in 1873 [1], although significantly contributed to identify many core features of AN, did not identify this aspect as a central element of the syndrome. Neither the French physician Ernest Charles Lasègue [2], who on the same year published one of the first series of AN cases in his paper entitled "*De l'Anorexie Hystérique,*" mentioned this feature specifically. The early clinical formulations of AN had the merit to identify several clinical cornerstones of the syndrome (e.g., the psychological nature of the disorder, the preference for female sex, the effects of prolonged starvation, the typical onset during adolescence/early adulthood, the role of family members, the typically chronic course, the refeeding therapeutic strategies). However, although reporting on the changes in body weight and shape induced by starvation, those descriptions did not unveil the psychological reverberations and the psychopathological underpinnings of such changes in terms of body image, along the course of the disease [3].

After a century, ED other than AN were identified and body image represented a crucial clinical feature of these syndromes. For example, Russell [4], when first

U. Volpe · A. M. Monteleone
Department of Psychiatry, University of Campania "L. Vanvitelli", Naples, Italy

P. Monteleone (✉)
Department of Psychiatry, University of Campania "L. Vanvitelli", Naples, Italy

Department of Medicine, Surgery and Dentistry "Scuola Medica Salernitana", University of Salerno, Salerno, Italy

M. Cuzzolaro, S. Fassino (eds.), *Body Image, Eating, and Weight*,
https://doi.org/10.1007/978-3-319-90817-5_4

describing the clinical picture of BN by the end of the twentieth century, posed as central diagnostic criteria the "irresistible urge to overeat, followed by self-inducing vomit," on the one hand, and the "morbid fear of becoming fat," on the other, heavily linking the essence of this ED to a disturbance of the body image. To date, all major ED have been widely recognized as to be intimately linked to body image disturbance, which serves both as a diagnostic and nosological criterion for ED.

4.2 Evolution of the Body Image Disturbance Construct in the ED Diagnosis

In order to explain why and how the body image disturbance in ED gained so much consensus as a diagnostic and classification element along the past century, it is probably necessary to take into account the seminal work on body image carried out in the first decades of last century by several psychopathologists, who probably provided the first proper conceptual framework to establish the centrality of the body image disturbance for the diagnosis of ED. Indeed, the tradition of transcendental phenomenology first posed specific attention to the analysis of the body, of the way people experience their own body ("embodiment") and of the "embodied subjectivity," clarifying the centrality of the function of the body when it comes to basic experience of self, other, and shape/space evaluations [5]. In more detail, Edmund Husserl started to supplement his theories on perception by including fundamental reflections on the relation between body and (inter-)subjectivity, with the greater aim to analyze systematically the intentional structure of consciousness. Indeed, he first put forward the notion of "kinaesthetic consciousness" seen as a form of "embodied subjectivity" in which the "lived body" (*leib*, differently from the physical body or *korper* and the object-body or *ding*) is conceived as a "center of experience," playing a key role in defining how we encounter other embodied agents in the explorable world and creating an essential link between subjectivity and perceptual experience [6]. In continuity with the original vision of the founder of phenomenology, Merleau-Ponty [7] also focused on the phenomenological reflection about the nature of perception and human embodiment for his entire life, contributing to a fundamental step towards a new ontology. In general, he conceived the entire human experience as the result of a unique relation between an embodied subject and that which shows itself to him/her at every instant, as an act of dialogic *connaissance* [8]. In more detail, Merleau-Ponty [9] conceptualized the objective/material body as already intentional and fully engaged in meaning constitution and the mind as an "incarnated" one, being these two levels of perception overlapping or rather naturally intertwined ("human embodiment"). Although he did not specifically focus on psychological disturbances of embodiment in humans, Merleau-Ponty [10] tied inextricably the reality of our corporeal existence, body image representation, and mental activity, providing a conceptual framework in which psychological motivations and bodily activity are woven together in the lived experience of existing in the world, being the external world seen as a natural setting of and field for all thoughts and explicit perceptions, the body as a "living envelope" of all our intentions and body scheme (*schéma corporel*) as a representation of the intuitive understanding of one's own the body in its relation to the external space/world [11]. Finally, Jean Paul Sartre [12] also significantly contributed to the psychopathological debate on body representation, focusing on the concept of "lived corporality" and more specifically by adding to the duality "body-subject/body-object" a third dimension, the "lived body for others." Sartre focused on the idea that one's body, when looked by another person, becomes an object for that person and that this external point of view also contributes to create our own body image, in the sense that our sense of identity is constructed also through the gaze of the others. To note that this specific feeling of "being an object for others" has been recently proposed as a specific aberrant feature for ED, conceptualized as disorders of lived corporality in which specific disturbances of embodiment constitute a core aspect of the syndromes, affect the sense of personal identity and determine the anomalies of eating behavior [13]. According to these theories, it has been recently proved that this embodiment disorder, in terms of exaggerated tendency to experience one's body from an external perspective, is associated with attachment experiences and mediates the relationship between attachment and ED psychopathology [14].

Given the vast echo that phenomenological interpretation of perception and subjectivity had in the field of psychopathology, it is plausible that such concepts influenced the way of conceptualizing body image disorders, with obvious reflections in ED psychopathology. In this sense, it is not surprising that, within the first modern descriptions of ED, the abnormalities in body image perception and processing were reported as a typical and constant feature of the clinical picture of ED. More than half a century ago, Hilde Bruch [15] was the first to clearly affirm that AN was intimately linked to a perceptual body image/concept disorder and to define AN and all severe ED as *self*-disorders in which developmental deficits of the organization of the self are manifested in aberrant body perception and inefficient control of bodily sensations [3]. Actually, Bruch, besides suggesting that a perceptual body disorder and the denial of thinness are pathognomonic for AN, clarified that the concept of "interoceptive confusion" is a part of a more general "self-disorder" typical of the disease (i.e., people with AN not only tend to perceive their body image as distorted but rather show a disturbance in the accuracy of perception and cognitive interpretation of all bodily sensations—such as hunger/satiety, fatigue, weakness, pain—and inner feelings), that the pursuit of a thin body is used by AN patients as a "camouflage" for other underlying problems (such as control of bodily sensations, confusion of emotional states, fear or social disapproval) and highlighted that the body image disorder may reach "delusional proportions" in most severe cases of the disease [16]. Also, Bruch [17] considered a correction of body image misperception to be an essential precondition for recovery from AN.

Since Bruch's seminal clinical descriptions, many other researchers focused on the definition and meaning of body image in ED, highlighting the relevance of the phenomenon in clinical (e.g., the degree of body overestimation was predictive of food preference/aversion; [18]), diagnostic (e.g., the more distorted body image, the more severe psychopathology; [19]), and prognostic (e.g., the more distorted body image, the poorer outcome; [20]) terms.

4.3 Body Image and Current Diagnostic Criteria for ED

Such seminal aspects of body distortion and denial of thinness have been built into current diagnostic criteria for AN as a key feature. Indeed, after a long series of studies that examined the topic of body image in AN (for a review, see: [21]), a general consensus about the idea that a disrupted body image constitutes a primordial element of the psychopathology of AN and BN has gradually spread. Thus, it is not surprising that both major current international diagnostic systems include this psychopathological feature as a diagnostic criterion. The tenth edition of the international classification of diseases (ICD-10; [22]) is particularly explicit about considering the alteration of body image of patients with ED as an *overvalued* idea: ICD-10 clearly specifies that a significant distortion of the body image exists in AN patients, while for BN patients the manual stresses that its central psychopathological features are very similar to those of AN and confirms that, within the BN clinical picture, the morbid fear of gaining weight and the choice of a lower body weight/thinner body shape than the premorbid ones stay as crucial diagnostic aspects. ICD-11 is expected to be released along the year 2018 although no significant changes concerning the specific role of body image distortion in ED in diagnostic terms are expected [23]. The DSM-IV [24] considered that during the course of AN a "disturbance in the way in which one's body weight or shape is experienced" and that "undue influence of body weight or shape on self-evaluation, and denial of the seriousness of the current body weight" are basic diagnostic features for AN; as for BN, DSM-IV was less explicit by stating only that "self-evaluation is unduly influenced by body shape and weight." With the fifth edition of the DSM [25], the basic diagnostic features of ED concerning body image distortion and body dissatisfaction were left unaltered. Indeed, in DSM-5, the idea that "experience and significance of body weight and shape are distorted in these individuals" was recognized in the diagnostic criterion C for AN, despite the attempt to reduce the "atipicality" of the syndromes and to ease the diagnostic process of ED (in order to avoid the inflation of the "unspecified" and "other specified" disorders' categories). Also for BN, the criterion D confirmed the excessive emphasis on body shape or weight for self-evaluation and self-esteem, remarking a close resemblance of subjects with BN and AN (for "their fear of gaining weight, in their desire to lose weight, and in the level of dissatisfaction with their bodies").

However, especially for disorders other than AN and BN, the current diagnostic definition of ED is far from being satisfactory, with particular reference to the role of body image abnormalities within ED psychopathology, and a number of issues have to be considered when evaluating the impact of body image disturbances on the current nosology of ED.

First, while in DSM-IV [24] binge eating disorder (BED) was listed as a "research category," DSM-5 included BED among fully fledged ED diagnosis [25]; furthermore, the DSM-5 has also introduced a revision of the frequency and duration of binge eating episodes (once weekly for past 3 months). However, BED is the only formal ED major diagnosis which does not require a criterion focusing on the cognition of body image, not paralleling the DSM-5 AN and BN diagnoses, both including disturbances in both eating behavior and in how the body is evaluated [25]. As noted by Grilo [25], the simple absence of a diagnostic criterion/specifier covering the presence of a disturbance in body image may imply the risk to reduce the BED-specific diagnosis to a mere "behavioral overeating construct". Actually, the DSM-5 admits only three behaviors (i.e., eating much more rapidly than normal, eating until feeling uncomfortably full, and eating large amounts of food when not feeling physically hungry) and two feelings (embarrassment by how much one is eating and disgust with oneself), besides the generic presence of distress. The lack of a reference to body image overvaluation is somehow surprising if one considers the research evidence that piled up over the last decades concerning the well-known psychopathological analogies that BED subjects shares with AN and BN ones about shape/weight concerns [27, 28]. Similarly, the absence of this feature in obese non-BED subjects (i.e., overvaluation of body image is unrelated to excess weight or other potential major demographic confounds; [29, 30]) and the relative stability of the construct (which is reported to be influenced by self-esteem rather than by mood fluctuations; [26]) seem to point to the same psychopathological aspects of body image perception. Furthermore, such body image abnormalities have been found to be significantly related to greater severity of eating disorder psychopathology [31], more severe levels of mood psychopathology [32] and of psychological problems [33], poorer outcome [34, 35] as well as to be able to predict remission from binge eating [36]. The omission of any reference to any body image-related cognitive criterion from the DSM-5 criteria for BED is even more puzzling, if one considers that the retention of criteria B and C is not supported by a substantial empirical evidence [37]. While the possibility that having body shape overvaluation listed as a diagnostic criterion for BED may imply a greater risk of false negatives (as it may exclude from the BED diagnosis many persons with clinically significant eating pathology; [31]), the recent suggestion of including it as a course specifier or a distinct subtype [26] is probably worth of thorough consideration because of its diagnostic and prognostic relevance.

Second, the recent inclusion of the avoidant/restricting food intake disorder (ARFID) within the DSM-5 group of "feeding and eating disorders" also deserves attention from a psychopathological viewpoint. The APA Task Force [25], when revising and updating the DSM-IV diagnostic criteria for eating and feeding disorders, explicitly aimed to reduce the prevalence of the residual diagnostic category of "eating disorders not otherwise specified" (EDNOS) and to combine together the diagnostic criteria for adult and infancy/early childhood EDs. However, the inclusion of ARFID within the section leaves behind some doubts and open some issues. A recent multi-center study on ARFID [38] confirmed that one of the main clinical features of the syndrome is food avoidance in the lack of any body image disorder although associated with a reduction of body weight. The latter condition may easily lead the clinician to think that ARFID and other restrictive ED share common aspects. However, along the past decades a robust evidence has proven that, in the case of AN, body weight loss is strictly linked to the drive for thinness and to a disturbed body image, and many specific psychological therapies for this disorder tend to include specific modules on body image psychopathology [39]. While DSM-5 Task Force aimed to improve clinical utility of their diagnostic criteria and to capture a population of children who had pathological eating habits, the simple inclusion of ARFID (and "pica," the other main ED of infancy/childhood) within a diagnostic class, whose all other diagnostic categories share the "abnormal body image" feature, cannot be evaluated as a simple and straightforward decision and probably deserves further consideration.

4.4 Complexity of Body Image Disturbance Definition

Some ambiguity concerning the concept of body image disturbance in ED is derived from its very same definition. One of its simplest definitions is the one provided by the DSM [25] for diagnostic purposes, which sounds as "disturbance in the way in which one's body weight or shape is experienced." However, the contemporary understanding of body image is a multidimensional construct, complex in its nature and including perceptual, affective, cognitive, evaluative, and behavioral components [40]. The relative role of each component in creating a clinically relevant body image disorder has been less than satisfactorily explored by empirical research. Historically, most attention has been devoted to the "perceptual" component of body image estimation while the negative thoughts and feelings towards one's own body (the so-called body dissatisfaction) gained more spotlight over the past decades. However, recent brain imaging evidence [41] seem to point to the presence of an abnormal connectivity in cortico-limbic circuitry of subjects with ED, involving abnormalities of complex brain functions (such as cognitive control, visual and homeostatic integration) in the genesis of body image disturbances. Such neurobiological evidence is in line with a more complex model of body image in which different components may play different roles in determining the clinical emergence of such disorder in ED. Another issue that is of great relevance for body image disturbance in ED is that of cultural influences over the body perception: it has been long demonstrated that body image represents an unstable construct and that many different (internal and external) factors may significantly influence it [42]. In particular, several studies have reported that body image distortion in ED seems to represent the result of an "acculturation process, spread through the therapeutic milieu and the mass media" [43]. Furthermore, recent evidence witnessed a cultural change in that male subjects also exhibit a significant degree of body image disturbances in adolescence [44], in young adulthood [45], middle-age, and in old-age [46].

However, the role of cultural factors in determining body image disturbances has been largely overlooked by current diagnostic systems and in order to fully understand this psychological construct and evaluate its impact in the diagnosis and the classification of ED a thorough rethinking of the concept within the clinical field is awaited.

4.5 Body Image Disturbance and Differential Diagnosis

The relevance of body image disturbances for ED diagnosis and classification is of particular relevance also in terms of differential diagnosis. Along the past decades, several other psychological and medical disorders have been demonstrated to be significantly associated to a disordered body image although with different degrees and charachteristics. Ranging from newer eating disorders such as "bigorexia" [47] to body dysmorphic disorder [48], a variety of psychiatric syndromes have been postulated to be strictly related to classical ED on the shared ground of a relevant body image distortion but, to date, none of such evidence has been properly considered within currently available diagnostic systems. A clearer differentiation between body dissatisfaction and body image disturbance should be established in clinical and nosological terms. Such lack of clarity will likely create a certain degree of diagnostic ambiguity and might pose relevant problems in the clinical field. Some examples of clinical situations in which body image disturbance may create diagnostic ambiguity possibly include patients with low weight who deny any body dissatisfaction at any point during the development of their disorder (e.g., due to spiritual concerns, fears of choking, selective aversion for certain foods, food allergies), somatoform disorders and delusions concerning body image representation (in which a dimensional rather than a categorical approach may seem more valuable), chronic acquired physical diseases, and traumatic injuries which imply rapid changes in physical appearance.

Moreover, some recent evidence also prompted the issue of body image representation in obese people [49] and confirmed that overweight and obese youth tend to underestimate their body shape, with associated behavioral and psychological distresses. Although this preliminary evidence seems to converge towards a common ground with ED, obesity is yet not considered as part of the ED spectrum.

Finally, the relevance of body image disorders for the diagnosis and classification of ED also lies in the little explored potential of psychological treatment programs focusing on this psychopathological feature. Although evidence exists concerning the positive clinical impact of such psychotherapeutic approaches, associated with distinct neurobiological changes in temporal and frontal areas (e.g., see [50]), the dissemination of psychological interventions specifically focused on body image approaches is still in its early phase. Same applies to early detection and prevention programs for ED based on early identification of body image distortion in "at risk" populations although the presence of body image distortion has been proved to have a clear prognostic value at least in AN [51].

Conclusions

It is evident from the above that the disturbance of body image is a key psychopathological feature of ED. Indeed, the aberrant eating behaviors of people with ED can be considered as epiphenomena secondary to a possible common deeper psychopathological core including body image disturbance that leads to persistent body weight and shape dissatisfaction [52, 53]. It has been reported that body image distortion precedes the onset of AN [54] and its persistence over the course of treatment may predict a poor outcome of AN and/or a relapse of EDs [55]. Therefore, addressing this component of the ED psychopathology is mandatory in the treatment of these disorders although successful interventions are still lacking. This is likely due to the complexity of the construct of body image, which includes several components whose individual contribution to the body image disturbance of people with ED still awaits to be fully elucidated.

Recently, studies employing functional magnetic resonance imaging techniques, which allow direct "in vivo" exploration of neuronal activity associated to specific mental activities, have been employed to investigate the brain processing of body image perception in patients with ED, and more knowledge on this topic is emerging. Indeed, evidence has been provided that body image disturbance in EDs might be associated with dysfunctional brain circuits involved in body-image-processing with concomitant involvement of affective structures although the direction of such dysfunctions and the brain areas involved were not consistent among the studies. Furthermore, the implications of those findings for the treatment of EDs still await to be defined.

In conclusion, the relevance of body image disturbance is widely recognized for both the diagnosis and the treatment of ED. However, several critical issues still remain in its conceptualization and application to the different ED categories. This should be an area of continuous revision in future studies.

References

1. Gull WW. Anorexia nervosa (apepsia hysterica, anorexia hysterica). Trans Clin Soc Lond. 1874;VII:22–8.
2. Lasègue C. De l'anorexie hystérique. Arch Gén Méd. 1873;1:384–403.
3. Pearce JMS. Richard morton: origins of anorexia nervosa. Eur Neurol. 2004;52:191–2.
4. Russell G. Bulimia nervosa: an ominous variant of anorexia nervosa. Psychol Med. 1979;9(3):429–48.
5. Zahavi D. Husserl's phenomenology of the body. Études Phénoménologiques. 1994;10(19):63–84.
6. Husserl E. Ideen zu einer reinen phaenomenologie und phaenomenologischen philosophie I. In: Schumann K, editor. Husserliana III. Den Haag: Martinus Nijhoff; 1913/1976.
7. Merleau-Ponty M. The visible and the invisible. Evanston, IL: Northwestern University Press; 1964/1968.
8. Carman T. The body in husserl and merleau-ponty. Philos Top. 1999;27(2):205–26.
9. Merleau-Ponty M. Sense and non-sense. Evanston, IL: Northwestern University Press; 1948/1964.
10. Merleau-Ponty M. Phenomenology of perception. London: Routledge; 1945/1962.
11. Bullington J. The expression of the psychosomatic body from a phenomenological perspective. Berlin: Springer; 2013. p. 19–37.
12. Sartre JP. Being and nothingness (*L'etre et le neant*). New York: Washington Square Press; 1943/1992.
13. Stanghellini G, Castellini G, Brogna P, Faravelli C, Ricca V. Identity and eating disorders (IDEA): a questionnaire evaluating identity and embodiment in eating disorder patients. Psychopathology. 2012;45(3):147–58.
14. Monteleone AM, Castellini G, Ricca V, Volpe U, De Riso F, Nigro M, Zamponi F, Mancini M, Stanghellini G, Monteleone P, Treasure J, Maj M. Embodiment mediates the relation-

ship between avoidant attachment and eating disorder psychopathology. Eur Eat Disord Rev. 2017;25(6):461–8.
15. Bruch H. Perceptual and conceptual disturbances in anorexia nervosa. Psychosom Med. 1962;24:187–94.
16. Skårderud F. Bruch revisited and revised. Eur Eat Disord Rev. 2009;17(2):83–8.
17. Bruch H. Eating disorders. Obesity, anorexia nervosa, and the person within. New York: Basic Books; 1973.
18. Garfinkel PE, Moldofsky H, Garner DM, Stancer HC, Coscina DV. Body awareness in anorexia nervosa: disturbances in "body image" and "satiety". Psychosom Med. 1978;40(6):487–98.
19. Garfinkel PE, Garner DM. Anorexia nervosa: a multidimensional perspective. New York: Brunner/Mazel; 1982.
20. Slade PD, Russell GF. Experimental investigations of bodily perception in anorexia nervosa and obesity. Psychother Psychosom. 1973;22(2):359–63.
21. Slade P. A review of body-image studies in anorexia nervosa and bulimia nervosa. J Psychiatr Res. 1985;19(2–3):255–65.
22. World Health Organization (WHO). International classification of mental and behavioral disorder: clinical descriptions and diagnostic guidelines, tenth edition (ICD-10). Geneva, WHO, 1992.
23. Uher R, Rutter M. Classification of feeding and eating disorders: review of evidence and proposals for ICD-11. World Psychiatry. 2012;11(2):80–92.
24. American Psychiatric Association. Diagnostic and statistical manual of mental disorders. 4th ed. Washington, DC: American Psychiatric Association; 1994.
25. American Psychiatric Association. Diagnostic and statistical manual of mental disorders. 5th ed. Washington, DC: American Psychiatric Association; 2013.
26. Grilo MC. Why no cognitive body image feature such as overvaluation of shape/weight in the binge eating disorder diagnosis? Int J Eat Disord. 2013;46:208–11.
27. Masheb RM, Grilo CM. Binge eating disorder: a need for additional diagnostic criteria. Compr Psychiatry. 2000;41:159–62.
28. Wilfley DE, Schwartz MB, Spurrell EB, Fairburn CG. Using the eating disorder examination to identify the specific psychopathology of binge eating disorder. Int J Eat Disord. 2000;27:259–69.
29. Grilo CM, Hrabosky JI, Allison KC, Stunkard AJ, Masheb RM. Overvaluation of shape and weight in binge eating disorder and overweight controls: refinement of a diagnostic construct. J Abnorm Psychol. 2008;117:414–9.
30. Grilo CM, Masheb RM, White MA. Significance of overvaluation of shape/weight in binge-eating disorder: comparative study with overweight and bulimia nervosa. Obesity. 2010;18:499–504.
31. Goldschmidt AB, Hilbert A, Manwaring JL, Wilfley DE, Pike KM, Fairburn CG, et al. The significance of overvaluation of shape and weight in binge eating disorder. Behav Res Ther. 2010;48:187–93.
32. Grilo CM, Crosby RD, Masheb RM, White MA, Peterson CB, Wonderlich SA, et al. Overvaluation of shape and weight in binge eating disorder, bulimia nervosa, and sub-threshold bulimia nervosa. Behav Res Ther. 2009;47:692–6.
33. Ojserkis R, Sysko R, Goldfein JA, Devlin MJ. Does the overvaluation of shape and weight predict initial symptom severity or treatment outcome among patients with binge eating disorder? Int J Eat Disord. 2012;45:603–8.
34. Hilbert A, Saelens B, Stein R, Mockus DS, Welch RR, Matt GE, et al. Pretreatment and process predictors of outcome in interpersonal and cognitive behavioral psychotherapy for binge eating disorder. J Consult Clin Psychol. 2007;75:645–51.
35. Sysko R, Hildebrandt T, Wilson GT, Wilfley DE, Agras WS. Heterogeneity moderates treatment response among patients with binge eating disorder. J Consult Clin Psychol. 2010;78:681–90.
36. Grilo CM, Masheb RM, Crosby RD. Predictors and moderators of response to cognitive behavioral therapy and medication for the treatment of binge eating disorder. J Consult Clin Psychol. 2012;80:186–95.

37. Mond JM. Classification of bulimic-type eating disorders: from DSM-IV to DSM-5. J Eat Disord. 2013;1:33.
38. Fisher MM, Rosen DS, Ornstein RM, Mammel KA, Katzman DK, Rome ES, Callahan ST, Malizio J, Kearney S, Walsh BT. Characteristics of avoidant/restrictive food intake disorder in children and adolescents: a "new disorder" in DSM-5. J Adolesc Health. 2014;55(1):49–52.
39. Zipfel S, Giel KE, Bulik CM, Hay P, Schmidt U. Anorexia nervosa: aetiology, assessment, and treatment. Lancet Psychiatry. 2015;2(12):1099–111.
40. Thompson JK, Heinberg LJ, Altabe M, Tantleff-Dunn S. Exacting beauty: theory, assessment, and treatment of body image disturbance. Washington, DC: American Psychological Association; 1999.
41. Gaudio S, Wiemerslage L, Brooks SJ, Schiöth HB. A systematic review of resting-state functional-MRI studies in anorexia nervosa: evidence for functional connectivity impairment in cognitive control and visuospatial and body-signal integration. Neurosci Biobehav Rev. 2016;71:578–89.
42. Gardner RM, Brown DL. Body size estimation in anorexia nervosa: a brief review of findings from 2003 through 2013. Psychiatry Res. 2014;219(3):407–10.
43. Gutierrez E, Carrera O. Anorexia nervosa and body-image disturbance. Lancet Psychiatry. 2016;3:e9–10.
44. Mitchison D, Hay P, Griffiths S, Murray SB, Bentley C, Gratwick-Sarll K, Harrison C, Mond J. Disentangling body image: the relative associations of overvaluation, dissatisfaction, and preoccupation with psychological distress and eating disorder behaviors in male and female adolescents. Int J Eat Disord. 2017;50(2):118–26.
45. Calzo JP, Horton NJ, Sonneville KR, Swanson SA, Crosby RD, Micali N, Eddy KT, Field AE. Male eating disorder symptom patterns and health correlates from 13 to 26 years of age. J Am Acad Child Adolesc Psychiatry. 2016;55(8):693–700.e2.
46. Mangweth-Matzek B, Kummer KK, Pope HG. Eating disorder symptoms in middle-aged and older men. Int J Eat Disord. 2016;49(10):953–7.
47. Suffolk MT, Dovey TM, Goodwin H, et al. Muscle dysmorphia: methodological issues, implications for research. Eat Disord. 2013;21:437–57.
48. Grant JE, Phillips KA. Is anorexia nervosa a subtype of body dysmorphic disorder? Harv Rev Psychiatry. 2004;12(2):123–6.
49. Sandoval JRG, Caracuel JC, Cocca A, Cocca M, Gurrola OC. Relation between body mass index and body image in spanish and mexican adolescents. Behav Med. 2017;23:1–9.
50. Vocks S, Schulte D, Busch M, Grönemeyer D, Herpertz S, Suchan B. Changes in neuronal correlates of body image processing by means of cognitive-behavioural body image therapy for eating disorders: a randomized controlled fMRI study. Psychol Med. 2011;41(8):1651–63.
51. Boehm I, Finke B, Tam FI, Fittig E, Scholz M, Gantchev K, Roessner V, Ehrlich S. Effects of perceptual body image distortion and early weight gain on long-term outcome of adolescent anorexia nervosa. Eur Child Adolesc Psychiatry. 2016;25(12):1319–26.
52. Bardone-Cone AM, Harney MB, Maldonado CR, Lawson MA, Robinson DP, Smith R. Defining recovery from an eating disorder: conceptualization, validation, and examination of psychosocial functioning and psychiatric comorbidity. Behav Res Ther. 2010;48:194–202.
53. Fairburn CG, Harrison PJ. Eating disorders. Lancet. 2003;361:407–16.
54. Jacobi C, Paul T, de Zwaan M, Nutzinger DO, Dahme B. Specificity of self-concept disturbances in eating disorders. Int J Eat Disord. 2004;35:204–10.
55. Keel PK, Dorer DJ, Franko DL, Jackson SC, Herzog DB. Postremission predictors of relapse in women with eating disorders. Am J Psychiatry. 2005;162:2263–8.

Body Dysmorphic Disorder and Muscle Dysmorphia

5

Massimo Cuzzolaro

5.1 From Morselli to DSM

The tormenting preoccupation with an imaginary or insignificant defect in one's physical appearance was recognized in 1891 by Enrico Morselli as a particular psychiatric disorder and named *dysmorphophobia* [1] (see Chap. 6 of the present volume). The Italian alienist classified it as an *insanity with fixed ideas* (*rudimentary paranoia*), highlighted the obsessive-compulsive features of this clinical picture and noted that some patients developed recognizable delusional thoughts about their body appearance. Therefore, Morselli's dysmorphophobia included both the non-delusional and the delusional variant. Nearly a century after that seminal paper, the expression *body dysmorphic disorder* officially replaced Morselli's neologism, but the term *dysmorphophobia* is still in use.

The old syndrome was very similar to the current descriptions of *body dysmorphic disorder* (BDD). A person with BDD may be terrified of being laughed at, rejected, humiliated, because of his/her physical aspect; conversely, in some cultures, he/she may be afraid to hurt others or to cause inconvenience to them for the same reason (*taijin-kyofu-sho*). A high-degree of self-consciousness is a typical feature of BDD and self-reference ideas are frequent.

These clinical pictures are difficult to classify, and during the last century, they have been categorized in very different ways: symptom or syndrome? A somatoform disorder like hypochondria or an obsessive-compulsive disorder? Obsession or delusion?

In 1930, the German psychiatrist Walther Jahrreiss emphasized the relationships with hypochondria and coined the expression *Schönheitshypochondrie* (beauty hypochondria) [2].

M. Cuzzolaro
Formerly Medical Pathophysiology Department, Eating Disorders and Obesity Unit, Sapienza University of Rome, Rome, Italy

M. Cuzzolaro, S. Fassino (eds.), *Body Image, Eating, and Weight*,
https://doi.org/10.1007/978-3-319-90817-5_5

The Diagnostic and Statistical Manual of Mental Disorders (DSM) did not use the term *dysmorphophobia* in the first two editions [3, 4]. In 1980, the third edition (DSM-III), revived the old term *dysmorphophobia* but not to indicate a distinct diagnostic category. *Dysmorphophobia* can be found in the group of *somatoform disorders*—which contained *hypochondriasis* as well—in the residual category *atypical somatoform disorder* (300.70). The "atypical" designation was similar to the "Not Otherwise Specified" category used in the subsequent editions of the diagnostic manual. Four lines describe the clinical picture:

> "An example of cases that can be classified here include those individuals who are preoccupied with some imagined defect in physical appearance that is out of proportion to any actual physical abnormality that may exist. This syndrome has sometimes been termed Dysmorphophobia" [5] (p. 252).

In 1987, the revised edition of the manual (DSM-III-R) introduced two specific psychiatric diagnostic categories for dysmorphic concerns and named them, respectively, *delusional disorder somatic type* (297.10) and *body dysmorphic disorder* (BDD) (300.70) [6]. BDD (non-delusional dysmorphophobia) was included in the group of *somatoform disorders*, together with *hypochondriasis*.

In 1994, also the DSM-IV classified BDD (300.70) within the section *somatoform disorders*, together with *hypochondriasis* [7]. However, in DSM-IV, the label BDD included the delusional cases too, with a double diagnosis:

> "individuals with BDD can receive an additional diagnosis of *delusional disorder, somatic type* (297.1), if their preoccupation with an imagined defect in appearance is held with a delusional intensity" [7] (p. 468).

This anodyne choice joined together the two clinical pictures and kept them apart at the same time, in an inconsistent way.

In their excellent analysis of 178 historical cases of dysmorphophobia [8], Berrios and Kan used the year 1985 as a cutoff point to compare cases published before and after DSM-III. They chose 1985 instead of 1980 because at least 5 years are needed to adopt a new taxonomy, design a research, and publish its results. From about 300 cases reported during the twentieth century, the authors selected 178 individuals (89 women and 89 men) by quality of data: 139 pre-DSM-III and 39 post-DSM-III. The main findings were the following:

- The pre-DSM-III group was more heterogeneous
- Included less male subjects (45% vs 69%)
- Included more sexual disorders
- Included more complaints about organs which were psychodynamically meaningful, such as nose and genitals
- Received less drug treatment
- Had a less good outcome

5.2 DSM-5 Diagnostic Criteria

In 2013, the fifth edition of the manual (DSM-5) classified BDD under the *obsessive-compulsive and related disorders* chapter [9].

DSM-5 requires two main phenomena to diagnose BDD:

- The individual is preoccupied about one or more perceived defects in his/her physical appearance.
- He/she repeatedly performs compulsive behaviors related to the appearance preoccupations.

Some words are desirable about the DSM-5 operational definitions of these symptoms.

Appearance preoccupation requires thinking about unreal or overvalued physical imperfections for at least an hour a day. Face and head (e.g., skin, hair, nose, eyes, chin, face shape) are the parts most commonly involved in BDD, but each segment and feature of the body can cause concern (e.g., too weak, insufficiently muscular). Males are more likely to be preoccupied with their genitals than females [10]. The uneasiness may also be indefinite as a general feeling of being unpleasant. It should be noted that DSM-IV referred to *imagined* defects while DSM-5 reads *perceived* defects.

Compulsivity means irresistible and repetitive behaviors (e.g., mirror checking, camouflaging, reassurance seeking, avoidance of situations or triggers that increase distress about the perceived physical defect) or mental acts (e.g., comparing one's physical features with those of other persons).

Furthermore, to diagnose BDD, both appearance preoccupations and compulsions must generate clinically significant distress and impairment in important areas of functioning.

DSM-5 provides two specifiers for identifying distinct subgroups of BDD:

- *Muscle dysmorphia*. If the appearance preoccupations focus on insufficient muscularity, the diagnosis should be *BDD, muscle dysmorphia form*
- *Insight*. How confident is the individual that the imaginary or insignificant aesthetic defects in his/her appearance are real and significant? This specifier is divided into three levels: "with good or fair insight" (recognition that one's beliefs are not true); "with poor insight"; "with absent insight/delusional beliefs".

It is worth noting that BDD with absent insight and delusional beliefs of reference is classified as BDD and not as a *delusional disorder*. In DSM-5, *the content* of this symptom seems to be pivotal.

In fact, his point and even the concept of insight are controversial issues.

In their conceptual and quantitative analysis of historical cases of dysmorphophobia [8], Berrios and Kan found relevant differences between delusional and non-delusional patients:

> "which suggests that the subsequent DSM-III-R subdivision between 'body dysmorphic disorder' and 'delusional disorder, somatic subtype' was justified. The types of differences found also suggest that these two groups are not just points on a continuum of severity, as has recently been suggested [11]" (p. 6).

On the contrary, during the DSM-5 development process, Katharine Phillips and the workgroup which was responsible for BDD affirmed that according to available evidence, delusional and non-delusional appearance preoccupations had "many more similarities than differences, including response to pharmacotherapy" [12] (p. 10).

Remarkable similarities were found across a broad range of antecedent and concurrent validators: sociodemographic factors, family history, risk factors, specific symptoms, comorbid psychiatric disorders, cognitive and emotional correlates, temperament and personality traits, functional impairment, quality of life, course of illness, and response to treatment. In particular, patients with delusional and non-delusional BDD responded to serotonin reuptake inhibitors (SRIs) monotherapy (e.g., fluoxetine, clomipramine) in the same way. Conversely, antipsychotic drugs did not show significant effects.

For that reason, the workgroup proposed the introduction of a *dimensional insight specifier* among the diagnostic criteria for BDD to indicate the *degree of delusionality*. Insight was defined as the level of a person's conviction in his/her disorder-relevant belief [12]. As a result, DSM-5 acknowledged that there is a continuum between the non-delusional and the delusional form of BDD.

Insight is a multidimensional concept with variable definitions in the psychiatric literature (see Chap. 1 of the present volume). It has been explored in many clinical conditions, including obsessive-compulsive disorder (OCD) and anorexia nervosa. The main components of insight are the following: (a) attribution of symptoms to a mental disorder; (b) awareness of illness, its effects, and need for treatment. Of course, *good, poor, absent* may be sketchy and preliminary evaluations.

As to insight in BDD, two studies found that, on average, persons with BDD had significantly poorer insight than individuals with OCD [13, 14]. In particular, in 2017 Toh et al. reexamined this issue in light of DSM-5 and suggested that appearance-related worries in many cases of BDD resemble delusional thoughts observed in psychotic disorders [14]. However, in BDD severity is associated with delusionality but not equivalent to it.

The two above-mentioned investigations used the Brown Assessment of Beliefs Scale (BABS) that assesses delusionality both dimensionally and categorically [15]. BABS is a semi-structured, clinician-administered, seven-item scale which evaluates insight/delusionality across a wide range of psychiatric disorders, including BDD [16] and eating disorders [17].

5.3 Muscle Dysmorphia

Beginning from the first decades of the twentieth century [18], the *drive for thinness* (desire to be thin) and the so-called *normative discontent* [19]—thinness-oriented body dissatisfaction—have become more and more common among girls and women, but rare among men. Most psychometric instruments and research procedures were designed to explore this female social and internalized thin ideal.

Only in the 1990s, some studies indicated that the male standard of physical attractiveness was a very muscular body and many boys and men tended to develop a *drive for muscularity* and reported a muscularity-oriented body dissatisfaction [20].

The *drive for muscularity* can be defined as the internalization of the muscular social ideal and the associated behaviors expected to increase the body muscle mass [21].

The expression *muscle dysmorphia* (MD) is currently used to describe people extremely concerned with their muscularity. This condition also received other names:

- *Reverse anorexia nervosa*: the individual feels his/her body is too small [20]
- *The Adonis complex*: in Greek mythology, the demigod Adonis was the utmost in masculine beauty [22]
- *Bigorexia*: the appetite for a big body [23]

A systematic review published in 2015 concluded that the current evidence does not ensure the validity and clinical utility of the inclusion of MD as a new mental disorder [24]. Some authors suggested that MD should be classified as a behavioral addiction [25].

However, as above-mentioned, DSM-5 identified MD as a psychiatric syndrome and classified it as a distinct subgroup of BDD: *BDD, muscle dysmorphia form* [9]. Its main features are the following:

- Unescapable appearance preoccupations focused on insufficient muscularity (extreme fear that one's own body is too small, like the proverbial *90-pound weakling*)
- Intense *drive for muscularity*
- Regular muscle-building behaviors: weight training and other anaerobic exercises; misuse of nutritional supplements, hormones, and hormone-like substances such as dehydroepiandrosterone (DHEA) and anabolic-androgenic steroids; dieting to gain weight and build muscle mass; *cheat meals*
- Significant distress and impairment in important areas of functioning.

Some findings support the notion that MD and anorexia nervosa (AN) share an ego-syntonic nature and several symptomatic similarities in the domains of body image disturbances and eating and exercise behaviors [26].

The divergence of body image worries towards a thin ideal (AN) or a muscular ideal (MD) appears, respectively, associated with the feminine or masculine gender role (see Chap. 19 of the present volume) affirmation. In a comparison study concerning gender role, men with MD reported elevated masculine gender role endorsement, whereas men with AN showed high adherence to feminine norms [27].

However, the divergence may be unstable. There is a high prevalence of premorbid AN among men with MD. The transition from a thinness-oriented to a muscularity-oriented disorder is a puzzling trans-diagnostic crossover and a clinical phenomenon that is often difficult to detect. It can be underestimated during treatment [28].

The so-called *cheat meals* represent an emerging dietary practice, in particular within pro-muscularity communities. A thematic content analysis found that *cheat meals* were associated with the idealization of overconsumption of large quantities of calorie-dense foods, the glorification of fitness and muscularity, and the function of a recurring reward [29]. A *cheat meal* sometimes appears as an objective binge eating episode.

In sum, muscularity-oriented disordered eating is frequent among people with MD, and it has been suggested that changes to current view and classification of ED are needed to amend the systematic underrepresentation of males in ED research [30, 31].

MD has been mostly studied in Western cultures where some interrelated risk factors are especially present:

- Physical size and strength are a customary measure of masculinity
- There is a decline in traditional male roles
- Visual media tend to present pictures of very muscular male bodies
- Video games and children's toys portray men in an hyper-muscular V-shape manner, with unrealistic height, bulk, and chest-to-waist ratio.

MD has also been described in non-Western countries, such as Samoa islands [32] and China [33]. The occurrence could be a universal sociobiological phenomenon but could also be due to the widespread penetration of Western media images of ideal male bodies [32]. There are differences, of course. For example, a study suggested that MD and anabolic steroid misuse are less severe problems in Taiwan than in Western nations [34].

MD is most prevalent in boys and men but not absent among girls and women, as some qualitative and case studies demonstrated [35]. Female bodybuilders seem to be at higher risk for MD and exercise dependence than female recreational weightlifters [36]. In both genders. The relationship between total television watched and drive for muscularity seems to be mediated by the internalization of athletic body shape ideals [37].

There is scant research on MD among sexual minorities (see Chap. 19 of the present volume).

In Australia and New Zealand, 2733 sexual minority men (gay and bisexual) recently completed a self-report survey. The research was aimed to explore the associations of some specific body features (height, muscularity, penis size, and body fat) dissatisfaction with quality of life (QoL) impairment [38]. Muscularity dissatisfaction had the most robust relationship with psychological QoL impairment, and penis size dissatisfaction the weakest.

The analysis of the same database showed that maladaptive use of image-centric social media platforms, such as Instagram, may be associated with muscularity dissatisfaction and disordered eating behaviors, also in sexual minority men [39]. Regarding body dissatisfaction, MD, ED, and anabolic steroid misuse, these platforms should receive greater attention than non-image-centric social media.

Several socio-environmental, cognitive, emotional, and behavioral factors contribute to the development of MD [40]. The drive for muscularity is associated with narcissism, negative affect, low self-esteem, perfectionism, parental and peer comments and teasing, media influences, ideal body internalization, self-objectification, social comparison, intra-sexual competition, and social physique anxiety [21, 41].

Medical and psychiatric comorbidities are frequent in both genders [42, 43]. MD is associated with greater psychopathology and higher attempted suicide rates than other forms of BDD [44]. Men at risk of MD appear more prone to social isolation than controls [45].

MD is a relatively new phenomenon. Furthermore, evaluating people's perceptions of their degree of body fat is more straightforward than examining perceptions of their muscularity [21]. Much research is needed in the areas of epidemiology, neurobiological underpinnings, assessment, and treatment of MD.

5.4 Differential Diagnoses According to DSM-5

Apart from BDD, in DSM-5, the new chapter on obsessive-compulsive and related disorders include two other body-focused repetitive behavior disorders: *trichotillomania* and *excoriation disorder*. The deliberate production of self-inflicted skin lesions is also named *dermatitis artefacta*. Thickening of the skin as a secondary process due to unpleasant sensations of pruritus and repetitive scratching or rubbing is called *Lichen simplex chronicus*.

BDD should be diagnosed rather than *trichotillomania* if the compulsive hair-pulling behavior is due to appearance preoccupations. Similarly, BDD should be diagnosed rather than *excoriation disorder* if the compulsive skin-picking behavior is due to appearance concerns.

If the main symptom is the firm belief that the body is infested with insects, the DSM-5 diagnosis should be *delusional disorder, somatic type*. Delusion of parasitosis and Ekbom's syndrome are other names, used in the past [46], for this uncommon body-focused psychotic disorder more often observed by dermatologists than by psychiatrists.

By the way, dermatologists frequently meet individuals with prominent obsessive-compulsive features focused on skin, hair, nails, AIDS phobia, and ideas of parasitosis. They often do not fulfill DSM-5 diagnostic criteria for *BDD*, *trichotillomania*, or *excoriation disorder*. A recent article proposed a novel classification, based on the degree of insight and named *obsessive-compulsive skin disorders* [47].

If an individual is worried about body weight and fat and meets diagnostic criteria for an eating disorder, then diagnosis should be *eating disorder* (ED). DSM-5 differentiates between BDD and ED and emphasizes the distinction (see Chap. 1 of the present volume). However, some patients have both an ED and BDD (appearance concerns other than body weight and shape). In fact, some authors think that comorbidity of BDD with an ED is underdiagnosed in the ED clinical units [48].

If social avoidance is due to appearance concerns, BDD should be diagnosed rather than *social anxiety disorder* (social phobia).

If a person is preoccupied with emitting an unpleasant smell, mostly from mouth, skin, vagina, and rectum, *olfactory reference syndrome* (ORS) should be diagnosed rather than BDD. ORS (also termed *bromidrosiphobia*) does not appear in ICD-10. In DSM-5, it is not a definite diagnosis, but the expression is mentioned in the section "Other specified obsessive-compulsive and related disorders" (300.2—F42) [9] (p. 837).

ORS has been described in the Western psychiatric literature, but a similar syndrome may be observed in other cultures too. In Japan, a patient preoccupied with a false belief that his/her body emits an unpleasant odor is recognized as *jiko-shu-kyofu*. This clinical picture is usually considered as a culture-bound syndrome, specific to Japan, but Suzuki et al. found that *jiko-shu-kyofu* and ORS may share most features. So, it should not be defined as a culture-bound disorder [49].

5.5 Taijin-Kyofu-Sho. Culture-Bound or Boundless Syndrome?

Jiko-shu-kyofu is a subtype of *taijin-kyofu-sho,* fear (*kyofu*) of interpersonal relationships (*taijin*). This syndrome was first described in Japan in the 1920s and defined "phobia of blushing and being ashamed" [50] (p. 146).

Later, the expression included other forms of social anxiety that, in some cases, presented delusional features. Nagata differentiated two subtypes of social anxiety: "offensive" (fear of embarrassing or offending others) and "non-offensive" (fear of being looked at by others with feelings of embarrassment and humiliation) [51]. He also underlined that the "offensive" subtype is not a culture-bound syndrome because it exists cross-nationally and has been described in Western cultures as well.

In the original Japanese classification of mental disorders, *taijin-kyofu-sho* was divided into four subtypes: *sekimen-kyofu* (phobia of blushing), *jiko-shu-kyofu* (phobia of one's own foul body odor), *shubo-kyofu* (phobia of a deformed body or face), and *jiko-shisen-kyofu* (phobia of one's own glance or eye-to-eye contact).

Table 5.1 Proposed diagnostic criteria for *taijin-kyofu-sho*

1	In the presence of others fear of (at least one): • Blushing • Stiffening of facial expression, trembling of the head, hands, feet, or voice, sweating • Physical deformities being noticed • Physical deformities being noticed • Line-of-sight becoming uncontrollable • Uncontrollable flatus in the presence of others
2	Because of the above fear, either of the following two. Fear of • Being looked at (noticed) by others • Offending or embarrassing others
3	The individual ***mostly*** recognizes that the fear is excessive or unreasonable
4	The symptoms significantly interfere with the person's well-being and psycho-social functioning
5	The symptoms must have been present for at least: • One year in adults • Six months in individuals younger than 18

In 1989, Takahashi proposed five diagnostic criteria (Table 5.1) for *taijin-kyofu-sho*, a disorder that the author first called *anthropophobia* [52] and then *social phobia syndrome* [53].

In DSM-5, *taijin-kyofu-sho* is listed under the label "Social anxiety disorder", and briefly described in the section "Culture-related diagnostic issues" [9].

However, in the Western taxonomies, the first three subtypes of *taijin-kyofu-sho,* respectively, correspond to *erythrophobia*, *body dysmorphic disorder,* and *olfactory reference syndrome*, whereas *jiko-shisen-kyofu* appears as a possible East Asian culture-related distinct syndrome [54].

A person with *jiko-shisen-kyofu* avoids personal interactions because he/she suffers from the preoccupation that his/her glance is offensive to others. It may be useful to remind that the Western cultures ascribe avoidance of eye contact to guilt, mendaciousness, shame. Conversely, in Japan making eye contact is considered offensive and rude, and the children "are taught to fix their gaze at the clavicular level of the people they are speaking to" [55] (p. 394).

Social withdrawal is, of course, a frequent after-effect of social anxiety, body appearance concerns, and *taijin-kyofu-sho*.

In the last two decades, *hikikomori*—severe occupational/social withdrawal for at least 6 months—has received increasing attention, first in Japan and then in Western countries as well [56–58]. Another phenomenon, widespread in the modern world and often intertwined with social anxiety and *hikikomori*, is called *NEET*: many young people in the contemporary world are Not in Education, Employment, or Training (NEET), and some of them show social anxiety and social withdrawal. The hen or the egg?

Also the Japanese categories *taijin-kyofu-sho*, with its four subtypes, and *hikikomori* let us see how much body appearance concerns and social anxiety involve personal, interpersonal, socioeconomic, and cultural factors that are always deeply interwoven in spite of any classification, inescapably restrictive (Fig. 5.1).

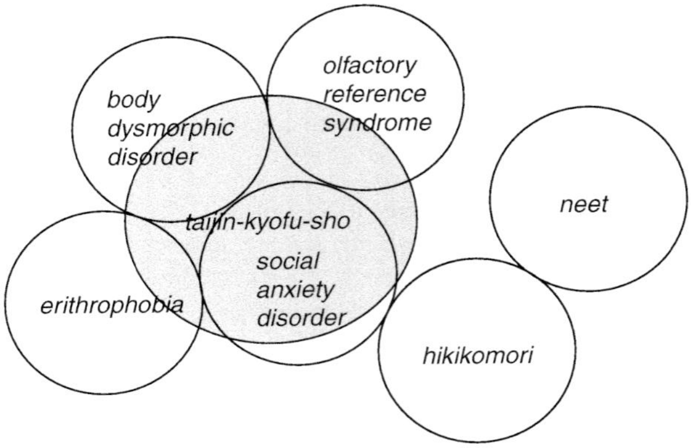

Fig. 5.1 *Taijin-kyo-fusho, hikikomori,* and Western nomenclature

5.6 BDD in the International Classification of Diseases (ICD)

The tenth edition of the International Classification of Diseases (ICD-10) did not follow DSM-III-R published 5 years before. In ICD-10, BDD is not a particular diagnostic category, but the term *dysmorphophobia* explicitly appears in the group of *somatoform disorders* (F45) to indicate a variant of the *hypochondriacal disorder* (F45.2) or—when it has delusional features—in the group of *other persistent delusional disorders* (F22.8) [59].

In fact, the ICD-10 offered at least four different possible diagnoses for BDD symptoms [60]: (a) *hypochondriacal disorder* (F45.2) for the non-delusional BDD; (b) *delusional disorder* or (c) *other persistent delusional disorder* (F22.0 or F22.8) for the delusional forms of BDD; and (d) *schizotypal disorder* (F21) for clinical pictures with ruminations and bizarre ideas with dysmorphophobic contents, not amounting to true delusions.

The WHO ICD-11 Working Group on the classification of *obsessive-compulsive and related disorders* has acknowledged that the absence of an autonomous category for BDD creates diagnostic confusion.

ICD-11, which is due by 2018, will probably contain a separate diagnostic category for BDD and will include it in the group of *obsessive-compulsive related disorders* like DSM-5 [61].

Table 5.2 synopsizes the DSM and ICD classifications of BDD that, during the last four decades, fluctuated from somatoform disorders to delusional disorders and obsessive-compulsive disorders. The unsteadiness reflects the rationale of current psychiatric classifications, which are grounded on descriptions of syndromes. As to most mental disorders, it is still impossible to identify true biological entities with natural boundaries like infectious diseases. Therefore, taxonomists pragmatically categorize collections of symptoms, correlated with each other, as concepts hopefully useful for epidemiologists and clinicians [62, 63].

Table 5.2 DSM and ICD classifications of the old *delusional* and *non-delusional dysmorphophobia* from 1952 to 2013

	Somatoform disorders (like hypochondriasis)	Delusional disorders	Obsessive-compulsive disorders
DSM-I (1952) DSM-II (1968)	The first two editions of the manual do not mention *dysmorphophobia*		
DSM-III (1980)	Non-delusional dysmorphophobia is not a distinct diagnostic category. It is included among the *Atypical somatoform disorders*	Delusional dysmorphophobia is not clearly identified (*Atypical somatoform disorder*, *Atypical psychosis*, *Atypical paranoid disorder*?)	
DSM-III-R (1987)	Non-delusional dysmorphophobia is a new distinct diagnostic category. It appears in the section of *Somatoform disorders* and is renamed *Body dysmorphic disorder* (BDD)	Delusional dysmorphophobia is considered to be different from BDD. It is not a distinct diagnostic category and is labeled as *Delusional disorder somatic type*	
ICD-10 (1992)	Non-delusional dysmorphophobia is not a distinct diagnostic category. It is considered to be a form of the *Hypochondriacal disorder*	Delusional dysmorphophobia is not a distinct diagnostic category and is labeled as *Delusional disorder* or *Other persistent delusional disorder* or *Schizotypal disorder*	
DSM-IV (1994)	Non-delusional and delusional dysmorphophobia are two distinct diagnostic categories in the section of somatoform disorders with the labels, respectively: *Body dysmorphic disorder*, *Body dysmorphic disorder* and *Delusional disorder somatic type*		
DSM-5 (2013)			Non-delusional and delusional dysmorphophobia are merged into a single diagnostic category in the group of *Obsessive-compulsive and related disorders*. The label is *Body dysmorphic disorder* with one of three possible levels of insight (good, poor, absent/delusional beliefs)

(continued)

Table 5.2 (continued)

	Somatoform disorders (like hypochondriasis)	Delusional disorders	Obsessive-compulsive disorders
ICD-11 (due by 2018)			ICD-11 will probably contain a separate diagnostic category for BDD that will be included in the group of *Obsessive-compulsive and related disorders*

5.7 BDD by Proxy

The expression *body dysmorphic disorder by proxy* (or *dysmorphophobia by proxy*) describes a variation on the BDD theme, that is a person who is preoccupied not with his/her appearance but how someone else might look. The person of concern may be a relative (child, partner, parent, etc.) or a stranger and the impact of this condition on the quality of life and the relationships may be heavy [64].

BDD by proxy is a form of *Münchausen syndrome by proxy*.

The term *Münchausen syndrome* is used to indicate a factitious disorder without a detectable concrete secondary gain. The patient invents symptoms and deliberately creates signs (e.g., cyanosis of a limb, blood in the urine) to get the attention usually given to a person with an actual disease.

The name *Münchausen syndrome by proxy* was coined to designate the feigning or the production of symptoms in another person. This clinical picture is mostly observed in mothers who fake or induce symptoms in their children. It is also defined *medical child abuse* [65].

As to eating disorders, it is possible to find in the medical literature case reports of *anorexia nervosa by proxy* [66] and *orthorexia nervosa by proxy* [67].

The American psychiatrist Katharine A. Phillips first called *BDD by proxy* a phenomenon characterized by

> "excessive worry about someone else's appearance" (p. 75).

In her 1996 book *The Broken Mirror*, Phillips reported the case of a woman who was very disappointed about her daughter's "crooked nose":

> "I worry that it doesn't look right, that it's crooked - she told me—even though everyone else says it looks fine. *She* doesn't worry about it, but *I* do! … I keep pushing on it to make it straight" [68] (p. 75).

A woman can decide to have a voluntary abortion because of nagging thoughts about possible aesthetic defects of her child. In 1997, Laugharne related that a woman in her mid-20s terminated three consecutive pregnancies:

> "she was preoccupied not with her own appearance but with the potential appearance of her babies" (short in stature, slanted eyes, big mouth) [69] (p. 266).

Jennifer Greenberg et al. tested the cognitive-behavior therapy in six adults with BDD by proxy and found some gains that were maintained at a very short (3-month) follow-up [70].

5.8 Is BDD Underdiagnosed?

BDD affects about 2% of the general population and more than 10% of psychiatric, plastic surgery, and dermatology patients. Therefore, it is more frequent than anorexia nervosa or schizophrenia. Probably it tends to occur a little bit more frequently in females.

In Germany, a representative nationwide survey using self-report questionnaires found that the prevalence of current BDD (DSM-IV criteria) was 1.8%. The subgroup with BDD reported significantly higher rates of suicidal ideation, suicide attempts, and cosmetic surgery [71].

BDD mostly begins in adolescence. An Australian study of 3149 adolescents (age 12–18) found that 1.7% self-reported symptoms of probable BDD according to DSM-IV, without sex differences. The prevalence was higher among older teens [72]. The prevalence of possible subthreshold BDD was 3.4% [73].

Another study of a nonclinical sample of German adolescents and young adults (age 15–21) found that 3.6% met DSM-5 criteria for BDD. This higher value might be due more to the different age range than to differences in methodology. In this research too, self-reported symptoms of BDD were associated with higher rates of appearance-related suicidal ideation and psychiatric comorbidity [74].

Phillips and colleagues found that 4% of people seeking medical treatment in an outpatient setting and 12% of psychiatric outpatients probably suffered from this disorder but the BDD diagnosis was missed in all cases:

> "BDD is often a secret disorder. The diagnosis isn't made because the symptoms aren't revealed" [68] (p. 43).

BDD is especially frequent among cosmetic surgery candidates and is a poor outcome predictor [75].

A 2017 systematic review with meta-analysis [76] found that:

- 15% of plastic surgery patients (range 2.2–56.7%; women 74%) had BDD.
- 13% of dermatology patients (range 4.5–35.2%; women 76%) had BDD.

Recent studies suggest that most aesthetic professionals have some knowledge of BDD but probably underestimate its prevalence in their clinical practice [77]. Routine screening and an accurate selection process are recommended [78].

Many persons with appearance concerns do not spontaneously talk about these worries with a clinician. Therefore, it is appropriate to investigate about symptoms of body uneasiness, especially in settings such as mental health units, eating disorders units, aesthetic medicine, and dermatology units [79].

5.9 A Brief Note on Treatment and Outcome

Treatment is difficult [80]. No medication has been formally approved for BDD, but some serotonin reuptake inhibitors (SRIs) have shown efficacy in controlled and open-label trials [81]. High doses may be needed. An antipsychotic can be added if insight is very weak and delusional thoughts are marked.

A manualized modular cognitive-behavior therapy for BDD (CBT-BDD) produced some significant improvements [82].

Treatment can also be delivered via the internet: a 12-week randomized controlled trial found that a therapist-guided internet-based CBT-BDD program could be usefully employed in a stepped care approach to individuals at low risk of suicide, with moderate symptoms [83].

A cognitive dissonance-based intervention demonstrated high acceptability and some efficacy in reducing ED and MD risk factors (e.g., body-ideal internalization, dietary restraint, bulimic symptoms, drive for muscularity) in men with body dissatisfaction [84].

BDD is a condition with a broad spectrum of severity, from a mild and transient disorder to an awful and long-lasting illness. In many cases, quality of life and social functioning are scanty. In an Australian survey, also adolescents with *subthreshold-BDD* reported significant difficulties in spite of fewer symptoms of depression and disordered eating [73].

Suicidal ideation is more common in individuals with BDD than in those with major depression. Nearly half of them consider suicide and suicide completion rates are much higher than in general population [85–87].

The *muscle dysmorphia* form of BDD is associated with poorer quality of life, higher rates of substance use disorders and suicidality than other forms of BDD [44].

References

1. Morselli E. Sulla dismorfofobia e sulla tafefobia, due forme non per anco descritte di pazzia con idee fisse. Bollettino della Regia Accademia Medica di Genova. 1891;6:110–9.
2. Jahrreiss W. Das hypochondrische Denken. Archiv der Psychiatrie und Nervenkrankheiten. 1930;92:686–823.
3. American Psychiatric Association. Diagnostic and statistical manual of mental disorders (DSM-I). Washington, DC: American Psychiatric Association Mental Hospital Service; 1952.
4. American Psychiatric Association. DSM-II. Diagnostic and statistical manual of mental disorders. 2nd ed. Washington, DC: American Psychiatric Association; 1968.

5. American Psychiatric Association. Diagnostic and statistical manual of mental disorders. DSM III. 3rd ed. Washington, DC: American Psychiatric Association; 1980.
6. American Psychiatric Association. Diagnostic and statistical manual of mental disorders. DSM IIIR, 3rd Revised, ed. Washington, DC: American Psychiatric Association; 1987.
7. American Psychiatric Association. Diagnostic and statistical manual of mental disorders, DSM-IV. 4th ed. Washington, DC: American Psychiatric Association; 1994.
8. Berrios GE, Kan CS. A conceptual and quantitative analysis of 178 historical cases of dysmorphophobia. Acta Psychiatr Scand. 1996;94(1):1–7.
9. American Psychiatric Association. Diagnostic and statistical manual of mental disorders, DSM-5. 5th ed. Arlington, VA: American Psychiatric Publishing; 2013.
10. Phillips KA. Body dysmorphic disorder. In: Cash TF, editor. Encyclopedia of body image and human appearance. 2nd ed. Amsterdam: Elsevier Academic Press; 2012. p. 74–81.
11. Phillips KA, McElroy SL, Keck PE Jr, Hudson JI, Pope HG Jr. A comparison of delusional and nondelusional body dysmorphic disorder in 100 cases. Psychopharmacol Bull. 1994;30(2):179–86.
12. Phillips KA, Hart AS, Simpson HB, Stein DJ. Delusional versus nondelusional body dysmorphic disorder: recommendations for DSM-5. CNS Spectr. 2014;19(1):10–20.
13. Phillips KA, Pinto A, Hart AS, Coles ME, Eisen JL, Menard W, et al. A comparison of insight in body dysmorphic disorder and obsessive-compulsive disorder. J Psychiatr Res. 2012;46(10):1293–9.
14. Toh WL, Castle DJ, Mountjoy RL, Buchanan B, Farhall J, Rossell SL. Insight in body dysmorphic disorder (BDD) relative to obsessive-compulsive disorder (OCD) and psychotic disorders: revisiting this issue in light of DSM-5. Compr Psychiatry. 2017;77:100–8.
15. Eisen JL, Phillips KA, Baer L, Beer DA, Atala KD, Rasmussen SA. The brown assessment of beliefs scale: reliability and validity. Am J Psychiatry. 1998;155(1):102–8.
16. Phillips KA, Hart AS, Menard W, Eisen JL. Psychometric evaluation of the brown assessment of beliefs scale in body dysmorphic disorder. J Nerv Ment Dis. 2013;201(7):640–3.
17. Konstantakopoulos G, Varsou E, Dikeos D, Ioannidi N, Gonidakis F, Papadimitriou G, et al. Delusionality of body image beliefs in eating disorders. Psychiatry Res. 2012;200(2–3):482–8.
18. Vigarello G. Histoire de la beauté. Le corps et l'art d'embellir XVIème XXème siècles. Paris: Seuil; 2004.
19. Rodin J, Silberstein L, Striegel-Moore R. Women and weight: a normative discontent. Neb Symp Motiv. 1984;32:267–307.
20. Pope HG Jr, Katz DL, Hudson JI. Anorexia nervosa and "reverse anorexia" among 108 male bodybuilders. Compr Psychiatry. 1993;34(6):406–9.
21. McCreary D. Muscularity and body image. In: Cash TF, editor. Encyclopedia of body image and human appearance. 2nd ed. Amsterdam: Elsevier Academic Press; 2012. p. 561–7.
22. Pope HG Jr, Phillips KA, Olivardia R. The Adonis complex. The secret crisis of male body obsession. New York: The Free Press; 2000.
23. Leone JE, Sedory EJ, Gray KA. Recognition and treatment of muscle dysmorphia and related body image disorders. J Athl Train. 2005;40(4):352–9.
24. Dos Santos Filho CA, Tirico PP, Stefano SC, Touyz SW, Claudino AM. Systematic review of the diagnostic category muscle dysmorphia. Aust N Z J Psychiatry. 2016;50(4):322–33.
25. Foster AC, Shorter GW, Griffiths MD. Muscle dysmorphia: could it be classified as an addiction to body image? J Behav Addict. 2015;4(1):1–5.
26. Murray SB, Rieger E, Hildebrandt T, Karlov L, Russell J, Boon E, et al. A comparison of eating, exercise, shape, and weight related symptomatology in males with muscle dysmorphia and anorexia nervosa. Body Image. 2012;9(2):193–200.
27. Murray SB, Rieger E, Karlov L, Touyz SW. Masculinity and femininity in the divergence of male body image concerns. J Eat Disord. 2013;1:11.
28. Murray SB, Griffiths S, Mitchison D, Mond JM. The transition from thinness-oriented to muscularity-oriented disordered eating in adolescent males: a clinical observation. J Adolesc Health. 2017;60(3):353–5.

29. Pila E, Mond JM, Griffiths S, Mitchison D, Murray SB. A thematic content analysis of #cheatmeal images on social media: characterizing an emerging dietary trend. Int J Eat Disord. 2017;50(6):698–706.
30. Griffiths S, Murray SB, Touyz S. Drive for muscularity and muscularity-oriented disordered eating in men: the role of set shifting difficulties and weak central coherence. Body Image. 2013;10(4):636–9.
31. Murray SB, Nagata JM, Griffiths S, Calzo JP, Brown TA, Mitchison D, et al. The enigma of male eating disorders: a critical review and synthesis. Clin Psychol Rev. 2017;57:1–11.
32. Lipinski JP, Pope HG Jr. Body ideals in young Samoan men: a comparison with men in North America and Europe. Int J Men's Health. 2002;1(2):163–71.
33. Jin X, Jin Y, Zhou S, Yang SN, Chang S, Li H. Attentional biases toward body images in males at high risk of muscle dysmorphia. Peer J. 2018;6:e4273.
34. Yang CF, Gray P, Pope HG Jr. Male body image in Taiwan versus the west: Yanggang Zhiqi meets the Adonis complex. Am J Psychiatry. 2005;162(2):263–9.
35. Leone JE. Muscle dysmorphia symptomatology and extreme drive for muscularity in a 23-year-old woman: a case study. J Strength Cond Res. 2009;23(3):988–95.
36. Hale BD, Diehl D, Weaver K, Briggs M. Exercise dependence and muscle dysmorphia in novice and experienced female bodybuilders. J Behav Addict. 2013;2(4):244–8.
37. Cramblitt B, Pritchard M. Media's influence on the drive for muscularity in undergraduates. Eat Behav. 2013;14(4):441–6.
38. Griffiths S, Murray SB, Mitchison D, Castle D, Mond JM. Relative strength of the associations of body fat, muscularity, height, and penis size dissatisfaction with psychological quality of life impairment among sexual minority men. Psychol Men Masculinity. 2018; Online First Publication, January 18, 2018. https://doi.org/10.1037/men0000149.
39. Griffiths S, Murray SB, Krug I, McLean SA. The contribution of social media to body dissatisfaction, eating disorder symptoms, and anabolic steroid use among sexual minority men. Cyberpsychol Behav Soc Netw. 2018;21(3):149–56.
40. Grieve FG. A conceptual model of factors contributing to the development of muscle dysmorphia. Eat Disord. 2007;15(1):63–80.
41. Harris M, Dunn M, Alwyn T. Intrasexual competition as a potential influence on anabolic-androgenic steroid use initiation. J Health Psychol. 2017: Online First Publication, February 1, 2017. https://doi.org/10.1177/1359105317692145.
42. Gruber AJ, Pope HG Jr. Psychiatric and medical effects of anabolic-androgenic steroid use in women. Psychother Psychosom. 2000;69(1):19–26.
43. Longobardi C, Prino LE, Fabris MA, Settanni M. Muscle dysmorphia and psychopathology: findings from an Italian sample of male bodybuilders. Psychiatry Res. 2017;256:231–6.
44. Pope CG, Pope HG, Menard W, Fay C, Olivardia R, Phillips KA. Clinical features of muscle dysmorphia among males with body dysmorphic disorder. Body Image. 2005;2(4):395–400.
45. Schneider C, Agthe M, Yanagida T, Voracek M, Hennig-Fast K. Effects of muscle dysmorphia, social comparisons and body schema priming on desire for social interaction: an experimental approach. BMC Psychol. 2017;5(1):19.
46. Lepping P, Freudenmann RW. Delusional parasitosis: a new pathway for diagnosis and treatment. Clin Exp Dermatol. 2008;33(2):113–7.
47. Zhu TH, Nakamura M, Farahnik B, Abrouk M, Reichenberg J, Bhutani T, et al. Obsessive-compulsive skin disorders: a novel classification based on degree of insight. J Dermatolog Treat. 2017;28(4):342–6.
48. Gruber M, Jahn R, Stolba K, Ossege M. 'Barbie doll Syndrome'. A case report of body dysmorphic disorder. Neuropsychiatrie. 2018;2(1):44–9.
49. Suzuki K, Takei N, Iwata Y, Sekine Y, Toyoda T, Nakamura K, et al. Do olfactory reference syndrome and jiko-shu-kyofu (a subtype of taijin-kyofu) share a common entity? Acta Psychiatr Scand. 2004;109(2):150–5. discussion 5.
50. Nakagami Y, Ii T, Russ TC, Marques JG, Riese F, Sonmez E, et al. Taijin kyofusho: a culture-bound diagnosis discussed by Japanese and international early career psychiatrists. Psychiatry Clin Neurosci. 2017;71(2):146.

51. Nagata T, Matsunaga H, van Vliet I, Yamada H, Fukuhara H, Yoshimura C, et al. Correlations between the offensive subtype of social anxiety disorder and personality disorders. Psychiatry Clin Neurosci. 2011;65(4):341–8.
52. Takahashi T. A social club spontaneously formed by ex-patients who had suffered from anthropophobia (Taijin kyofu (sho)). Int J Soc Psychiatry. 1975;21(2):137–40.
53. Takahashi T. Social phobia syndrome in Japan. Compr Psychiatry. 1989;30(1):45–52.
54. Iwata Y, Suzuki K, Takei N, Toulopoulou T, Tsuchiya KJ, Matsumoto K, et al. Jiko-shisen-kyofu (fear of one's own glance), but not taijin-kyofusho (fear of interpersonal relations), is an east Asian culture-related specific syndrome. Aust N Z J Psychiatry. 2011;45(2):148–52.
55. Lim L. Taijin-Kyofu-Sho: a subtype of social anxiety. Open J Psychiatry. 2013;3:393–8.
56. Nagata T, Yamada H, Teo AR, Yoshimura C, Nakajima T, van Vliet I. Comorbid social withdrawal (hikikomori) in outpatients with social anxiety disorder: clinical characteristics and treatment response in a case series. Int J Soc Psychiatry. 2013;59(1):73–8.
57. Teo AR, Fetters MD, Stufflebam K, Tateno M, Balhara Y, Choi TY, et al. Identification of the hikikomori syndrome of social withdrawal: psychosocial features and treatment preferences in four countries. Int J Soc Psychiatry. 2015;61(1):64–72.
58. Watts J. Public health experts concerned about "hikikomori". Lancet. 2002;359(9312):1131.
59. World Health Organization. The ICD-10 classification of mental and behavioural disorders. Clinical descriptions and diagnostic guidelines. Geneva: World Health Organization; 1992.
60. Veale D, Matsunaga H. Body dysmorphic disorder and olfactory reference disorder: proposals for ICD-11. Rev Bras Psiquiatr. 2014;36(Suppl 1):14–20.
61. Stein DJ, Kogan CS, Atmaca M, Fineberg NA, Fontenelle LF, Grant JE, et al. The classification of obsessive-compulsive and related disorders in the ICD-11. J Affect Disord. 2016;190:663–74.
62. Kendell R, Jablensky A. Distinguishing between the validity and utility of psychiatric diagnoses. Am J Psychiatry. 2003;160(1):4–12.
63. McHugh PR, Slavney PR. Mental illness--comprehensive evaluation or checklist? N Engl J Med. 2012;366(20):1853–5.
64. Greenberg JL, Falkenstein M, Reuman L, Fama J, Marques L, Wilhelm S. The phenomenology of self-reported body dysmorphic disorder by proxy. Body Image. 2013;10(2):243–6.
65. Ali-Panzarella AZ, Bryant TJ, Marcovitch H, Lewis JD. Medical child abuse (Munchausen syndrome by proxy): multidisciplinary approach from a pediatric gastroenterology perspective. Curr Gastroenterol Rep. 2017;19(4):14.
66. Katz RL, Mazer C, Litt IF. Anorexia nervosa by proxy. J Pediatr. 1985;107(2):247–8.
67. Cuzzolaro M, Donini LM. Orthorexia nervosa by proxy? Eat Weight Disord. 2016;21(4):549–51.
68. Phillips KA. The broken mirror. Understanding and treating body dysmorphic disorder. New York: Oxford University Press; 1996.
69. Laugharne R, Upex T, Palazidou E. Dysmorphophobia by proxy. J R Soc Med. 1998;91(5):266.
70. Greenberg JL, Mothi SS, Wilhelm S. Cognitive-behavioral therapy for body dysmorphic disorder by proxy. Behav Ther. 2016;47(4):515–26.
71. Buhlmann U, Glaesmer H, Mewes R, Fama JM, Wilhelm S, Brahler E, et al. Updates on the prevalence of body dysmorphic disorder: a population-based survey. Psychiatry Res. 2010;178(1):171–5.
72. Schneider SC, Turner CM, Mond J, Hudson JL. Prevalence and correlates of body dysmorphic disorder in a community sample of adolescents. Aust N Z J Psychiatry. 2017;51(6):595–603.
73. Schneider SC, Mond J, Turner CM, Hudson JL. Subthreshold body dysmorphic disorder in adolescents: prevalence and impact. Psychiatry Res. 2017;251:125–30.
74. Mollmann A, Dietel FA, Hunger A, Buhlmann U. Prevalence of body dysmorphic disorder and associated features in German adolescents: a self-report survey. Psychiatry Res. 2017;254:263–7.
75. Sweis IE, Spitz J, Barry DR Jr, Cohen M. A review of body dysmorphic disorder in aesthetic surgery patients and the legal implications. Aesthet Plast Surg. 2017;41(4):949–54.
76. Ribeiro RVE. Prevalence of body dysmorphic disorder in plastic surgery and dermatology patients: a systematic review with meta-analysis. Aesthet Plast Surg. 2017;41(4):964–70.

77. Bouman TK, Mulkens S, van der Lei B. Cosmetic professionals' awareness of body dysmorphic disorder. Plast Reconstr Surg. 2017;139(2):336–42.
78. Joseph J, Randhawa P, Hannan SA, Long J, Goh S, O'Shea N, et al. Body dysmorphic disorder in patients undergoing septorhinoplasty surgery: should we be performing routine screening? Clin Otolaryngol. 2017;42(3):508–13.
79. Koblenzer CS. Body dysmorphic disorder in the dermatology patient. Clin Dermatol. 2017;35(3):298–301.
80. Krebs G, de la Cruz LF, Mataix-Cols D. Recent advances in understanding and managing body dysmorphic disorder. Evid Based Ment Health. 2017;20(3):71–5.
81. Phillips KA. Pharmacotherapy for body dysmorphic disorder. Psychiatr Ann. 2010;40(7):325–32.
82. Wilhelm S, Phillips KA, Didie E, Buhlmann U, Greenberg JL, Fama JM, et al. Modular cognitive-behavioral therapy for body dysmorphic disorder: a randomized controlled trial. Behav Ther. 2014;45(3):314–27.
83. Enander J, Andersson E, Mataix-Cols D, Lichtenstein L, Alstrom K, Andersson G, et al. Therapist guided internet based cognitive behavioural therapy for body dysmorphic disorder: single blind randomised controlled trial. BMJ. 2016;352:i241.
84. Brown TA, Forney KJ, Pinner D, Keel PK. A randomized controlled trial of the body project: more than muscles for men with body dissatisfaction. Int J Eat Disord. 2017;50(8):873–83.
85. Angelakis I, Gooding PA, Panagioti M. Suicidality in body dysmorphic disorder (BDD): a systematic review with meta-analysis. Clin Psychol Rev. 2016;49:55–66.
86. Phillips KA. Suicidality in body dysmorphic disorder. Prim Psychiatry. 2007;14(12):58–66.
87. Phillips KA, Menard W. Suicidality in body dysmorphic disorder: a prospective study. Am J Psychiatry. 2006;163(7):1280–2.

Enrico Morselli and the Invention of Dysmorphophobia

6

Massimo Cuzzolaro and Umberto Nizzoli

6.1 Enrico Morselli

The Italian physician, psychiatrist, and anthropologist Enrico Agostino Morselli was born in Modena on 17 July 1852 and died in Genova on 13 February 1929. Therefore, he was a contemporary of turn-of-the-century alienists such as Valentin Magnan (1835–1916), Hippolyte Bernheim (1840–1919), Emil Kraepelin (1856–1926), Sigmund Freud (1856–1939), and Pierre Janet (1859–1947).

Morselli graduated doctor of medicine, in 1874, worked in several mental hospitals (Reggio Emilia, Florence, Macerata, Turin, Genoa), held positions at the medical faculty of Turin, and became a full professor of psychiatry at the university of Genoa in 1889. In Florence, he worked with Paolo Mantegazza, a famous physiognomist. That training probably contributed to the subsequent interest in physical anthropology and body shape.

In 1875, Carlo Livi, Augusto Tamburini, and Enrico Morselli founded, in Reggio Emilia, the *Rivista sperimentale di freniatria e di medicina legale in relazione con l'antropologia e le scienze giuridiche e sociali* (Experimental review of psychiatry and legal medicine in relation with anthropology and legal and social sciences), a scientific journal that is still getting published.

Morselli was importantly influenced by positivism of the nineteenth century, with its emphasis on the *positive* knowledge, imposed on the mind by experience and grounded on verified data. In 1881, he founded and edited the *Rivista di filosofia*

M. Cuzzolaro (✉)
Formerly Medical Pathophysiology Department, Eating Disorders and Obesity Unit, Sapienza University of Rome, Rome, Italy

U. Nizzoli
Eating Disorders and Addictions Services of Reggio Emilia, Reggio Emilia, Italy

Italian Society for the Study of Eating Disorders (SISDCA), Reggio Emilia, Italy

M. Cuzzolaro, S. Fassino (eds.), *Body Image, Eating, and Weight*,
https://doi.org/10.1007/978-3-319-90817-5_6

scientifica (Review of scientific philosophy), destined to become the official organ of Italian positivism.

Furthermore, Morselli introduced some reforms to renew and humanize the Italian mental asylums but, on the other hand, some of his writings seem to support eugenics and pseudoscientific views about the classification of human populations into discrete racial categories.

As a curious scientist, Morselli was interested in exploring unusual phenomena such as hypnosis and mediumism, and he used photography to document the actions of the famous medium Eusapia Paladino and tackle the problem of subjectivity or objectivity of apparitions during spiritual séances [1].

As regards hypnotism, he embraced Bernheim's (*école de Nancy*) psychological interpretation based on the concept of suggestion, rather than Charcot's (*école de la Salpêtrière*) neurological vision. Unlike Charcot, Bernheim assumed that suggestion was the key to all hypnotic phenomena, and the hypnotic state was not a neurosis [2].

In 1926, 3 years before dying, Morselli published *La psicanalisi. Studii ed appunti critici* (The psychoanalysis, studies, and critical notes). In spite of some doubts and critical remarks that the author raised from a medical point of view, these two volumes were one of the first attempts to introduce Sigmund Freud's theory into the Italian culture [3].

Morselli wrote many articles and books on clinical and forensic psychiatry, experimental psychology, sociology, and anthropology. However, in the history of psychiatry, he is known primarily for having coined the word *dysmorphophobia* in the last years of the nineteenth century.

6.2 Birth of the Neologism *Dysmorphophobia*

On April 1891, Enrico Morselli published, in the *Bollettino della Regia Accademia Medica di Genova*, an article with the title 'Sulla Dismorfofobia e sulla Tafefobia due forme non per anco descritte di Pazzia con idee fisse' (Fig. 6.1) [4]. Some authors incorrectly reported 1886 as the publication date of that seminal paper [5, p. 257].

In his article, Morselli created 'due denominazioni nuove' (two neologisms): 'tafefobia' and 'dismorfofobia'. The word *tafefobia* (in English 'taphephobia') was invented to indicate the abnormal fear of being buried alive. It is derived from the Greek τάφος (grave) and φόβος (flight, fear, anxiety, concern, horror). The other neologism, *dismorfofobia* (in English 'dysmorphophobia'), was coined to describe a condition in which a person is tortured by the preoccupation with some imagined or negligible defects in his/her physical appearance. It is derived from the Greek δύσμορφος (misshapen) and φόβος.

In his paper, Morselli did not attach more importance to dysmorphophobia than to taphephobia.

> Alle varie forme sintomatiche assunte dalla Pazzia con idee fisse e il cui carattere fondamentale consiste nella fobia che le accompagna, sono da aggiungerne, secondo le mie osservazioni di questi ultimi anni, due non ancora descritte da alcun alienista o, per lo

Sulla Dismorfofobia e sulla Tafefobia
due forme non per anco descritte di Pazzia con idee fisse.

Nota del Socio ordinario Prof. ENRICO MORSELLI, **Direttore della Clinica delle malattie mentali.**

Alle varie forme sintomatiche assunte dalla Pazzia con idee fisse e il cui carattere fondamentale consiste nella fobia che le accompagna, sono da aggiungerne, secondo le mie osservazioni di questi ultimi anni, due non ancora descritte da alcun alienista, o, per lo meno, poco conosciute. Esse sarebbero la *dismorfofobia* e la *tafefobia*, due denominazioni nuove che io mi permetto di proporre per la prima volta, ma che sono costrutte secondo le norme generalmente adottate dai migliori trattatisti.

La prima consiste nell'insorgere improvviso e nello stabilirsi davanti alla coscienza dell'idea della propria deformità; l'individuo teme di essere divenuto o di poter divenire deforme (δύσμορφος, deforme) e prova a questa rappresentazione una angoscia indicibile (φόβος, timore). La seconda, o *tafefobia*, consiste, invece, in ciò che l'ammalato è incolto dal dubbio di potere essere seppellito ancora vivo quando gli avverrà di avvicinarsi alla morte (ταφή, sepoltura), ed il dubbio gli occasiona pure un'angustia terribilmente penosa. Parmi inutile dare una descrizione particolareggiata delle due nuove forme di paranoia rudimentaria da me scoperte e denominate; non farei che ripetere quanto si trova lungamente scritto intorno alle loro consorelle, che son già tanto numerose e svariate, nei libri e nei

Non indico naturalmente nulla degli altri caratteri clinici, sui quali reputo inutile insistere; ma per ispiegar meglio il mio concetto dirò che il dismorfofobico sta all'ipocondriaco, che investiga lo stato fisico del proprio organismo, e il tafefobico sta al melanconico, che teme la morte, negli stessi identici rapporti che il rupofobiaco ha col pazzo affetto da delirio di avvelenamento.

Per rispetto alla patogenesi di queste forme, diviene per me sempre più evidente che essa deve porsi in rapporto colle leggi psicologiche dell'associazione, o meglio della sistemazione degli stati psichici, cui io avevo accennato in altra mia nota precedente (1). Gli ultimi studi sull'ipnotismo e le speculazioni d'alcuni distinti psicologi (Ribot, Paulhan, Pietro Janet, W. James, ecc.) ci conducono al concetto che la personalità sia una sintesi sistematica di rappresentazioni e di tendenze. La pazzia, in tutte le sue forme, è da riguardarsi come un'anomala sistemazione o come una disintegrazione degli elementi fisico-psichici che compongono la personalità: del che spero poter dare una dimostrazione in altri miei scritti ulteriori (2). Ma egli è specialmente nella pazzia con idee fisse che noi assistiamo al morboso disassociarsi di codesti elementi: lo stato psichico che la caratterizza, sia esso una rappresentazione, o un sentimento, o una tendenza, irrompe dal fondo dell'incosciente, e portandosi con veemenza e somma vivacità nel campo appercettivo giunge a dominare nella coscienza e ne inibisce l'ingresso ad ogni altro stato psichico che si trovi con esso in antagonismo.

Genova, aprile 1891.

(1) Morselli, *Paranoia rudimentale impulsiva*, « Riv. sperim. di freniatria e medicina legale », 1886.

(2) Nel secondo volume del mio *Manuale di Semeiottica delle Malattie mentali*, che è ora sotto stampa, e in un prossimo *Trattato clinico di Psichiatria* cui attendo da più anni.

Fig. 6.1 First and last pages of Morselli's article on taphephobia and dysmorphophobia [4]

meno, poco conosciute. Esse sarebbero la *dismorfofobia* e la *tafefobia*, due denominazioni nuove che io mi permetto di proporre per la prima volta, ma che sono costrutte secondo le norme generalmente adottate dai migliori trattatisti [4, p. 110].

According to some observations I made in the last few years, two new varieties should be added to the various forms of Insanity with fixed ideas, whose essential feature is the phobia that underlies them. They are still undescribed or, at least, not very well-known. *Dysmorphophobia* and *taphephobia* are the two new terms I take the liberty of putting forward, following the lexical rules usually adopted by outstanding writers of treatises.

In an interesting historical review, Berrios remarks that sometimes the creation of the neologism *dysmorphophobia* was mistakenly attributed to the famous German alienist Emil Kraepelin [6]. For example, in 1962, the French psychiatrist Cyrille Koupernik—who named dysmorphophobia '*psychose de la laideur*' (ugliness psychosis)—indicated Kraepelin as the minter of the new expression [7, p. 321].

In fact, Kraepelin never named the new syndrome in the first three editions of his classic handbook *Psychiatrie. Ein Lehrbuch für Studierende und Ärzte* (Psychiatry. A manual for students and physicians) [8–10]. He introduced the term *Dysmorphophobie* in the German language only in the 1915 edition [11] (p. 1861, line 15), without citing Morselli's work (Fig. 6.2).

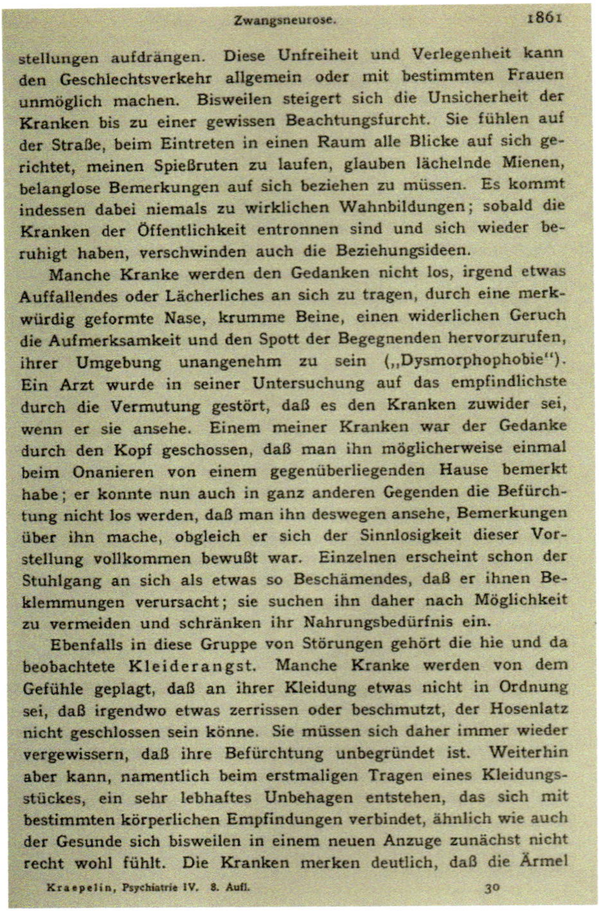

Zwangsneurose. 1861

stellungen aufdrängen. Diese Unfreiheit und Verlegenheit kann den Geschlechtsverkehr allgemein oder mit bestimmten Frauen unmöglich machen. Bisweilen steigert sich die Unsicherheit der Kranken bis zu einer gewissen Beachtungsfurcht. Sie fühlen auf der Straße, beim Eintreten in einen Raum alle Blicke auf sich gerichtet, meinen Spießruten zu laufen, glauben lächelnde Mienen, belanglose Bemerkungen auf sich beziehen zu müssen. Es kommt indessen dabei niemals zu wirklichen Wahnbildungen; sobald die Kranken der Öffentlichkeit entronnen sind und sich wieder beruhigt haben, verschwinden auch die Beziehungsideen.

Manche Kranke werden den Gedanken nicht los, irgend etwas Auffallendes oder Lächerliches an sich zu tragen, durch eine merkwürdig geformte Nase, krumme Beine, einen widerlichen Geruch die Aufmerksamkeit und den Spott der Begegnenden hervorzurufen, ihrer Umgebung unangenehm zu sein („Dysmorphophobie"). Ein Arzt wurde in seiner Untersuchung auf das empfindlichste durch die Vermutung gestört, daß es den Kranken zuwider sei, wenn er sie ansehe. Einem meiner Kranken war der Gedanke durch den Kopf geschossen, daß man ihn möglicherweise einmal beim Onanieren von einem gegenüberliegenden Hause bemerkt habe; er konnte nun auch in ganz anderen Gegenden die Befürchtung nicht los werden, daß man ihn deswegen ansehe, Bemerkungen über ihn mache, obgleich er sich der Sinnlosigkeit dieser Vorstellung vollkommen bewußt war. Einzelnen erscheint schon der Stuhlgang an sich als etwas so Beschämendes, daß er ihnen Beklemmungen verursacht; sie suchen ihn daher nach Möglichkeit zu vermeiden und schränken ihr Nahrungsbedürfnis ein.

Ebenfalls in diese Gruppe von Störungen gehört die hie und da beobachtete Kleiderangst. Manche Kranke werden von dem Gefühle geplagt, daß an ihrer Kleidung etwas nicht in Ordnung sei, daß irgendwo etwas zerrissen oder beschmutzt, der Hosenlatz nicht geschlossen sein könne. Sie müssen sich daher immer wieder vergewissern, daß ihre Befürchtung unbegründet ist. Weiterhin aber kann, namentlich beim erstmaligen Tragen eines Kleidungsstückes, ein sehr lebhaftes Unbehagen entstehen, das sich mit bestimmten körperlichen Empfindungen verbindet, ähnlich wie auch der Gesunde sich bisweilen in einem neuen Anzuge zunächst nicht recht wohl fühlt. Die Kranken merken deutlich, daß die Ärmel

Kraepelin, Psychiatrie IV. 8. Aufl. 30

Fig. 6.2 In 1915, the word *Dysmorphophobie* appears in an Emil Kraepelin's book [11]

6.3 Morselli's Concept of *Dysmorphophobia*

In 1885, Morselli published the first volume of his *Manuale di semejotica di malattie mentali* (Handbook of semiotics of mental disorders), mainly devoted to the anthropological and physiological evaluation of the patients [12]. Nine years later, the second volume appeared in which the author underlined the uncertainties of the neuropathological explanations of mental symptoms and gave great significance to the psychological aspects, particularly to the role of the emotions [13]. The paper on dysmorphophobia and taphephobia was written between these two phases. It introduced two new words and, above all, investigated a psychopathological concept.

In the 1891 article, Morselli did not present clinical vignettes of patients with dysmorphophobia. He probably collected his sample of persons with that enigmatic symptom—the fear of deformity—during the 1880s, mainly in his private practice [6]. But how many patients with dysmorphophobia did he see?

Katharine Phillips, in her excellent book *The broken mirror*, wrote that 'In the late 1800s, Morselli saw 78 patients with Body Dysmorphic Disorder (BDD)' [14, p. 20]. This figure appears exaggeratedly high. In fact, Morselli spoke, in his article, of 78 cases, but he referred to the total number of cases of *Insanity with fixed ideas* he had seen in his private practice. The list of symptoms he observed included:

- First, *agoraphobia* (fear of open spaces), *acrophobia* (fear of heights), *aichmophobia* (fear of pointed objects), *belonephobia* (fear of needles and pins), *claustrophobia* (fear of narrow spaces and tunnels), *dysmorphophobia* (fear of deformity), *hyalophobia* (fear of fragments of glass that might be present in foods), *mysophobia* or *rhypophobia* (fear of dirt), *taphephobia* (fear of apparent death and premature entombment);
- Secondly, the clinical pictures that the German psychiatrist Rudolf Gottfried Arndt (1835–1900) called *questioning paranoias* such as *arithmomania* (number madness) and *onomatomania* (name madness);
- Thirdly, the irresistible need to act in some singular manner such as *coprolalia* (outburst of obscene words), *dipsomania* (craving for alcohol), *kleptomania* (urge for stealing), *oniomania* (compulsion to buy), *pyromania* (impulse to start fires);
- And to finish, the *antivivisectionist insanity* (obsessional preoccupation with the suffering of animals subjected to experiments in scientific laboratories) first described by the French psychiatrist Valentin Magnan (1835–1916).

> Generalmente queste sindromi psicopatiche si attribuiscono alla influenza ereditaria e si considerano come psicosi degenerative: esse, cioè, per la maggioranza degli alienisti, sono forme della psicosi degli ereditarii (Morel). Ma io ho da qualche anno insistito sul fatto, da me osservato e confermato, che non tutte le pazzie con idee fisse, incoercibili ed impulsive, sono indizio o stigmata psichica di degenerazione. Avendo ormai raccolto nella mia clientela privata circa *ottanta* casi di questa singolare condizione psicopatica (più esattamente *settantotto*), posso riaffermare quanto dissi fino dal 1882 al Congresso Medico di Modena: che, cioè, in un certo numero di casi non è possibile scoprire il benché menomo indizio di eredità psico- o neuro-patica, ma solo uno stato neurastenico qualche volta transitorio [4, p. 115].
>
> These psychopathic syndromes are usually attributed to hereditary factors and are regarded as degenerative psychoses: in other words, for most alienists they are forms of Morel's hereditary psychoses. However, for some years, I have insisted upon the fact I have observed and confirmed, that not all varieties of insanity with fixed, uncontrollable and impulsive ideas are the sign or the psychic stigma of degeneration. I have now collected, among my private clients, nearly *eighty* cases of this particular psychopathic condition (*seventy-eight*, to be precise), and I can confirm what I said ever since 1882 at the Medical Congress of Modena: namely that, in a certain number of cases, it is impossible to detect the minimum sign of a psycho- or neuro-pathic inheritance, but only a neurasthenic state, sometimes temporary.

The above passage shows that Morselli contrasted in his article the causal theory of *degeneration* developed by Bénédict Augustin Morel (1809–1873) and, later, by

Valentin Magnan (1835–1916). That deterministic model dominated European psychiatry for some decades, particularly in France. It regarded many mental disorders—such as delusional and obsessional states—as *inherited degenerative illnesses* with an inexorable negative outcome. On the contrary, Morselli considered dysmorphophobia, at least in some cases, as an acquired state of *neurasthenia* which may be transitory. Furthermore, he underlined the psychological aspects of insanity with fixed ideas and, in the last lines of his article, he used the word *unconscious*:

> lo stato psichico che la caratterizza, sia esso una rappresentazione, o un sentimento, o una tendenza, irrompe dal fondo dell'incosciente, e portandosi con somma vivacità nel campo appercettivo giunge a dominare nella coscienza e ne inibisce l'ingresso ad ogni altro stato psichico che si trovi con esso in antagonismo [4, p. 119].

> the typical psychic state of the insanity with fixed ideas—representation, or feeling, or tendency—breaks with great vivacity from the depths of the unconscious into the apperceptive field, dominates the consciousness and prevents the entry into it of any other antagonist psychic state.

As regards taxonomy, generally speaking, an alienist of the late nineteenth century could consider a clinical phenomenon as an alteration of a *cognitive*, *emotional*, or *volitional* faculty (e.g. fixed ideas, fears, impulses). Otherwise, he could classify a psychopathological symptom on the basis of its *content* (e.g. anorexia nervosa, hypochondria) [6, 15].

Morselli defined dysmorphophobia primarily by the *content* of the complaint: disliking some parts of the physical body. As Berrios and Kan marked, in doing so the author founded 'a narrow view of dysmorphophobia' as a distinct mental disorder [6, p.1]. In addition, he attached much more importance to the *ideational* component of dysmorphophobia (fixed idea of deformity) than to the *emotional* (fear, anxiety, shame) and *volitional* (avoidant behaviours, compulsive checking) elements.

As to the second part of the neologism, Morselli used the term *phobia* in a broad sense that was very common in the nineteenth century and included obsessive thoughts [15]. He always regarded dysmorphophobia as a form of 'vera pazzia del dubbio' (true madness of doubts) with 'idee fisse che moltissime volte danno origine ad azioni coatte' (fixed ideas that very often give rise to compulsive actions) [13, p. 441].

In the 1891 article, he wrote:

> Il dismorfofobico è, infatti, un vero infelice: egli, in mezzo alle sue occupazioni, ai discorsi, alla lettura, durante il pranzo, ovunque insomma e a tutte le ore del giorno, è incolto dal dubbio di una deformità, che possa essersi sviluppata nel suo corpo e a sua insaputa: teme di avere o di *potere avere* la *fronte depressa e schiacciata*, il *naso ridicolo*, le *gambe torte*, ecc. e però si guarda ripetutamente allo specchio, si frega la fronte, si misura la lunghezza del naso, esamina le più piccole macchie della pelle, o investiga su se stesso le proporzioni del tronco e la direzione delle membra, e solo dopo un certo tempo, convincendosi del contrario, si libera dallo stato penoso in cui l'accesso lo ha posto [16, p. 111]

> The dysmorphophobic, indeed, is a really miserable individual; in the middle of his daily affairs, while talking, while reading, during meals, in short everywhere and at any time, he is suddenly caught by the doubt of some deformity, that might have developed in his body without his knowing it: he is afraid he has, or he might develop a squashed and flattened

> forehead, a ridiculous nose, bandy legs, etc., so he looks at himself in the mirror repeatedly, feels his forehead, measures the length of his nose, scrutinizes the smallest specks in his skin, or inspects the proportions of his trunk and the straightness of his limbs, and only after a period of time, he can to be reassured and free himself from the painful state the attack put him in.

Three years after, in the second volume of the *Manuale di semejotica,* Morselli mentioned dysmorphophobia only once, in the section 'Il linguaggio dell'alienato' (The language of the alienated person). He catalogued this disorder among the 'Idee morbose' (morbid ideas), in the general cluster 'Rappresentazioni verbali di idee fisse, incoercibili e coartanti' (Verbal representations of fixed, invincible, and compulsive ideas).

In particular, the author classified dysmorphophobia in the subgroup 'Ipotesi egoistiche per lo più relative alla conservazione e integrità dell'io personale e ai suoi rapporti col mondo esterno' (egoistic hypotheses that mainly concern the preservation of the subject and his relationships with the external world) [13, p. 440].

Morselli placed dysmorphophobia among *insanities with fixed ideas* and highlighted the obsessional features of that clinical picture. He observed that persons suffering from dysmorphophobia showed all the symptoms contemporary alienists used to describe for the *insanity with fixed ideas*, a condition that Rudolf Gottfried Arndt (1835–1900) also called 'paranoia rudimentaria' (rudimentary—or partial or primitive—paranoia) [17, p. 534].

Morselli reported in his article (Fig. 6.3) a summary of the main signs of this group of insanities, according to the school of Jacques Joseph Valentin Magnan (1835–1916). It is possible to find the original schema in a French book published in 1886 by Paul Maurice Legrain (1860–1939) [18, p. 70]. It is exactly alike.

The concept of *insanity with fixed ideas* was widely shared in those years.

Fig. 6.3 Summary of the main signs of *insanity with fixed ideas* or *rudimentary paranoia*. From E. Morselli, 1891 (p. 115)

il Magnan ci ha dato il seguente prospetto:

a	1. Ossessione 2. Impulso	3. Irresistibilità
b	4. Coscienza completa dello stato morboso 5. Angoscia concomitante	
c	6. Soddisfazione consecutiva.	

Magnan proposed the following table:

a	1. obsession 2. impulse	3. irresistibility
b	4. consciousness of the morbid state 5. accompanying anguish	
c	6. subsequent relief	

Gabriele Buccola (1854–1885) was a brilliant psychiatrist who worked with Morselli in Turin from 1881 to 1885 when he prematurely died. He defined the fixed ideas as 'mental representations that arise and persist in the consciousness in a coercive way and that German alienists call by a very expressive word, *Zwangsvorstellungen*' [19, p. 155]. Buccola included under that label phobias, obsessions, impulsions, and delusions.

A classification arranges together phenomena that are like and separates those which appear unlike. Subsequently, nosology studies linkages among different diagnostic categories of a taxonomy. So Morselli explored similarities and differences between dysmorphophobia and other mental disorders.

He noted that some patients with dysmorphophobia were first aware of the absurdity of their ideas but later and gradually lost this critical ability and developed a distinctly recognizable delusion.

Furthermore, he indicated the affinities with certain melancholic and hypochondriacal states but affirmed that the emotional disturbance of dysmorphophobia comes in bouts and is not a stable mood alteration. Fig. 6.4 graphically schematizes the relationships among dysmorphophobia, delusional, hypochondriacal, and melancholic states according to Morselli's way of thinking.

As regards eating disorders, neither Lasègue's *anorexie histérique* [20] nor Gull's *anorexia nervosa* [21] was mentioned by Morselli in his article on dysmorphophobia. As a matter of fact, Gull and Lasègue did never report in their clinical vignettes the presence of a body image disturbance. The first medical description of a severe body uneasiness associated with eating disordered behaviours appeared 12 years after Morselli's work (see Chap. 1 of the present book). In 1903, Pierre Janet described the case of Nadia, a girl with anorexic symptoms due to the obsession of body shame ('obsession de la honte du corps') [22, pp. 33–40].

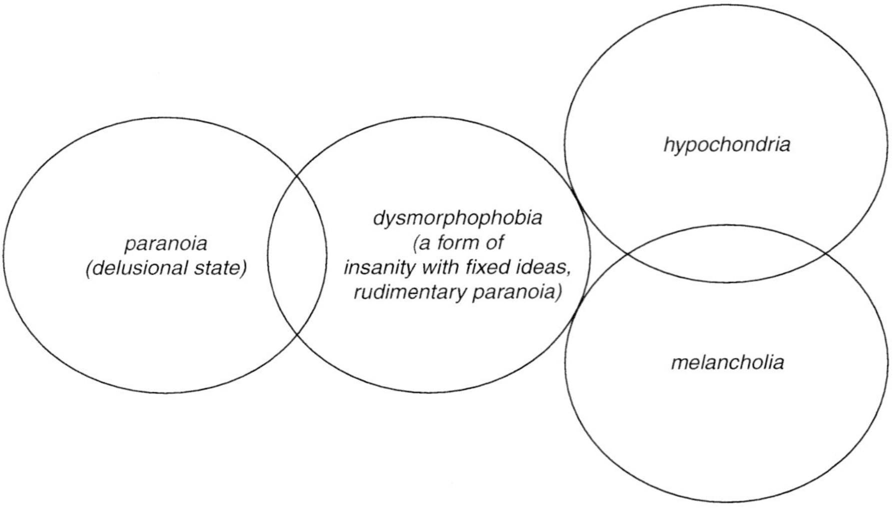

Fig. 6.4 Relationships among dysmorphophobia, delusional, hypochondriacal, and melancholic states according to Enrico Morselli's thought, 1891

6.4 Use of the Term *Dysmorphophobia* After Morselli

For some decades, the medical literature on dysmorphophobia was poor and scattered, and the new word appeared only in a small number of European publications, mostly of anecdotal nature [5].

In 1905, the Italian psychiatrist Eugenio Tanzi described in his treatise on mental disorders [23] three beautiful young women suffering from dysmorphophobia. He cited Morselli's work and, like Morselli, regarded this clinical picture as a fixed idea, using the term *phobia* in the old broad sense that included obsessional thoughts.

However, it is not without interest that Tanzi considered this clinical picture as 'the teratological chapter of pathophobia' (p. 508), highlighting the relationship with hypochondria. In Tanzi's book, dysmorphophobia was classified as one of the possible psychic symptoms of *neurasthenia*, defined as 'a persistent state of valetudinary, without definite objective abnormalities' (p. 497). *Valetudinarian* is a person whose chief concern is his/her physical health and, indeed, also in dysmorphophobia the body is the central focus of the obsessional thoughts.

In 1909, Robertson and MacKenzie translated Tanzi's textbook and the word '*dysmorphophobia*' appeared in the English language [24, p. 150]. A century later Laurence Jerome provided the first readily available English translation of Morselli's classic paper. It appeared in the journal *History of Psychiatry* with the title 'Dysmorphophobia and taphephobia: two hitherto undescribed forms of insanity with fixed ideas' [16].

In 1915, Emil Kraepelin mentioned, very briefly, some patients who were obsessed by the idea they had a strange nose, or had bandy legs, or smelt bad and, consequently, attracted attention and became an object of derision. Like Morselli, Kraepelin considered '*Dysmorphophobie*' as a '*Zwangsneurose*' (obsessive-compulsive neurosis) and described this condition together with '*Ereuthophobie*' (a nagging fear of blushing) [11, pp. 1860–1861].

In the tenth edition of the International Classification of Diseases (ICD-10), *dysmorphophobia* is not a specific diagnostic category, but the term still appears to indicate a variant of the *hypochondriacal disorder* (F45.2) or—when it has delusional features—one of the *other persistent delusional disorders* (F22.8) [25].

As regards the Diagnostic and Statistical Manual of Mental Disorders (DSM), the term *dysmorphophobia* was not used in the first two editions [26, 27].

On the contrary, in the DSM-III [28], the word *dysmorphophobia* occurred in the residual category *atypical somatoform disorder* (300.70). The 'atypical' designation was similar to the 'Not Otherwise Specified' category used in the subsequent editions of the diagnostic manual. Four lines described the clinical picture:

> An example of cases that can be classified here include those of individuals who are preoccupied with some imagined defect in physical appearance that is out of proportion to any actual physical abnormality that may exist. This syndrome has sometimes been termed 'Dysmorphophobia' (p. 252).

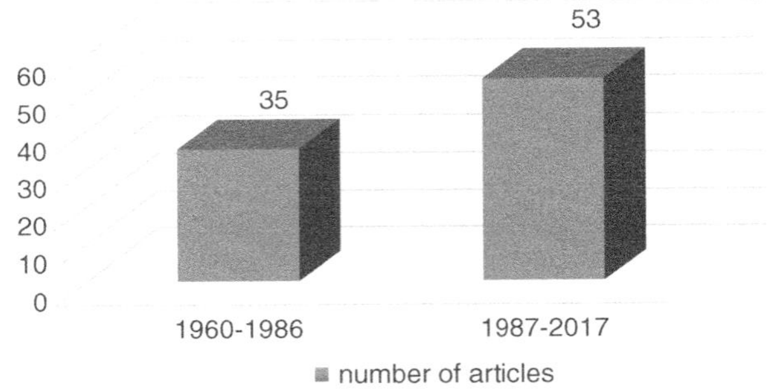

Fig. 6.5 *PubMed* articles with a title that contains the word *dysmorphophobia*

Seven years after, in 1987, the revised edition DSM-III-R [29] introduced the expressions *delusional disorder somatic type* (297.10) and *body dysmorphic disorder* (BDD) (300.70) to indicate two distinct psychiatric diagnostic categories (see Chap. 5 of the present book). BDD was included in the group of somatoform disorders together with hypochondriasis. *Dysmorphophobia* was officially replaced by the new terms.

However, the old word did not disappear (Fig. 6.5).

6.5 Final Note

In 1891, Morselli coined an Italian neologism that is still being used, '*dismorfofobia*' (English: *dysmorphophobia*; French: *dysmorphophobie*; German: *Dysmorphophobie* or *Körperdysmorphophobie*; Spanish: *dismorfofobia*). Morselli applied the concept of phobia in its broad pre-Freudian sense that did not distinguish phobias from obsessions. He considered dysmorphophobia as an *insanity with fixed ideas*, a group of mental disorders that included phobias, obsessions, compulsive behaviours, and delusional thoughts. To construct this new diagnostic category, he attached more clinical importance to the *content* of the symptom (imagined or negligible imperfections in body appearance) and its *cognitive* component (obsessional or, sometimes, delusional ideas) than to the associated emotions (anxiety, shame). As to aetiology and prognosis, Morselli refused the concept of dysmorphophobia as a *degenerative* (inherited) *illness* and sustained that, at least in some cases, it may be an acquired and transitory state of *neurasthenia*.

References

1. Morselli E. Psicologia e spiritismo. Impressioni e note critiche sui fenomeni medianici di Eusapia Paladino. Torino: Bocca; 1908.
2. Nicolas S. L'hypnose: Charcot face à Bernheim: L'école de la Salpêtrière face à l'école de Nancy. Paris: L'Harmattan; 2004.
3. Morselli E. La psicanalisi. Studii ed appunti critici. Torino: Bocca; 1926.
4. Morselli E. Sulla dismorfofobia e sulla tafefobia, due forme non per anco descritte di pazzia con idee fisse. Bollettino della Regia Accademia Medica di Genova. 1891;6:110–9.

5. Frank OS. Dysmorphophobia. In: Galnd RN, Fawzy FI, Hudson BL, Pasnau RO, editors. Current themes in psychiatry. London: Macmillan Education UK; 1985. p. 257–78.
6. Berrios GE, Kan CS. A conceptual and quantitative analysis of 178 historical cases of dysmorphophobia. Acta Psychiatr Scand. 1996;94(1):1–7.
7. Koupernik C. La psychose de laideur ou dysmorphophobie. Entretiens de Bichat-Médecine. 1962:321–6.
8. Kraepelin E. Psychiatrie Ein Lehrbuch für Studierende und Ärzte, vol. 1. Leipzig: Johann Ambrosius Barth; 1899.
9. Kraepelin E. Psychiatrie. Ein Lehrbuch für Studierende und Ärzte, vol. 2. Lipzig: Johann Ambrosius Barth; 1910.
10. Kraepelin E. Psychiatrie. Ein Lehrbuch für Studierende und Ärzte, vol. 3. Leipzig: Johann Ambrosius Barth; 1913.
11. Kraepelin E. Psychiatrie. Ein Lehrbuch für Studierende und Ärzte, vol. 4. Leipzig: Johann Ambrosius Barth; 1915.
12. Morselli E. Manuale di semejotica delle malattie mentali. Guida alla diagnosi della pazzia per i medici, i medico-legisti e gli studenti. Volume I. Generalità. Esame anamnestico, antropologico e fisiologico degli alienati. Milano: Vallardi; 1885.
13. Morselli E. Manuale di semejotica delle malattie mentali. Guida alla diagnosi della pazzia per i medici, i medico-legisti e gli studenti. Volume II. Esame psicologico degli alienati. Milano: Vallardi; 1894.
14. Phillips KA. The broken mirror. Understanding and treating body dysmorphic disorder. New York: Oxford University Press; 1996.
15. Berrios GE. The history of mental symptoms. Descriptive psychopathology since the 19th century. Cambridge: Cambridge University Press; 1996.
16. Morselli E, Jerome L. Dysmorphophobia and taphephobia: two hitherto undescribed forms of Insanity with fixed ideas. Hist Psychiatry. 2001;12(45):103–7.
17. Arndt RG. LeLehrbuch der Psychiatrie für Ärzte und Studirende. Wien: Urban & Schwarzenberg; 1883.
18. Legrain PM. Du délire chez les dégénérés: observations prises à l'asile Sainte-Anne, 1885-1886 (service de M. Magnan). In Publications du Progrès Médical. Paris; 1886.
19. Buccola G. Sulle idee fisse e sulle loro condizioni fisiopatologiche. Rivista sperimentale di freniatria e di medicina legale. 1882;VI(1–2):155–81.
20. Lasègue C. De l'anorexie hystérique. Archives Générales de Médecine. 1873;21:385–403.
21. Gull WW. Anorexia nervosa (apepsia hysterica, anorexia hysterica). Trans Clin Soc London. 1874;7:22–8.
22. Janet P. Les obsessions et la psychasthénie (1903). Tome I: Analyse des symptômes. Tome II: Études générales. Paris: L'Harmattan; 2005.
23. Tanzi E. Trattato delle malattie mentali. Milano: Società Editrice Libraria; 1905.
24. Tanzi E. A textbook of mental diseases (translated by W. F. Robertson and T. C. MacKenzie). London: Rebman; 1909.
25. World Health Organization. The ICD-10 Classification of Mental and Behavioural Disorders. Diagnostic criteria for research (ICD-10: DCR-10). Geneva: World Health Organization; 1993.
26. American Psychiatric Association. Diagnostic and statistical manual of mental disorders (DSM-I). Washington, DC: American Psychiatric Association Mental Hospital Service; 1952.
27. American Psychiatric Association. DSM-II. Diagnostic and statistical manual of mental disorders. 2nd ed. Washington, DC: American Psychiatric Association; 1968.
28. American Psychiatric Association. Diagnostic and statistical manual of mental disorders. DSM III. 3rd ed. Washington, DC: American Psychiatric Association; 1980.
29. American Psychiatric Association. Diagnostic and statistical manual of mental disorders. DSM IIIR. 3rd Revised ed. Washington, DC: American Psychiatric Association;1987.

Neuroscience, Brain Imaging, and Body Image in Eating and Weight Disorders

7

Santino Gaudio, Antonios Dakanalis, Giuseppe Fariello, and Giuseppe Riva

7.1 Introduction

Several neuroscientific strides over the past two decades have significantly improved our understanding of the pathophysiology of various psychiatric disorders. The increased use of advanced brain-imaging techniques (e.g. functional magnetic resonance imaging, positron emission tomography, and single photon emission computed tomography) has also allowed the elucidation of cerebral regions and brain networks involved in eating and weight-related disorders (EWDs), characterized, among others, by body image disturbance [1].

Before presenting neuroimaging findings related to body image disturbance in EWDs, it is useful to briefly introduce the nature and complexity of the

S. Gaudio (✉)
Department of Neuroscience, Functional Pharmacology, Uppsala University, Uppsala, Sweden

Area of Diagnostic Imaging, Departmental Faculty of Medicine and Surgery, Università "Campus Bio-Medico di Roma", Rome, Italy

A. Dakanalis
Department of Medicine and Surgery, University of Milano Bicocca, Milan, Italy

Department of Brain and Behavioral Sciences, University of Pavia, Pavia, Italy

Department of Clinical Psychology and Psychobiology, University of Barcelona, Barcelona, Spain

Applied Technology for Neuro-Psychology Lab, Istituto Auxologico Italiano, Milan, Italy

G. Fariello
Department of Diagnostic Imaging, Ospedale San Pietro Fatebenefratelli, Rome, Italy

G. Riva
Centro Studi e Ricerche di Psicologia della Comunicazione, Università Cattolica del Sacro Cuore, Milan, Italy

Applied Technology for Neuro-Psychology Lab, Istituto Auxologico Italiano, Milan, Italy

M. Cuzzolaro, S. Fassino (eds.), *Body Image, Eating, and Weight*,
https://doi.org/10.1007/978-3-319-90817-5_7

dysfunctional body image experience in EWDs, which has been made the focus of multi-decade research through the use of different assessment tools [2, 3]. Although it is widely accepted that body image disturbance is a core feature of EWDs (e.g. anorexia nervosa, bulimia nervosa, binge-eating disorder, and obesity) (e.g. [2, 4]), there is still not consensus on its constituent components or dimensions [3]. Consistent with prior research (e.g. [1, 2, 5]), in this chapter, we use the term "body image distortion," as a comprehensive definition of body image disturbance. Considering the most studies EWDs (i.e. anorexia nervosa and bulimia nervosa), behavioural studies highlighted that body image distortion is a multidimensional symptom [2, 3]. In brief, although the different components cannot be completely disentangled, body image distortion can be considered as a multidimensional construct consisting of three main components: perceptive, affective, and cognitive. Namely, EWD patients show an overestimation of own body size, body dissatisfaction, and self-ideal discrepancies, respectively [2]. The perceptive component of body image distortion is primarily related to the identification, detection, and estimation of one's own body size and is defined as the inaccuracy of the subjects' judgement of their shape, and weight relative to their actual size [6, 7]; the affective component principally comprises the satisfaction/dissatisfaction of one's own body and the feelings that subjects develop towards their body forms [8]; the cognitive component mainly includes the mental representation of one's own body built through the beliefs about body shape and appearance [8]. Some studies have suggested a behavioural component as an additional component [3], which is characterized by the behaviours aimed to change one's own body. Such component is not widely accepted because some authors argue that these behaviours may be an effect of the above reported affective and cognitive components of body image distortion [9, 10]. In this chapter, explaining the neural substrate of body image distortion, we will also consider body image distortion as a multidimensional symptom composed by the three main accepted (perceptive, affective, and cognitive) components [1].

The goal of this chapter is to give an overview of (a) the neural basis of visual body perception and body awareness in humans and of (b) the findings of structural and functional neuroimaging studies related to body image distortion in EWDs, and (c) to discuss neural substrates of body image distortion in EWDs.

7.2 Body in the Human Brain

Several research groups have explored the neural basis of visual body perception (referring to the detection and identification of one's own body and of other human bodies) [11] and body awareness (referring to the perception, knowledge, and evaluation of one's own body and of other bodies and including proprioception and interoception as well) [12]. Although these two concepts are interconnected, the debate on the terms and the concepts of body perception and body awareness is still open; here, we try to give an overview of the main findings without discussing the controversies about this matter (e.g. [12]).

The investigation of the visual processing of the human body has been initially performed with functional magnetic resonance imaging (fMRI) [13] and subsequently with additional methods, e.g. evoked potentials, intracranial recordings, and transcranial magnetic stimulation (for a review, see [11]).

There is evidence that two specific brain areas are specialized for the encoding of human bodies: the extrastriate body area (EBA) and the fusiform body area (FBA) [11]. In particular, fMRI studies revealed that the EBA, which is located in the posterior inferior temporal sulcus/middle temporal gyrus, is specifically activated by images of human bodies and body parts (e.g. [11, 13]). In addition, fMRI studies have identified a second brain area that specifically responds to images of human bodies and body parts: the FBA, which is located in the fusiform gyrus [11]. Although these two brain regions are involved in the detection and identification of human bodies, the distinction between self-body-identification and other-body-identification seems to be a more complex process [14–16].

A first study of Hodzic and colleagues [14] investigated the neural correlates of three different levels of visual body perception/identification: processing of unknown human bodies (body-detection), discrimination between familiar and unknown bodies (body-identification) and distinction of one's own body from a familiar body (self-identification). These authors confirmed that the body-detection involves the EBA in both hemispheres, and the FBA in the right hemisphere, also showing the involvement of the right inferior parietal lobe. Hodzic and colleagues [14] also pointed out that the body-identification involves a network of brain areas that comprises, in addition to the right FBA and the right inferior parietal lobe, the inferior frontal gyrus of both hemispheres and the right medial frontal gyrus, the right cingulate gyrus, and the right central and the post-central sulcus. Finally, the self-identification was characterized by the involvement of a partially different network of areas, which includes the right inferior parietal lobe, the right inferior parietal sulcus, the left posterior orbital gyrus, and the left lateral occipital gyrus.

A second study of Hodzic and colleagues [15] confirmed the role of the EBA and parietal lobes in encoding of human bodies and highlighted a different brain network involved in the identification of one's own body, which partially overlapping in the parietal areas with the previous one and also comprises the right FBA and the middle frontal gyrus.

These findings seem to indicate that the EBA does not have a key role in the distinction between self and others. However, a subsequent study of Vocks and colleagues [16] pointed out an increased activation of the right EBA and FBA in response to one's own body images compared to other female's body images, suggesting a role of the EBA in the distinction between self and others.

Furthermore, a transcranial magnetic stimulation study focused on the right EBA and temporoparietal junction suggests a role of the EBA in the perceptions of one's own body [17]. To date, although the role of the EBA is still under debate, we can assume that a fronto-parietal network, which mainly includes the inferior parietal lobe, is involved in the visual identification of one own's body [14].

The consciousness of one's body and oneself goes beyond visual body perception including proprioceptive, tactile, and interoceptive information received and processed by the brain [12]. In other words, integration of different stimuli (i.e. visual, proprioceptive, tactile, and interoceptive) is needed to develop a realistic and correct perception of one's own body, and the relations between one's own body and physical environment.

Several neuroimaging studies have shed more light on neural substrates of body awareness also considering the proprioceptive-tactile and interoceptive perception of the body (for a review, see [12]). In particular, interoception comprises feelings such as hunger, visceral sensations, temperature, and pain, and it can be viewed as a sense of the homeostatic state of the body [12].

Regarding interoception, the insula is considered to be the key brain area for integrating homeostatic state and subjective sensations related to the body into self-consciousness and emotions [12, 18]. Proprioception is considered as the sense of knowing where body and limb position is in space [19]. Namely, perception and detection of body position and orientation are allowed by integration of multiple sensory and motor mechanisms, which involve the highest levels of cognitive functions [19].

The right parietal lobe has been considered to be involved in self-generated actions as well as in disownership phenomena related to brain lesions [12]. In particular, the inferior parietal cortex seems to be involved in the distinction of self-generated actions and actions of others, whereas the anterior insula seems to play a role in the integration of multisensory reactions related to voluntary movements.

In addition, two other brain regions (i.e. EBA and temporal-parietal junction) seem to be involved in the distinction between self-generated actions and actions generated by others [20, 21].

On the other hand, out-of-body experiences and autoscopic phenomena seem to be related to an altered multisensory integration in the right temporoparietal cortex, also including the posterior insula and frontal areas and fronto-parietal altered connections [22, 23].

Interestingly, the posterior parietal cortex (i.e. parietal lobes and precuneus), as part of the default mode network ([24]; for details on the network, see also Sect. 8.4.2), seems to be involved in self-awareness and conscious experience [25].

In summary, although the complexity of brain areas/networks involved in body perception and awareness need to be better defined by future research, it can be assumed that visual perception, proprioception, and interoception work together to provide the brain with a complete information about body, and those specific brain areas (i.e. EBA, FBA, parietal cortex, and insula) are mainly involved in processing of self-body experiences.

7.3 Structural Neural Correlates of Body Image Distortion in Eating and Weight-Related Disorders (EWDs)

Several research groups have used structural neuroimaging techniques to investigate anatomical brain differences in EWD patients. In the last decade, the development of the automated voxel-based morphometry (VBM) technique, which allows a voxel-by-voxel analysis of differences across the whole brain without a priori hypotheses, enable us to investigate the global and regional alterations of grey matter (GM), white matter (WM), and cerebral spinal fluid (CSF) volume and concentration [26].

As regards anorexia nervosa (AN), VBM studies, confirming previous MRI studies (e.g. [27]), revealed that acute AN patients, due to their specific symptomatology (i.e. malnutrition and starvation), had global GM and WM decreases and CSF increases (for a meta-analysis, see [28]). These alterations seem to be partially [29] or completely [30] restored after AN recovery.

Regarding regional neural changes in AN patients, a recent meta-analysis has shown that AN patients mainly have specific GM decreases in the inferior parietal lobe and hypothalamus of the left hemisphere and in the right caudate and lentiform nucleus of the right hemisphere [28]. Considering that these regions are also involved in somatosensory perception and appetite, the authors suggested that enduring food restriction may support an altered feeling/perception of the body in response to eating and abnormal reward responses [28].

Due to the number of available VBM studies, the authors were unable to take into account AN duration in their analyses. However, it is worth noting that alteration of the inferior parietal lobe and precuneus have been found in both the early stages of AN [29, 31] and in recovered AN patients [32]. These areas are involved in self-body identification and self-consciousness ([14, 15, 25]; see also Sect. 8.2) and maybe a vulnerability trait marker of body image distortion in AN.

A limited number of studies have investigated structural brain changes in EWDs, other than AN. In particular, VBM studies on patients with bulimia nervosa (BN) indicated GM increases in frontal and ventral striatal areas [33]. Interestingly, a GM volume increase has been found bilaterally in the somatosensory regions, precuneus and paracentral lobule in BN patients with a long duration of the disease [34]. On the other hand, obese patients (men included) revealed grey matter alterations in brain areas mainly involved in reward and taste regulation (i.e. post-central gyrus, frontal operculum, putamen, and middle frontal gyrus) [35] and working memory (e.g. dorsolateral prefrontal cortex) [36].

Regarding WM investigations, a new neuroimaging technique has been developed in the last years: diffusion tensor imaging (DTI). This allows exploring microstructural integrity of WM tracts that cannot be detected using volumetric approaches (e.g. VBM) [37]. In particular, DTI assesses WM diffusion parameters: fractional anisotropy, mean diffusivity, radial diffusivity, and axial diffusivity (for details, see [38]). Some DTI studies have investigated WM alterations in EWDs.

DTI studies on patients with current or past AN have mainly shown WM microstructural alterations in superior longitudinal fasciculus [39–44], fornix [40–46], and corona radiata [39, 40, 43, 44].

In particular, the superior longitudinal fasciculus mainly connects parietal, and prefrontal cortices, brain areas involved in self-body perception (for details, see Sect. 8.2), and could sustain body image distortion of AN [42, 44]. Few studies have been performed with BN patients [47] and obese subjects [48] but superior longitudinal fasciculus alterations have also been evidenced in obese subjects [49].

In summary, according to structural MRI studies AN patients seem to have a GM vulnerability of the posterior parietal areas and a WM vulnerability of the superior longitudinal fasciculus. Although the structural abnormalities can be due to malnutrition and starvation, it is worth noting that these structures are involved in visual self-body perception and could be related to body image distortion. To date, the MRI studies on BN and obesity are few, but they evidence some similar results.

7.4 Functional Neural Correlates of Body Image in EWDS

7.4.1 Event-Related fMRI Studies: Body Image Distortion in EWDs Brain

To date, fMRI, allows us investigating brain activity in response to specific tasks or at rest, has been the most frequently used technique in EWDs [50]. Several fMRI studies have examined brain activity in response to body-related tasks in AN (for a review, see [1]), while a limited number of fMRI studies have investigated the neural basis of body image distortion in BN using body-related paradigms [50].

The fMRI studies which used the AN patient's own body image as visual stimulus showed partially consistent results [51–54]. In particular, AN patients had a decreased activation or an absence of activation in response to the self-body image in the inferior parietal lobule [51, 52] and in the precuneus [51], as compared to healthy controls. Interestingly, research has also revealed that BN subjects had lower activation in the inferior parietal lobe in response to the one's own body photograph, as compared to controls [52].

Two studies with a longitudinally design pointed out that in the pre- vs. post-therapy comparison, AN patients had an increased activation of the left middle temporal gyrus (including the extrastriate body area) and a decreased activation in a widely distributed network also including precuneus and inferior parietal lobe [53, 54].

Recently, a research group used video clips of AN patient's own body and another's body and pointed out that AN patients showed a higher activity in the dorsal posterior cingulate cortex during the video clip of their own body and a lower activity in the precuneus and ventral posterior cingulate cortex during the video clip of another's body [55].

Using line drawings of female (underweight, normal, and overweight) bodies compared to line drawings of houses, Uher and colleagues [56] showed that AN and BN patients had lower activation in the parietal cortex and in the lateral fusiform gyrus, as compared to controls. Furthermore, Mohr and colleagues [57] revealed lack of modulation of the precuneus activity during a specific body size estimation task (i.e. subjects were required to choose the image from thinner to fatter that most closely resembles the subject's real body image) in the AN subjects, as compared to controls.

Overall, considering the multidimensionality of body image distortion ([2]; see also Sect. 8.1), the studies mentioned above used visual tasks, which predominantly involved the perceptive component of visual body perception, highlighted the involvement of the posterior parietal areas. These findings suggest that specific brain areas (i.e. inferior parietal lobe and precuneus) may be involved in the perceptive component of body image distortion in AN and BN patients [1].

Some fMRI studies used distorted own and other's body image as body-related tasks. Five studies using a self-distorted fat body image in AN patients mainly found functional alterations in the prefrontal cortex [58–60] and amygdala [59, 61]. In particular, Miyake and colleagues [59] indicated a higher activation in the prefrontal cortex in patients with AN-binge-purging type and healthy women, but not in AN-restrictive type and BN patients. Interestingly, using the task mentioned above, significantly greater activation was found in the medial prefrontal cortex in BN patients, as compared to controls [62].

A research group adopted a more complex body-related task, during which AN patients were asked to choose their ideal body shape viewing images with different degrees of body size distortion (from thinner to fatter), and revealed a higher activation of the insula and the lateral anterior prefrontal cortex in the satisfaction rating for the thinner self images [57]. This research group, using the same task, also showed the involvement of the anterior insula in BN patients [63]. In response to self-distorted thin body images, a stronger activation of the right dorsolateral prefrontal cortex and parietal cortex and of the occipito-temporal cortex has been found in AN patients and controls [59]. Furthermore, a research group, using images of slim fashion model bodies, showed increased activation of the insula and premotor cortex and reduced activation of the anterior cingulate cortex (ACC) in AN patients, as compared to controls [64].

Overall, the studies above used body-related tasks that primarily involved the affective component of body image distortion [2]. Namely, participants were exposed to unpleasant (e.g. self-distorted fat body photograph) or/and pleasant (e.g. self-distorted thin body photograph) stimuli that mainly involve satisfaction/dissatisfaction of one's own body.

It can be suggested that prefrontal cortex and insula alterations may sustain the affective component of body image distortion [1]. In particular, unpleasant stimuli (self-distorted fat image) are mainly related to altered prefrontal cortex activations, and pleasant stimuli (self-distorted thin image) are mainly related to insula alterations.

Interestingly, Miyake and colleagues [65], using unpleasant words concerning body, showed a stronger activation in the left inferior parietal lobe in AN patients as compared to controls, in the left medial prefrontal cortex in AN-binge-purging type and BN patients as compared to controls and of right amygdala in AN patients as compared to controls and BN patients. This task, following the multidimensional construct of body image distortion [2], mainly involves both the affective and cognitive component of body image distortion. Thus, these latter results seem to confirm the involvement of the prefrontal cortex in the affective/cognitive component of body image distortion. On the other hand, the role of the amygdala in the affective/cognitive component of body image distortion remains under debate [1].

In summary, the fMRI studies which used body-related tasks showed specific neural correlates for each of the main components of body image distortion in AN. Namely, the posterior parietal areas alterations (i.e. inferior parietal lobe and precuneus) seem to sustain the perceptive component of body image distortion, and the prefrontal cortex and insula alterations seem to be related to the affective component of body image distortion.

These latter findings seem to be also consistent in BN even though the studies performed with BN patients are few. To date, neural correlates of body image disturbance remain poorly studies in binge-eating disorder [66] and obesity [67].

7.4.2 Resting-State fMRI Studies: Neural Correlates of Body Image Distortion in the Brain at Rest

In the recent years, several fMRI studies have investigated functional brain connectivity at rest in EWDs. Although resting-state fMRI studies do not directly explore body image disturbance, some resting-state networks/areas are also related to self-regulation and visuospatial and somatosensory processing (for details on resting-state networks, see [68]).

Therefore, it can be of interest to have an overview of networks and brain areas specifically affected in EWD patients and related to body image disturbance. Several resting-state fMRI studies have explored functional connectivity in AN patients (for a review, see [69]). These studies, using different resting-state approaches, have mainly shown alterations in the corticolimbic circuitry (for details, see [69]). In particular, AN patients showed functional connectivity alterations in the insula [70–73] and in a subnetwork including the thalamus and posterior insula [71–73] which overlapped between methods.

The insula is primarily implicated in interoception of bodily feelings and sensorimotor integration ([74]; for details on insula functions, see also Sects. 7.2 and 7.4.1) and the aforementioned subnetwork has been considered involved in affected integration between visuospatial and somatosensory signals in AN patients [71–73].

In addition, resting-state studies that used independent component analysis-based approach showed alterations within the visual, somatosensory [75], and occipital networks [76] and between the visual and somatosensory networks [77]. Taken as a whole, these resting-state results may indicate that several brain regions involved in body image distortion are affected at rest in AN patients and may be involved in altered visual and homeostatic integration [69].

Some resting-state fMRI studies have explored brain at rest in obesity and have mainly found functional connectivity alterations in networks and/or brain areas involved in reward-related brain regions and prefrontal and feeding circuits [78, 79] as well as interoception and cognitive control [80]. These latter findings suggest an alteration of the insula, which is an area specifically affected in AN and involved in visual and body-signal integration [69].

One fMRI study has investigated resting-state functional connectivity in BN patients [81]. It showed a decreased functional connectivity within the somatosensory network, posterior cingulate cortex, and two visual areas (one of them comprises the EBA), suggesting that altered connectivity between the somatosensory cortex and the EBA may be involved in altered body image processing in BN.

In summary, regarding neural correlates of body image distortion, the resting-state fMRI studies on AN patients showed functional alterations in the networks (i.e. visual and somatosensory) and areas (insula and thalamus) involved in processing and integration of visual and somatosensory perceptual information. These alterations may be related and sustain body image distortion in AN. Interestingly, the studies on obese subjects and the few data on BN patients showed partially similar results.

Conclusions

In the last decades, neuroimaging studies have shed more light on the neural basis of body image distortion and on the complexity of this puzzling EWD feature (Fig. 7.1). The event-related fMRI studies that used body-related tasks mainly showed that posterior parietal areas are involved in the perceptive component (overestimation, misperception) of body image distortion and that prefrontal areas and the insula are involved in the affective component (dissatisfaction) of body image distortion in AN [1].

The few event-related fMRI studies, which have explored the neural basis of body image distortion in BN, have also shown alterations of the insula in response to body-related affective stimuli. On the other hand, neural correlates of body image distortion have been poorly investigated via event-related fMRI in both obesity and binge-eating disorder.

Interestingly, AN structural studies also showed regional GM and microstructural WM vulnerability in posterior parietal areas and tracts, respectively. Furthermore, resting-state fMRI studies on AN patients showed altered functional connectivity in areas (i.e. insula and thalamus) and networks (e.g. visual,

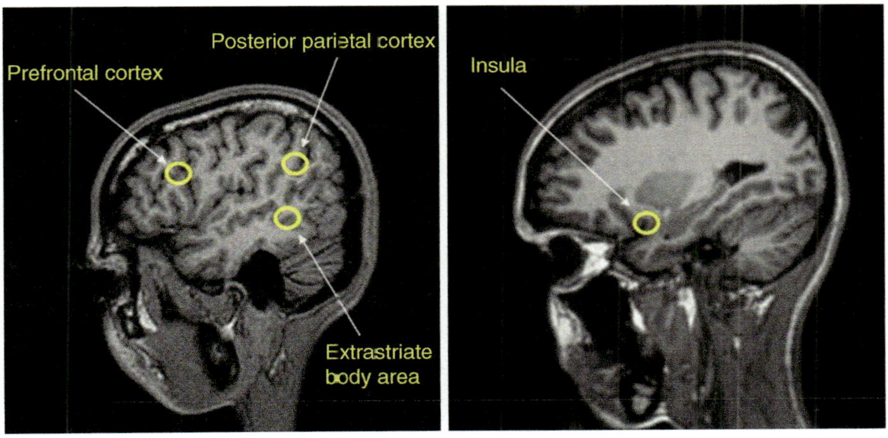

Fig. 7.1 The figure highlights the main brain areas involved in body image distortion. The left image shows the prefrontal cortex, the extrastriate body area, and the posterior parietal cortex which comprises inferior parietal lobe and precuneus. The right image shows the insula. For the specific and/or interconnected role of each area also see Sects. 7.3, 7.4.1, and 7.4.2 of the chapter.

somatosensory) also involved in processing and integration of visual and interoceptive/somatosensory signals. Interestingly, some similar results have also been found in BN and obese patients.

Overall, it can be suggested that posterior parietal areas, insula, prefrontal cortex, and EBA have a specific and interconnected role in body image distortion in AN. In particular, the alterations of the posterior parietal areas may sustain altered visual body perception, and the insula alterations may be involved in altered body awareness and negative attitudes towards the body.

Interestingly, a novel hypothesis (i.e. allocentric lock theory, see also Chap. 24 in this book) suggests linking body image distortion to the neuropsychological research related to spatial reference frames (egocentric vs. allocentric). Specifically, the egocentric network seems to involve the precuneus primarily, and the allocentric network also seems to include the occipito-temporal areas and the right superior parietal lobe (e.g. [82]).

Recently, an impairment in the processing of reference frames has been pointed out in ED patients [83]. Although there are not neuroimaging studies which directly investigated neural correlates of spatial reference frame, the above-mentioned findings suggest that posterior parietal areas alterations could sustain an impairment in the egocentric (perceptual)—allocentric (memory) transformation processing producing body image distortion [84–86]. Namely, unpleasant memories of the body are not modified by real-time perceptual information, and EWDs patients can be locked to an allocentric (observer view) negative representation of one's own body.

Although some findings are consistent across EWDs, neural correlates of body image distortion remain poorly studied in BN, obesity and binge-eating disorder. More neuroimaging research is needed to improve our knowledge of the neural correlates of body image distortion in EWDs and enhance the efficacy of the extant treatment approaches and strategies for EWDs. Finally, taking into account the complexity of body image distortion, the current findings suggest that further neuroimaging studies should also explore spatial reference frames in EWDs.

References

1. Gaudio S, Quattrocchi CC. Neural basis of a multidimensional model of body image distortion in anorexia nervosa. Neurosci Biobehav Rev. 2012;36(8):1839–47.
2. Cash TF, Deagle EA. The nature and extent of body-image disturbances in anorexia nervosa and bulimia nervosa: a meta-analysis. Int J Eat Disord. 1997;22:107–25.
3. Banfield SS, McCabe MP. An evaluation of the construct of body image. Adolescence. 2002;37:373–93.
4. Dakanalis A, Carrà G, Calogero R, Zanetti MA, Gaudio S, Caccialanza R, Riva G, Clerici M. Testing the cognitive behavioural maintenance models across DSM-5 bulimic-type eating disorder diagnostic groups: a multistudy. Eur Arch Psychiatry Clin Neurosci. 2015;265(8):663–76.
5. Dakanalis A, Clerici M, Carrà G, Riva G. Dysfunctional bodily experiences in anorexia nervosa: where are we? Eat Weight Disord. 2016;21(4):731–2.

6. Cash TF, Wood KC, Phelps KD, Boyd K. New assessments of weight related body image derived from extant instruments. Percept Mot Skills. 1991;73:235–41.
7. Slade PD. What is body image? Behav Res Ther. 1994;32:497–502.
8. Cash TF, Green GK. Body weight and body image among college women: perception, cognition, and affect. J Pers Assess. 1986;50:290–3017.
9. Gleaves DH, Williamson DA, Eberenz KP, Sebastian SB, Barker SE. Clarifying body-image disturbance: analysis of a multidimensional model using structural modeling. J Pers Assess. 1995;64:478–93.
10. Dakanalis A, Carrà G, Timko A, Volpato C, Pla-Sanjuanelo J, Zanetti A, Clerici M, Riva G. Mechanisms of influence of body checking on binge eating. Int J Clin Health Psychol. 2015;152:93–104.
11. Peelen MV, Downing PE. The neural basis of visual body perception. Nat Rev Neurosci. 2007;8:636–48.
12. Berlucchi G, Aglioti SM. The body in the brain revisited. Exp Brain Res. 2010;200(1):25–35.
13. Downing PE, Jiang Y, Shuman M, Kanwisher N. A cortical area selective for visual processing of the human body. Science. 2001;293:2470–3.
14. Hodzic A, Kaas A, Muckli L, Stirn A, Singer W. Distinct cortical networks for the detection and identification of human body. Neuroimage. 2009;45:1264–71.
15. Hodzic A, Muckli L, Singer W, Stirn A. Cortical responses to self and others. Hum Brain Mapp. 2009;30:951–62.
16. Vocks S, Busch M, Gronemeyer D, Schulte D, Herpertz S, Suchan B. Differential neuronal responses to the self and others in the extrastriate body area and the fusiform body area. Cogn Affect Behav Neurosci. 2010;10:422–9.
17. Cazzato V, Mian E, Serino A, Mele S, Urgesi C. Distinct contributions of extrastriate body area and temporoparietal junction in perceiving one's own and others' body. Cogn Affect Behav Neurosci. 2015;15(1):211–28.
18. Craig AD. How do you feel-now? The anterior insula and human awareness. Nat Rev Neurosci. 2009;10:59–70.
19. Blanke O. Multisensory brain mechanisms of bodily self-consciousness. Nat Rev Neurosci. 2012;13(8):556–71.
20. David N, Jansen M, Cohen MX, Osswald K, Molnar-Szakacs I, Newen A, Vogeley K, Paus T. Disturbances of self-other distinction after stimulation of the extrastriate body area in the human brain. Soc Neurosci. 2008;21:1–9.
21. Spengler S, von Cramon DY, Brass M. Was it me or was it you? How the sense of agency originates from ideomotor learning revealed by fMRI. Neuroimage. 2009;46:290–8.
22. Blanke O, Metzinger T. Full-body illusions and minimal phenomenal selfhood. Trends Cogn Sci. 2009;13:7–13.
23. Aspell JE, Lenggenhager B, Blanke O. Multisensory perception and bodily self-consciousness. In: Murray MT, Wallace MM, editors. The neural bases of multisensory processes. Boca Raton: CRC Press; 2012. p. 467–84.
24. Raichle ME, MacLeod AM, Snyder AZ, Powers WJ, Gusnard DA, Shulman GL. A default mode of brain function. Proc Natl Acad Sci U S A. 2001;98:676–82.
25. Cavanna AE, Trimble MR. The precuneus: a review of its functional anatomy and behavioural correlates. Brain. 2006;129:564–83.
26. Ashburner J, Friston KJ. Voxel-based morphometry – the methods. Neuroimage. 2000;11:805–21.
27. Kohn MR, Ashtari M, Golden NH, Schebendach J, Patel M, Jacobson MS, Shenker IR. Structural brain changes and malnutrition in anorexia nervosa. Ann N Y Acad Sci. 1997;817:398–9.
28. Titova OE, Hjorth OC, Schiöth HB, Brooks SJ. Anorexia nervosa is linked to reduced brain structure in reward and somatosensory regions: a meta-analysis of VBM studies. BMC Psychiatry. 2013;13:110.
29. Castro-Fornieles J, Bargallo N, Lazaro L, Andres S, Falcon C, Plana MT, Junqué C. A cross-sectional and follow-up voxel-based morphometric MRI study in adolescent anorexia nervosa. J Psychiatr Res. 2009;43:331–40.

30. Lázaro L, Andrés S, Calvo A, Cullell C, Moreno E, Plana MT, Falcón C, Bargalló N, Castro-Fornieles J. Normal gray and white matter volume after weight restoration in adolescents with anorexia nervosa. Int J Eat Disord. 2013;46(8):841–8.
31. Gaudio S, Nocchi F, Franchin T, Genovese E, Cannatà V, Longo D, Fariello G. Gray matter decrease distribution in the early stages of Anorexia Nervosa restrictive type in adolescents. Psychiatry Res. 2011;191:24–30.
32. Joos A, Hartmann A, Glauche V, Perlov E, Unterbrink T, Saum B, Tuscher O, Tebartz van Alst L, Zeeck A. Grey matter deficit in long-term recovered anorexia nervosa patients. Eur Eat Disord Rev. 2011;19:59–63.
33. Van den Eynde F, Suda M, Broadbent H, Guillaume S, Van den Eynde M, Steiger H, Israel M, Berlim M, Giampietro V, Simmons A, Treasure J, Campbell I, Schmidt U. Structural magnetic resonance imaging in eating disorders: a systematic review of voxel-based morphometry studies. Eur Eat Disord Rev. 2012;20:94–105.
34. Amianto F, Caroppo P, D'Agata F, Spalatro A, Lavagnino L, Caglio M, Righi D, Bergui M, Abbate-Daga G, Rigardetto R, Mortara P, Fassino S. Brain volumetric abnormalities in patients with anorexia and bulimia nervosa: a voxel-based morphometry study. Psychiatry Res. 2013;213(3):210–6.
35. Pannacciulli N, Del Parigi A, Chen K, Le DSN, Reiman EM, Tataranni PA. Brain abnormalities in human obesity: a voxel-based morphometric study. Neuroimage. 2006;31(4):1419–25.
36. Brooks SJ, Benedict C, Burgos J, Kempton MJ, Kullberg J, Nordenskjöld R, Kilander L, Nylander R, Larsson EM, Johansson L, Ahlström H, Lind L, Schiöth HB. Late-life obesity is associated with smaller global and regional gray matter volumes: a voxel-based morphometric study. Int J Obes (Lond). 2013;37(2):230–6.
37. Le Bihan D, Mangin JF, Poupon C, Clark CA, Pappata S, Molko N, Chabriat H. Diffusion tensor imaging: concepts and applications. J Magn Reson Imaging. 2001;13:534–46.
38. Soares J, Marques P, Alves V, Sousa N. A hitchhiker's guide to diffusion tensor imaging. Front Neurosci. 2013;7:31.
39. Frieling H, Fischer J, Wilhelm J, Engelhorn T, Bleich S, Hillemacher T, Dörfler A, Kornhuber J, de Zwaan M, Peschel T. Microstructural abnormalities of the posterior thalamic radiation and the mediodorsal thalamic nuclei in females with anorexia nervosa-a voxel based diffusion tensor imaging (DTI) study. J Psychiatr Res. 2012;46:1237–42.
40. Frank GK, Shott ME, Hagman JO, Yang TT. Localized brain volume and white matter integrity alterations in adolescent anorexia nervosa. J Am Acad Child Adolesc Psychiatry. 2013;52:1066–75.
41. Yau WY, Bischoff-Grethe A, Theilmann RJ, Torres L, Wagner A, Kaye WH, Fennema-Notestine C. Alterations in white matter microstructure in women recovered from anorexia nervosa. Int J Eat Disord. 2013;46:701–8.
42. Via E, Zalesky A, Sánchez I, Forcano L, Harrison BJ, Pujol J, Fernández-Aranda F, Menchón JM, Soriano-Mas C, Cardoner N, Fornito A. Disruption of brain white matter microstructure in women with anorexia nervosa. J Psychiatry Neurosci. 2014;39:367–75.
43. Travis KE, Golden NH, Feldman HM, Solomon M, Nguyen J, Mezer A, Yeatman JD, Dougherty RF. Abnormal white matter properties in adolescent girls with anorexia nervosa. Neuroimage Clin. 2015;9:648–59.
44. Gaudio S, Quattrocchi CC, Piervincenzi C, Zobel BB, Montecchi FR, Dakanalis A, Riva G, Carducci F. White matter abnormalities in treatment-naive adolescents at the earliest stages of anorexia nervosa: a diffusion tensor imaging study. Psychiatry Res. 2017;266:138–45.
45. Kazlouski D, Rollin M, Tregellas J, Shott M, Jappe L, Hagman J, Pryor T, Yang TT, Frank GK. Altered fimbria-fornix white matter integrity in anorexia nervosa predicts harm avoidance. Psychiatry Res. 2011;192:109–16.
46. Nagahara Y, Nakamae T, Nishizawa S, Mizuhara Y, Moritoki Y, Wada Y, Sakai Y, Yamashita T, Narumoto J, Miyata J, Yamada K, Fukui K. A tract-based spatial statistics study in anorexia nervosa: abnormality in the fornix and the cerebellum. Prog Neuropsychopharmacol Biol Psychiatry. 2014;51:72–7.

47. He X, Stefan M, Terranova K, Steinglass J, Marsh R. Altered white matter microstructure in adolescents and adults with bulimia nervosa. Neuropsychopharmacology. 2015;41(7):1841–8.
48. Kullmann S, Schweizer F, Veit R, Fritsche A, Preissl H. Compromised white matter integrity in obesity. Obes Rev. 2015;16(4):273–81.
49. Kullmann S, Callaghan MF, Heni M, Weiskopf N, Scheffler K, Häring HU, Fritsche A, Veit R, Preissl H. Specific white matter tissue microstructure changes associated with obesity. Neuroimage. 2016;125:36–44.
50. Frank GKW, Kaye WH. Current status of functional imaging in eating disorders. Int J Eat Disord. 2013;45:723–36.
51. Sachdev P, Mondraty N, Wen W, Gulliford K. Brains of anorexia nervosa patients process self-images differently from non-self-images: an fMRI study. Neuropsychologia. 2008;46: 2161–8.
52. Vocks S, Busch M, Gronemeyer D, Schulte D, Herpertz S, Suchan B. Neural correlates of viewing photographs of one's own body and another woman's body in anorexia and bulimia nervosa: an fMRI study. J Psychiatry Neurosci. 2010;35:163–76.
53. Vocks S, Busch M, Schulte D, Grönermeyer D, Herpertz S, Suchan B. Effects of body image therapy on the activation of the extrastriate body area in anorexia nervosa: an fMRI study. Psychiatry Res. 2010;183:114–8.
54. Vocks S, Schulte D, Busch M, Gronemeyer D, Herpertz S, Suchan B. Changes in neuronal correlates of body image processing by means of cognitive behavioural body image therapy for eating disorders: a randomized controlled fMRI study. Psychol Med. 2011;41:1651–63.
55. Via E, Goldberg X, Sánchez I, Forcano L, Harrison BJ, Davey CG, Pujol J, Martínez-Zalacaín I, Fernández-Aranda F, Soriano-Mas C, Cardoner N, Menchón JM. Self and other body perception in anorexia nervosa: the role of posterior DMN nodes. World J Biol Psychiatry. 2016;22:1–15.
56. Uher R, Murphy T, Friederich HC, Dalgleish T, Brammer MJ, Giampietro V, Phillips ML, Andrew CM, Ng VW, Williams SC, Campbell IC, Treasure J. Functional neuroanatomy of body shape perception in healthy and eating disordered women. Biol Psychiatry. 2005;58:990–7.
57. Mohr HM, Zimmermann J, Roder C, Lenz C, Overbeck G, Grabhorn R. Separating two components of body image in anorexia nervosa using fMRI. Psychol Med. 2010;40:1519–29.
58. Wagner A, Ruf M, Braus DF, Schmidt MH. Neuronal activity changes and body image distortion in anorexia nervosa. Neuroreport. 2003;14:2193–7.
59. Miyake Y, Okamoto Y, Onoda K, Kurosaki M, Shirao N, Yamawaki S. Brain activation during the perception of distorted body images in eating disorders. Psychiatry Res. 2010;181: 183–92.
60. Castellini G, Polito C, Bolognesi E, D'Argenio A, Ginestroni A, Mascalchi M, Pellicanò G, Mazzoni LN, Rotella F, Faravelli C, Pupi A, Ricca V. Looking at my body. Similarities and differences between anorexia nervosa patients and controls in body image visual processing. Eur Psychiatry. 2013;28(7):427–35.
61. Seeger G, Braus DF, Ruf M, Goldberger U, Schmidt MH. Body image distortion reveals amygdala activation in patients with anorexia nervosa – a functional magnetic resonance imaging study. Neurosci Lett. 2002;326:25–8.
62. Spangler DL, Allen MD. An fMRI investigation of emotional processing of body shape in bulimia nervosa. Int J Eat Disord. 2012;45(1):17–25.
63. Mohr HM, Röder C, Zimmermann J, Hummel D, Negele A, Grabhorn R. Body image distortions in bulimia nervosa: investigating body size overestimation and body size satisfaction by fMRI. Neuroimage. 2011;56(3):1822–31.
64. Friederich HC, Brooks S, Uher R, Campbell IC, Giampietro V, Brammer M, Williams SC, Herzog W, Treasure J. Neural correlates of body dissatisfaction in anorexia nervosa. Neuropsychologia. 2010;48:2878–85.
65. Miyake Y, Okamoto Y, Onoda K, Shirao N, Otagaki Y, Yamawaki S. Neural processing of negative word stimuli concerning body image in patients with eating disorders: an fMRI study. Neuroimage. 2010;50:1333–9.

66. Kessler RM, Hutson PH, Herman BK, Potenza MN. The neurobiological basis of binge-eating disorder. Neurosci Biobehav Rev. 2016;63:223–38.
67. Carnell S, Gibson C, Benson L, Ochner CN, Geliebter A. Neuroimaging and obesity: current knowledge and future directions. Obes Rev. 2012;13(1):43–56.
68. Smith SM, Fox PT, Miller KL, Glahn DC, Fox PM, Mackay CE, Filippini N, Watkinsa KE, Torod R, Laird AR, Beckmann CF. Correspondence of the brain's functional architecture during activation and rest. Proc Natl Acad Sci U S A. 2009;106:13040–5.
69. Gaudio S, Wiemerslage L, Brooks SJ, Schiöth HB. A systematic review of resting-state functional-MRI studies in anorexia nervosa: evidence for functional connectivity impairment in cognitive control and visuospatial and body-signal integration. Neurosci Biobehav Rev. 2016;71:578–89.
70. Boehm I, Geisler D, King JA, Ritschel F, Seidel M, Deza Araujo Y, Petermann J, Lohmeier H, Weiss J, Walter M, Roessner V, Ehrlich S. Increased resting state functional connectivity in the fronto-parietal and default mode network in anorexia nervosa. Front Behav Neurosci. 2014;8:346.
71. Ehrlich S, Lord AR, Geisler D, Borchardt V, Boehm I, Seidel M, Ritschel F, Schulze A, King JA, Weidner K, Roessner V, Walter M. Reduced functional connectivity in the thalamo-insular subnetwork in patients with acute anorexia nervosa. Hum Brain Mapp. 2015;36: 1772–81.
72. Geisler D, Borchardt V, Lord AR, Boehm I, Ritschel F, Zwipp J, Clas S, King JA, Wolff-Stephan S, Roessner V, Walter M, Ehrlich S. Abnormal functional global and local brain connectivity in female patients with anorexia nervosa. J Psychiatry Neurosci. 2015;41: 6–15.
73. Lord A, Ehrlich S, Borchardt V, Geisler D, Seidel M, Huber S, Murr J, Walter M. Brain parcellation choice affects disease-related topology differences increasingly from global to local network levels. Psychiatry Res Neuroimaging. 2016;249:12–9.
74. Simmons WK, Rapuano KM, Kallman SJ, Ingeholm JE, Miller B, Gotts SJ, Avery JA, Hall KD, Martin A. Category-specific integration of homeostatic signals in caudal but not rostral human insula. Nat Neurosci. 2013;16:1551–2.
75. Favaro A, Santonastaso P, Manara R, Bosello R, Bommarito G, Tenconi E, DiSalle F. Disruption of visuospatial and somatosensory functional connectivity in anorexia nervosa. Biol Psychiatry. 2012;72:864–70.
76. Amianto F, D'Agata F, Lavagnino L, Caroppo P, Abbate-Daga G, Righi D, Scarone S, Bergui M, Mortara P, Fassino S. Intrinsic connectivity networks within cerebellum and beyond in eating disorders. Cerebellum. 2013;12:623–31.
77. Phillipou A, Abel LA, Castle DJ, Hughes ME, Nibbs RG, Gurvich C, Rossell SL. Resting state functional connectivity in anorexia nervosa. Psychiatry Res Neuroimaging. 2016;251: 45–52.
78. Hogenkamp PS, Zhou W, Dahlberg LS, Stark J, Larsen AL, Olivo G, Wiemerslage L, Larsson EM, Sundbom M, Benedict C, Schiöth HB. Higher resting-state activity in reward-related brain circuits in obese versus normal-weight females independent of food intake. Int J Obes (Lond). 2016;40(11):1687–92.
79. Geha P, Cecchi G, Todd Constable R, Abdallah C, Small DM. Reorganization of brain connectivity in obesity. Hum Brain Mapp. 2017;38(3):1403–20.
80. Moreno-Lopez L, Contreras-Rodriguez O, Soriano-Mas C, Stamatakis EA, Verdejo-Garcia A. Disrupted functional connectivity in adolescent obesity. Neuroimage Clin. 2016;12: 262–8.
81. Lavagnino L, Amianto F, D'Agata F, Huang Z, Mortara P, Abbate-Daga G, Marzola E, Spalatro A, Fassino S, Northoff G. Reduced resting-state functional connectivity of the somatosensory cortex predicts psychopathological symptoms in women with bulimia nervosa. Front Behav Neurosci. 2014;8:270.
82. Zaehle T, Jordan K, Wustenberg T, Baudewig J, Dechent P, Mast FW. The neural basis of the egocentric and allocentric spatial frame of reference. Brain Res. 2007;1137:92–103.

83. Serino S, Dakanalis A, Gaudio S, Carrà G, Cipresso P, Clerici M, Riva G. Out of body, out of space: impaired reference frame processing in eating disorders. Psychiatry Res. 2015;230(2):732–4.
84. Riva G, Gaudio S. Allocentric lock in anorexia nervosa: new evidences from neuroimaging studies. Med Hypotheses. 2012;79(1):113–7.
85. Riva G, Gaudio S, Dakanalis A. I'm in a virtual body: a locked allocentric memory may impair the experience of the body in both obesity and anorexia nervosa. Eat Weight Disord. 2014;19(1):133–4.
86. Dakanalis A, Gaudio S, Serino S, Clerici M, Carrà G, Riva G. Body-image distortion in anorexia nervosa. Nat Rev Dis Primers. 2016;2:16026.

Body Image Disturbances in Anorexia Nervosa

8

Enrica Marzola and Giovanni Abbate-Daga

8.1 Introduction

Anorexia nervosa (AN) is a severe mental illness with typical onset in female adolescents and largely unknown etiology. It is characterized by aberrant patterns of eating behaviors, extremely low body weight, restriction of energy consumption, and fear of gaining weight. Body image is also severely distorted so patients tend to perceive themselves as fat even when emaciated to death. A distorted body image is therefore a hallmark of this disorder. Body image disturbances in AN are defined as "a disturbance in the way in which one's body weight or shape is experienced" [1]. However, body image has been theorized as a multidimensional construct [2] with attitudinal aspects and perceptual dimensions of body image as entrenched aspects in determining and evaluating one's own body size and shape.

In AN, body image disturbances are a key aspect with respect to both etiology [3] and relapse prevention [4]; during the 1960s, Bruch described AN as a "disturbance in body image of delusional proportions" [5]. About 50% of patients with AN recover while about 20% develop a severe and enduring disorder [6]; however, outcome rates vary also depending on the inclusion of patients' overestimation of their body size. Body image distortions are crucial in AN with relevant consequences from a development, prognosis, and maintenance point of view [7–10]. Body image concerns have been linked to relapse as well; this is of interest given the unsatisfactory outcomes that characterize this disorder [11]. The available therapeutic armamentarium mainly relies on the modifications of body-related cognitions and behaviors rather than on the multisensory factors of patients' body image.

A number of different components of body image play a role in body image disturbances in AN: affective, i.e., subjective feelings towards their body's appearance and satisfaction/dissatisfaction and subjective preoccupations with body size

E. Marzola · G. Abbate-Daga (✉)
Eating Disorders Center, Department of Neuroscience, University of Turin, Turin, Italy
e-mail: giovanni.abbatedaga@unito.it

M. Cuzzolaro, S. Fassino (eds.), *Body Image, Eating, and Weight*,
https://doi.org/10.1007/978-3-319-90817-5_8

or shape; cognitive, i.e., thoughts on body shape and body mental representation [12]; and perceptual, i.e., the accurate identification and estimation of one's own body size, shape, and weight and behavioral aspects [13, 14]. Overall, literature on AN showed that such dimensions are characterized by an overall overestimation of body size coupled with greater body dissatisfaction. However, data are overall mixed about accuracy in estimating body size in AN since a whole variety of assessments has been performed to date in order to reliably capture this complex and multifaceted construct. For example, assessments vary (e.g., asking participants to evaluate their total body versus some specific body parts) as well as assessment tools (pen-and-paper versions of silhouettes versus virtual reality), and phase of the illness (hospitalization, extreme versus mild body mass index) alike. On the other hand, the aforementioned multiple components of body image directly hamper a straightforward evaluation of this construct thus yielding inconsistent results and jeopardizing the overall generalizability of the study results from a methodological point of view [15, 16].

8.2 Sensory Modalities Involved in Body Image Disturbances in Anorexia Nervosa

As stated earlier, a number of different methods have been performed to measure perceptual dimension of body image disturbances in AN, including silhouette methods [17], distorting mirrors [18], and photograph and video techniques altering pictures of one's own body [19–22]. However, research tried to expand the assessment of body image in AN across different sensory modalities.

In fact, different classifications and hierarchical assessments of the different sub-representations needed when experiencing our body exist [23–26]; for example, body schema refers to motor actions while body image to body representations [27–29]. All in all, these models highlight the variety of sensory modalities that come into play when our body is experienced. For example, it remains unclear as to whether individuals with AN have a perceptual disturbance biasing their own body experience. In addition to body size estimation tasks, several other methods of assessment have been performed. Therefore, literature on AN tried to expand the available knowledge on the analysis of the different senses that are involved in body representations, including haptic perception [30, 31], altered interoceptive awareness [32, 33], integration of visual and proprioceptive information [34–36], and tactile stimuli [37, 38]. For a review on this topic, see Gaudio and Quattrocchi [39].

For example, the rubber hand illusion paradigm has been used in order to study visuo-tactile abilities in AN. Such an experimental setting induces participants to experience a fake body part generating a visuo-tactile conflict, that is touching at the same time both actual and fake body parts. As a result, the brain is required to put together two different inputs [40, 41]. In AN, currently ill and recovered individuals showed greater likelihood of experiencing the rubber hand illusion than healthy controls did [34, 35, 42] and also that the overestimation of their hand width lowered over time [35], entailing potentially therapeutic effects.

Relatedly, in order to address the multisensory components of body image distortions in AN, virtual reality and full body illusions have also been performed [43, 44–47]. In these experimental conditions, participants can experience a modification of their body size, depending on the avatar. In AN, Keizer and collaborators [48] showed that patients with AN reported more marked alterations of the estimation of their body size and body circumference than healthy controls did. However, since patients could reliably describe and measure other parameters (including their height) a general bias in the assessment of body dimensions has been excluded. All in all, in line with everyday clinical practice, patients with AN tend to experience as "fat" those body parts which trigger more their body obsessions (e.g., abdomen, thighs).

8.3 State-of-the-Art of Body Image Distortions in Anorexia Nervosa

An earlier review was conducted on the published papers on body image distortions in AN by Farrell and collaborators [16]. The authors included in their review only those works recruiting more than 10 participants, and included a total number of 52 papers. Considering the different assessments performed, mixed results were collected and contrasting data were finally available. A half of the included studies showed AN sufferers as overestimating their body when compared to healthy controls thus providing support to the difficulty of patients with AN in accurately evaluate their own body. However, in two studies [49, 50] only specific body parts were evaluated as overestimated. Relatedly, one study [51] highlighted that only those patients with AN and a history of bulimia nervosa reported an overestimation of their body size. In contrast, two studies showed both patients with AN and healthy controls as underestimating their body size [16, 52]. With respect to selected body sizes, patients with AN overestimated certain body parts thus providing a more accurate description of their body than healthy controls did; however, in other studies no differences emerged between patients with AN and healthy controls in the accuracy of one's own body estimation [16]. All in all, although the majority of papers confirmed that AN patients tend to overestimate their body, data are far from being conclusive on this topic.

Subsequently, Gardner and Brown [53] reviewed the available literature on body size estimation in individuals with AN analyzing papers published from 2002 to 2014 and, on the basis of the available data, the authors concluded that AN sufferers overestimated their body size more than healthy controls did with two studies [54, 55] failing to reach statistical significance for such a difference. However, when effect sizes were calculated in order to overcome the bias of small sample sizes of some studies, the mainly large effect sizes obtained provided support to the reliability of overestimation of body size in AN. With more detail, shoulders, hips, waist, and thighs resulted as particularly oversized according to two studies [56, 57].

More recently, Caspi and collaborators [58] used a computerized assessment of body image to ascertain as to whether different diagnosis of eating disorders differ in body image. The authors confirmed that those with an eating disorder show greater body disturbances than healthy controls; moreover, they found that patients with AN overestimated more than those with bulimia nervosa their own body size. Such a difference remained significant when other confounders were controlled for (e.g., age and body mass index) with respect to both perceptual and affective dimensions of body image, thus providing support to the role of body image distortion as maintaining factor for eating disorders. Additionally, the difference in body size overevaluation between patients with eating disorder and healthy controls remained significant also after controlling for anxiety and depression [58].

Finally, studies on recovered individuals show that body image disturbances persist also after recovery from both AN [59] and bulimia nervosa [60].

8.4 Body Size Estimation of Others in Anorexia Nervosa

It remains unclear as to whether the disturbance in body perception refers only to patients' own body or not. The available body of evidence showed that patients with AN can detect earlier than healthy controls the transition from thin to obese of a woman during a morphing video [61]. Also, patients with AN are known to consider thin bodies as more attractive when compared to normal weight bodies; still, the more the observer is underweight the more the body size is perceived as larger [62]. When observing a whole body, patients with AN paid more attention to the different body areas than face regions [63].

Biological motion, the ability of the visual system to perceive a biological entity while performing a recognizable activity, has also been used as a technique to assess body size estimation of others in AN. Poor emotion perception has been found in autism spectrum disorder [64] and schizophrenia [65] using this technique. Individuals with AN showed poorer identification of sad stimuli while recovered individuals reported results comparable to those of healthy controls [66]. More recently, Phillipou and collaborators [67] performed human biological motion in order to assess body size estimation of others in AN. The authors concluded that patients with AN can judge the body size of others as accurately as healthy controls do; nevertheless, patients with AN showed different ocular behavior with "hyperscanning," namely heightened fixations, of the presented stimuli.

8.5 Body Image Disturbances in Anorexia Nervosa and Body Dysmorphic Disorder

Body image disturbances are a common feature of body dysmorphic disorder (BDD) as well. In BDD, the main diagnostic psychopathology feature is preoccupation with perceived defects in appearance, which are unnoticeable, or slight, to others [1]. Both disorders share body image disturbance [68–70] with dysfunctional compensatory strategies and maladaptive cognitive processes as reinforcing and maintaining behavioral symptoms. Relatedly, patients with AN and BDD place much emphasis on physical attractiveness in turn over-evaluating eventual bodily imperfections. A vicious cycle is generated since rituals and avoidance of stressful situations provide patients with temporary relief from anxiety and other negative emotions but in turn reinforce symptom-related dysfunctional cognitions and behaviors, namely fasting and binge-purging behaviors in AN and mirror checking in BDD. Nevertheless, the models of AN include also other components rather than focusing on avoidance and checking behaviors, more typical of BDD. The available body of evidence on the comparison of individuals with AN and BDD found comparable body image dissatisfaction across diagnoses but more marked avoidance and negative self-evaluation in BDD compared with AN [71]. Also, patients with BDD were found to report a greater variety of bodily concerns (e.g., hair, nose) while patients with AN and bulimia nervosa reported typical preoccupations with shape and weight [71]. More recent research using multidimensional assessments [72] showed patients with AN, bulimia nervosa, and BDD as more body dissatisfied than healthy controls. Consistently with previous findings, patients with BDD were found to show more severe body image disturbances and poorer quality of life than the other groups with an eating disorder [71]. Finally, a recent study by Kollei and collaborators [73] provided further support to marked body image dissatisfaction in BDD and AN, with the BDD group showing more compulsive checking and manipulation of physical appearance than those with AN. In line with the aforementioned researches, also Hartmann and colleagues [74] confirmed that individuals with AN and BDD report significantly higher body dissatisfaction and more dysfunctional coping strategies than healthy controls. However, differently from previous research [72] individuals with AN showed more marked body image dissatisfaction than BDD individuals. Methodological differences can be responsible for such differences but future studies are needed to shed light on these aspects in order to draw more firm conclusions on this topic.

8.6 Neural Bases of Body Image in AN

A growing body of evidence is accumulating on the neurobiology of AN [75] but literature is overall sparse on the neural basis of body image disturbances in AN. The neurobiology of body image distortion in AN is far from being clarified. However, posterior parietal regions have been linked to perceptive body attitudes while prefrontal and insula regions are mainly involved in affective body attitudes [39]. Favaro and collaborators [76] conducted a resting state functional magnetic resonance imaging study to investigate the functional connectivity of networks involved in visuospatial and somatosensory processing. The authors showed that both groups reported hypoconnectivity in the ventral visual network while currently ill patients displayed also hyperconnectivity in the somatosensory network.

Consistently with clinical research, also neuroimaging studies began using tasks based on photograph and video techniques altering pictures of one's own body instead of silhouettes and drawings in order to stimulate more the neurological underpinning of interoceptive, emotive, and motivational networks [77]. Pietrini and collaborators [78] showed how dorsolateral prefrontal cortex (DLPFC), supplementary motor, insular, inferior parietal, fusiform, occipito-temporal, and cingulate regions are involved in body image processing in AN. Also, patients with AN when presented with body image stimuli, reported heightened activation of the amygdala and frontal, striatal, and insular cortices, namely those areas involved in the processing of emotions. In contrast, parietal cortices, involved in the visuospatial processing of the body were poorly active.

When presented with pictures of underweight individuals, patients with AN showed increased activation of the ventral striatum providing support to the reinforcing and rewarding value of emaciation for affected individuals [79]. The DLPFC as well as insula and putamen were more active in patients with AN than in healthy controls during a task comparing participants' body with idealized female bodies, highlighting the involvement of emotive and reward and decision making response in this regard [77, 80].

Via and collaborators [81] showed that the posterior cingulate cortex/precuneus play a role in body evaluation of both self and others in AN. It has been shown a hyperactivation of the dorsal posterior cingulate cortex while patients with AN process their own body image; in contrast, affected individuals failed to activate both precuneus and ventral posterior cingulate cortex while processing others' body. Patients with AN also reported increased connectivity in the dorsal posterior cingulate cortex when processing their own images and in mid-temporal areas then processing others' body image. During resting state, connectivity between posterior cingulate cortex and the angular gyrus was reported as well.

Amygdala [82] and DLPFC [83] have been found to be active when patients with AN saw oversized images of their own body. Still, patients with AN showed hyperactivation in the mesolimbic reward network when presented with underweight female stimuli; in contrast, healthy controls were mainly stimulated by normal weight female stimuli.

8.7 Body Image Distortions and Treatment Approaches and Outcome in Anorexia Nervosa

AN is currently characterized by poor outcomes with a standardized mortality ratio of about 6 [84] and a long-term mortality rate of 10% [85]. A better understanding of the core features of this disorder is needed in order to develop more effective treatments. Body image disturbances represent both a key clinical aspect of AN and a core element of psychological models of AN [15, 86]. With more detail, body image disturbance is a persistent symptom predicting relapse [87, 88] with recovered individuals still reporting overestimation of their own body [59, 60].

Body image disturbances tend to persist also after treatment even when other symptoms have improved [59, 89]. Nevertheless, scant attention has been paid to body image disturbances in treatment so far. Such an intervention is likely to increase anxiety in both patients and therapists [90]. Nevertheless, novel approaches have been pioneered. Mirror exposure with inpatients after weight restoration significantly reduced body dissatisfaction [91]; such intervention was then revised yielding to a significantly improved body image in weight-restored patients [92]. Relatedly, Grant and Cash [93] had previously developed a cognitive behavioral body image treatment for patients with BDD, using mirror exposure and desensitization leading to improved body satisfaction in women not affected by eating disorders [93, 94]. Since then, mirror exposure has been included in therapeutic interventions for eating disorders, mostly focused on cognitive behavioral techniques [95, 96].

In fact, cognitive behavioral therapy (CBT) also provided evidence of effectiveness in patients with eating disorders including AN from a body image standpoint. CBT with mirror exposure delivered in a group format was helpful in reducing negative emotionality elicited by looking in a mirror [96]. Outpatient CBT reduced body dissatisfaction and body image dysphoria [97] and, more recently, an eight-session CBT group with in vivo exposure has been described as effective for patients with AN [98]. Also cognitive behavior therapy-enhanced (CBT-E) [99] reported a specific focus on body image.

More recently, BodyWise, a low-intensity group treatment, has been developed for patients with AN at low weights in order to avoid the challenging activities of therapeutic interventions designed for weight-restored patients [100]. Such an intervention showed preliminary effectiveness in improving weight and shape concerns and body checking.

A pilot study on the ten session body image therapy (BAT-10) has also been conducted [101]. The BAT-10 is a group therapy with a behavioral framework; sessions are delivered in a group format over a 10-week timeframe. Elements of psycho-education, motivational enhancement therapy, self-help, cognitive therapy, and mindfulness are included in the intervention that showed encouraging preliminary results in promoting affective and cognitive changes in body dissatisfaction and core beliefs of eating disorders [101].

Interestingly, body size estimation has been taken into account also from an outcome perspective. In fact, body image disturbances are hallmarks of eating disorders and represent diagnostic criteria for both AN and bulimia nervosa [1]. Also, body image concerns are of relevance from a treatment standpoint. In fact, the detrimental effects of body image disturbance for the long-term outcome of patients with AN were highlighted since the 1970s when Slade and Russell [88] showed that relapse was more likely for those patients whose body concerns persisted after weight restoration and that overestimation of body size tended to decrease with weight gain. Also, patients with more severe overestimation of their own body report heightened denial of illness, improve weight to a lesser extent during hospitalizations [102, 103], and tend to be re-hospitalized more over time [104]. A significant correlation between body size concern after mirror exposure and clinical improvement has been demonstrated in AN [105]; relatedly, body size overestimation has been linked to relapse as well [106, 107]. Other lines of research showed that persistent body dissatisfaction predicts relapse at follow-up [4, 86, 108]. More recently, Boehm and collaborators [109] showed that low body image dissatisfaction is predictive of a more positive long-term outcome in AN. Nevertheless, contrasting findings are also available; for example, body size concern has been found to be unrelated to treatment outcome in a sample of patients with eating disorders using the video distortion techniques [110].

Conclusions

In closing, body image disturbances are a key element in AN with respect to development, maintenance, and relapse of this severe mental disorder that benefits from a limited therapeutic armamentarium [111, 112] and entails a heavy burden on sufferers [113]. Patients with AN tend to overestimate the perception of their own body also in the light of the multiple components (e.g., affective, cognitive, behavioral, and perceptual) of body image. In contrast, affected individuals can reliably assess other's body size. Research on the neurobiology of body image disturbances in AN is in its infancy; however, several brain regions have been found to be involved during tasks eliciting patients' body image perception including dorsolateral prefrontal cortex, supplementary motor, insular, inferior parietal, fusiform, occipito-temporal, and cingulate regions. The available therapeutic approaches showed encouraging results although larger controlled studies are needed to replicate the available findings. At now, mainly cognitive behavioral interventions exist, delivered in both individual and group setting also including mirror exposure. The detrimental effects of body image disturbance for the long-term outcome of patients with AN had been highlighted since the 1970s and subsequently confirmed by recent research. Therefore, further clinical and research efforts are needed to expand the knowledge on body image in AN and its therapeutic implications.

References

1. American Psychiatric Association, editor. Diagnostic and statistical manual for mental disorders, (DSM-5). 5th ed. Washington, DC: American Psychiatric Association; 2013.
2. Banfield SS, McCabe M. An evaluation of the construct of body image. Adolescence. 2002;37(146):373–93.
3. Jacobi C, Hayward C, de Zwaan M, Kraemer HC, Agras WS. Coming to terms with risk factors for eating disorders: application of risk terminology and suggestions for a general taxonomy. Psychol Bull. 2004;130(1):19–65.
4. Keel PK, Dorer DJ, Franko DL, Jackson SC, Herzog DB. Postremission predictors of relapse in women with eating disorders. Am J Psychiatry. 2005;162(12):2263–8.
5. Bruch H. Perceptual and conceptual disturbances in anorexia nervosa. Psychosom Med. 1962;24:187–94.
6. Steinhausen HC. The outcome of anorexia nervosa in the 20th century. Am J Psychiatry. 2002;159(8):1284–93. Review. PubMed PMID: 12153817.
7. Killen JD, Taylor CB, Hayward C, Haydel KF, Wilson DM, Hammer L, et al. Weight concerns influence the development of eating disorders: a 4-year prospective study. J Consult Clin Psychol. 1996;64(5):936–40. https://doi.org/10.1037//0022-006x.64.5.936. Epub 1996/10/01. PMID: 8916622.
8. Stice E. Risk and maintenance factors for eating pathology: a meta-analytic review. Psychol Bull. 2002;128(5):825–48. https://doi.org/10.1037//0033-2909.128.5.825. Epub 2002/09/11. PMID: 12206196.

9. Farrell C, Shafran R. Empirically evaluated treatments for body image disturbance: a review. Eur Eat Disord Rev. 2006;14:289–300. https://doi.org/10.1002/erv.693.
10. Carter JC, Blackmore E, Sutandar-Pinnock K, Woodside DB. Relapse in anorexia nervosa: a survival analysis. Psychol Med. 2004;34(4):671–9. https://doi.org/10.1017/S0033291703001168. Epub 2004/04/22. S0033291703001168 [pii]. PMID: 15099421.
11. Espeset EM, Nordbo RH, Gulliksen KS, Skarderud F, Geller J, Holte A. The concept of body image disturbance in anorexia nervosa: an empirical inquiry utilizing patients' subjective experiences. Eat Disord. 2011;19(2):175–93. https://doi.org/10.1080/10640266.2011.551635. Epub 2011/03/02. 933979760 [pii]. PMID: 21360367.
12. Cash TF, Green GK. Body weight and body image among college women: perception, cognition, and affect. J Pers Assess. 1986;50:290–301.
13. Cash TF, Wood KC, Phelps KD, Boyd K. New assessments of weight related body image derived from extant instruments. Percept Mot Skills. 1991;73:235–41.
14. Slade PD. What is body image? Behav Res Ther. 1994;32:497–502.
15. Cash TF, Deagle EA. The nature and extent of body-image disturbances in anorexia nervosa and bulimia nervosa: a meta-analysis. Int J Eat Disord. 1997;22:107–25.
16. Farrell C, Lee M, Shafran R. Assessment of body size estimation: a review. Eur Eat Disord Rev. 2005;13:75–88.
17. Bell C, Kirkpatrick SW, Rinn RC. Body image of anorexic, obese, and normal females. J Clin Psychol. 1986;42:431–9.
18. Traub AC, Orbach J. Psychophysical studies of body-image: 1. The adjustable body-distorting mirror. Arch Gen Psychiatry. 1964;11(1):53.
19. Gardner RM, Moncrieff C. Body image distortion in anorexics as a non-sensory phenomenon: a signal detection approach. J Clin Psychol. 1998;44:101–7.
20. Garner DM, Garfinkel PE, Stancer HC, Moldofsky H. Body image disturbances in anorexia nervosa and obesity. Psychosom Med. 1976;38:327–36.
21. Probst M, Vandereycken W, Van Coppenolle H, Pieters G. Body size estimation in eating disorder patients: testing the video distortion method on a life-size screen. Behav Res Ther. 1995;33:985–90.
22. Shafran R, Fairburn CG. A new ecologically valid method to assess body size estimation and body size dissatisfaction. Int J Eat Disord. 2002;32:458–65.
23. de Vignemont F. Body schema and body image—pros and cons. Neuropsychologia. 2010;48(3):669–80. https://doi.org/10.1016/j.neuropsychologia.2009.09.022. Epub 2009/09/30. S0028-3932(09)00373-9 [pii]. PMID: 19786038.
24. Longo MR. Implicit and explicit body represenations. Eur Psychol. 2015;20(1):6–15. https://doi.org/10.1027/1016-9040/a000198.
25. Longo MR, Azanon E, Haggard P. More than skin deep: body representation beyond primary somatosensory cortex. Neuropsychologia. 2010;48(3):655–68. https://doi.org/10.1016/j.neuropsychologia.2009.08.022. Epub 2009/09/02. S0028-3932(09)00339-X [pii]. PMID: 19720070.
26. Longo MR, Haggard P. Implicit body representations and the conscious body image. Acta Psychol. 2012;141(2):164–8. https://doi.org/10.1016/j.actpsy.2012.07.015. Epub 2012/09/12. S0001-6918(12) 00129-1 [pii]. PMID: 22964057.
27. Dijkerman HC, de Haan EH. Somatosensory processes subserving perception and action. Behav Brain Sci. 2007;30(2):189–201. https://doi.org/10.1017/S0140525X07001392; discussion 201–39. Epub 2007/08/21. S0140525X07001392 [pii]. PMID: 17705910.
28. Haggard P, Wolpert DM. Disorders of body scheme. In: Freund HJ, Jeannerod M, Hallett M, Leguarda R, editors. Higher-order motor disorders. Oxford: Oxford University Press; 2005.
29. Gallagher S. How the body shapes the mind. Oxford: Oxford University Press; 2005.
30. Grunwald M, Ettrich C, Assmann B, Dahne A, Krause W, Busse F, et al. Deficits in haptic perception and right parietal theta power changes in patients with anorexia nervosa before and after weight gain. Int J Eat Disord. 2001;29(4):417–28. https://doi.org/10.1002/eat.1038. Epub 2001/04/04. PMID: 11285579.

31. Guardia D, Cottencin O, Thomas P, Dodin V, Luyat M. Spatial orientation constancy is impaired in anorexia nervosa. Psychiatry Res. 2012;195(1–2):56–9. https://doi.org/10.1016/j.psychres.2011.08.003. Epub 2011/08/30. S0165-1781(11)00575-0 [pii]. PMID: 21872340.
32. Miller SP, Redlich AD, Steiner H. The stress response in anorexia nervosa. Child Psychiatry Hum Dev. 2003;33(4):295–306. Epub 2003/05/02. PMID: 12723902.
33. Strigo IA, Matthews SC, Simmons AN, Oberndorfer T, Klabunde M, Reinhardt LE, et al. Altered insula activation during pain anticipation in individuals recovered from anorexia nervosa: evidence of interoceptive dysregulation. Int J Eat Disord. 2013;46(1):23–33. https://doi.org/10.1002/eat.22045. Epub 2012/07/28. PMID: 22836447; PubMed Central PMCID: PMC3507323.
34. Eshkevari E, Rieger E, Longo MR, Haggard P, Treasure J. Increased plasticity of the bodily self in eating disorders. Psychol Med. 2012;42(4):819–28. https://doi.org/10.1017/S0033291711002091. Epub 2011/10/25. S0033291711002091 [pii]. PMID: 22017964.
35. Keizer A, Smeets MA, Postma A, van Elburg A, Dijkerman HC. Does the experience of ownership over a rubber hand change body size perception in anorexia nervosa patients? Neuropsychologia. 2014;62:26–37. https://doi.org/10.1016/j.neuropsychologia.2014.07.003. Epub 2014/07/23. S0028-3932(14)00223-1 [pii]. PMID: 25050852.
36. Case LK, Wilson RC, Ramachandran VS. Diminished size-weight illusion in anorexia nervosa: evidence for visuo-proprioceptive integration deficit. Exp Brain Res. 2012;217(1):79–87. https://doi.org/10.1007/s00221-011-2974-7. Epub 2011/12/21. PMID: 22183754.
37. Keizer A, Smeets MA, Dijkerman HC, van den Hout M, Klugkist I, van Elburg A, et al. Tactile body image disturbance in anorexia nervosa. Psychiatry Res. 2011;190(1):115–20. https://doi.org/10.1016/j.psychres.2011.04.031. Epub 2011/05/31. S0165-1781(11)00362-3 [pii]. PMID: 21621275.
38. Keizer A, Smeets MA, Dijkerman HC, van Elburg A, Postma A. Aberrant somatosensory perception in anorexia nervosa. Psychiatry Res. 2012;200(2–3):530–7. https://doi.org/10.1016/j.psychres.2012.05.001. Epub 2012/06/01. S0165-1781(12)00248-X [pii]. PMID: 22648006.
39. Gaudio S, Quattrocchi CC. Neural basis of a multidimensional model of body image distortion in anorexia nervosa. Neurosci Biobehav Rev. 2012;36:1839–47.
40. Botvinick M, Cohen J. Rubber hands 'feel' touch that eyes see. Nature. 1998;391(6669):756. https://doi.org/10.1038/35784. Epub 1998/03/05. PMID: 9486643.
41. Ehrsson HH, Spence C, Passingham RE. That's my hand! Activity in premotor cortex reflects feeling of ownership of a limb. Science. 2004;305(5685):875–7. https://doi.org/10.1126/science.1097011. Epub 2004/07/03. PMID: 15232072.
42. Guardia D, Lafargue G, Thomas P, Dodin V, Cottencin O, Luyat M. Anticipation of body-scaled action is modified in anorexia nervosa. Neuropsychologia. 2010;48(13):3961–6. https://doi.org/10.1016/j.neuropsychologia.2010.09.004. Epub 2010/09/14. S0028-3932(10)00384-2 [pii]. PMID: 20833193.
43. Slater M, Spanlang B, Sanchez-Vives MV, Blanke O. First person experience of body transfer in virtual reality. PLoS One. 2010;5(5):e10564. https://doi.org/10.1371/journal.pone.0010564. Epub 2010/05/21. PMID: 20485681; PubMed Central PMCID: PMC2868878.
44. Banakou D, Groten R, Slater M. Illusory ownership of a virtual child body causes overestimation of object sizes and implicit attitude changes. Proc Natl Acad Sci U S A. 2013;110(31):12846–51. https://doi.org/10.1073/pnas.1306779110. Epub 2013/07/17. 1306779110 [pii]. PMID: 23858436; PubMed Central PMCID: PMC3732927.
45. Normand JM, Giannopoulos E, Spanlang B, Slater M. Multisensory stimulation can induce an illusion of larger belly size in immersive virtual reality. PLoS One. 2011;6(1):e16128. https://doi.org/10.1371/journal.pone.0016128. Epub 2011/02/02. PMID: 21283823; PubMed Central PMCID: PMC3023777.
46. Maister L, Slater M, Sanchez-Vives MV, Tsakiris M. Changing bodies changes minds: owning another body affects social cognition. Trends Cogn Sci. 2015;19(1):6–12. https://doi.org/10.1016/j.tics.2014.11.001. Epub 2014/12/20. S1364-6613(14)00234-4 [pii]. PMID: 25524273.

47. Osimo SA, Pizarro R, Spanlang B, Slater M. Conversations between self and self as Sigmund Freud—a virtual body ownership paradigm for self counselling. Sci Rep. 2015;5:13899. https://doi.org/10.1038/srep13899. Epub 2015/09/12. srep13899 [pii]. PMID: 26354311; PubMed Central PMCID: PMC4564809.
48. Keizer A, van Elburg A, Helms R, Dijkerman HC. A virtual reality full body illusion improves body image disturbance in anorexia nervosa. PLoS One. 2016;11(10):e0163921. https://doi.org/10.1371/journal.pone.0163921. eCollection 2016. PubMed PMID: 27711234; PubMed Central PMCID: PMC5053411.
49. Fichter MM, Meister I, Koch HJ. The measurement of body image disturbances in anorexia nervosa: experimental comparison of different methods. Br J Psychiatry. 1986;148:453–61.
50. Sunday SR, Halmi KA, Werdann L, Levey C. Comparison of body size estimation and eating disorder inventory scores in anorexia and bulimia patients with obese, and restrained and unrestrained controls. Int J Eat Disord. 1992;11:133–49.
51. Freeman RJ, Thomas CD, Solyom L, Koopman RF. Clinical and personality correlates of body size overestimation in anorexia nervosa and bulimia nervosa. Int J Eat Disord. 1985;4:439–56.
52. Bowden PK, Touyz SW, Rodriguez PJ, Hensley R, Beumont PJ. Distorting patient or distorting instrument? Body shape disturbance in patients with anorexia nervosa and bulimia. Br J Psychiatry. 1989;155:196–201.
53. Gardner RM, Brown DL. Body size estimation in anorexia nervosa: a brief review of findings from 2003 through 2013. Psychiatry Res. 2014;219(3):407–10. https://doi.org/10.1016/j.psychres.2014.06.029. Epub 2014 Jun 26. Review. PubMed PMID:25023364.
54. Urdapilleta I, Cheneau C, Masse L, Blanchet A. Comparative study of body image among dancers and anorexic girls. Eat Weight Disord. 2007;12:140–6.
55. Benninghoven D, Tetsch N, Jantschek G. Patients with eating disorders and their siblings: an investigation of body image perception. Eur Child Adolesc Psychiatry. 2008;17(2):118–26.
56. Gila A, Castro J, Cesena J, Toro J. Anorexianervosainmaleadolescents: body image, eating attitudes and psychological traits. J Adolesc Health. 2005;36:221–6.
57. Schneider N, Frieler K, Pfeiffer E, Lehmkuhi U, Salbach-Andrae H. Comparison of body size estimation in adolescents with different types of eating disorders. Eur Eat Disord Rev. 2009;17:468–75.
58. Caspi A, Amiaz R, Davidson N, Czerniak E, Gur E, Kiryati N, Harari D, Furst M, Stein D. Computerized assessment of body image in anorexia nervosa and bulimia nervosa: comparison with standardized body image assessment tool. Arch Womens Ment Health. 2017;20(1):139–47. https://doi.org/10.1007/s00737-016-0687-4. Epub 2016 Oct 29. PubMed PMID: 27796596.
59. Bachner-Melman R, Zohar AH, et al. An examination of cognitive versus behavioral components of recovery from anorexia nervosa. J Nerv Ment Dis. 2006;194(9):697–703.
60. Stein D, Kaye WH, et al. Pain perception in recovered bulimia nervosa patients. Int J Eat Disord. 2003;34(3):331–6.
61. Smeets MAM. Body size categorization in anorexia nervosa using a morphing instrument. Int J Eat Disord. 1999;25(4):451–5.
62. Tovée MJ, Emery JL, Cohen–Tovée EM. The estimation of body mass index and physical attractiveness is dependent on the observer's own body mass index. Proc Biol Sci. 2000;267(1456):1987–97.
63. Watson KK, Werling DM, Zucker NL, Platt ML. Altered social reward and attention in anorexia nervosa. Front Psych. 2010;1(36):1–8.
64. Parron C, Da Fonseca D, Santos A, Moore D, Monfardini E, Deruelle C. Recognition of biological motion in children with autistic spectrum disorders. Autism. 2008;12(3):261–74.
65. Couture SM, Penn DL, Losh M, Adolphs R, Hurley R, Piven J. Comparison of social cognitive functioning in schizophrenia and high functioning autism: more convergence than divergence. Psychol Med. 2010;40(4):569–79.
66. Zucker NL, Moskovich A, Bulik CM. Merwin R, Gaddis K, Losh M, et al. Perception of affect in biological motion cues in anorexia nervosa. Int J Eat Disord. 2013;46(1):12–22.

67. Phillipou A, Rossell SL, Gurvich C, Castle DJ, Troje NF, Abel LA. Body image in anorexia nervosa: body size estimation utilising a biological motion task and eyetracking. Eur Eat Disord Rev. 2016;24(2):131–8. https://doi.org/10.1002/erv.2423. Epub 2015 Dec 1. PubMed PMID: 26621427.
68. Fairburn CG. Cognitive behavior therapy and eating disorders. New York: The Guilford Press; 2008.
69. Veale D, Neziroglu F. Body dysmorphic disorder: a treatment manual. West Sussex: John Wiley & Sons Ltd; 2010.
70. Wilhelm S, Phillips KA, Steketee G. Cognitive-behavioral therapy for body dysmorphic disorder. New York: The Guilford Press; 2013.
71. Rosen JC, Ramirez E. A comparison of eating disorders and body dysmorphic disorder on body image and psychological adjustment. J Psychosom Res. 1998;44:441–9.
72. Hrabosky JI, Cash TF, Veale D, Neziroglu F, Soll EA, Garner DM, Phillips KA. Multidimensional body image comparisons among patients with eating disorders, body dysmorphic disorder, and clinical controls: a multisite study. Body Image. 2009;6:155–63.
73. Kollei I, Brunhoeber S, Rauh E, de Zwaan M, Martin A. Body image, emotions and thought control strategies in body dysmorphic disorder compared to eating disorders and healthy controls. J Psychosom Res. 2012;72:321–7.
74. Hartmann AS, Thomas JJ, Greenberg JL, Elliott CM, Matheny NL, Wilhelm S. Anorexia nervosa and body dysmorphic disorder: a comparison of body image concerns and explicit and implicit attractiveness beliefs. Body Image. 2015;14:77–84. https://doi.org/10.1016/j.bodyim.2015.03.013. Epub 2015 Apr 28. PubMed PMID:25920044.
75. Kaye WH, Wierenga CE, Bailer UF, Simmons AN, Bischoff-Grethe A. Nothing tastesas good as skinny feels: the neurobiology of anorexia nervosa. Trends Neurosci. 2013;36(2):110–20. https://doi.org/10.1016/j.tins.2013.01.003. Epub 2013 Jan 18. Review. PubMed PMID: 23333342; PubMed Central PMCID: PMC3880159.
76. Favaro A, Santonastaso P, Manara R, Bosello R, Bommarito G, Tenconi E, et al. Disruption of visuospatial and somatosensory functional connectivity in anorexia nervosa. Biol Psychiatry. 2012;72:864–70.
77. Friederich HC, Brooks S, Uher R, Campbell IC, Giampietro V, Brammer M, Williams SC, Herzog W, Treasure J. Neural correlates of body dissatisfaction in anorexia nervosa. Neuropsychologia. 2010;48:2878–85.
78. Pietrini F, Castellini G, Ricca V, Polito C, Pupi A, Faravelli C. Functional neuroimaging in anorexia nervosa: a clinical approach. Eur Psychiatry. 2011;26:176–82.
79. Fladung AK, Gron G, Grammer K, Herrnberger B, Schilly E, Grasteit S, Wolf RC, Walter H, von Wietersheim J. A neural signature of anorexia nervosa in the ventral striatal reward system. Am J Psychiatry. 2010;167:206–12.
80. Mohr HM, Zimmermann J, Roder C, Lenz C, Overbeck G, Grabhorn R. Separating two components of body image in anorexia nervosa using fMRI. Psychol Med. 2010;40:1519–29.
81. Via E, Goldberg X, Sánchez I, Forcano L, Harrison BJ, Davey CG, Pujol J, Martínez-Zalacaín I, Fernández-Aranda F, Soriano-Mas C, Cardoner N, Menchón JM. Self and other body perception in anorexia nervosa: the role of posterior DMN nodes. World J Biol Psychiatry. 2016;22:1–15. https://doi.org/10.1080/15622975.2016.1249951.
82. Miyake Y, Okamoto Y, Onoda K, Kurosaki M, Shirao N, Okamoto Y, Yamawaki S. Brain activation during the perception of distorted body images in eating disorders. Psychiatry Res. 2010;181:183–92.
83. Castellini G, Polito C, Bolognesi E, D'Argenio A, Ginestroni A, Mascalchi M, Pellicanò G, Mazzoni LN, Rotella F, Faravelli C, Pupi A, Ricca V. Looking at my body. Similarities and differences between anorexia nervosa patients and controls in body image visual processing. Eur Psychiatry. 2013;28:427–35.
84. Arcelus J, Mitchell AJ, Wales J, Nielsen S. Mortality rates in patients with anorexia nervosa and other eating disorders. A meta-analysis of 36 studies. Arch Gen Psychiatry. 2011;68(7):724–31. https://doi.org/10.1001/archgenpsychiatry.2011.74. PubMed PMID: 21727255.

85. Berkman ND, Lohr KN, Bulik CM. Outcomes of eating disorders: a systematic review of the literature. Int J Eat Disord. 2007;40:293–309.
86. Fairburn CG, Cooper Z, Shafran R. Cognitive behaviour therapy for eating disorders: a "transdiagnostic" theory and treatment. Behav Res Ther. 2003;41:509–28.
87. Channon S, DeSilva W. Psychological correlates of weight gain in patients with anorexia nervosa. J Psychiatr Res. 1985;19 267–71.
88. Slade P, Russell G. Awareness of body dimensions in anorexia nervosa: cross-sectional and longitudinal studies. Psychol Med. 1973;3:188–99.
89. Federici A, Kaplan AS. The patient's account of relapse and recovery in anorexia nervosa: a qualitative study. Eur Eat Disord Rev. 2008;16:1–10.
90. Turner H, Tatham M, Lant M, Mountford VA, Waller G. Clinicians' concerns about delivering cognitive-behavioural therapy for eating disorders. Behav Res Ther. 2014;57:38–42.
91. Key A, George CL, Beattie D, Stammers K, Lacey H, Waller G. Body image treatment within an inpatient program for anorexia nervosa: the role of mirror exposure in the desensitization process. Int J Eat Disord. 2002;31:185–90.
92. Morgan JF, Lazarova S, Schelhase M, Saedi S. 10 session body image therapy: efficacy of a manualised body image therapy. Eur Eat Disord Rev. 2013;22:66–71.
93. Grant JR, Cash TF. Cognitive-behavioral bodyimage therapy, comparative efficacy of group and modestcontact treatments. Behav Res Ther. 1995;26:69–84.
94. Rosen JC, Reiter J, Orosan P. Cognitive behavioural body image therapy for body dysmorphic disorder. J Consult Clin Psychol. 1995;63:263–9.
95. Jansen A, Nederkoorn C, Mulkens S. Selective visual attention for ugly and beautiful body parts in eating disorders. Behav Res Ther. 2005;43:183–96.
96. Vocks S, Wächter A, Chter A, Wutherer M, Kosfelder J. Look at yourself, can body image therapy affect the cognitive and emotional response to seeing oneself in the mirror in eating disorders? Eur Eat Disord Rev. 2008;16:147–54.
97. Nye S, Cash TF. Outcomes of manualised cognitivebehavioural body image therapy with eating disorders women treated in private clinical practice. Eat Disord. 2006;14:31–40.
98. Bhatnagar KAC, Wisniewski L, Solomon M, Heinberg L. Effectiveness and feasibility of a cognitive-behavioral group intervention for body image disturbance in women with eating disorders. J Clin Psychol. 2013;69:1–13.
99. Fairburn CG, Cooper Z, Doll HA. O'Connor ME, Palmer RL, Dalle Grave R. Enhanced cognitive behaviour therapy for adults with anorexia nervosa: a UK-Italy study. Behav Res Ther. 2013;51(1):R2–8. https://doi.org/10.1016/j.brat.2012.09.010. Epub 2012 Oct 22. PubMed PMID: 23084515; PubMed Central PMCID: PMC3662032.
100. Mountford VA, Brown A, Bamford B, Saeidi S, Morgan JF, Lacey H. BodyWise: evaluating a pilot body image group for patients with anorexia nervosa. Eur Eat Disord Rev. 2015;23(1):62–7. https://doi.org/10.1002/erv.2332. Epub 2014 Nov 9. PubMed PMID: 25382845.
101. Morgan JF, Lazarova S, Schelhase M, Saeidi S. Ten session body image therapy: efficacy of a manualised body image therapy. Eur Eat Disord Rev. 2014;22(1):66–71. https://doi.org/10.1002/erv.2249. Epub 2013 Sep 5. PubMed PMID: 24006359.
102. Skrzypek S, Wehmeier P, Remschmidt H. Body image assessment using body size estimation in recent studies on anorexia nervosa. A brief review. Eur Child Adolesc Psychiatry. 2001;10(4):215–21.
103. Casper RC, Halmi KA, Goldberg SC, Eckert E, Davis J. Disturbances in body image estimation as related to other characteristics and outcome in anorexia nervosa. Br J Psychiatry. 1979;134(1):60–6.
104. Castro J, Gila A, Puig J, Rodriguez S, Toro J. Predictors of re-hospitalization after total weight recovery in adolescents with anorexia nervosa. Int J Eat Disord. 2004;36(1):22–30.
105. Norris DL. The effects of mirror confrontation on self-estimation of body dimensions in anorexia nervosa, bulimia and two control groups. Psychol Med. 1984;14:835–42.
106. Button EJ, Fransella F, Slade PD. A reappraisal of body perception disturbance in anorexia nervosa. Psychol Med. 1977;7:235–43.

107. Crisp AH, Kalucy RS. Aspects of the perceptual disorder in anorexia nervosa. Br J Med Psychol. 1974;47:349–61.
108. Fairburn CG, Stice E, Cooper Z, Doll HA, Norman PA, O'Connor ME. Understanding persistence in bulimia nervosa, a five year naturalistic study. J Consult Clin Psychol. 2003;71:173–90.
109. Boehm I, Finke B, Tam FI, Fittig E, Scholz M, Gantchev K, Roessner V, Ehrlich S. Effects of perceptual body image distortion and early weight gain on long-term outcome of adolescent anorexia nervosa. Eur Child Adolesc Psychiatry. 2016;25(12):1319–26. Epub 2016 May 7. PubMed PMID: 27154049.
110. Fernandez-Aranda F, Dahme B, Meermann R. Body image in eating disorders and analysis of relevance: a preliminary study. J Psychosom Res. 1999;47:419–28.
111. Marzola E, Desedime N, Giovannone C, Amianto F, Fassino S, Abbate-Daga G. Atypical antipsychotics as augmentation therapy in anorexia nervosa. PLoS One. 2015;10(4):e0125569. https://doi.org/10.1371/journal.pone.0125569. eCollection 2015. PubMed PMID: 25922939; PubMed Central PMCID: PMC4414549.
112. Abbate-Daga G, Marzola E, Amianto F, Fassino S. A comprehensive review of psychodynamic treatments for eating disorders. Eat Weight Disord. 2016;21(4):553–80. Epub 2016 Mar 15. Review. PubMed PMID: 26980319.
113. Abbate-Daga G, Facchini F, Marzola E, Delsedime N, Giovannone C, Amianto F, Fassino S. Health-related quality of life in adult inpatients affected by anorexia nervosa. Eur Eat Disord Rev. 2014;22(4):285–91. https://doi.org/10.1002/erv.2302. Epub 2014 May 29. PubMed PMID: 24888791.

Body Image Disturbances in Bulimia Nervosa

9

Daniela Degortes, Paolo Santonastaso, and Angela Favaro

9.1 Introduction

Bulimia nervosa (BN) is characterized by recurrent and uncontrollable episodes of binge eating, inappropriate compensatory behaviors to prevent weight gain (e.g., self-induced vomiting, strict dieting, fasting or excessive exercise), and undue influence of body weight and shape on self-evaluation.

Although Professor Gerald Russell [1], in the first diagnostic definition of this disease, included "a morbid fear of becoming fat" among the diagnostic criteria of BN, for decades the body image of patients with BN has received little attention in the literature. In the mid-1980s, preoccupations with shape and body size were considered among the relevant factors for the risk of developing BN [2], and some early studies clearly demonstrated that body image distortion and strong drive for thinness are not only a characteristic of anorexia nervosa (AN), but also a "core feature" of BN [3, 4].

According to some assumptions proposed in those years, an increase in the prevalence of BN was observable, and it was at least partially attributable to changes in social pressures towards an ideal of thinness and a consequent stigmatization of obesity. Striegel-Moore [5] suggested that women at high risk of developing BN are those who have accepted and internalized the socio-cultural standards of thinness and physical appearance.

Since 1987, the American Psychiatric Association has included in subsequent editions of the Diagnostic and Statistical Manual for Mental Disorders (DSM) a "persistent overconcern with body shape and weight" as one criterion for bulimia nervosa; this psychological dimension was maintained in the DSM 5 diagnostic criteria as "self-evaluation is unduly influenced by body shape and weight" (Criterion D), while the ICD 10 reported that "the psychopathology consists of a

D. Degortes · P. Santonastaso · A. Favaro (✉)
Department of Neurosciences, University of Padova, Padua, Italy
e-mail: angela.favaro@unipd.it

M. Cuzzolaro, S. Fassino (eds.), *Body Image, Eating, and Weight*,
https://doi.org/10.1007/978-3-319-90817-5_9

morbid dread of fatness and the patient sets herself or himself a sharply defined weight threshold" [6].

Individuals with BN usually exhibit intense body dissatisfaction, fear of getting fat, and overevaluation of body weight and shape, and these psychological dimensions do not seem to be simple correlates of the eating psychopathology, but stable "core" traits with a role in the pathogenesis and maintenance of the disorder [7]. Besides the cognitive/emotional components of body image dysfunction (feelings and thoughts about one's own body), perceptual distortions (overestimation of one's own body dimensions), and behavioral components (avoidance of body-related situations and body checking rituals) have often been described in bulimia nervosa patients [8].

The dual-pathway model of bulimic pathology [9] incorporates body dissatisfaction in the etiology and maintenance of BN. According to this model, initial pressure to be thin and the internalization of thinness ideals contribute to body dissatisfaction. The latter is also strengthened by pressures towards thinness exerted by family, peers, and media.

According to the cognitive-behavioral theory [10], the overevaluation of body weight and shape is the "core psychopathology" of BN, and it is the main factor of maintenance of the disorder. Dysfunctional thoughts about body image lead to dysfunctional behaviors, such as strict dieting, excessive exercise, self-induced vomiting or misuse of laxatives, diuretics, or enemas. Self-worth is strictly influenced by body weight and shape cognitions, while other life domains (e.g., interpersonal relationships, school, job performance, family, hobbies) seem to play a less relevant role in building a solid and balanced self-esteem.

Furthermore, body image disturbance is a persistent symptom in BN and is an important factor from a prognostic perspective, but still little is known about its pathogenesis, clinical correlates, and neurobiological underpinnings [7].

9.2 Body Image in Bulimia Nervosa

There is still no agreement on the nature and definition of body image disturbances in BN. Inconsistencies may be due to the use of different definitions of the body image construct, to non-homogeneous samples, and to different methods of assessment [11]. Clinical observations suggest that BN patients tend to overestimate their body widths, perceiving their body to be fatter than is objectively true, and increasing the size of specific parts of the body, such as waist, abdomen, hips, and thighs. Moreover, women with BN showed consistently greater discrepancy between ideal and estimated body size in comparison to healthy controls [12, 13].

A meta-analysis of 66 studies (from 1974 to 1993) by Cash and Deagle [14], considering perceptual body-size distortion, showed that women with eating disorders exhibit greater overestimation than controls—with larger effects for whole-body than for body part size estimation—whereas AN and BN women do not differ in their perceptual distortion.

Sepulveda et al. [15] updated the previous meta-analysis [14], reporting a significant difference between anorexia and BN, with a greater perceptual body distortion in BN. In addition, the authors found that techniques for assessing body parts showed an effect size significantly greater than whole-body measures in both eating disorder groups.

An interesting research by Vocks et al. [16] recognized that the perceptual component of a disturbed body image in BN patients is not only limited to the overestimation of one's own body dimensions (static body image), but it may be extended to a misperception of one's own motion patterns (dynamic body image). According to this study, the overestimation of their own body dimensions among BN subjects might be due to a stronger activation of negative body-related self-schemes when they look at the picture of their body, so that cognitive attitudes and expectations affect the mental representation of misperception of one's own body dimension and motion patterns.

A variety of alternative explanations for body size estimation in BN have been proposed. Subjects with BN do not seem to have a generalized sensory-perceptual deficit since there is no significant difference in comparison to controls in their size estimation of neutral objects [14]. It has been hypothesized that body image distortion in BN may be related to cognitive and emotional factors: internalization of an ideal of thinness leads to an attentional bias and a negative evaluation of one's body or body parts that are perceived as bigger than in reality [8]. Those studies that found an extreme distortion of body image more frequently in AN than BN, and in the latter group in patients with a previous history of AN, suggested a possible causal link between body image distortion and starvation [7]. An inability to update one's own body concept was clinically observed in AN, and this inflexibility tends to be exacerbated with weight loss, leading to dangerous vicious cycle of pathological behavior [17]. BN subjects have not undergone a significant change in body size and they are not emaciated, so it is possible that this phenomenon is less intense than in AN subjects.

In summary, as for AN, the origin of body image distortion in BN remains unclear. In addition, little is known about which clinical and temperamental factors are associated with body image distortion in these patients. In BN women, body size overestimation seems to correlate with the duration and severity of the eating disorder [18], and with a higher body weight [19]. Counts and Adams [20] reported that a history of childhood obesity seemed to significantly affect body size estimation. Moreover, BN overestimation has been associated with depression [11]. A more recent study [7] revealed that high anticipatory anxiety and lack of interoceptive awareness were the main clinical correlates of body image distortion in both AN and BN. The close association between body image distortion and interoceptive awareness highlights the relative importance of both visual and proprioceptive functions as the putative neural basis of body image disturbance [17].

Most studies on the emotional and cognitive dimensions of body image have shown that women with BN exhibited a significantly intense bodily dissatisfaction or disparagement and wanted to be thinner than healthy controls [14, 21]. Cash and Deagle [14] considered the body image disturbance of BN patients more in terms of cognitive-affective disparagement than in terms of perceptual body image distortion. Higher body dissatisfaction in BN than AN could be explained by the fact that AN women have reached their ideal of severe thinness, and thus they could be more satisfied with their weight and shape, whereas BN subjects who are usually of normal weight, strive desperately to achieve their idealized thin body, alternating restriction, fasting, binge eating, and purging behaviors [22]. Indeed, higher levels of body dissatisfaction in BN were associated with greater feelings of fatness, dieting behavior, higher current weight, higher maximum lifetime weight and low self-esteem [23], depression, drive for thinness [24], and with general psychological distress [22].

Studies on correlation between body affect and body perception yielded mixed results. Hsu and Sobkiewicz [21], in their review, reported that some studies found a correlation between emotional and perceptual measures, whereas others did not.

Although relatively less attention has been given to ideal body size in BN, several studies using silhouette cards have found that women with BN selected a smaller ideal body than controls [20, 25, 26]. Similar findings were found with visual distorting techniques, in which BN subjects selected thinner ideal size relative to perceived size in comparison to controls [27]. On the other hand, using more sophisticated techniques of assessing ideal body image (i.e., a software image warping system that uses biometric data based on real body shapes), no significant differences were found between BN and healthy controls in their ideal body shape [28].

As we have previously stated, high current societal standards for physical appearance play an important role in the development of body dissatisfaction; however, the mechanisms by which this process occurs in BN are not yet fully understood. An interesting point of view has been proposed by Blechert et al. [29], who have investigated the role of social comparison for body dissatisfaction in BN using eye-tracking methodology. The findings of their study suggest that BN women preferred upward social comparisons (comparisons to superior peers), and this disadvantageous strategy might be related to a reduction of self-esteem and body satisfaction in the short term, but aim at long-term self-enhancement by preferring more attractive others.

Despite the important role of the family in the development and consolidation of internalized ideals and self-esteem, little evidence so far exists about the body image of family members, especially the mother, of patients with BN. Benninghoven et al. [30] compared BN and AN patients and their mothers in relation to family functioning, perceptual body size distortion and body dissatisfaction; the study found that BN patients exhibited more body dissatisfaction than AN patients, whereas AN showed a greater overestimation of their body than BN. A positive correlation was found between the body dissatisfaction of mothers and daughters with BN, whereas no significant correlation was found between mothers and AN daughters. Moreover, in families of BN patients, there was a significant relationship between body dissatisfaction and family dysfunction.

The main findings of most recent (last 10 years) studies about body image in BN are reported in Table 9.1.

Table 9.1 Summary of body image disturbances studies in Bulimia Nervosa published in the last 10 years

Authors	Aim of the study	Participants	Measures/ techniques	Main findings
Benninghoven et al. [30]	To investigate body image (body dissatisfaction and body size distortion) in patients with eating disorders and their mother and to explore the relationship between their body image and family functioning	20 BN (+ their mothers) 29 AN (+ their mothers)	– Somatomorphic program (computer program to assess muscularity and body fat) – Family assessment measure, beck depression inventory (BDI)	Body dissatisfaction was higher in BN than AN, whereas overestimation of one's own body was higher in AN group. No differences were found between the two groups of mothers (both of them underestimated their body and wished to be thinner). Mother of BN patients underestimate their daughter's body size and wanted them to be slightly bigger. In BN group a positive association of body dissatisfaction was found between patients and their mothers
Blechert et al. [29]	To investigate the role of social comparison for body dissatisfaction in BN	20 BN 22 healthy controls	– Eye-tracking methodology (measuring eye movements during presentation of digitized body image of participants comparison bodies with higher or lower BMI) – Eating disorder examination-questionnaire, body image avoidance questionnaire, body checking questionnaire, physical appearance comparison scale, body image state scale	Whilst healthy controls showed comparable time of fixation for bodies with higher and lower BMI, BN patients fixated longer the pictures with lower BMI, suggesting disadvantageous social comparison strategies

(continued)

Table 9.1 (continued)

Authors	Aim of the study	Participants	Measures/ techniques	Main findings
Freeman et al. [18]	To assess perceived actual body size and ideal size and to examine clinical and personality correlates of body image distortion in AN and BN	23 BN with previous AN 24 BN without previous AN 17 AN 18 phobic controls 33 healthy controls	– VDT – Eating attitudes test, beck depression inventory, anorexic behavioral scale, rotter's internal-external control scale, mosher forced choice guilt inventory, MMPI	BN patients with previous AN significantly overestimated their actual body size than AN patients and control groups (phobic and healthy subjects), moreover the former group had significantly higher body dissatisfaction than other groups. In BN with previous AN, body size overestimation and body dissatisfaction were significantly related with the duration and severity of illness
Garfinkel et al. [23]	To explore the extent of body dissatisfaction in BN and to determine the relationship between the severity of body dissatisfaction and some clinical and psychometric features	524 BN 770 college women (population norms)	– Distorting photograph technique – Berscheid body satisfation test, feelings of fatness scale EAT-26, SCL-90, restraint scale, BDI, rosenberg self esteem scale, janis-field feelings of inadequacy scale	BN women showed higher frequency of severe levels of body dissatisfaction relative to a population of college women. BN with high body dissatisfaction showed higher severity of eating and psychiatric psychopathology than BN with moderate and low body dissatisfaction. High levels of body dissatisfaction were also related to high concerns regarding weight and shape

Table 9.1 (continued)

Authors	Aim of the study	Participants	Measures/ techniques	Main findings
Goldfein et al. [31]	To compare three different measures of excessive shape and weigh concerns in BN: influence of shape and weight, overconcern with shape and weight, and dissatisfaction with shape and weight	120 BN 27 restrained eaters with no history of eating disorders 28 normal controls	– Three-factor eating questionnaire, eating disorder examination, body shape questionnaire, beck depression inventory, symptom checklist-90-R	BN patients reported significantly greater influence and overconcern, but not dissatisfaction, than normal controls; while no significant difference was found between BN and restrained eaters
Hrabosky et al. [32]	To examine the presence and severity of body image disturbance in individuals with AN, BN and body dysmorphic disorder (BDD)	26 BN 35 AN 56 BBD 34 female psychiatric controls 36 male psychiatric controls	– Multidimensional body-self relations questionnaire appearance scales – Situational inventory of body-image dysphoria-short form – Appearance schemas inventory-revised – Body image coping strategies inventory – Body image disturbance questionnaire – Body image quality-of-life inventory	AN, BN and BBD showed greater body image dissatisfaction relative to their gender-matched clinical controls. AN and BN groups reported greater dissatisfaction with almost all physical characteristics than female controls; BBD reported more discontent with their face and hair. AN and BN showed greater concern with their weight than BBD or female controls
Laporta-Herrero et al. [33]	To analyze the body dissatisfaction in 204 adolescent with eating disorders and to explore the relationship between body dissatisfaction and certain aesthetic body shape model influence and psychological variables	35 BN 72 AN-R 28 AN-P 21 BED 45 EDNOS	– Self report questionnaires: Spanish children's depression questionnaire, rosenberg self-esteem scale, eating attitudes test, body shape questionnaire, questionnaire of influences of aeshtetic body shape model	BN group showed the highest level of body dissatisfaction compared with other eating disorders groups. In all patients, a greater level of body dissatisfaction is related to lower self-esteem, more depression, higher frequency of disordered eating attitudes and more influence of the aesthetic body shape model

(continued)

Table 9.1 (continued)

Authors	Aim of the study	Participants	Measures/ techniques	Main findings
Ortega-Roldán et al. [34]	To explore the emotional and attentional impact of exposure to one's own body in BN	30 BN 30 healthy controls	– Startle-defense paradigm: physiological measures (eye-blink startle, cardiac defense, skin conductance) – Self-report measures (bulimic investigatory test edinburgh, body shape questionnaire, self-assessment manikin)	When viewing their own bodies, BN women compared to healthy controls perceives their own body as unpleasant and uncontrollable. Moreover, they showed (1) greater inhibition of the startle reflex, (2) higher cardiac acceleration in the first component of the defence reaction, and (3) larger skin conductance
Schneider et al. [35]	To examine differences in body image distortion in adolescent girls with AN and BN	34 adolescent BN 69 adolescent AN-R 26 adolescent AN-BP 354 healthy adolescent girls	– EDI 2 (drive for thinness and body dissatisfaction subscales) – Body image distortion in children and adolescent (BID-CA)	BN adolescent girls showed higher scores on EDI-DT and BD than healthy girls and AN-R. The 30% of eating disorder patients overestimated their body parts, while healthy adolescent girls showed an average overestimation of 8 (thigh)- 16% (arm and waist). No significant differences were found between AN and BN regarding body image distortion

Table 9.1 (continued)

Authors	Aim of the study	Participants	Measures/ techniques	Main findings
Stewart et al. [36]	To test three-dimensional (3D) body scanning in eating disorder patients	12 BN 9 AN 1 EDNOS 22 controls	Visual screening: – Two-dimensional (2D) digital photography (to assess perception and dissatisfaction) – 3D full-body scanning	Patients and controls perceived themselves to be fatter and wished to be thinner than their true 2D size. BN had greater body dissatisfaction and perceived their shape less well than AN group. Considering body scanner, AN group significantly underestimated the size of their torso relative to frontal area
Vocks et al. [16]	To assess the static and dynamic body image in BN	30 BN 55 normal controls	– Photo distortion technique (static body image) – Motion distortion technique (dynamic body image) – EDE-Q, EDI-2, body image avoidance questionnaire	BN patients overestimated their "actual" and "felt" body dimensions (static body image) and they also perceived their own motion patterns to be more heavier than controls (dynamic body image). In BN group static body image significantly correlated with shape and weight concerns and drive for thinness; dynamic body image correlated with social insecurity and body image avoidance

(continued)

Table 9.1 (continued)

Authors	Aim of the study	Participants	Measures/ techniques	Main findings
Vossbeck-Elsebusch et al. [37]	To examine the association between misperception of one's own body and body-related behaviour in BN	31 BN 47 EDNOS	– Digital photo distortion technique – Weight and shape concern EDE-Q subscales – "Clothing" and "Social Activities" subscales of body image avoidance-behavior questionnaire (BIAQ)	BN and EDNOS participants overestimated their body size by 4.4% on average, no differences were found between the two groups. Body-related avoidance behavior is associated with body size estimation
Zanetti et al. [7]	To analyse the correlations of aspects of body image disturbance with psychopathological and temperamental characteristics in eating disorder patients	750 BN 538 AN	– EDI, tridimensional personality questionnaire – Several aspects of BID (body image distortion, body dissatisfaction, fear of weight gain, weight checking) were assessed by specific questions during the clinical interview	BN group showed the highest level of fear of weight gain and body dissatisfaction, while the binge eating/purging type AN group reported the highest frequency of body image distortion. In both groups anticipatory anxiety and interoceptive awareness were significantly and independently associated with BID, whereas ineffectiveness was associated to weight checking

9.3 Neural Correlates of Body Image Disturbances in Bulimia Nervosa

The neurobiology of BN is poorly understood and brain imaging studies usually focus on dysfunctional self-regulation and reward processing. These studies found alterations in fronto-striatal circuit function in women with BN, and these were assumed to be involved in the core symptomatology of BN, such as binge eating, purging behaviors, and inappropriate weight and body shape concern and dissatisfaction [38].

Although cognitive bias and distortions concerning body weight and shape are well documented among BN patients, functional magnetic resonance imaging (fMRI) studies are few and inconclusive due to the different definitions used for body image disturbances and the different tasks and stimuli employed.

Brain imaging techniques such as fMRI have been used to investigate whether BN patients might have functional abnormalities in those brain systems involved in body size or image processing.

Uher et al. [39] measured the brain responses to line drawings of female bodies in women with BN or AN and in healthy controls. They found that in all groups of participants, the left and right lateral fusiform gyrus, inferior parietal cortex, and lateral prefrontal cortex (PFC) were activated in response to line drawings of body shape, in comparison to the control condition (drawings of houses). However, in comparison to healthy women, women with AN and BN exhibited lower activation during exposure to body shape in the posterior parietal and occipito-temporal cortex. This effect was stronger in AN women compared to both BN women and healthy controls, whereas BN women showed activation in the right lateral fusiform gyrus that was intermediate between the AN group and healthy controls, while they did not differ significantly from the latter in parietal activation. This study suggests that a lower activation of the posterior parietal cortex might be associated with difficulties in body perception and seems to support the putative role of this brain area in the development of body image disturbances.

Different findings were reported by Miyake et al. [40], who reported that the right amygdala, the left medial prefrontal cortex (MPFC), and the right dorsolateral prefrontal cortex (DLPFC) were significantly less activated in BN patients than in healthy women during processing of their own fat-image. Weaker activation of the medial prefrontal cortex in response to body stimuli has also been found by other fMRI studies [41] although differences in brain activation patterns between BN women and healthy controls were observed in several brain regions (temporal, parietal, and occipital).

Vocks et al. [42], compared neural correlates of viewing photographs of one's own body and another woman's body in patients with BN or AN and healthy women. When viewing their own body, participants with BN exhibited lower activation in the left inferior temporal gyrus and in the left middle temporal gyrus in comparison to healthy women. Additionally, weaker activation in BN patients compared with controls was found in the right inferior parietal lobule and right middle frontal gyrus. By direct comparison of women with BN and those with AN, a stronger activation in the right medial frontal gyrus was exhibited in BN. When looking at images of another woman's body, participants with AN showed a stronger amygdala activation compared to those with BN and healthy controls, whereas BN participants did not exhibit any alteration in brain activation patterns. The authors speculated that pronounced limbic activity stimulated by looking at another female body might be due to an enhanced emotional activation and a higher level of vigilance, probably resulting from social comparison processes.

Other fMRI studies supported the hypothesis of insula dysfunction in individuals with eating disorders [43] since this brain area is involved in interoceptive awareness and thus in body perception. Van den Eynde et al. [38] investigated brain activation patterns related to processing of food stimuli and body image in a group of

BN and healthy controls. The brain activation patterns in response to food stimuli did not differ between groups, whereas significant between-group differences emerged in the comparison of exposure to images of one's own body against images of the body of a slim woman: compared to controls, BN women activated the insula more and the fusiform gyrus less. This suggests that an alteration of insula function might have a role during integration of emotional and interoceptive information processes.

Despite the need for further studies to deepen the neural correlates of body image disturbances in BN, all these data support the idea of developing targeted treatment strategies and cognitive techniques to encourage a more adequate and realistic image of one's own body also in patients with BN. There is some evidence that cognitive behavioral interventions might modify brain activation patterns in response to visual body stimuli in patients with AN and BN [44]; furthermore, future research will clarify whether innovative interventions such as transcranial brain stimulation might have some effects on body image distortions [38].

In conclusion, most studies observed negative body attitudes and marked body dissatisfaction in BN. Less consistent findings are available regarding perceptual (body-size distortion) and behavioral (body checking and avoidance) aspects of body image. These findings highlight the importance of considering the body image construct, in its complexity and multidimensionality, in the assessment of patients with BN. It is common practice to pay more attention to characteristic symptoms of bulimia nervosa, such as binge eating and purging behaviors, while the disparagement of one's own body could be underestimated or taken for granted. However, it is essential to investigate this aspect as a potential risk factor for relapses or non-response to treatment. Cognitive-behavioral treatment in BN not only aims at regularizing eating and the cessation of binge eating and purging behaviors, but also at improving body image disturbance from both a cognitive and emotional point of view. Therefore, further research is warranted to explore treatment paradigms that address the thoughts and cognitive processes underlying body image disturbance in BN.

References

1. Russell G. Bulimia nervosa: an ominous variant of anorexia nervosa. Psychol Med. 1979;9:429–48.
2. Fairburn CG, Garner DM. The diagnosis of bulimia nervosa. Int J Eat Disord. 1986;5:403–19.
3. Willmuth ME, Fondacaro KM, Gross J, Leitenberg H, Rosen JC. Body size distortion in bulimia nervosa. Int J Eat Disord. 1985;4:71–8.
4. Huon GF, Brown LB. Body images in anorexia nervosa and bulimia nervosa. Int J Eat Disord. 1986;5:421–39.
5. Striegel-Moore RH, Silberstein LR, Rodin J. Toward an understanding of risk factors for bulimia. Am Psychol. 1986;41(3):246–63.
6. World Health Organisation. ICD-10 classifications of mental and behavioural disorder: clinical descriptions and diagnostic guidelines. Geneva: World Health Organisation; 1992.
7. Zanetti T, Santonastaso P, Sgaravatti E, Degortes D, Favaro A. Clinical and temperamental correlates of body image disturbance in eating disorders. Eur Eat Disord. 2013;21:32–7.

8. Crowther JH, Williams NM. Body image and bulimia nervosa. In: Cash TF, Smolak L, editors. Body image: a handbook of science, practice, and prevention. New York: Guilford; 2011. p. 288–95.
9. Stice E. A prospective test of the dual pathway model of bulimic pathology: mediating effects of dieting and negative affect. J Abnorm Psychol. 2001;110:124–35.
10. Fairburn CG, Cooper Z, Shafran R. Cognitive behaviour therapy for eating disorders: a "transdiagnostic" theory and treatment. Behav Res Ther. 2003;41:509–28.
11. Cash TF, Brown TA. Body image in anorexia nervosa and bulimia nervosa. A review of the literature. Behav Modif. 1987;11:487–521.
12. Szymanski LA, Seime RJ. A re-examination of body image distortion: evidence against a sensory explanation. Int J Eat Disord. 1997;21:175–80.
13. Peterson CB, Wimmer S, Ackard DM, Crosby R, Cavanagh LC, Engbloom S, Mitchell JE. Changes in body image during cognitive-behavioral treatment in women with bulimia nervosa. Body Image. 2004;1:139–53.
14. Cash TF, Deagle EA III. The nature and extent of body-image disturbances in anorexia nervosa and bulimia nervosa: a meta-analysis. Int J Eat Disord. 1997;22:107–25.
15. Sepulveda AR, Botella J, León JA. Body-image disturbance in eating disorders: a meta-analysis. Psychol Spain. 2002;6:83–95.
16. Vocks S, Legenbauer T, Rüddel H, Troje NF. Static and dynamic body image in bulimia nervosa: mental representation of body dimensions and biological motion patterns. Int J Eat Disord. 2007;40:59–66.
17. Favaro A, Santonastaso P, Manara R, Bosello R, Bommarito G, Tenconi E, Di Salle F. Disruption of visuospatial and somatosensory functional connectivity in anorexia nervosa. Biol Psychiatry. 2012;72:864–70.
18. Freeman RJ, Thomas CD, Solyom L, Koopman RF. Clinical and personality correlates of body size overestimation in anorexia nervosa and bulimia nervosa. Int J Eat Disord. 1985;4:439–56.
19. Birtchnell SA, Lacey JH, Harte A. Body image distortion in bulimia nervosa. Br J Psychiatry. 1985;147:408–12.
20. Counts CR, Adams HE. Body image in bulimic, dieting, and normal females. J Psychopathol Behav Assess. 1985;7:289–300.
21. Hsu LK, Sobkiewicz TA. Body image disturbance: time to abandon the concept for eating disorders? Int J Eat Disord. 1991;10:15–30.
22. Ruuska J, Kaltiala-Heino R, Rantanen P, Koivisto AM. Are there differences in the attitudinal body image between adolescent anorexia nervosa and bulimia nervosa? Eat Weight Disord. 2005;10:98–106.
23. Garfinkel PE, Goldbloom D, Davis R, Olmsted MP, Garner DM, Halmi KA. Body dissatisfaction in bulimia nervosa: relationship to weight and shape concerns and psychological functioning. Int J Eat Disord. 1992;11:151–61.
24. Wiederman MW, Pryor TL. Body dissatisfaction, bulimia, and depression among women: the mediating role of drive for thinness. Int J Eat Disord. 2000;27:90–5.
25. McKenzie SJ, Williamson DA, Cubic BA. Stable and reactive body image disturbances in bulimia nervosa. Behav Ther. 1993;24:195–207.
26. Williamson DA, Davis CJ, Goreczny AJ, Blouin DC. Body-image disturbances in bulimia nervosa: influences of actual body size. J Abnorm Psychol. 1989;98:97–9.
27. Probst M, Vandereycken W, van Coppenolle H, Pieters G. Body size estimation in eating disorder patients: testing the video distortion method on a life-size screen. Behav Res Ther. 1995;33:985–90.
28. Tovée MJ, Benson PJ, Emery JL, Mason SM, Cohen-Tovée EM. Measurement of body size and shape perception in eating-disordered and control observers using body-shape software. Br J Psychol. 2003;94:501–16.
29. Blechert J, Nickert T, Caffier D, Tuschen-Caffier B. Social comparison and its relation to body dissatisfaction in bulimia nervosa: evidence from eye movements. Psychosom Med. 2009;71:907–12.

30. Benninghoven D, Tetsch N, Kunzendorf S, Jantschek G. Body image in patients with eating disorders and their mothers, and the role of family functioning. Compr Psychiatry. 2007;48:118–23.
31. Goldfein JA, Walsh BT, Midlarsky E. Influence of shape and weight on self-evaluation in bulimia nervosa. Int J Eat Disord. 2000;27:435–45.
32. Hrabosky JI, Cash TF, Veale D, et al. Multidimensional body image comparisons among patients with eating disorders, body dysmorphic disorder, and clinical controls: a multisite study. Body Image. 2009;6:155–63.
33. Laporta-Herrero I, Jáuregui-Lobera I, Barajas-Iglesias B, et al. Body dissatisfaction in adolescents with eating disorders. Eat Weight Disord. 2018;23(3):339–47. https://doi.org/10.1007/s40519-016-0353-x.
34. Ortega-Roldán B, Rodríguez-Ruiz S, Perakakis P, et al. The emotional and attentional impact of exposure to one's own body in bulimia nervosa: a physiological view. PLoS One. 2014;9(7):e102595. https://doi.org/10.1371/journal.pone.0102595.
35. Schneider N, Frieler K, Pfeiffer E, et al. Comparison of body size estimation in adolescents with different types of eating disorders. Eur Eat Disord Rev. 2009;17:468–75.
36. Stewart AD, Klein S, Young J, et al. Body image, shape, and volumetric assessments using 3D whole body laser scanning and 2D digital photography in females with a diagnosed eating disorder: preliminary novel findings. Br J Psychol. 2012;103:183–202.
37. Vossbeck-Elsebusch AN, Waldorf M, Legenbauer T, et al. Overestimation of body size in eating disorders and its association to body-related avoidance behavior. Eat Weight Disord. 2015;20:173–8.
38. Van den Eynde F, Giampietro V, Simmons A, Uher R, Andrew CM, Harvey PO, Campbell IC, Schmidt U. Brain responses to body image stimuli but not food are altered in women with bulimia nervosa. BMC Psychiatry. 2013;13:302.
39. Uher R, Murphy T, Friederich HC, Dalgleish T, Brammer MJ, Giampietro V, Phillips ML, Andrew CM, Ng VW, Williams SC, Campbell IC, Treasure J. Functional neuroanatomy of body shape perception in healthy and eating-disordered women. Biol Psychiatry. 2005;58:990–7.
40. Miyake Y, Okamoto Y, Onoda K, Kurosaki M, Shirao N, Okamoto Y, Yamawaki S. Brain activation during the perception of distorted body images in eating disorders. Psychiatry Res. 2010;181:183–92.
41. Spangler DL, Allen MD. An fMRI investigation of emotional processing of body shape in bulimia nervosa. Int J Eat Disord. 2012;45:17–25.
42. Vocks S, Busch M, Grönemeyer D, Schulte D, Herpertz S. Neural correlates of viewing photographs of one's own body and another woman's body in anorexia and bulimia nervosa: an fMRI study. J Psychiatry Neurosci. 2010;35:163–76.
43. Mohr HM, Röder C, Zimmermann J, Hummel D, Negele A, Grabhorn R. Body image distortions in bulimia nervosa: investigating body size overestimation and body size satisfaction by fMRI. NeuroImage. 2011;56:1822–31.
44. Vocks S, Schulte D, Busch M, Grönemeyer D, Herpertz S, Suchan B. Changes in neuronal correlates of body image processing by means of cognitive-behavioural body image therapy for eating disorders: a randomized controlled fMRI study. Psychol Med. 2011;48:1–9.

Body Image and Binge Eating Disorder

10

Federico Amianto and Secondo Fassino

10.1 Introduction

10.1.1 Diagnostic Criteria of Binge Eating Disorder

The recently published fifth revision of the Diagnostic and Statistical Manual of Mental Disorders (DSM-5) includes binge eating disorder (BED) for the first time as a diagnostic category in the Eating Disorders section, while before it was listed as an Eating Disorder not Otherwise Specified (EDNOS) needing future definition. According to the criteria, which are basically in line with the former research criteria of the DSM-IV-TR, BED is characterized by recurring episodes of binge eating over the course of at least 3 months with one binge episode on average per week (DSM-IV-TR: duration of 6 months with two binge episodes per week), in which a large amount of food is consumed in a distinct amount of time, often accompanied by a feeling of loss of control. To measure the severity of the disorder, the DSM-5 proposes binge eating frequency as a specifying criterion. In contrast to other prominent eating disorders, such as anorexia nervosa (AN) or bulimia nervosa (BN), no regular inappropriate compensatory behaviors are undertaken to avoid weight gain, e.g., self-induced vomiting, abuse of laxatives, or excessive sport or exercise. Binge eating is often associated with eating quickly and to the point of feeling uncomfortably full, along with feelings of disgust and shame, leading to the individual mostly eating alone.

Whereas in the diagnostic criteria for AN and BN, body image disturbance is a required criterion for diagnosis, it is not included in the criteria for BED. However, there is growing evidence that body image disturbance might be characteristic for BED as well even though only a limited number of studies have addressed body image disturbance in BED [1].

F. Amianto (✉) · S. Fassino
Eating Disorders Center for Treatment and Research, Department of Neuroscience, University of Turin, Turin, Italy
e-mail: federico.amianto@unito.it; secondo.fassino@unito.it

M. Cuzzolaro, S. Fassino (eds.), *Body Image, Eating, and Weight*,
https://doi.org/10.1007/978-3-319-90817-5_10

10.1.2 Epidemiology and Comorbidity of BED

BED is a relatively common disorder, with an estimated lifetime prevalence in general population around 1.4%. This disease is of particular interest for its frequency in primary care, its link with obesity and its medical and psychiatric comorbidities, leading to high socio-economic impact due to reduced quality of life and increased health service utilization [2, 3]. As a consequence of the excessive food intake, the most frequent comorbidity in BED is obesity, with about 40–70% of people with BED also suffering from severe overweight. Prevalence is likely to increase, especially because of the rising incidence that both obesity and EDs show worldwide rather than for the widening of diagnostic criteria introduced in DSM-5 [1, 4, 5].

Furthermore, BED is associated with elevated eating disorder psychopathology, increased body dissatisfaction and decreased self-esteem. Clinical studies indicate that among obese individuals, those with BED experience greater eating disorder psychopathology, psychiatric and medical comorbidity, impairment in social and occupational functioning, and reduced quality of life than those without BED [6–8].

Despite the fact that obese subjects with and without BED do not differ in degree of overweight, binge eaters show considerable more eating, weight, and shape concerns, and also lower levels of self-reported physical appearance and global self-worth. Dietary restraint is generally assumed to be a core characteristic of binge eating among individuals with eating disorders and a pathogenic element of the binge behavior itself [9]. It remains unclear to what extent dietary restraint has a function in the binge eating problems among obese subjects [10].

10.1.3 Assessment of BED

The diagnosis of BED is eminently clinical and should be performed by an expert psychiatrist, possibly using a semi-structured interview such as the SCID (Structured Clinical Interview) for the DSM 5 criteria. Nevertheless in clinical studies the BED is quantified through various tools:

- Eating Disorder Examination-Questionnaire (EDE-Q) [11], a self-report questionnaire that assesses the frequency of key eating disorder behaviors, differentiating between the various forms of overeating and providing the determination of binge eating as defined in the fourth edition of the Diagnostic and Statistical Manual of Mental Disorders (DSM-IV) [10, 12];
- Binge Eating subscale of the Minnesota Eating Behavior survey [13], which assesses the presence or absence of binge eating symptoms, such as feeling out of control while eating and eating when upset, not captured by the EDE-Q binge eating frequency item [6];
- Dutch Eating Behavior Questionnaire (DEBQ) [14], auto administered, designed to investigate disordered eating behaviors in three different sub-domains: restrained eating, emotional eating, external eating.

10.2 Body Image and the Concept of Self

The self, according to the model proposed by Amianto and coworkers [15], may be understood as an integrative structure of the mind that organizes and coordinates different functions (affective, cognitive, social, sensorimotor, and vegetative) with regard to interoceptive and exteroceptive stimuli from one's own body and the environment. In this model, the self is the cognitive, conative, and affective representation of one's subjective experience and one's identity. Thus, the self plays an integral part in human motivation, cognition, affect, and social identity. The self also implies a temporal concept. It extends across time from the past over the present and to the future. In contrast to the concept of identity, which describes the diachronic sameness of a person over time, the concept of self is synchronic, that is, it concerns the experience of an individual as him or herself, and allows him or her to attribute specific experiences, persons, or objects at a particular point in time. This entails a self-specific organization of both neural and psychological activity [16].

According to Higgins [17], our behavior is guided by three different domains of the self: the "actual" self (what we think we are), the "ideal" self (what we want to be), and the "ought" self (what we think we ought to be with regard to social norms). The actual self represents our core self-concept. It describes the person we think we are, with all its attributes and traits. The ideal and ought selves are self-guides, in that they drive us to seek new self-states. Whereas the ideal self represents what we would ideally like to be and contains the traits and characteristics of that ideal person, the ought self represents the kind of person we think we need to become if we are to comply with social norms. The ought self therefore contains traits and characteristics that are highly normative and socially constrained. Higgins' theory suggests that people are motivated to achieve a certain match between their self-concept and their self-guides. Any perceived discrepancy between the self-concept and a self-guide leads to different negative emotional and motivational states, depending on the type of discrepancy. Actual/ideal self-discrepancies result in disappointment or dissatisfaction, while actual/ought self-discrepancies lead more to feelings of fear and threat. Self-discrepancies, assessed with Higgins' method are related to body dissatisfaction and disordered eating, with the actual/ideal discrepancy being related to bulimia and the actual/ought discrepancy to anorexia. High self-discrepancies are also associated with low self-esteem and emotional vulnerability [18].

Often in the BED subjects, it emerges another problem relating the self and body image: the body image is not completely integrated in the self. BED and in general obese subject do not completely or stably diachronically perceive their body image. It may happen that even openly recognizing of being overweight they intimately deny their body shape and pretend to be thinner than they really are [19]. Thus they may also engage in activities that are not adequate for their body shape or weight (such as dressing inappropriately, trying to pass through small spaces or attempting risky sports). In particular, when they are overwhelmed by emotional eating they completely loose the contact with their sense of being fat and the need to contain their impulses and this reduces the ability to contain their behaviors. Also after their binging they do not perceive the need in engaging in compensatory behaviors as BN subjects. They protect themselves for the painful feeling of being overweight removing the perception of the body self, sometimes refusing to face with the mirrors, to speak about the fat as a serious problem, and in general escaping from the awareness of their condition.

At a deeper layer, the BED body image perception may be significantly hampered by the difficulty of these subjects of setting, perceiving, and maintaining the boundaries of their self. They in general express poor skills in setting and respecting the limits in general, also with respect to emotions, relationships, social cues, and requests. BED individuals often shift towards an attitude of requesting unlimited emotional expression, relational gratification, love, and social recognition. This is expressed by their unlimited attitudes towards food and visualized by their limitless growth in body shape [20–23].

10.2.1 Overvaluation of Weight and Shape

Overvaluation of body shape/weight refers to one's preoccupation with shape and weight and using one's shape and weight as a major source of self-esteem [24]. In the transdiagnostic cognitive-behavioral model of eating disorders [25], overvaluation is the core psychopathology that maintains eating disorder symptoms and behaviors. According to Fairburn, shape/weight concerns, such as feelings of fatness (feeling fat or that a specific body part is fat) and fat phobia (fear of becoming fat), are conceptualized as distinct constructs that emanate from overvaluation of shape/weight [26].

It has been shown that overvaluation of weight and shape seems to occur to a comparable degree in BED as in AN and BN. When comparing obese persons with BED to individuals with obesity without an eating disorder a number of studies reported significantly higher weight and shape concerns in the first (it is present in 60% of BED patients, a level which is significantly higher than in non-BED obese patients, even though it is lower than in AN and BN, where it is nearly universal). Even if this feature is present only in a subgroup of BED patients, and so it is not included among the official diagnostic criteria, it is related to higher psychosocial impairment and worse quality of life [27].

A stronger overvaluation of shape and weight also seems to be associated with a more pronounced eating disorder pathology in general as well as with higher levels of depression in BED and is shown to act as a mediator between weight bias internalization and self-esteem. Overvaluation of shape and weight can be thus considered either a diagnostic specifier or a dimensional severity rate, with a primary relevance for diagnosis, treatment choice, global impairment and outcome, and it can also be considered as a specific target for psychological therapies [1, 27–29]. Furthermore, it has been shown that overvaluation of body shape and weight predicts lower rates of remission from binge eating and higher frequency of binge eating at 12-month follow-ups after completing treatments [28].

10.2.2 How Overvaluation of Weight and Shape May Lead to Binge Eating

The manner by which overvaluation of body shape and weight maintains eating disorders is complex. Many models have been proposed, among these the most relevant link overvaluation of weight and binge eating with the presence of restrictive eating behavior and with a deficit in managing negative emotions.

According to the transdiagnostic cognitive-behavioral model of eating disorders, as seen above, overvaluation of shape/weight is the driving force that propels engagement in non-compensatory weight-control behaviors, such as engagement in restrictive eating and compulsive exercise that is independent of the amount of food intake and presence of binge eating episodes [1, 26].

According to this model, low self-esteem, body image-related, generates anxiety and negative emotions resulting in excessive diet restrictions, in turn triggering binging.

Popular weight loss strategies among adolescents include dieting and calorie restriction. However, these weight loss techniques put individuals at risk for eating disorders including anorexia nervosa at first, then bulimia nervosa [30] and finally also binge eating behavior. It has been proposed that binge eating is largely a product of the particular way that these patients attempt to restrict their eating (i.e., their form of dietary restraint), whether or not there is an actual energy deficit. Rather than adopting general guidelines about how they should eat, they try to adhere to multiple extreme, and highly specific, dietary rules. Accompanying these dietary rules is a tendency to react negatively to the (almost inevitable) breaking of them with even minor dietary slips being interpreted as evidence of their lack of self-control, the result being that they respond by temporarily abandoning their efforts to restrict their eating. Patient reports indicate that this is a major trigger of binge eating with an overcompensation of diet restrictions [31].

The peculiar food choice that patients make during binge episodes, in fact—e.g., fats, carbohydrates, sweets and snacks—has been related to the hypothesis of a "hedonic deprivation," were eating impulsiveness can be triggered by restrictions on palatable foods during everyday life, even if at more recent findings the presence of this clinical feature seems controversial [1, 32]. Increased engagement in these behaviors leads to binge eating which, in turn, reinforces overvaluation of shape/weight and consequent personal devaluation which rises unpleasant emotions [26].

This therefore maintains the core psychopathology by magnifying patients' concerns about their ability to control their eating, shape and weight. This encourages yet greater dietary restraint, thereby further increasing the risk of binge eating. In the original cognitive-behavioral formulation, it was noted that these patients' dietary slips and binges do not happen at random; rather, they are particularly likely to occur in response to acute changes in mood (typically adverse mood states) since these appear to interfere with the ability to maintain dietary restraint. These patients tend to be extremely self-critical, they set themselves demanding standards in terms of their eating, shape and weight, and control. When they cannot meet them, they see themselves as being at fault rather than their standards as being too harsh. The result is a secondary negative self-evaluation. This too maintains the eating disorder since it leads patients to strive even harder to achieve "success" in the area of life that is most important to them; that is, controlling their eating, shape and weight. In this way, a further vicious circle serves to maintain the eating disorder [31].

On the other hand, in addition to dietary restraint, deficitary negative emotion managing and emotional eating appear to be involved in development and maintenance of BED. Obese individuals with BED may lack effective strategies for managing negative emotions, and it has been hypothesized that eating is undertaken as a strategy to regulate or change negative emotions [33]. Recent studies describe binge eating in BED as the possible result of an immediate breakdown of emotion and impulse regulation caused by sudden increases of negative affect and tension, and/or rapid decrease of positive affect [1].

External emotional eating has been identified as forms of disordered eating behaviors. External eating involves reacting to external cues for food intake (e.g., eating because other people are eating, eating during meal preparation or in response to the sight or smell of food) rather than relying on internal cues, such as hunger. Emotional eating refers to excessive eating in response to emotional experiences such as anxiety or anger. This pattern, linked to attempts to improve one's mood through the consumption of food, has been identified as a precursor to binge eating [30].

It was recognized in the original cognitive-behavioral theory that adverse mood states can be a trigger of binge eating, and it was suggested that their primary effect was to disrupt dietary restraint [24]. It is now clear that in some patients there is a more complex relationship between emotional states and binge eating. Usually, this intolerance is of adverse mood states, such as anger, anxiety, or depression, but in some cases there is intolerance of all intense mood states including positive ones (e.g., excitement). Instead of accepting changes in mood and dealing appropriately with them, these patients engage in what may be termed "dysfunctional mood modulatory behavior." This reduces their awareness of the triggering mood state (and the associated cognitions), and also neutralizes it, but at a personal cost. The dysfunctional mood modulatory behavior may take the form of self-injury (e.g., cutting, punching, or burning themselves) which has the effect of rapidly dissipating the initial mood state, or it may involve taking psychoactive substances (e.g., alcohol, tranquillizers) to directly modify how they feel. In patients with bulimia nervosa, binge eating, self-induced vomiting, and intense exercising may also be used as forms of mood modulatory behavior, binge eating most commonly serving this purpose. Among these patients (i.e., those with an eating disorder and mood intolerance), such forms of behavior (i.e., binge eating, vomiting, intense exercising) can become habitual means of mood modulation [31, 34].

It has to be remembered that triggers of binge eating are commonly of interpersonal nature. It can be argued that this reflects a short-term intensification of their need for a sense of "control," a need which is displaced onto dietary self-control. Second, it is obvious that certain interpersonal environments magnify concerns about controlling eating, shape and weight. These include families in which there are other members with an eating disorder, and occupations in which there is pressure to be slim [31].

The relationship between interpersonal dynamics and binge behavior is complex and polymorphic, and appears to be strictly related to personality traits and anger. In particular, it has recently enlightened the role of the personality trait cooperativeness in mediating such relationship. Low cooperativeness, which strictly correlates with the severity of a personality disorder, has been evidenced as a relevant predictor of dropout. Studies demonstrated that cooperativeness not only influence adherence to treatment but is related to binge eating and impulse regulation. In fact, many authors underline a strong relationship between anger feelings and interpersonal difficulties, in particular, with regard to interpersonal boundaries and aspects of the experience of the self. Temperamental shyness and sensibility to criticism related to Harm Avoidance may favor anger feelings towards others, which may impair the relational coping skills expressed by Cooperativeness. Social interactions with low Cooperativeness may consequently foster anger feelings and these elicit binge eating and impulsive behaviors when the patient faces with conflicting situations. Therefore, it appears fundamental to address cooperativeness in treating BED: this may rise social skills and social adaptation and help to control anger and, eventually, significantly reduce impulse-related binge symptoms [35].

In conclusion, overvaluation and engagement in non-compensatory weight-control behaviors mutually reinforce each other in a reciprocal manner [26].

10.2.3 Body Dissatisfaction in BED

Body dissatisfaction is widespread among girls and women throughout Western cultures, with approximately 60% of 13–15-year-old girls, 90% of 18–30-year-old women, and 80% of middle-aged women reporting dissatisfaction with their appearance. Body dissatisfaction appears to be a major risk factor for the development of eating disorders [36, 37]. Of these individuals who are dissatisfied with their body and wish to alter their appearance, approximately one-third engage in unhealthy body change practices, such as forcing themselves to purge, deliberately abusing laxatives or diuretics, or strict dieting or fasting. Surprisingly, body dissatisfaction is also related to binge eating, and this relationship is not simply driven by shared association with other eating disorder symptoms. The act of binging typically occurs amid a general effort to restrict eating to achieve a slim figure [30, 38].

Teasing related to appearance has been one of the most empirically well-supported links to body dissatisfaction and some research supports a causal link between teasing and body dissatisfaction. A meta-analysis suggests that teasing during adolescence may be a risk factor for body dissatisfaction during adulthood [39] and may play a role in the development of body image disturbance and possibly related disordered eating outcomes [40].

It has been shown that subjective perceptions of body weight and, to a lesser extent, body shape, play a greater role in disordered eating and body image concerns than do objective measures of BMI and WHR. In other words, the extent to which someone perceives himself or herself as being overweight is a much better predictor of body dissatisfaction, body esteem, and disordered eating, than the actual BMI [41].

Moreover, body dissatisfaction can be evaluated by Digital Photo Distortion Technique, based on an individual photograph of one's own body. The discrepancy scores between the "actual" and "ideal" as well as the "actual" and "felt" body dimensions are higher in obese BED patients compared to non-BED obese patients, indicating a higher degree of discontent with one's own body size and a greater wish to be thinner than those without an eating disorder.

According to the objectification theory, body dissatisfaction is at least partially linked to the role and position of women in society. Women, particularly in Western cultures, are commonly viewed as objects by society, with their bodies being attended to in a sexual, objectifying manner. Given the pervasiveness of this objectification, it is argued that many women adopt a third-person perspective of their own appearance (self-objectification), which, in turn, leads to a preoccupation with outward appearance, more frequent engagement in self-monitoring, and subsequent body dissatisfaction [38].

10.2.4 How Body Dissatisfaction May Lead to Binge Eating

Many theories have been proposed on how body dissatisfaction can contribute to cause and maintain binge eating disorder. Broadbent and colleagues [38] have compared three different models: a dual pathway model involving negative affectivity and dietary restraint, a model considering binge eating as a self-distraction maladaptive coping strategy and a third model based on interoceptive deficits.

The dual pathway model proposes that body dissatisfaction may induce general and intense states of negative affect or depressed mood, which are resolved through distraction and/or comfort through food consumption. Individuals who experience difficulties regulating this emotional arousal may thus use binge eating as a means to distract themselves.

Alternatively, dietary restraint may be used in attempts to reduce body dissatisfaction, but this too leads to overeating as sustained food restriction increases hunger levels, appetitive response to food and, ultimately, increases the likelihood of food over-consumption to restore energy levels after a period of deprivation. The proposed pathways of negative affect and dietary restraint have received extensive support in both eating disordered and non-eating disordered samples of women. Negative mood, depressive symptoms, and emotional regulation difficulties have been shown to be more common among individuals with eating disorders, and in non-clinical populations, these mood disturbances are positively associated with severity of disordered eating symptomatology.

Heatherton and Baumeister's escape from awareness model propose instead that binge eating is a consequence of successful self-distraction attempts [42].

Negative affectivity, a generic feeling of depressed mood or negative mood in relation to body dissatisfaction, may induce some individuals to respond by shifting attention away from considerations of meaning and consequences, and instead move towards emphasis on concrete aspects of stimuli, such as smell, sight, feel, and taste of stimuli in their environment. The focus on these concrete aspects of food (when present) coupled with reduced consideration of the consequences of food consumption may have the effect of temporarily suspending any self-imposed prohibitions on food consumption. Consistent with the escape from awareness model, binge episodes are typically preceded by heightened negative affect, and subsequent to the binge episode, individuals exhibit poor recall of amount of food consumed. Individuals with body dissatisfaction are also more likely to adopt coping strategies involving self-distraction from, and avoidance of, aversive self-criticism. Moreover, escape from awareness could be favored by a deficit in internal awareness, or interoceptive awareness. According to the Objectification theory, individuals with poor interoceptive awareness are unaware of satiety signals that prevent overeating. Extant literature provides evidence for a link between self-objectification and interoceptive awareness, with lack of awareness being correlated with greater eating disorder symptoms [38].

10.2.5 Internal Weight Bias and Self-Esteem

Weight-biased attitudes and resulting weight-stigmatization are prevalent in all domains of society, and individuals with obesity who internalize this bias apply negative stereotypes to themselves and base their self-evaluation on these stigmatizing attitudes. Weight bias internalization among individuals with obesity is associated with a host of negative mental and physical health outcomes such as low self-esteem, weight and shape concerns, body dissatisfaction, and unhealthy eating behaviors including binge eating. Weight bias internalization is distinct from overvaluation of shape and weight because it includes applying negative weight stereotypes to oneself. Low self-esteem, frequently found in BED patients, may contribute to the internalization of weight bias through the process of basing one's self-evaluation strongly in shape and weight [43, 44].

The complexity of interactions between body weight and shape, self-esteem, body dissatisfaction, ideal weight, and internal weight bias is reflected in the findings that show that such interactions are bi-directional. Accordingly, Bucholz and colleagues demonstrated that internalization of the thin ideal and the muscular ideal, in females and males, respectively, has emerged as an important risk factor for the development of body image concerns and eating disorders. Such internalization is culturally dependent and largely influenced by media, especially in adolescents [30, 45]. Moreover, overweight/obese college women with binge eating showed more distress and preoccupation regarding their shape and weight and lower overall appearance satisfaction and self-esteem in comparison to women without binge eating [6].

10.2.6 How Internal Weight Bias and Low Self-Esteem May Lead to Binge Eating

Body esteem and internal weight bias are important factors to consider in understanding the relationship between internalization of the ideal body figure and disordered eating. Body self-esteem can be conceptualized as composed by weight-esteem and appearance-esteem. Studies have shown the latter to be a strong mediator in the relationship between internalization of the ideal body shape and both emotional and external eating. Appearance-esteem also resulted in a significant predictor for both emotional eating and external eating in males and females adolescents. Because neuroticism has been linked with emotional and external eating [46, 47] it could be that poor appearance-esteem and internalization of the muscular ideal are more likely to occur among males who experience negative affect and emotional instability [48, 49].

Furthermore, weight-esteem emerged as a mediator in the relationship between internalization of the ideal body shape and emotional eating in adolescents females but not in adolescents males. On the contrary, it appeared to be a major predictor of restrained eating both in adolescents females and males [30].

Low self-esteem is not to be considered only as a causative factor, but also a maintenance factor. According to the transdiagnostic cognitive-behavioral model of eating disorders, low self-esteem tends to obstruct change through two main mechanisms. First, it creates in patients hopelessness about their capacity to change, thereby undermining their compliance with treatment; and second, it results in them pursuing, with particular determination, achievement in their valued domains (in this case, the pursuit of control over eating, shape and weight) thereby making change in these areas all the more difficult. The state is also self-perpetuating since these patients show particularly pronounced negative cognitive processing biases, coupled with over-generalization, with the result that any perceived "failure" is interpreted as confirmation that they are failures as people thereby reaffirming their overall negative view of themselves [31].

10.3 The Role of Body Image in the Prevention and Treatment of Eating Disorders

Negative body image is an important risk factor which increases the probability of developing other key components of eating pathology: dietary restraint, binge eating, and negative affect. Stice [50] conducted a meta-analytic review: data from these studies confirm that negative body image is an independent predictor of disordered eating. Therefore, it is possible to state that, if negative body image could be prevented, the incidence of eating pathology would be reduced [51].

Self-compassion is, on the other hand, a psychological dimension that can be protective against the development of binge eating disorder. It is a multi-dimensional construct based on the recognition that suffering, failure, and inadequacy are part of the human condition, and that all people—oneself included—are worthy of compassion. It can be considered as an "adaptive affect regulation" and a coping strategy. Self-compassion may directly mitigate the maladaptive outcomes of poor body image or eating pathology and may prevent the initial occurrence of a risk factor (e.g., thin-ideal internalization) of a maladaptive outcome (e.g., eating pathology), disrupting the vicious circle through which risk factors operate. A recent review conducted by Tosca and colleagues strongly supports a role for self-compassion as a protective factor in relation to negative body image and ED and may foster other protective factors and potentiate body- and ED-related outcomes. This finding can be implemented in treatment: self-compassion training may directly or indirectly foster increased interoceptive awareness, and/or be particularly helpful at inducing self-soothing and non-reactivity during unpleasant emotional or endogenous hunger and satiety cues that may otherwise be suppressed or misinterpreted [45].

Acknowledgement Dott. Gabriela Dorati contributed to this chapter.

References

1. Amianto F, Ottone L, Abbate Daga G, Fassino S. Binge-eating disorder diagnosis and treatment: a recap in front of DSM-5. BMC Psychiatry. 2015;15:70. https://doi.org/10.1186/s12888-015-0445-6. PMCID: PMC4397811.
2. Amianto F, Lavagnino L, Abbate-Daga G, Fassino S. The forgotten psychosocial dimension of the obesity epidemic. Lancet. 2011;378(9805):e8. https://doi.org/10.1016/S0140-6736(11)61778-9.
3. Wang YC, McPherson K, Marsh T, Gortmaker SL, Brown M. Health and economic burden of the projected obesity trends in the USA and the UK. Lancet. 2011;378(9793):815–25. https://doi.org/10.1016/S0140-6736(11)60814-3.
4. Hudson JI, Coit CE, Lalonde JK, Pope HG Jr. By how much will the proposed new DSM-5 criteria increase the prevalence of binge eating disorder? Int J Eat Disord. 2010;45(1):139–41. https://doi.org/10.1002/eat.20890.
5. Trace SE, Thornton LM, Root TL, Mazzeo SE, Lichtenstein P, Pedersen NL, Bulik CM. Effects of reducing the frequency and duration criteria for binge eating on lifetime prevalence of bulimia nervosa and binge eating disorder: implications for DSM-5. Int J Eat Disord. 2012;45(4):531–6. https://doi.org/10.1002/eat.20955.
6. Herbozo S, Schaefer LM, Thompson JK. A comparison of eating disorder psychopathology, appearance satisfaction, and self-esteem in overweight and obese women with and without binge eating. Eat Behav. 2015;17:36–9. https://doi.org/10.1016/j.eatbeh.2015.01.007.
7. Bulik CM, Sullivan PF, Kendler KS. Medical and psychiatric morbidity in obese women with and without binge eating. Int J Eat Disord. 2002;32(1):72–8.
8. Wilfley DE, Wilson GT, Agras WS. The clinical significance of binge eating disorder. Int J Eat Disord. 2003;34(Suppl):S96–106.
9. Heatherton TF, Polivy J, Herman CP, Baumeister RF. Self-awareness, task failure, and disinhibition: how attentional focus affects eating. J Pers. 1993;61(1):49–61.
10. Decaluwé V, Braet C, Fairburn CG. Binge eating in obese children and adolescents. Int J Eat Disord. 2003;33(1):78–84.
11. Fairburn CG, Beglin SJ. Assessment of eating disorders: interview or self-report questionnaire? Int J Eat Disord. 1994;16(4):363–70.
12. American Psychiatric Association. Diagnostic and statistical manual of mental disorders. 4th ed. Washington, DC: American Psychiatric Association; 1994.
13. von Ranson KM, Klump KL, Iacono WG, McGue M. The Minnesota Eating Behavior Survey: a brief measure of disordered eating attitudes and behaviors. Eat Behav. 2005;6(4):373–92.
14. Van Strien T, Rookus MA, Bergers GP, Frijters JE, Defares PB. Life events, emotional eating and change in body mass index. Int J Obes. 1986;10(1):29–35.

15. Amianto F, Northoff G, Abbate Daga G, Fassino S, Tasca GA. Is anorexia nervosa a disorder of the self? A psychological approach. Front Psychol. 2016;7:849. https://doi.org/10.3389/fpsyg.2016.00849. PMCID: PMC4906654.
16. Schaefer M, Northoff G. Who am I: the conscious and the unconscious self. Front Hum Neurosci. 2017;11:126. https://doi.org/10.3389/fnhum.2017.00126.
17. Higgins ET. Self-discrepancy: a theory relating self and affect. Psychol Rev. 1987;94(3):319–40.
18. Arciszewski T, Berjot S, Finez L. Threat of the thin-ideal body image and body malleability beliefs: effects on body image self-discrepancies and behavioral intentions. Body Image. 2012;9(3):334–41. https://doi.org/10.1016/j.bodyim.2012.04.007.
19. Valtolina GG. Body-size estimation by obese subjects. Percept Mot Skills. 1998;86(3):1363–74.
20. Glasofer DR, Haaga DA, Hannallah L, Field SE, Kozlosky M, Reynolds J, Yanovski JA, Tanofsky-Kraff M. Self-efficacy beliefs and eating behavior in adolescent girls at-risk for excess weight gain and binge eating disorder. Int J Eat Disord. 2013;46(7):663–8. https://doi.org/10.1002/eat.22160.
21. Pisetsky EM, Haynos AF, Lavender JM, Crow SJ, Peterson CB. Associations between emotion regulation difficulties, eating disorder symptoms, non-suicidal self-injury, and suicide attempts in a heterogeneous eating disorder sample. Compr Psychiatry. 2017;73:143–50.
22. Mason TB, Lavender JM, Wonderlich SA, Crosby RD, Engel SG, Strauman TJ, Mitchell JE, Crow SJ, Le Grange D, Klein MH, Smith TL, Peterson CB. Self-discrepancy and eating disorder symptoms across eating disorder diagnostic groups. Eur Eat Disord Rev. 2016;24(6):541–5. https://doi.org/10.1002/erv.2483.
23. Monell E, Högdahl L, Mantilla EF, Birgegård A. Emotion dysregulation, self-image and eating disorder symptoms in University Women. J Eat Disord. 2015;3:44. https://doi.org/10.1186/s40337-015-0083-x.
24. Cooper Z, Fairburn CG. Refining the definition of binge eating disorder and nonpurging bulimia nervosa. Int J Eat Disord. 2003;34(Suppl):S89–95.
25. Fairburn CG, Cooper Z, Doll HA, O'Connor ME, Bohn K, Hawker DM, Wales JA, Palmer RL. Transdiagnostic cognitive-behavioral therapy for patients with eating disorders: a two-site trial with 60-week follow-up. Am J Psychiatry. 2009;166(3):311–9. https://doi.org/10.1176/appi.ajp.2008.08040608.
26. Tabri N, Murray HB, Thomas JJ, Franko DL, Herzog DB, Eddy KT. Overvaluation of body shape/weight and engagement in non-compensatory weight-control behaviors in eating disorders: is there a reciprocal relationship? Psychol Med. 2015;45(14):2951–8. https://doi.org/10.1017/S0033291715000896.
27. Grilo CM, Crosby RD, Masheb RM, White MA, Peterson CB, Wonderlich SA, Engel SG, Crow SJ, Mitchell JE. Overvaluation of shape and weight in binge eating disorder, bulimia nervosa, and sub-threshold bulimia nervosa. Behav Res Ther. 2009;47(8):692–6. https://doi.org/10.1016/j.brat.2009.05.001.
28. Grilo CM, White MA, Gueorguieva R, Wilson GT, Masheb RM. Predictive significance of the overvaluation of shape/weight in obese patients with binge eating disorder: findings from a randomized controlled trial with 12-month follow-up. Psychol Med. 2013;43(6):1335–44. https://doi.org/10.1017/S0033291712002097.
29. Ojserkis R, Sysko R, Goldfein JA, Devlin MJ. Does the overvaluation of shape and weight predict initial symptom severity or treatment outcome among patients with binge eating disorder? Int J Eat Disord. 2012;45(4):603–8. https://doi.org/10.1002/eat.20981.
30. Flament MF, Hill EM, Buchholz A, Henderson K, Tasca GA, Goldfield G. Internalization of the thin and muscular body ideal and disordered eating in adolescence: the mediation effects of body esteem. Body Image. 2012;9(1):68–75. https://doi.org/10.1016/j.bodyim.2011.07.007.
31. Fairburn CG, Cooper Z, Shafran R. Cognitive behaviour therapy for eating disorders: a "transdiagnostic" theory and treatment. Behav Res Ther. 2003;41(5):509–28.
32. Wolfe BE, Baker CW, Smith AT, Kelly-Weeder S. Validity and utility of the current definition of binge eating. Int J Eat Disord. 2009;42(8):674–86. https://doi.org/10.1002/eat.20728.

33. Gianini LM, White MA, Masheb RM. Eating pathology, emotion regulation, and emotional overeating in obese adults with binge eating disorder. Eat Behav. 2013;14(3):309–13. https://doi.org/10.1016/j.eatbeh.2013.05.008.
34. Cooper PJ, Fairburn CG. The depressive symptoms of bulimia nervosa. Br J Psychiatry. 1986;148:268–74.
35. Amianto F, Siccardi S, Abbate-Daga G, Marech L, Barosio M, Fassino S. Does anger mediate between personality and eating symptoms in bulimia nervosa? Psychiatry Res. 2012;200(2–3):502–12. https://doi.org/10.1016/j.psychres.2012.07.036.
36. Polivy J, Herman CP. Causes of eating disorders. Annu Rev Psychol. 2002;53:187–213.
37. Stice E, Schupak-Neuberg E, Shaw HE, Stein RI. Relation of media exposure to eating disorder symptomatology: an examination of mediating mechanisms. J Abnorm Psychol. 1994;103(4):836–40.
38. Holmes M, Fuller-Tyszkiewicz M, Skouteris H, Broadbent J. Understanding the link between body image and binge eating: a model comparison approach. Eat Weight Disord. 2015;20(1):81–9. https://doi.org/10.1007/s40519-014-0141-4.
39. Grilo CM, Wilfley DE, Brownell KD, Rodin J. Teasing, body image, and self-esteem in a clinical sample of obese women. Addict Behav. 1994;19(4):443–50.
40. Menzel JE, Schaefer LM, Burke NL, Mayhew LL, Brannick MT, Thompson JK. Appearance-related teasing, body dissatisfaction, and disordered eating: a meta-analysis. Body Image. 2010;7(4):261–70. https://doi.org/10.1016/j.bodyim.2010.05.004.
41. Wilson JM, Tripp DA, Boland FJ. The relative contributions of subjective and objective measures of body shape and size to body image and disordered eating in women. Body Image. 2005;2(3):233–47.
42. Heatherton TF, Baumeister RF. Binge eating as escape from self-awareness. Psychol Bull. 1991;110(1):86–108.
43. Pearl RL, White MA, Grilo CM. Overvaluation of shape and weight as a mediator between self-esteem and weight bias internalization among patients with binge eating disorder. Eat Behav. 2014;15(2):259–61. https://doi.org/10.1016/j.eatbeh.2014.03.005.
44. Lewer M, Nasrawi N, Schroeder D, Vocks S. Body image disturbance in binge eating disorder: a comparison of obese patients with and without binge eating disorder regarding the cognitive, behavioral and perceptual component of body image. Eat Weight Disord. 2016;21(1):115–25. https://doi.org/10.1007/s40519-015-0200-5.
45. Braun TD, Park CL, Gorin A. Self-compassion, body image, and disordered eating: a review of the literature. Body Image. 2016;17:117–31. https://doi.org/10.1016/j.bodyim.2016.03.003.
46. Heaven PC, Mulligan K, Merrilees R, Woods T, Fairooz Y. Neuroticism and conscientiousness as predictors of emotional, external, and restrained eating behaviors. Int J Eat Disord. 2001;30(2):161–6.
47. Steptoe A, Pollard TM, Wardle J. Development of a measure of the motives underlying the selection of food: the food choice questionnaire. Appetite. 1995;25(3):267–84.
48. Amianto F, Dorati G, Spalatro A, Abbate-Daga G, Fassino S. Homosexuality and anorexia nervosa: an explorative study on personality traits. Acta Psychopathol. 2016;2:42. https://doi.org/10.4172/2469-6676.100068.
49. Fassino S, Abbate-Daga G, Leombruni P, Amianto F, Rovera G, Rovera GG. Temperament and character in italian men with anorexia nervosa: a controlled study with the temperament and character inventory. J Nerv Ment Dis. 2001;189(11):788–94.
50. Stice E. Risk and maintenance factors for eating pathology: a meta-analytic review. Psychol Bull. 2002;128(5):825–48.
51. Levine MP, Piran N. The role of body image in the prevention of eating disorders. Body Image. 2004;1(1):57–70.

Body Image Disturbances in Other Specified Feeding and Eating Disorders (OSFED)

11

Patrizia Todisco

11.1 Introduction

Body image disturbance is clinically widespread among eating disorders (ED) even though in the latest edition of the Diagnostic and Statistical Manual for Mental Disorders (DSM-5) [1] isn't an essential criterion for all of them and the comprehensive category of Feeding and Eating Disorders (FED). Formerly categorized as Eating Disorders Not Otherwise Specified (EDNOS), the Other Specified Feeding and Eating Disorder (OSFED) category includes warning signs and related medical/psychological conditions that are similar to and sometimes just as severe as those of the other ED even though frequently individuals satisfying the criteria for these syndromes are considered less critical. This condition is also termed Feeding or Eating Disorders Not Elsewhere Classified (FED-NEC).

In the newly defined OSFED category, the disturbance of body image is not explicitly mentioned or required, but it's implicit in the definition of some of the disorders included in the category. In fact, OSFED criteria apply to presentations in which symptoms characteristic of a feeding and eating disorder that cause clinically significant distress or impairment in social, occupational, or other important areas of functioning predominate but do not meet the full criteria for any of the disorders in the FED diagnostic class [1]. The OSFED category is used in situations in which the clinician chooses to communicate the precise reason that the presentation does not meet the criteria for any distinct feeding and eating disorder [1]. In such a case, the DSM-5 record is OSFED followed by the exact reason (e.g. "bulimia nervosa of low frequency") [1]. According to DSM-5 [1], examples of presentations that can be defined using the "other specified" description include the following:

P. Todisco
Eating Disorders Unit, Villa Margherita, Vicenza, Italy
e-mail: patrizia.todisco@casadicuravillamargherita.it; ptodis@tin.it

M. Cuzzolaro, S. Fassino (eds.), *Body Image, Eating, and Weight*,
https://doi.org/10.1007/978-3-319-90817-5_11

- Atypical anorexia nervosa (AAN): All of the criteria for anorexia nervosa are met, except that, despite significant weight loss, the individual's weight is within or above the normal range.
- Subthreshold bulimia nervosa (SBN): All of the criteria for bulimia nervosa are met, except that the binge eating and inappropriate compensatory behaviours occur, on average, less than once a week or for less than 3 months.
- Subthreshold binge-eating disorder (SBED): All of the criteria for binge-eating disorder are met, except that the binge eating occurs, on average, less than once a week or for less than 3 months.
- Purging disorder (PD): Recurrent purging behaviour to influence weight or shape (e.g. self-induced vomiting; misuse of laxatives, diuretics, or other medications) in the absence of binge eating.
- Night eating syndrome (NES): Recurrent episodes of night eating, as manifested by eating after awakening from sleep or by excessive food consumption after the evening meal. There are awareness and recall of the eating. The night eating is not better explained by external influences such as changes in the individual's sleep-wake cycle or by local social norms. The night eating causes significant distress and impairment in functioning. The disordered pattern of eating is not better explained by binge-eating disorder or another mental disorder, including substance use, and is not attributable to another medical disorder or an effect of a medication.

In addition to OSFED, the DSM-5 created another residual category—Unspecified Feeding or Eating Disorder (UFED)—that applies to presentations in which symptoms are clinically significant but do not meet criteria for any other diagnostic category. This diagnosis does not require detailing why the criteria are not met for a specific disorder. It includes presentations in which there is insufficient information to make a more straightforward diagnosis [1].

11.2 DSM-5 OSFED and UFED: Epidemiological and Clinical Data

Because of its recent definition we have a small number of data expressly addressing OSFED characteristics so we refer to studies mainly analysing EDNOS, the DSM-IV residual category which included all patients that cannot be recognized in the main categories Anorexia Nervosa and Bulimia Nervosa, and also to general population's studies.

The 2-stage survey performed by Mustelin and colleagues gives an idea of the epidemiological impact of the DSM-5 changes [2]. They examined a cohort of almost 3000 Finnish twin women (age 22–27 years) with a screening questionnaire and a diagnostic interview and found that 21% of women with an eating disorder fell in the residual OSFED and UFED categories. The lifetime prevalence of DSM-IV EDNOS (including BED) in their sample was 3.9% (3.3% excluding BED) whereas the lifetime prevalence of OSFED-UFED was 1.5%. Therefore, they observed a 62% reduction in the size of the residual diagnostic category. They also reported that only 37% of the residual category could be diagnosed as OSFED (13% AAN; 10% SBN; 11% SBED; 3% PD) whereas 63% were UFED (subthreshold/atypical ED different from presentations suggested in DSM-5) [2].

This crude prevalence estimate was in line with data obtained in Australia (1–1.4%) [3], the Netherlands (0.8%) [4], and Portugal (2.0%) [5]. However, some other studies found different values in the USA (11.5% FED-NEC; 2.8% AAN, 4.4% SBN, 3.6% SBED, 3.4% purging disorder) [6] and in Australia (9.7%, 5% OSFED and 4.7% UFED) [7, 8].

In an Italian study [9], the application of DSM-5 criteria to 206 patients (age 15–56 years), previously studied and classified according to DSM-IV, produced a decrease in EDNOS by 17%, and 30.8% was reclassified as OSFED.

Applying DSM-5 criteria to 1654 subjects (female and male adolescents) through a structured inventory, Hammerle and colleagues [10] found a prevalence of 3.6% for AAN, 0% for SBN, 0% for SBED, and 1.9% for PD. They also used a hierarchical approach to obtain the prevalence rates of partial syndromes (satisfying only the main criteria for a disorder, but not all the ones required; 10.9% for AN, 0.2% for BN, and 2.1% for BED) and of subthreshold syndromes (for reasons different from low duration or low frequency; 0.8% for AN, 0.3% for BN, and 0.2% for BED), and they acquired discordant data [10].

A review on PD [11] revealed a lifetime prevalence between 1.1 and 5.3%. These results were recently confirmed in a community sample of female twins (3.77%) [12]. A 9-years follow-up study performed in Germany with a PD inpatient population [13] observed a crude mortality rate of 5.0% and a standardized mortality ratio of 3.9 (95% CI; 2.05; 7.21). In that sample, the age at admission and the presence of one or more comorbid somatic illnesses at admission were negative outcome factors [13]. Using a large naturalistic Swedish ED database [14], 2233 adult women were diagnosed using DSM-5. Few meaningful differences emerged among AN binge/purge type, PD and BN [14], and PD did not appear to constitute a distinct diagnosis. The same study [14] also showed that the DSM-5 distinction between atypical AN and PD requires clarification. As far as the biological factors that may contribute to purging disorder, Keel and colleagues [15] investigated the satiety peptide YY (PYY) and the hunger peptide ghrelin. These authors discovered that PD subjects had: (1) a significantly greater postprandial PYY response compared to BN-purging (BNp) patients and controls; (2) Ghrelin levels significantly higher compared to control and similar to BNp individuals. Findings support the physiological distinction between PD and BN.

In the Finnish investigation cited before [2], the incidence rate per 100,000 person-years among women aged 10–24 years was 270 for EDNOS including BED (230 excluding BED) and 92 for OSFED/UFED, the mean age of onset of OSFED-UFED was 18 (range 14–25) years, the median duration of symptoms was 2 years (ranging from a few months to 10 years), and the 5-year probability of recovery was 60% (95% CI 43–77%).

In a community sample of adolescent females [6], lifetime prevalence by age 20 was 2.8% for AAN, 4.4% for SBN, 3.6% for SBED, 3.4% for PD. The peak age of onset was 18–20 for PD and overall FED-NEC [6]. Youth with these ED typically reported greater functional impairment, distress, suicidality, mental health treatment, and unhealthy BMI, though effect sizes were relatively smaller for AAN, SBN, and PD [6]. Average episode duration in months ranged from 2.9 for BN to 11.2 for AAN [6]. One-year remission rates ranged from 71% for AAN to 100% for BN, SBN, and BED [6]. Recurrence rates ranged from 6% for PD to 33% for BED and SBED [6]. Diagnostic progression from subthreshold to threshold ED was higher for BN and BED (32 and 28%) than for AN (0%), suggesting some escalation mechanism for binge eating [6].

Mustelin et al. [2] discovered also that DSM-5 residual category was difficult to detect by clinicians and that there were no significant differences between OSFED and UFED as far as mean age of onset (18 vs. 19 years, $p = 0.09$), median duration of illness (3 vs. 2 years, $p = 0.57$), or proportion recovered at the time of the interview (57% vs. 63%, $p = 0.74$). The authors [2] ascribed the differences among studies to the diagnostic methods applied, the characteristics of the samples, and the unclear separation between OSFED and UFED that seems of doubtful utility and needs at least the definition of a minimal level of psychopathology for UFED [14].

Subjects belonging to OSFED category mimic the clinical characteristics of main disorders (at a low level or a low frequency) so have similar clinical manifestations and complications [6, 7]. They usually show disturbed eating habits and intense fear of gaining weight; some have distorted body image, are seriously concerned about their weight and body shape and exhibit high level of anxiety or agitation approaching meals.

From a conceptual point of view, some authors believe that there is a continuum from altered eating behaviours and concerns about body shape and weight to typical anorexic and bulimic disorders; others classify them as subcategories of full or mixed disorders [6, 7, 10].

OSFED is sometimes misinterpreted as a "subclinical" or "subthreshold" diagnosis in terms of severity, and frequently they don't receive clinical attention (only 11% of them) [2]. Individuals with OSFED have poor Quality of Life and impairment increases with illness severity, particularly in the presence of binge/purge behaviours [16]. They often require the same level of treatment and support as those with major ED, and without treatment, a significant number of individuals with OSFED may go on to meet full criteria for AN, BN, or BED at some point during their illness [10].

In an analysis of results of ED treatment, Keel and Brown [17] found similar 5-year outcomes for patients with BN and EDNOS. They also reported that 75% of EDNOS patients recovered; however, the other 25% had chronic courses of disease [17].

In many women with OSFED-UFED, symptoms are quite long-standing, and over a third suffers from comorbid psychiatric disorders, which means that psychiatric comorbidity is nearly as common as among individuals with full-syndrome ED [6, 7, 18]. In particular [2], among subjects meeting criteria for OSFED, 43% has a lifetime diagnosis of major depressive disorder and 21% diagnosis of obsessive-compulsive disorder. Other psychiatric symptoms reported by OSFED patients refer to post-traumatic stress disorder, phobias, and psychosis.

Comorbidity with personality disorders in a meta-analysis [18] was noteworthy reaching a proportion of 0.38 for any personality disorders, 0.38% for cluster C (avoidant 0.18, obsessive-compulsive 0.11) and 0.25 for cluster B (borderline 0.12). One study [19] found that 75% of individuals with EDNOS had co-occurring psychiatric disorders and 25% had suicidal thoughts; moreover, adolescents with subthreshold AN (SAN) endorsed more anxiety than AN ($p < 0.05$), and adolescents and adults with SAN reported more suicidal plans than AN (p's < 0.05) [19]. Comparisons between BN and SBN didn't demonstrate significant differences in general psychopathology and personality traits [20].

Sawyer et al. [21] compared adolescents affected by AAN (not underweight in spite of significant weight loss) with full-threshold AN patients and reported that the formers were more likely to be overweight or obese before the onset of ED symptoms (71% vs. 12%), and had lost more weight (17.6 vs. 11.0 kg) over a more extended period (13.3 vs. 10.2 months). The frequency of psychiatric comorbidities (38% vs. 45%) and suicidal ideation (43% vs. 39%) was no different in the two groups. Distress related to eating and body image was more severe in AAN patients than in those with full-syndrome AN [21]. Despite having a healthier weight, the atypical group was as severely affected by dysfunctional metacognitions and drive for thinness as the typical group [22].

Le Grange and colleagues [23] investigated AAN and full-syndrome AN through a momentary ecological assessment and reported higher rates of checking thighs and joints in the former compared to the second.

Nakai et al. [24] reported in a Japanese sample that atypical AN may be distinguished in two subtypes in terms of fat phobia and body image disturbance: Nonfat-phobic AN (NFP-AN) (22.5% of the entire sample) and AN with fat phobia but no evidence of distortions related to body shape and weight (AN-NED) (25.3% of the whole sample). Interestingly, all the participants who at the beginning fulfilled all the diagnostic criteria for AN except Criterion B, subsequently admitted that they had fat phobia. These two subtypes had a shorter duration of illness compared to the typical AN group and didn't report any transition to the full syndrome during the 2- to 7-year follow-up period. Compared to those with typical AN: NFP-AN patients had less psychopathology, but the outcome resulted not different or rather worse; the AN-NED group reported significantly lower scores in most psychometric variables, but higher scores in most psychiatric variables than the NFP-AN group. Patients with NFP-AN or AN-NED never went on a diet for slimness: NFP-AN started to lose weight due to somatic or psychiatric disorders such as infectious diseases, gastrointestinal diseases, and depression; AN-NED refused to eat due to poor skills of social adaptation. These results suggest that the NFP-AN and AN-NED groups may not represent early stages of the typical AN group [24].

Silén et al. [25] discovered that AAN patients were significantly older ($p = 0.03$), heavier (minimum body mass index 16.7 vs. 15.1 kg/m^2, $p = 0.003$), and less prone to comorbidities (38% vs. 71%, $p = 0.04$) and had shorter, less intensive, and less costly treatments than typical AN patients. The only significant predictor of treatment success was the diagnosis: recovery from AAN was 4.3 times as likely as recovery from typical AN.

A recent study [26] demonstrated that patient with AN and AAN with a history of overweight/obesity are less likely to receive inpatient medical care, despite greater degree of weight loss and no difference in duration of illness, due to presenting at a higher weight.

Wade and O'Shea [8] reported data about UFED in adolescents comparing subjects with no-ED, AN and AAN. They found that individuals with UFED were in the overweight range while striving to lose weight, placed a high degree of importance on weight and shape in their self-evaluation, were indistinguishable from the two eating disorder groups on measures of global eating disorder severity, and demonstrated significantly elevated impairment and distress compared to the no-ED group commensurate with the ED groups.

Stice et al. [27] collected data from three prevention trials that targeted young women with body dissatisfaction ($N = 1272$; Mean age = 18.5, SD = 4.2) over a 3-year follow-up to identify predictors of subthreshold/threshold AN, BN, BED, and PD. Negative affect and functional impairment predicted the onset of all ED. Thin-ideal internalization, body dissatisfaction, dieting, overeating, and mental health care predicted the onset of subthreshold/threshold BN, BED, and PD. Positive thinness expectations, denial of the cost of pursuing the thin ideal, and fasting predicted the onset of two of these three disorders. Low BMI and dieting specifically predicted the onset of subthreshold/threshold AN Results provide support for the theory that pursuit of the thin ideal and the resulting body dissatisfaction, dieting, and unhealthy weight control behaviours increase the risk for binge/purge spectrum ED, and suggest that youth who are inherently lean, rather than purposely pursuing the thin ideal, are at risk for AN.

The Thought-Shape Fusion Body Questionnaire (TSF-B) [28] was developed and validated to assess the trait susceptibility to the experience of body-related cognitive distortions associated with ED and the imagination of thin ideals. Both the total scale and its two subscales (Imagination of thin ideals and Striving for own thin ideal) showed good ability to discriminate between individuals with subthreshold/clinical ED and healthy controls. The possibility that TSF-B is predictive for the development and course of ED is under study [28].

The OSFED category includes night eating syndrome (NES), a disorder characterized by evening hyperphagia and nocturnal ingestions in addition to sleep and mood disturbances. Associations between NES, eating disorder behaviours and attitudes (e.g. elevated shape concerns), poor physical and psychosocial functioning, and maladaptive coping have been found [29].

The prevalence of NES using proposed diagnostic criteria was reported as 4–5.7% in university samples [29, 30], 1% in the general population, 6–14% in individuals seeking treatment related to obesity [31], and 22.4% in a psychiatric outpatient population [32]. NES among psychiatric outpatients is associated with depression, impulse control disorder, nicotine dependency, body dissatisfaction, and higher symptom severity [32].

Compared to controls, non-obese persons with NES reported significantly different circadian distribution of food intake, greater depressed mood, sleep disturbance, disordered eating and body image concerns, perceived stress, decreased quality of life, and more frequent Axis I comorbidity, specifically anxiety, mood, and substance use disorders [33].

11.3 DSM-IV EDNOS, DSM-5 OSFED, and Body Image

Taken as a whole, ED patients are over-concerned with their body image and weight (see Chap. 4 of this book). Body image is a multidimensional construct consisting of a mental picture of one's physical body (including size, shape, and appearance) and one's attitude toward the physical self (e.g. thoughts, feelings, and beliefs about one's body) [34, 35], laying on a continuum from healthy body perceptions (i.e. accurate and mostly positive) to unhealthy body perceptions (i.e. inaccurate and mostly negative) (see Chap. 1 of this book).

Body image incorporates perceptual, affective, and cognitive components as well as behavioural features [36] and focuses on evaluations (i.e. dissatisfaction with the size or shape of the stomach, arms, etc.) or body image perceptions (i.e. believing that one's body is larger or smaller than one's perceived ideal) [37].

Having distorted oversized body image leads the patients with an ED to body dissatisfaction, resulting in negative thoughts and feelings about their own body, reinforces the fear of gaining weight or becoming fat and may have negative consequences (e.g. depression, anxiety, poor self-esteem, eating behaviour, sexual behaviour, and emotional stability) and is influenced by specific life context and quality of life [37]. These concerns usually are intrusive and pervasive and represent a risk factor in the development, persistence, and relapses of ED, having thus a prognostic value [36, 37].

The mechanisms underlying a distorted body image in ED patients remain unclear [38], but the development of neurocognitive sciences produced studies that evoked a primary impairment in the processing of spatial reference frames along with an inability to update stored representations of body shape [39]. EDs may be the outcome of impairment in the ability to update a negative body representation stored in autobiographical memory (allocentric) with real-time sensorimotor and proprioceptive data (egocentric) [40]. Recent behavioural and neuroimaging evidence from non-clinical and clinical populations (e.g. ED patients) suggests that basic interoceptive processes and interoceptive awareness may crucially contribute to the complex formation of body image, as well as to its disturbances. In particular, lower interoceptive accuracy and awareness are associated with body-image concerns [41].

Objectification theory [42] is another way to explain body dissatisfaction, and it posits that women internalize the societal message that their bodies are objects, valuable only for their potential use by others. As a result, women come to view their bodies as objects (self-objectification) and engage in habitual body monitoring. This self-objectification, in turn, is hypothesized to be associated with negative psychological consequences, such as depression, anxiety, body dissatisfaction, and disordered eating [43].

According to Brogna and Caroppo [44], people with EDNOS perceive their bodies in the presence of other people mainly as body-for-others (how one experiences one's own body when someone else is looking at it, and the subject-body being can become conscious of being a body-object for others). Therefore, EDNOS could be conceived as an anthropological configuration vulnerable to ED rather than a diagnostic category. ED appear as an "identity disorder" characterized by a suspension of the experiential polarity between self and other-than-self.

Some studies that aimed to develop empirically based classifications established that body image disturbance might distinguish categorically distinct disorders of eating [45]. In particular, the single indicator that characterizes an eating disorder latent group with no weight phobia from healthy controls and the other eating disorder groups (AN, BN, BED) is level of body image disturbance [45]. These findings may underline some of OSFED characteristics.

Body Dysmorphic Disorder (BDD) (see Chap. 5 of this book) and ED commonly co-occur (when BDD consists of other appearance concerns that do not involve weight or body fat, as specified by BDD's DSM-5 criterion D) and the most difficult differentiation is between BDD and OSFED [38]. In samples of patients with BDD lifetime prevalence rates of OSFED are 17.5% and, conversely, 38.5% of OSFED reported a BDD [46].

Mitchison et al. [47] investigated two non-clinical cohorts of women, symptomatic and asymptomatic of EDs, to assess if symptoms theoretically associated with Body Dysmorphic Disorder are experienced by, predictive of, and associated with impairment in women with probable EDs. Participants with probable EDs reported more severe BDD symptoms than healthy controls and the items on which BDD and ED subjects scored similarly tended to measure the frequency of mental and behavioural acts such as appearance checking, reassurance-seeking, camouflaging, comparison-making, and social avoidance. These authors [47] discovered that the vast majority of items on the Body Dysmorphic Disorder Examination Self Report (BDDE-SR) had high specificity in predicting probable ED cases. Conversely fewer items (particularly those items measuring checking, camouflaging, and comparison-making behaviours; as well as preoccupation and dissatisfaction with appearance) had high sensitivity to ED cases, meaning that not all people with EDs experience BDD-type features. All of these items also had reasonably high specificity, and thus there is a strong case that these symptoms are particularly predictive of people with EDs. The presence of clinical BDD symptoms was also associated with greater impairment in quality of life and greater psychological distress in participants with EDs [47]. Subthreshold-BDD individuals reported significantly lower ED and hyperactivity than probable-BDD subjects [48].

In clinical and non-clinical samples of individuals with ED has been demonstrated a co-presence of altered body image and alexithymia as well as feelings of shame [49]. Shame seems to hold a prevalent role in the structuring of body-image disorder, and the link between feelings of shame and the perception of an adverse body image is aggravated by previous threatening events like traumatic experiences. Alexithymia may be a consequence of previous traumatic experiences and feelings of shame that have remained unelaborated. It seems partially associated with adverse image disorders; it appears as though alexithymia is mostly a covariant of other psychopathologic traits or experiences, at least in bulimic patients [49].

In a study investigating body dissatisfaction (BD) in adolescents with different diagnostic categories of ED [50], EDNOS presented 8.3% of the dissatisfaction group according to Body Shape Questionnaire-34 (BSQ-34). Considering BSQ-34 total scores, four categories were established with respect to body image concerns, and EDNOS patients distributed in the different categories as follow: no-concern group 10.3%; mild concern group 2%; moderate concern group 7.8%; extreme concern group 0%. The correlation between BD and depression was significant and positive, while that between BD and self-esteem was significant and negative. The results demonstrate that patients showing more BD have more depressive symptoms and that a poor body image is usually associated with low self-esteem (at least one-third of the self-esteem is linked to positive or negative self-image). According to this study, an individual cannot appreciate personal qualities as dexterity, intelligence, or work regardless of his/her body appreciation, especially in women, who usually subordinate many of these qualities to the physical appeal. Laporta-Herrero and colleagues also reported that BD is directly related to sociocultural influences that contribute to the internalization of the current aesthetic body shape model (extreme thinness). Patients who show higher BD usually have more abnormal eating attitudes, especially those related to the fear of gaining weight, drive for thinness, and restrictive eating patterns [50].

In a registry-based Swedish sample of ED patients, negative self-image variables were associated with prior suicide attempts in ANR and EDNOS (SAN, SBN, and PD) [51].

In a study comparing healthy controls and ED patients as far as the relevance of social and self-standards, Gunnard et al. [52] found that high self-standards in physical appearance were more relevant in BN and EDNOS. The treatment of body image disturbances is considered a relevant facet of the therapeutic approach to ED [53] because BD represents one of the most consistent risk factors for developing and maintaining an ED that can be modified [50].

A recent meta-analysis suggested that the effect sizes of the principal treatments for body image disturbance were relatively small [54] and we need to ameliorate them.

Moreover, studies regarding OSFED patients are lacking. A novel adaptation of a cognitive bias training programme [55] was applied to women with AAN, and they recalibrated the body size judgements and reduced their body size and eating-disordered concerns. Data suggest that the response to CBT in terms of reduction in weight and shape concerns is not influenced by distinction between threshold and subthreshold AN [56], BN and SBN [20], BED and SBED [57]. Furthermore, the shape concern level at baseline seems to represent the main risk factor for recovery and treatment resistance [56].

References

1. American Psychiatric Association. Diagnostic and statistical manual of mental disorders. 5th ed. Arlington: American Psychiatric Publishing; 2013.
2. Mustelin L, Lehtokari V-L, Keski-Rahkonen A. Other specified and unspecified feeding or ED among women in the community. Int J Eat Disord. 2016;49:1010–7. https://doi.org/10.1002/eat.22586.
3. Hay P, Girosi F, Mond J. Prevalence and sociodemographic correlates of DSM-5 ED in the Australian population. J Eat Disord. 2015;3:19. https://doi.org/10.1186/s40337-015-0056-0.

4. Smink FRE, van Hoeken D, Oldehinkel AJ, Hoek HW. Prevalence and severity of DSM-5 ED in a community cohort of adolescents. Int J Eat Disord. 2014;47:610–9. https://doi.org/10.1002/eat.22316.
5. Machado PPP, Gonçalves S, Hoek HW. DSM-5 reduces the proportion of ednos cases: evidence from community samples. Int J Eat Disord. 2013;46:60–5. https://doi.org/10.1002/eat.22040.
6. Stice E, Marti CN, Rohde P. Prevalence, incidence, impairment, and course of the proposed DSM-5 eating disorder diagnoses in an 8-year prospective community study of young women. J Abnorm Psychol. 2013;122(2):445–7. https://doi.org/10.1037/a0030679.
7. Fairweather-Schmidt AK, Wade TD. DSM-5 ED and other specified eating and feeding disorders: is there a meaningful differentiation? Int J Eat Disord. 2014;47:524–33. https://doi.org/10.1002/eat.22257.
8. Wade TD, O'Shea A. DSM-5 unspecified feeding and ED in adolescents: what do they look like and are they clinically significant? Int J Eat Disord. 2015;48:367–74. https://doi.org/10.1002/eat.22303.
9. Gualandi M, Simoni M, Manzato E, Scanelli G. Reassessment of patients with ED after moving from DSM-IV towards DSM-5: a retrospective study in a clinical sample. Eat Weight Disord. 2016;21:617–24. https://doi.org/10.1007/s40519-016-0314-4.
10. Hammerle F, Huss M, Ernst V, Bürger A. Thinking dimensional: prevalence of DSM-5 early adolescent full syndrome, partial and subthreshold ED in a cross-sectional survey in German schools. BMJ Open. 2016;6(5):e010843.
11. Keel PK. Purging disorder: subthreshold variant or full-threshold eating disorder? Int J Eat Disord. 2007;40:S89–94. https://doi.org/10.1002/eat.20453.
12. Munn-Chernoff MA, Keel PK, Klump KL, Grant JD, Bucholz KK, Madden PAF, Heath AC, Duncan AE. Prevalence of and familial influences on purging disorder in a community sample of female twins. Int J Eat Disord. 2015;48:601–6. https://doi.org/10.1002/eat.22378.
13. Koch S, Quadflieg N, Fichter M. Purging disorder: a pathway to death? A review of 11 cases. Eat Weight Disord. 2014;19(1):21–9. https://doi.org/10.1007/s40519-013-0082-3.
14. Ekeroth K, Clinton D, Norring C, Birgegård A. Clinical characteristics and distinctiveness of DSM-5 eating disorder diagnoses: findings from a large naturalistic clinical database. J Eat Disord. 2013;1:31. https://doi.org/10.1186/2050-2974-1-31.
15. Keel PK, Eckel LA, Hildebrandt BA, Haedt-Matt AA, Appelbaum J, Jimerson DC. Disturbance of gut satiety peptide in purging disorder. Int J Eat Disord. 2018;51:53–61. https://doi.org/10.1002/eat.22806.
16. DeJong H, Oldershaw A, Sternheim L, Samarawickrema N, Kenyon MD, Broadbent H, et al. Quality of life in anorexia nervosa, bulimia nervosa and eating disorder not-otherwise-specified. J Eat Disord. 2013;1:43. https://doi.org/10.1186/2050-2974-1-43.
17. Keel PK, Brown TA. Update on course and outcome in ED. Int J Eat Disord. 2010;43:195–204. https://doi.org/10.1002/eat.20810.
18. Friborg O, Martinussen M, Kaiser S, Øvergård KT, Martinsen EW, Schmierer P, Rosenvinge JH. Personality disorders in eating disorder not otherwise specified and binge eating disorder: a meta-analysis of comorbidity studies. J Nerv Ment Dis. 2014;202(2):119–25.
19. Le Grange D, Swanson SA, Crow SJ, Merikangas KR. Eating disorder not otherwise specified presentation in the US population. Int J Eat Disord. 2012;45(5):711–8. https://doi.org/10.1002/eat.22006.
20. Krug I, Casasnovas C, Granero R, Martinez C, Jiménez-Murcia S, Bulik C, Fernández-Aranda F. Comparison study of full and subthreshold bulimia nervosa: personality, clinical characteristics, and short-term response to therapy. Psychother Res. 2008;18(1):37–47.
21. Sawyer SM, Whitelaw M, Le Grange D, Yeo M, Hughes EK. Physical and psychological morbidity in adolescents with atypical anorexia nervosa. Pediatrics. 2016;137(4):e20154080. https://doi.org/10.1542/peds.2015-4080.
22. Davenport E, Rushford N, Soon S, McDermott C. Dysfunctional metacognition and drive for thinness in typical and atypical anorexia nervosa. J Eat Disord. 2015;3:24. https://doi.org/10.1186/s40337-015-0060-4.

23. Le Grange D, Crosby RD, Engel SG, Cao L, Ndungu A, Crow SJ, et al. DSM-IV-defined anorexia nervosa versus subthreshold anorexia nervosa (EDNOS-AN). Eur Eat Disord Rev. 2013;21(1):1–7. https://doi.org/10.1002/erv.2192.
24. Nakai Y, Nin K, Teramukai S, Taniguchi A, Fukushima M, Wonderlich SA. Typical and atypical anorexia nervosa in a Japanese sample. Int J Eat Disord. 2014;47:130–7. https://doi.org/10.1002/eat.22208.
25. Silén Y, Raevuori A, Jüriloo E, Tainio V-M, Marttunen M, Keski-Rahkonen A. Typical versus atypical anorexia nervosa among adolescents: clinical characteristics and implications for ICD-11. Eur Eat Disord Rev. 2015;23:345–51. https://doi.org/10.1002/erv.2370.
26. Kennedy GA, Forman SF, Woods ER, Hergenroeder AC, Mammel KA, Fisher MM, et al. History of overweight/obesity as predictor of care received at 1-year follow-up in adolescents with anorexia nervosa or atypical anorexia nervosa. J Adolesc Health. 2017;60(6):674–9.
27. Stice E, Gau JM, Rohde P, Shaw H. Risk factors that predict future onset of each DSM-5 eating disorder: predictive specificity in high-risk adolescent females. J Abnorm Psychol. 2017;126(1):38–51. https://doi.org/10.1037/abn0000219.
28. Wyssen A, Debbeler LJ, et al. Cognitive distortions associated with imagination of the thin ideal: validation of the thought-shape fusion body questionnaire (TSF-B). Front Psychol. 2017;8:2194.
29. Runfola CD, Allison KC, Hardy KK, Lock J, Peebles R. Prevalence and clinical significance of night eating syndrome in university students. J Adolesc Health. 2014;55(1):41–8. https://doi.org/10.1016/j.jadohealth.2013.11.012
30. Nolan LJ, Geliebter A. Night eating is associated with emotional and external eating in college students. Eat Behav. 2012;13(3):202–5. https://doi.org/10.1016/j.eatbeh.2012.02.002.
31. Milano W, De Rosa M, Milano L, Capasso A. Night eating syndrome: an overview. J Pharm Pharmacol. 2012;64:2–10. https://doi.org/10.1111/j.2042-7158.2011.01353.x.
32. Saraçlı Ö, Atasoy N, Akdemir A, Güriz O, Konuk N, Sevinçer GM, Ankaralı H, Atik L. The prevalence and clinical features of the night eating syndrome in psychiatric out-patient population. Compr Psychiatry. 2015;57:79–84. https://doi.org/10.1016/j.comppsych.2014.11.007.
33. Lundgren JD, Allison KC, O'Reardon JP, Stunkard AJ. A descriptive study of non-obese persons with night eating syndrome and a weight-matched comparison group. Eat Behav. 2008;9(3):343–51. https://doi.org/10.1016/j.eatbeh.2007.12.004.
34. Cash TF. Cognitive-behavioral perspectives on body image. In: Cash TF, Pruzinsky T, editors. Body image: a handbook of theory, research, and clinical practice. New York: Guilford Press; 2002. p. 38–46.
35. Thompson JK, Heinberg LJ, Altabe M, Tantleff-Dunn S. Exacting beauty: theory, assessment, and treatment of body image disturbance. Washington, DC: American Psychological Association; 1999.
36. Thompson JK. The (mis)measurement of body image: ten strategies to improve assessment for applied and research purposes. Body Image. 2004;1:7–14.
37. Hrabosky JI, Cash TF, Veale D, Neziroglu F, Soll EA, Garner DM, et al. Multidimensional body image comparisons among patients with ED, body dysmorphic disorder, and clinical controls: a multisite study. Body Image. 2009;6:155–63. https://doi.org/10.1016/j.bodyim.2009.03.001.
38. Gailledrat L, Rousselet M, Venisse J-L, Lambert S, Rocher B, Remaud M, Guilleux A, Sauvaget A, Eyzop E, Grall-Bronnec M. Marked body shape concerns in female patients suffering from ED: relevance of a clinical sub-group. PLoS One. 2016;11(10):e0165232. https://doi.org/10.1371/journal.pone.0165232.
39. Serino S, Dakanalis A, Gaudio S, Carra G, Cipresso P, Clerici M, et al. Out of body, out of space: impaired reference frame processing in ED. Psychiatry Res. 2015;230(2):732–4. https://doi.org/10.1016/j.psychres.2015.10.025.
40. Riva G. Out of my real body: cognitive neuroscience meets ED. Front Human Neurosci. 2014;8:236. https://doi.org/10.3389/fnhum.2014.00236.
41. Badoud D, Tsakiris M. From the body's viscera to the body's image: is there a link between interoception and body image concerns? Neurosci Biobehav Rev. 2017;77:237–46. https://doi.org/10.1016/j.neubiorev.2017.03.017.

42. Fredrickson B, Roberts T. Objectification theory: toward understanding women's lived experiences and mental health risks. Psychol Women Q. 1997;21:173–206.
43. Mitchell KS, Mazzeo SE. Evaluation of a structural model of objectification theory and eating disorder symptomatology among European American and African American undergraduate women. Psychol Women Q. 2009;33(4):384–95. https://doi.org/10.1111/j.1471-6402.2009.01516.x.
44. Brogna P, Caroppo E. The body as a simulacrum of identity: the subjective experience in the ED. Ann Ist Super Sanita. 2010;46(4):427–35.
45. Keel PK, Holm-Denoma J, Crosby RD, Haedt AA, Gravener JA, Joiner TE. Latent structure of bulimic syndromes: an empirical approach utilizing latent profile analyses and taxometric analyses. In: Striegel-Moore RH, Wonderlich SA, Walsh BT, Mitchell JE, editors. Developing an evidence-based classification of ED: scientific findings for DSM-5. Washington, DC: American Psychiatric Association; 2011. p. 145–64.
46. Grant JE, Leppink EW, Redden SA. The relationship between body dysmorphic disorder and eating disorder. In: Phillips KA, editor. Body dysmorphic disorder: advances in research and clinical practice (chap. 36). Oxford: Oxford University Press; 2017.
47. Mitchison D, Crino R, Hay P. The presence, predictive utility, and clinical significance of body dysmorphic symptoms in women with ED. J Eat Disord. 2013;1:20. https://doi.org/10.1186/2050-2974-1-20.
48. Schneider SC, Mond J, Turner CM, Hudson JL. Subthreshold body dysmorphic disorder in adolescents: prevalence and impact. Psychiatry Res. 2017;251:125–30.
49. Franzoni E, Gualandi S, Caretti V, Schimmenti A, Di Pietro E, Pellegrini G, et al. The relationship between alexithymia, shame, trauma, and body image disorders: investigation over a large clinical sample. Neuropsychiatr Dis Treat. 2013;9:185–93. https://doi.org/10.2147/NDT.S34822.
50. Laporta-Herrero I, Jáuregui-Lobera I, Barajas-Iglesias B, Santed-Germán MÁ. Body dissatisfaction in adolescents with ED. Eat Weight Disord. 2016;30:1–9. https://doi.org/10.1007/s40519-016-0353-x.
51. Runfola CD, Thornton LM, Pisetsky EM, Bulik CM, Birgegård A. Self-image and suicide in a Swedish national ED clinical register. Compr Psychiatry. 2014;55(3):439–49. https://doi.org/10.1016/j.comppsych.2013.11.007.
52. Gunnard K, Krug I, Jiménez-Murcia S, Penelo E, Granero R, Treasure J, Tchanturia K, Karwautz A, Collier D, Menchón JM, Fernández-Aranda F. Relevance of social and self-standards in ED. Eur Eat Disord Rev. 2012;20(4):271–8. https://doi.org/10.1002/erv.1148.
53. Cash TF, Hrabosky JI. Treatment of body image disturbances. In: Thompson JK, editor. Handbook of ED and obesity. Hoboken: Wiley; 2004. p. 515–41.
54. Alleva JM, Sheeran P, Webb TL, Martijn C, Miles E. A meta-analytic review of stand- alone interventions to improve body image. PLoS One. 2015;10:e0139177. https://doi.org/10.1371/journal.pone.0139177.
55. Gledhill LJ, Cornelissen KK, Cornelissen PL, Penton-Voak IS, Munafò MR, Tovée MJ. An interactive training programme to treat body image disturbance. Br J Health Psychol. 2017;22(1):60–76.
56. Ricca V, Castellini G, Lo Sauro C, Mannucci E, Ravaldi C, Rotella F, Faravelli C. Cognitive-behavioral therapy for threshold and subthreshold anorexia nervosa: a three-year follow-up study. Psychother Psychosom. 2010;79(4):238–48.
57. Friederich H-C, Schild S, Wild B, De Zwaan M, Quenter A, Herzog W, Zipfel S. Treatment outcome in people with subthreshold compared with full-syndrome binge eating disorder. Obesity. 2007;15:283–7. https://doi.org/10.1038/oby.2007.545.

Orthorexia Nervosa and Body Image 12

Anna Brytek-Matera and Lorenzo M. Donini

The term orthorexia nervosa (ON) was introduced by Steven Bratman in 1997 [1] to describe a "condition" characterised by a pathological fixation with healthy eating and proper nutrition. Differently by anorexia nervosa (AN) or bulimia nervosa (BN), the primary concern is not the quantity of food consumed, but the quality of food [2, 3]. ON has not yet been recognised as an eating disorder (ED) (and it has not been included in the DSM-5), and there is an ongoing discussion concerning its definition and the characterisation of diagnostic criteria. The link with other ED is under debate since ON is considered by some Authors as a socially acceptable method of weight control for individuals with AN and BN (coping strategy) or a risk factor for a "classical" ED when patients switch from an obsession with the quality of food to an obsession with its quantity [4, 5]. In any case, a growing number of PubMed articles refer to the word *orthorexia* as a keyword (83 papers on 18.02.2018; https://www.ncbi.nlm.nih.gov/pubmed/?term=orthorexia) with a tendency to an increase in publications in the last years [6].

Orthorexia nervosa is characterised by a desire to consume a healthy diet. The classification of food as healthy or harmful is autonomously given by the subject with ON and it doesn't coincide in most cases with any real risk [2]. Consequently, individuals suffering from ON eliminate from their diet food that is, individually, perceived as impure or not suitable. Their diet may be therefore very restrictive with a high risk of insufficient intake of certain nutrients [7]. Besides, the obsessive pre-occupation with food and its source is characterised by a pathological level of concern and stress regarding food [8] that may lead to a significant amount of time (more than 3 h per day) spent on seeking, examining, and preparing meal [7].

A. Brytek-Matera
SWPS University of Social Sciences and Humanities, Katowice, Poland

L. M. Donini (✉)
Sapienza University of Rome, Rome, Italy
e-mail: lorenzomaria.donini@uniroma1.it

M. Cuzzolaro, S. Fassino (eds.), *Body Image, Eating, and Weight*,
https://doi.org/10.1007/978-3-319-90817-5_12

Due to certain similarities between ON and AN, some Authors have focused their research on factors that have been implicated in the development and maintenance of EDs (body image, perfectionism, attachment style, self-esteem) [9–11] to verify their role in ON.

The term body image represents a global conceptualisation of perceptions, attitudes, and behaviours. The characteristics of the body image concept are presented in Table 12.1.

Concern about body image and internalisation of the thin ideal are dominant in eating disorders (EDs) [13]. Behaviours and psychopathology related to body image in EDs are presented in Fig. 12.1.

Table 12.1 Main characteristics of body image (adapted from Cash and Pruzinsky, 1990) [12]

• Components of body image
Perceptions (size and shape of various aspect of the body)
Cognitions (thoughts, beliefs, and self-statements concerning body)
Emotions (experiences of (dis)comfort, (dis)satisfaction associated to appearance)
• Body image experiences are linked to feelings towards the "self"
• Body image is a construct determined by socio-cultural factors
• Body image is changeable
• Body image influences the information processing (people who are schematic with respect to their physical appearance process the information in terms of competence in body attractiveness)
• Body image influences behaviour
• Body image concept is multifaceted (body experiences encompasses the perceptions and attitudes towards appearance, body shape and size, aspect relating to physical condition, health, and disease)

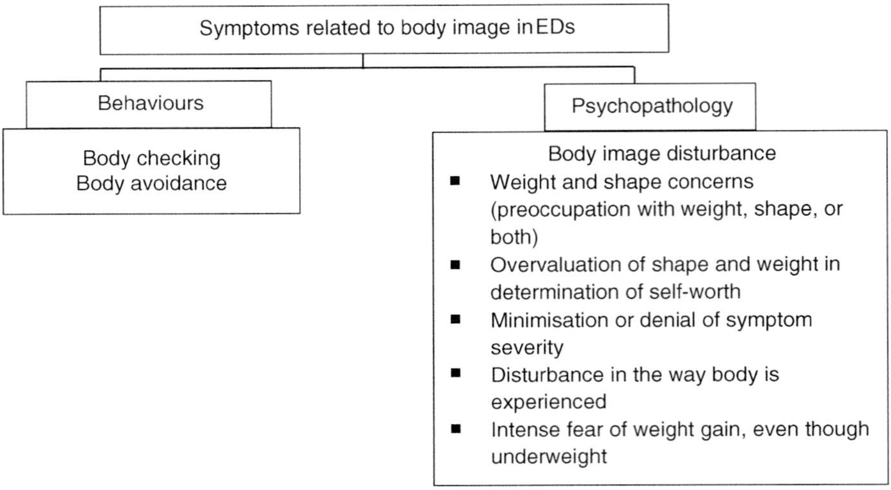

Fig. 12.1 Symptoms related to body image in eating disorders

ON did not include the most characteristic symptoms of EDs such as fear of becoming fat and overestimation of body size. The literature suggests that individuals with ON are not concerned with weight loss, while the presence of body dissatisfaction is not universally accepted. Some studies found no clear and significant association between ON and negative body image attitudes [14], while in other studies the concern about body image was found to be present in ON.

The latest research has shown that ON involves both the associations related to disturbed eating-related behaviours and cognitive preoccupations about body shape and weight [4]. In ED patients, orthorexic behaviour was negatively predicted by eating pathology, weight concern, health orientation, and appearance evaluation and body areas satisfaction [15].

In a paper published by Brytek-Matera et al., the Authors found that in female students with ON "low body areas (parts) satisfaction, high fitness orientation, high overweight preoccupation, and high appearance orientation were independent predictors of greater fixation on eating healthy food" [16].

These data are consistent with another study where it was found that fitness participants who displayed orthorexic tendencies showed internalisation of a thin ideal as well as social physique anxiety associated with body image dissatisfaction and disordered eating [17].

ON, as well as other EDs, seems to be connected with social pressures. EDs are influenced by the thin-ideal standard of beauty, whereas ON is affected by the requirement for the healthy living [18]. Maintaining a healthy diet and having control over their own desires seems to be in ON more fulfilling and important than possible concerns about body image.

Self-esteem, which may be associated with body dissatisfaction, has been found to be lower among individuals suffering from AN and BN [19]. The literature suggests that self-esteem is associated with ON, but the results are not univocal.

The previous research has shown that self-esteem seems to be higher in ON than in non-orthorexic subjects [20] and adherence to dietary restriction may become linked to self-esteem individuals with ON tendency [21]. However, in another study [22] the results demonstrated a relationship between ON and lower self-esteem. The link between ON and self-esteem has not been confirmed in latest studies: self-esteem was not significantly correlated with ON [5].

Eating disorders (following the DSM-5 classification), muscle dysmorphia (see Chap. 4 of this book), and ON are different conditions affecting above all adolescents and young adults, with a relatively high prevalence and an important social impact.

These attitudes seem to be frequently associated, particularly in certain cohorts. It has been hypothesised that some students could choose a university course oriented on healthy food (e.g. school of Dietetics) and healthy body (e.g. Exercise and Sport Sciences school) because they have a pre-existent peculiar eating behaviour or pre-existing muscle dysmorphia traits. Anyway, individuals with traits of any of these disorders are more frequently on a diet, are highly concerned with body image, and are more frequently at risk of another disorder [23].

Cultural ideals of beauty strongly influence the behaviours of those who most desire to be socially accepted. Today's adolescents are bombarded with images of extreme thinness which represents, in Western culture, beauty, happiness, wealth, and popularity.

Social media contribute significantly to the promotion of these ideals. They can influence psychological well-being and behaviours by amplifying messages, which are bounced through the various communication modes, suggesting controversial or dangerous behaviours to achieve these goals (e.g. pro-ana blogs), and promoting negative social comparison in particular with media celebrities. Finally, a negative role on body image/dissatisfaction and disordered eating has been attributed to them in particular among young adults. In a recent online survey conducted on media users ($N = 680$) following health food accounts, and investigating eating behaviours and ON the Authors found that healthy eating community on Instagram has a high prevalence of orthorexia symptoms, with higher Instagram use being linked to increased symptoms [24, 25].

In conclusion, although body image dissatisfaction is not required at the moment for the diagnosis of ON, the discussion is going on, and this particular concern has been proposed among the possible diagnostic criteria or specifiers [6].

References

1. Bratman S. Orthorexia nervosa. Yoga J. 1997;136:42–50. http://www.orthorexia.com/original-orthorexia-essay/. Accessed May 2015.
2. Donini LM, Marsili D, Graziani MP, Imbriale M, Cannella C. Orthorexia nervosa: a preliminary study with a proposal for diagnosis and an attempt to measure the dimension of the phenomenon. Eat Weight Disord. 2004;9(2):151–7. https://doi.org/10.1007/BF03325060.
3. Segura-Garcia C, Ramacciotti C, Rania M, Aloi M, Caroleo M, Bruni A, Gazzarrini D, Sinopoli F, De Fazio P. The prevalence of orthorexia nervosa among eating disorder patients after treatment. Eat Weight Disord. 2015;20(2):161–6. https://doi.org/10.1007/s40519-014-0171-y.
4. Tremelling K, Sandon L, Vega GL, McAdams CJ. Orthorexia nervosa and eating disorder symptoms in registered dietitian nutritionists in the United States. J Acad Nutr Diet. 2017;117(10):1612–7. https://doi.org/10.1016/j.jand.2017.05.001. pii: S2212-2672(17)30448-3.
5. Barnes MA, Caltabiano ML. The interrelationship between orthorexia nervosa, perfectionism, body image and attachment style. Eat Weight Disord. 2017;22(1):177–84. https://doi.org/10.1007/s40519-016-0280-x.
6. Cuzzolaro M, Donini LM. Orthorexia nervosa by proxy? Eat Weight Disord. 2016;21(4):549–51.
7. Bratman S, Knight D. Health food junkies. Orthorexia nervosa: overcoming the obsession with healthful eating. New York: Brodways Books; 2000.
8. Koven NS, Abry AW. The clinical basis of orthorexia nervosa: emerging perspectives. Neuropsychiatr Dis Treat. 2015;11:385–94. https://doi.org/10.2147/NDT.S61665.
9. Brown AJ, Parman KM, Rudat DA, Craighead LW. Disordered eating, perfectionism, and food rules. Eat Behav. 2012;13(4):347. https://doi.org/10.1016/j.eatbeh.2012.05.011.
10. Zachrisson HD, Skårderud F. Feelings of insecurity: review of attachment and eating disorders. Eur Eat Disord Rev. 2010;18(2):97–106. https://doi.org/10.1002/erv.999.
11. Bardone-Cone AM, Wonderlich SA, Frost RO, Bulik CM, Mitchell JE, Uppala S, Simonich H. Perfectionism and eating disorders: current status and future directions. Clin Psychol Rev. 2007;27(3):384–405. https://doi.org/10.1016/j.cpr.2006.12.005.

12. Cash TF, Pruzinsky T, editors. Body images: development, deviance, and change. New York: Guilford Press; 1990.
13. Keel PK, Dorer DJ, Franko DL, Jackson SC, Herzog DB. Postremission predictors of relapse in women with eating disorders. Am J Psychiatry. 2005;162(12):2263–8. https://doi.org/10.1176/appi.ajp.162.12.2263.
14. Aksoydan E, Camci N. Prevalence of orthorexia nervosa among Turkish performance artists. Eat Weight Disord. 2009;14(1):33–7.
15. Brytek-Matera A, Rogoza R, Gramaglia C, Zeppegno P. Predictors of orthorexic behaviours in patients with eating disorders: a preliminary study. BMC Psychiatry. 2015;15:252. https://doi.org/10.1186/s12888-015-0628-1.
16. Brytek-Matera A, Donini LM, Krupa M, Poggiogalle E, Hay P. Erratum to: Orthorexia nervosa and self-attitudinal aspects of body image in female and male university students. J Eat Disord. 2016;4:16. https://doi.org/10.1186/s40337-016-0105-3. eCollection 2016.
17. Eriksson L, Baigi A, Marklund B, Lindgren EC. Social physique anxiety and sociocultural attitudes toward appearance impact on orthorexia test in fitness participants. Scand J Med Sci Sports. 2008;18(3):389–94. https://doi.org/10.1111/j.1600-0838.2007.00723.x.
18. Martins MCT, Alvarenga MS, Vargas SVA, Sato KSCJ, Scagliusi FB. Ortorexia nervosa: reflexões sobre um novo conceito. Rev Nutr. 2011;24(2):345–57.
19. Gual P, Pérez-Gaspar M, Martínez-González MA, Lahortiga F, Irala-Estévez JD, Cervera-Enguix S. Self-esteem, personality, and eating disorders: baseline assessment of a prospective population-based cohort. Int J Eat Disord. 2002;31(3):261–73. https://doi.org/10.1002/eat.10040.
20. Kinzl JF, Hauer K, Traweger C, Kiefer I. Orthorexia nervosa in dieticians. Psychother Psychosom. 2006;75(6):395–6. https://doi.org/10.1159/000095447.
21. Bundros J, Clifford D, Silliman K, Neyman Morris M. Prevalence of orthorexia nervosa among college students based on Bratman's test and associated tendencies. Appetite. 2016;101:86–94. https://doi.org/10.1016/j.appet.2016.02.144.
22. Barthels F, Meyer F, Pietrowsky R. Orthorexic eating behavior. A new type of disordered eating. Ernährungs Umschau. 2015;62:156–61.
23. Bo S, Zoccali R, Ponzo V, Soldati L, De Carli L, Benso A, Fea E, Rainoldi A, Durazzo M, Fassino S, Abbate-Daga G. University courses, eating problems and muscle dysmorphia: are there any associations? J Transl Med. 2014;12:221. https://doi.org/10.1186/s12967-014-0221-2.
24. Turner PG, Lefevre CE. Instagram use is linked to increased symptoms of orthorexia nervosa. Eat Weight Disord. 2017;22(2):277–84. https://doi.org/10.1007/s40519-017-0364-2.
25. Cartwright MM. Eating disorder emergencies: understanding the medical complexities of the hospitalized eating disordered patient. Crit Care Nurs Clin North Am. 2004;16(4):515–30.

13 Obesities: Controversies in Diagnosis and Classification

Ottavio Bosello, Angiola Vanzo, Maria Pia Donataccio, and Massimo Cuzzolaro

13.1 Introduction

The work has the purpose of elucidating the origin and current use of the concepts of metabolically healthy obesity (MHO), metabolically obese normal-weight (MONW), and obesity-survival paradox (OP), taking into account the most recent literature contributions on this subject.

This chapter is an updating of a previous article [1] of the same authors used with permission (Springer Nature and Copyright Clearance Center, License Number 4293160192587, License date Feb 20, 2018).

Obesity is described as an excess accumulation of body fat, but there is no accepted definition of it linked to body fat, and it is still diagnosed by an anthropometric concept, body mass index (BMI) [2].

Tomiyama et al. [3] studied the misclassification of cardio-metabolic health when using BMI categories in NHANES 2005–2012. They found that nearly half of overweight individuals, 29% of obese individuals, and even 16% of obesity type 2/3 individuals were metabolically healthy. Moreover, over 30% of normal-weight individuals were cardio-metabolically unhealthy. Using BMI categories as the primary indicator of health, an estimated significant proportion of US adults are misclassified as cardio-metabolically unhealthy or cardio-metabolically healthy. Authors suggest that we should consider the unintended consequences of relying solely on BMI, and researchers should seek to improve diagnostic tools related to weight and cardio-metabolic health.

O. Bosello · M. P. Donataccio
Department of Medicine, University of Verona, Verona, Italy

A. Vanzo
Department of Food Hygiene and Nutrition, ULSS 8 Berica, Vicenza, Italy

M. Cuzzolaro (✉)
Formerly Medical Pathophysiology Department, Eating Disorders and Obesity Unit, Sapienza University of Rome, Rome Italy

M. Cuzzolaro, S. Fassino (eds.), *Body Image, Eating, and Weight*,
https://doi.org/10.1007/978-3-319-90817-5_13

Batsis et al. [4] suggest that accurate measurements of adiposity must be considered especially in older adults. This procedure can eliminate the challenges observed by using BMI as a clinical tool with its lack of diagnostic accuracy.

Many incongruities weaken the value of BMI as the cornerstone of the current classification system for obesity [5], but the reliance upon this easy and cheap tool goes on. Why?

Although other anthropometric measures (e.g., waist circumference, waist-to-hip ratio, waist-to-height ratio, sagittal depth) could well add extra information to BMI, BMI in itself is accepted by and large as a strong predictor of overall mortality.

Multiple studies demonstrated that the relationship between BMI and mortality follows a J-shaped [6] or a U-shaped curve [6, 7]. In white adults, overweight and obesity (and possibly underweight) are associated with increased all-cause mortality that is lowest with a BMI of 20.0–24.9 [3] with an apparent optimum at about 22.5–25 kg/m^2 [8].

Eugenia E. Calle and colleagues, in a prospective study of more than one million adults in the United States, found the nadir of the curve for BMI and mortality at a BMI of 23.5–24.9 in men and 22.0–23.4 in women. They found that obesity doubled the risk of death in general and cardiovascular death in particular [9].

From a 2013 Centers for Disease Control and Prevention (CDC) systematic review and meta-analysis of 97 studies with a combined sample size of more than 2.88 million individuals emerged that, using the BMI cut-off points, grades 2 and 3 obesity were associated with significantly higher all-cause mortality but surprisingly grade 1 was not associated with higher mortality and overweight was associated with significantly lower all-cause mortality [10].

Several long-term prospective studies have suggested that BMI in itself is a reliable and independent predictor of coronary artery disease (CAD) and overall mortality, both above and below the apparent optimum of about 22.5–25 kg/m^2 [8, 11].

Among many other similar reports, the Framingham study found that excessive weight is associated with coronary disease, heart failure (HF), stroke, and cardiovascular death, with an age-adjusted relative risk (RR) for cardiovascular disease (CVD) increased by about 20% for the overweight and by 40–60% for the obese [12].

There is more limited information on the incidence of coronary heart disease (CHD) in women across a wide range of BMI, but recently a large prospective study showed that CHD incidence in women increased progressively with BMI [13, 14].

Countless surveys have proved that excess body weight is a significant risk factor for diabetes, musculoskeletal disorders, non-alcoholic fatty liver disease, psychiatric problems, functional limitations, and disabilities as well [15–17].

An extensive longitudinal study on BMI and cancer recently confirmed that a higher BMI increases the risk for the majority of cancers [18].

The increased morbidity and premature mortality in individuals with obesity are thought to be mediated in some measure by a cluster of interconnected factors that Gerald Reaven initially called syndrome X [19] and later renamed metabolic syndrome (MetS) [20].

Several attempts have been made to define the MetS as a diagnostic category [21].

However, in 2001 Reaven himself wrote [22]: "Not all overweight individuals are insulin resistant, nor are all insulin resistant individuals overweight. Syndrome X is not a disease. It cannot be defined by an arbitrary collection of abnormalities." The concept of MetS remains controversial [23–26].

There is a lot of misinformation about desirable body weight, appropriate weight loss and health, and false and unproven beliefs are still widespread [27–29]. As a consequence, it has not been obvious to consider obesity as a disease in itself.

For longtime, obesity has been characterized only as a major and modifiable risk factor for premature mortality, morbidity, and disability [11, 30]. But recently, in 2011, the American Association of Clinical Endocrinologists (AACE) and, 2 years later, the American Medical Association (AMA) officially declared that obesity is a disease per se and requires treatment [31–33]. Also according to the guidelines released by the American Heart Association (AHA), American College of Cardiology, and The Obesity Society in November 2013, doctors should consider obesity a disease and treat obese patients for weight loss [34, 35].

Nevertheless, there is no universal consensus about calling BMI-based obesity a disease [36]. In fact, the AMA did so against the advice of its Council on Science and Public Health [37]. The Council concluded that recognizing obesity as a disease, opposed to a condition or disorder, is problematic and will not necessarily lead to improved health outcomes.

To sum up, because of the documented health risks and increases in prevalence, obesity is currently recognized as a major health and public health challenge, and according to many medical associations, it should be called a disease.

On the other hand, in the 2000s a growing number of studies have complicated the picture of obesity through the notions of metabolically healthy obesity, metabolically obese normal-weight, and obesity paradox.

This chapter is an overview of the origin and current use of these three concepts. Starting from our paper mentioned above [1], we used as sources MEDLINE/PubMed, CINAHL, EMBASE, and Cochrane Library, from inception to December 2017.

Also, we hand-searched references from the retrieved articles and explored some related websites. After discussion, we chose 137 relevant papers.

13.2 Obesity Paradox (OP)

Obesity is associated with premature mortality but, in a substantial number of studies, overweight or obese adults have demonstrated a survival advantage compared with leaner adults. This counterintuitive association has been termed the obesity-survival paradox (OP).

The phenomenon was first described in 1999 in patients undergoing hemodialysis. Fleischmann et al. studied 1346 patients attending limited-care hemodialysis units across the state of Mississippi and found that, compared with the normal-weight, the 1-year survival rate was significantly higher in the overweight patients (BMI >27.5) and lower in the underweight patients (BMI <20) [38].

About this, larger body size with more muscle mass appears associated with a higher survival rate in long-term hemodialysis patients [39] this apparent paradox might be explained by the loss of muscle mass. Also Kalantar-Zadeh et al. suggest that a considerable proportion of the obesity paradox in these patients might be justified by the amount of decline in muscle mass [40].

BMI should not be used as an implicit adiposity index, and weight loss and fat loss may have independent effects on mortality rate.

An interesting paper was published by Allison DB and coworkers, in 1999, on two prospective population-based cohort studies, the Tecumseh Community Health Study and the Framingham Heart Study. David Allison et al. found that, in both studies, among individuals that were not severely obese, weight loss was associated with an increased, and fat loss with a decreased, mortality rate [41].

After the Fleischmann's seminal study, the survival advantage of overweight/obesity has been described in many other clinical settings, e.g., CVDs, hypertension, stroke, diabetes, chronic obstructive pulmonary disease, surgery [38].

The expression obesity paradox (OP) was first used in 2002 by Luis Gruberg et al. on the impact of obesity on the short-term and long-term outcomes after percutaneous coronary intervention [42].

In studies on the association between obesity and premature mortality, weight history and smoking are two principal sources of bias [43].

Also, many papers have discussed the interactions of OP with aging and cardiorespiratory fitness. Aging seems very important in shifting the predictive value of adiposity from negative to positive, and some studies have shown that the association between obesity and mortality risk weakens with age.

Bender et al. made an extensive study (6193 obese patients) with a long mortality follow-up (median follow-up time of 14.8 years) of a cohort of obese patients, including a considerable number of subjects with obesity (BMI of 32–40 kg/m^2) and morbid obesity (BMI >40 kg/m^2). They found that the excess mortality associated with obesity declined considerably with age for both sexes in all degrees of obesity [44].

However, controversy persists about the potential harms of obesity in the elderly [45]. The debate is focused on the relation between obesity in old age and total or disease-specific mortality, the definition of obesity in the elderly, its clinical relevance, and the need for its treatment.

Knowledge of age-related body composition and fat distribution changes should help us to better understand the relationships between obesity, morbidity, and mortality in the elderly.

At length, cardiorespiratory fitness (CRF) has been overlooked as a potential modifier of the OP. However in recent times, a growing number of studies confirm that: (a) mortality risk is lower for both obese and nonobese individuals who are fit; (b) only overweight and obese persons with high CRF have increased longevity; (c) low fitness and central obesity are independently and cumulatively associated with increased mortality; (d) the paradoxically higher mortality risk observed with lower BMI is likely the result of unhealthy reduction in body weight and, perhaps most importantly, considerable loss of lean body mass [46–49].

Sahakyan et al. examined the risk of total and cardiovascular mortality associated with central obesity but normal BMI. They found that persons with normal-weight central obesity had the worst long-term survival and concluded that normal-weight central obesity defined by WHR is associated with higher mortality than BMI-defined obesity, mainly when obesity is in the absence of central fat distribution [50].

CRF significantly impact the relationship between adiposity and subsequent prognosis in patients with CVD, as suggested by two recent reviews: an obesity paradox is only present with low CRF [51, 52].

Substantial health benefits may be achieved by reasonably small increases in physical activity (e.g., 20-min brisk walk each day).

Ekelund et al., using data from The European Prospective Investigation into Cancer and Nutrition Study (EPIC), showed that within each stratum for BMI and waist circumference, the hazard of all-cause mortality was substantially reduced when the inactive group was compared with the moderately inactive group [53]. Improving levels of CRF may be even more important than improving BMI/BF (Body Fat) in patients with CVD [54, 55].

13.3 Metabolically Healthy Obesity (MHO)

A formal definition of metabolically healthy obesity (MHO) does not exist, and this obesity phenotype is sometimes called metabolically benign obesity [56–59]. MHO may be described as a phenotype having BMI >30, but not having any metabolic syndrome component and having a homeostasis model assessment (HOMA) of insulin resistance <2.5 [60].

Half of overweight and a third of obese individuals of a cross-sectional survey of 5440 participants of the National Health and Nutrition Examination Surveys (NHANES-III 1999–2004) had a low burden of cardio-metabolic abnormalities [60]. Two reviews suggest that the prevalence of this phenotype varies from 10 to 30% among obese individuals [61, 62].

MHO was more prevalent in women than in men and decreased with age in both sexes in a collaborative analysis of ten large European cohort studies. However, there was considerable variability in the prevalence of healthy obesity across the different populations (from 7 to 28% in women and from 2 to 19% in men) [63].

Gutierrez-Repiso et al. studied patterns of obesity and cardio-metabolic phenotypes and their association with lifestyle factors. They found that prevalence rates of metabolically healthy obese (MHO) subjects vary depending on the adopted criteria [64]. Furthermore, they found that smoking, physical activity level, and alcohol intake contribute to the explanation of the prevalence of cardio-metabolic abnormalities in the Spanish population, as in the US population. However, in Spain, olive oil intake contributes significantly to the explanation of the variance in the prevalence of cardio-metabolic abnormalities.

From a recent systematic review emerged the heterogeneity of MHO prevalence estimates and the need for a commonly established definition of metabolic health [65].

A Korean study demonstrated that waist circumference and waist-to-height ratio provide useful indicators for diagnosing MHO, and are more accurate than BMI and fat percentage [66].

Peterson et al., using the data of NHANES 2003–2006, estimated the degree of obesity misclassification, between BMI and BF percentage, in adults with functional mobility impairment, to determine cardio-metabolic risk profiles, They observed that obesity misclassification and cardio-metabolic risk is prevalent among individuals with functional mobility impairments, and thus diagnostic screening for obesity should be modified to account for %BF and/or waist circumference. They suggested some behavioral interventions to decrease sedentary behavior, increase activity, and reduce abdominal obesity [67].

In a recent review, the differences between MHO and metabolically unhealthy obese individuals and some possible underlying mechanisms have been discussed as adipocyte differentiation, immune regulation, and cellular energy metabolism [62].

Hansen et al., in a 10-year follow-up, investigated the association of MHO and ischemic heart disease (IHD). They found that metabolically healthy obese men had increased risk of IHD compared with metabolically healthy normal-weight. Being metabolically healthy but overweight was not associated with higher risk of IHD, but a substantial proportion of metabolically healthy individuals became metabolically unhealthy after 5 years of follow-up [68].

Mark Hamer and Emmanuel Stamatakis [69] examined the association between metabolically healthy obesity and risk of cardiovascular disease (CVD) and all-cause mortality in 22,203 men and women, aged 54.1, without a known history of CVD at baseline. They concluded that metabolically healthy obese participants were not at increased risk of CVD and all-cause mortality over 7 years.

In a comment to this paper, Després [70] argues that obesity assessed by the BMI cannot correctly estimate CVD and all-cause mortality risk. He furthermore affirms that the therapeutic objective of achieving a normal BMI to prevent/manage cardiometabolic diseases may also be questioned by the emerging evidence. Vigorous physical activity to reduce visceral adiposity/ectopic fat and to maintain a proper level of insulin sensitivity may be more important than achieving a "healthy" body weight defined by the BMI.

However, many studies have shown that MHO is not always a harmless condition. Several studies have provided evidence that the MHO phenotype may not be a benign condition [71–75].

From a 13-year longitudinal study has emerged that variations in BMI alone poorly reflected the risk of ischemic heart disease [76].

Koko Aung et al. discovered that MHO individuals had an increased risk for diabetes and CVD in comparison to metabolically healthy normal-weight persons [77].

Häring described phenotypes observed in a population with increased risk for type 2 diabetes, from data collected at the University Hospital of Tübingen [78]. They used imaging to characterize subphenotypes of fat distribution, metabolically healthy obesity and metabolically unhealthy obesity. Haring discussed the role of genetic predisposition, ectopic fat stores in liver and pancreas in determining the phenotype of metabolically healthy and unhealthy fatty liver and the recently recognized phenotype of fatty pancreas, with particular attention to metabolic impact of perivascular adipose tissue, in the development of the different prediabetes phenotypes. He concluded that both genetic predisposition and ectopic fat distribution seems to contribute to these phenotypes and the progression from prediabetes to diabetes.

Another study found that almost half of the MHO participants had ultrasonographic fatty liver (FL) [79].

Yoosoo Chang et al. found that MHO individuals had a higher prevalence of subclinical coronary atherosclerosis than metabolically healthy normal-weight individuals [59].

Another survey of 4009 asymptomatic Korean subjects confirmed that MHO individuals had substantial subclinical coronary atherosclerotic burden compared with metabolically healthy nonobese subjects [80].

Overweight and obesity were associated with an increased incidence of chronic kidney disease in metabolically healthy young and middle-aged participants in an extensive 5-year prospective cohort study [81].

For mental health, a recent pooled analysis revealed that obese persons with a favorable metabolic profile had a slightly increased risk of depressive symptoms compared with nonobese, but the risk was higher when obesity was combined with an adverse metabolic profile [82].

There are still open questions about predictors, biological determinants, and mechanisms underlying MHO and whether MHO represents a transient phenotype changing with aging, behavioral and environmental factors [83].

Many studies have rejected the concept that the MHO phenotype is a benign condition at long-term (follow-up 10–30 years) [71, 72, 84–86]. Caroline Kramer et al., in a systematic review and meta-analysis, found that MHO individuals were at increased risk for adverse long-term outcomes compared with metabolically healthy normal-weight individuals when only studies with 10 or more years of follow-up were considered [84].

Hwang et al. aimed a study to determine prospectively the frequency of conversion of MHO to MUO and the clinical variables that independently predicted this conversion, with a particular focus on the role of body composition [87]. They observed that MHO was a transient state, with nearly two-thirds developing MUO over 10 years, with higher conversion to MUO independently associated with VAT, female sex, higher fasting insulin level, and lower baseline HDL cholesterol level. They concluded that visceral abdominal fat accumulation predicts the conversion of metabolically healthy obese subjects to an unhealthy phenotype.

From a recent meta-analysis emerged that metabolically healthy overweight (MHOW) and obese (MHOB) individuals, compared with healthy normal-weight individuals, showed an increased risk for CVD events, which appeared much stronger during the long-term follow-up period of 15 years. Metabolically abnormal obese individuals were at the highest risk for CVD and mortality [85].

The English Longitudinal Study of Ageing showed that the MHO phenotype was relatively unstable over 8 years and transition to an unhealthy state was not fully explained by lifestyle risk factors [88]. Furthermore, the prognostic value of the MHO phenotype may depend on the health outcome being examined.

Hinnouho et al., using the Whitehall II cohort study, remember that metabolically healthy obese (MHO) phenotype refers to obese individuals with a favorable metabolic profile, but that prognostic value is unclear and may depend on the health outcome being examined. The authors examined the association of MHO phenotype with incident cardiovascular disease (CVD) and type 2 diabetes. Their study seems to permit the conclusion that for type 2 diabetes, the MHO phenotype is associated with lower risk than the metabolically unhealthy obese, but for CVD the risk is as elevated in both obesity phenotypes [89].

A narrative review concluded that the impact of MHO on future morbidity and mortality is to date unquestionably controversial even conflicting [90]. In a 2015 commentary on the public health implications of the MHO phenotype, Rey-Lopez et al. argued that it is not benign and has very limited relevance as a public health target [91]. In the opinion of Bradshaw and Stevens, the utility of this concept remains unresolved [92].

Muñoz-Garach et al. [93] asked themselves if the metabolically healthy obesity exists. They confirm that MHO is common among the obese population and constitutes a unique subset of characteristics that reduce metabolic and cardiovascular risk factors despite the presence of excessive fat mass. But authors remember that the protective factors that grant a healthier profile to individuals with MHO are being elucidated.

Individuals with MHO did not significantly improve their cardio-metabolic risk upon weight loss interventions, Matthias Bluher underlined [83].

Dobson et al. [94] also raised the question of metabolically healthy and unhealthy obesity, aiming at differential effects on myocardial function, according to the metabolic syndrome rather than obesity. They classified metabolically healthy or unhealthy obese according to the presence or absence of metabolic syndrome. They found that unhealthy (lean or obese) individuals had higher liver fat and decreased early diastolic strain rate, early diastolic tissue velocity and systolic strain indicative of subclinical systolic and diastolic dysfunction. The magnitude of dysfunction correlated with the number of components of metabolic syndrome but not with BMI or with the degree of ectopic (visceral or liver) fat deposition. They concluded that myocardial dysfunction appears to be related to poor metabolic health rather than merely BMI or fat mass and that these data may partly explain the epidemiological evidence on CVD risk about the different obesity phenotypes.

Bluher and Schwarz suggested that an internationally accepted definition of the MHO phenotype should at least include inflammatory markers as well as features of the non-alcoholic fatty liver disease (NAFLD), but it is missing to date [90].

Current knowledge on the prognosis of MHO phenotype is limited due to the exclusive use of the BMI to define obesity and the lack of information on cardiorespiratory fitness (CRF). A large Swedish study found that: (a) higher CRF should be considered a characteristic of MHO phenotype; (b) once CRF is accounted for, the MHO phenotype is a benign condition, with a better prognosis for mortality and morbidity than metabolically abnormal obese individuals [95].

13.4 Metabolically Obese Normal-Weight (MONW)

The existence of a subgroup of normal-weight individuals displaying obesity-related phenotypic characteristics was first proposed in 1981 when Neil Ruderman and colleagues wrote a brief review about patients with type 2 diabetes, hypertension, and hypertriglyceridemia who were not obese but who responded favorably to caloric restriction. They introduced the concept of metabolically obese normal-weight individual (MONW) [96], just the opposite of the obesity paradox. This phenotype is also called metabolically abnormal but normal-weight (MANW) [97], metabolically unhealthy normal-weight (MUH-NW) [77], or normal-weight obesity [98].

A formal definition of MONW has not yet been developed and officially approved [98, 99]. However, research on the MONW phenotype could help to understand the obesity paradox and the relationship between BMI and metabolic syndrome.

In the United States, the NHANES-III study made available data that bore out the MONW concept.

Hamer et al. affirm that the association between obesity—defined by BMI—and mortality in the general population is controversial. Their study in a large sample of the general adult population showed that waist measurement is a stronger predictor of death than BMI [100].

St-Onge et al. observed that men and women in the upper end and just above the normal BMI range (BMI 25.0–26.9 kg/m^2) were more likely to have the metabolic syndrome—defined according to National Cholesterol Education Program Adult Treatment Panel III criteria [101]—and its single components, in comparison with those with BMI 18.5–20.9 kg/m^2 [102].

Wildman et al. found that the MONW prevalence in NHANES-III data was high: 23.5% of normal-weight adults were metabolically abnormal [60]. Another study from the NHANES-III showed that individuals with normal BMI but high BF content (MONW-like) had higher cardiovascular mortality, particularly in women [103].

A survey on men and women Korean found that the MONW phenotype, compared to metabolically healthy normal-weight individuals and MHO individuals, are burdened by increased arterial stiffness and carotid atherosclerosis, even after adjusting for confounding factors [97].

From a meta-analysis of 14 prospective cohort studies was emerged that MONW individuals-compared with healthy normal-weight individuals were at increased risk for CVD, and all-cause death [85].

Lassale et al., in a pan-European case-cohort analysis ("EPIC-CVD"), studied the separate and combined associations of obesity and metabolic health with coronary heart disease. The study demonstrated that irrespective of BMI, metabolically unhealthy individuals had higher CHD risk than their healthy counterparts. Conversely, regardless of metabolic health, overweight, and obese people had higher CHD risk than lean people. The authors suggested that these findings challenge the concept of "metabolically healthy obesity," encouraging population-wide strategies to tackle obesity [104].

An analysis of prospective data (median follow-up 7.4 years) of a population-based study among Mexican-Americans and non-Hispanic whites was performed by Koko Aung. MONW individuals were defined as BMI\25 kg/m^2 with two or more metabolic abnormalities. They had an increased risk for diabetes and CVD in comparison to metabolically healthy normal-weight individuals [76]. An intriguing example of the MONW phenotype is new-onset type 2 diabetes (DM2) in normal-weight adults (BMI <25), which has become increasingly common over time, with uncertain consequences for mortality. A pooled analysis of five longitudinal cohort studies found that the proportion of adults who were normal-weight at the time of incident diabetes ranged from 9 to 21% (overall 12%). After adjustment for demographic characteristics, waist circumference, lipid levels, blood pressure, and smoking status, hazard ratios comparing normal-weight participants with overweight/obese participants for total, cardiovascular, and noncardiovascular mortality were 2.08 (95% CI 1.52–2.85) [105]. Jennifer Logue et al. studied the association between BMI measured within a year after diagnosis of T2DM and mortality and observed a J-shaped association between BMI and mortality among all participants [106].

The critical role of white adipose tissue (WAT) depots, immune cell infiltration, and adipokine production in the development of MONW and MHO phenotypes has been highlighted by Badoud et al. [107].

Using the components of the ATP III definition of the metabolic syndrome, Unab Khan et al. found that at-risk normal-weight women (MONW) had higher leptin and lower adiponectin levels (a less favorable profile) compared to metabolically healthy normal-weight women. On the other hand, metabolically benign overweight/obese women (MHO) had an intermediate adipokine profile (between at-risk obese and metabolically benign normal-weight women). Adiponectin is a BMI independent adipokine, and it may have a role in the etiological pathway of these phenotypes [108].

A study of Stefan et al. on metabolically healthy obesity questioned if a little effort is useful in obesity treatment. They remember that accumulating evidence suggests that, although the risk of all-cause mortality and cardiovascular events might be higher in people with metabolically healthy obesity compared with metabolically healthy people of a normal-weight, the risk is substantially lower than in individuals with metabolically unhealthy obesity [109]. Therefore, every person with obesity should be motivated to achieve a moderate weight loss sufficient for the transition from metabolically unhealthy obesity to metabolically healthy obesity and lower the risk of adverse outcomes. They concluded that this transition might be supported by lifestyle factors—such as the Mediterranean diet—that affect cardiovascular risk, independent of body fat.

13.5 Beyond BMI

There is broad agreement that BMI is a simple tool to estimate the risks to health at the population level. A recent commentary by Rey-Lopez et al. argued that "more efforts must be allocated to reducing the distal and actual causal agents that lead to weight gain, instead of the current disproportionate scientific interest in the biological processes that explain the heterogeneity of obesity" [91] (p. 737).

Many authors affirm that the protective effect of obesity among individuals with cardiovascular disease can be attributed to a form of selection bias known as collider-stratification bias (unmeasured confounding induced by selection bias, e.g., smoking) [110, 111]. However, an inverse association between BMI and mortality (OP) has been reported in patients with many different disease states [112]. Sperrin et al. have recently emphasized that collider bias can only be a partial explanation of the OP and alternative hypotheses should continue to be explored [113].

The puzzling phenomenon of the obesity paradox, together with MONW and MHO, challenges the value of BMI as a marker for obesity [97], influences clinical attitudes, and affects treatment and prevention models. It is not to forget that the BMI is a single number that combines different biomarkers possibly associated with both disease and health [114, 115]: subcutaneous and visceral fat, fat mass and fat-free mass, eutopic and ectopic fat (i.e., fat into non-adipose tissues).

The suggestive hypothesis of adipose tissue expandability seems to indicate that the capacity of adipose tissue to expand maintaining its role of storage organ is not unlimited and varies between individuals [116, 117].

Bays [118, 119] argues that during a positive caloric balance, if subcutaneous adipose tissue (SAT) can activate the proliferation and differentiation of the adipocytes, this can slow down an excess of energetic flow towards other fat deposits. Conversely, if during a positive caloric balance the SAT is not able to proliferate and differentiate adequately, the energy overflow can promote the accumulation of fat in other fat deposits (first, visceral adipose tissue, VAT; then, pericardial fat, perivascular fat and within various organs and systems), contributing to multiple metabolic abnormalities, and increasing cardiovascular risk.

The new concept of functional body composition integrates body components into regulatory systems relating the mass of organs and tissues to corresponding in vivo functions and metabolic processes. During weight gain and loss, the between organ/tissue mass relationships are associated with and explained by crosstalks between organs and tissues mediated by cytokines, hormones, and metabolites, as observed in obesity and cancer cachexia.

Combining individual body components with their related functional aspects (e.g., the endocrine, metabolic and inflammatory profiles) will provide a suitable basis for future definitions of metabolically healthy or unhealthy body composition [120, 121].

Wellen and Hotamisligil discussed on obesity-associated chronic, low-grade inflammation with the adipose tissue characterized by macrophage infiltration. They concluded for a significant role for macrophages in the molecular changes that occur in adipose tissue in obesity [122].

Are now available more accurate measures of adiposity and fat distribution but even though the joint contribution of CRF and obesity on mortality in diverse populations is still uncertain-using only adiposity measures to assess mortality risk may be misleading unless CRF is considered [51, 123].

Notwithstanding, in 2016 has been made a meta-analysis of 239 prospective studies in four continents on BMI and all-cause mortality. The conclusion was that the associations of both overweight and obesity with higher all-cause mortality were broadly worldwide consistent [124].

Furthermore, longitudinal studies have shown that the duration of obesity is an important and independent risk factor and many initially healthy obese individuals undergo adverse obesity-related metabolic changes over time [125]. Also, changes in weight have been observed carry over a relative risk of disease in women [126]. Moreover, Bangalore et al. [127] recently noted that fluctuation in body weight was associated with higher mortality and a higher rate of cardiovascular events.

Nevertheless, MHO seems to be an important phenotype with health risks between healthy normal-weight and unhealthy obese individuals [128].

Also, lifestyle factors should be considered: physical activity and compliance with food pyramid recommendations increase the likelihood of MHO [129, 130].

Furthermore, psychological and behavioral variables such as food craving/addiction and binge eating, with their neural correlates, play an essential role [131, 132].

13.6 Phenotyping the Obesities. Conclusive Remarks

At the end of this overview, we think that observations on the so-called obesity paradox and healthy obesity cannot be easily dismissed as just a myth [133, 134].

OP, MHO, and MONW appear intrinsically linked to the frail BMI-based diagnostic definition of obesity that includes too many different anatomical, physiological, and psychological phenotypes. For the same reasons, it remains conceptually problematic to label a condition as a disease per se, till it is defined by a simple index of weight for height.

The Edmonton Obesity Staging System (EOSS) is a recent classification using obesity-related comorbidities or functional limitations [135]. EOSS is a practical tool that could help identify obese individuals at higher mortality risk [136] and predict differences in treatment outcomes [137]. However, its sensitivity, specificity, reliability, and clinical utility have not yet been sufficiently evaluated. In addition, as the authors partly acknowledge [135], it suffers from substantial limitations: (a) criteria and cutoffs are not always well defined, and some of them are subjective parameters; (b) it is often uncertain whether or not a condition is caused or merely aggravated by obesity; (c) EOSS does not consider body composition, fat distribution, weight history, lifestyle, and eating behaviors; (d) EOSS includes MHO (stage 0), but fails to capture MONW individuals.

Table 13.1 [1] recaps current definitions of different obesity phenotypes. According to this review, they are controversial. A commonly established new characterization and classification of obesities, based on some specific variables, is an essential goal but probably it is not near.

Table 13.1 Current definitions of some adult obesity phenotypes [1]

	Diagnostic criteria
Overweight	• Body mass index 25–29.9
Obesity	• Body mass index ≥30
Metabolically healthy obesity (MHO)	• Body mass index ≥30 • Not having any metabolic syndrome component • Homeostasis model assessment (HOMA) of insulin resistance <2.5
Metabolically obese normal weight (MONW)	• Body mass index 18.5–24.9 • Having at least one metabolic syndrome component
Edmonton obesity staging system (EOSS)	• Body mass index ≥30 • Stage 0: no apparent obesity-related risk factors, no physical symptoms, no psychopathology, no functional limitations • Stage 1: obesity-related subclinical risk factors (e.g. borderline hypertension), mild symptoms/limitations • Stage 2: established obesity-related chronic disease (e.g. type 2 diabetes), moderate symptoms/limitations • Stage 3: established end-organ damage (e.g. myocardial infarction), significant symptoms/limitations • Stage 4: severe (potentially end-stage) disabilities from obesity-related chronic diseases, severe symptoms/limitations

References

1. Bosello O, Donataccio MP, Cuzzolaro M. Obesity or obesities? Controversies on the association between body mass index and premature mortality. Eat Weight Disord. 2016;21(2):165–74. https://doi.org/10.1007/s40519-016-0278-4. Review. PMID:27043948.
2. World Health Organization. Obesity and overweight. Fact sheet no 311. Updated January 2015. 2015. http://www.who.int/mediacentre/factsheets/fs311/en/. Accessed 1 Nov 2015.
3. Tomiyama AJ, Hunger JM, Nguyen-Cuu J, Wells C. Misclassification of cardio-metabolic health when using body mass index categories in NHANES 2005–2012. Int J Obes. 2016;40(5):1–4. https://doi.org/10.1038/ijo.2016.17.
4. Batsis JA, et al. Diagnostic accuracy of body mass index to identify obesity in older adults: NHANES 1999–2004. Int J Obes. 2016;40(5):761–7. https://doi.org/10.1038/ijo.2015.243.
5. Prentice AM, Jebb SA. Beyond body mass index. Obes Rev. 2001;2(3):141–7.
6. Berrington de Gonzalez A, Hartge P, Cerhan JR, Flint AJ, et al. Body-mass index and mortality among 1.46 million white adults. N Engl J Med. 2010;363(23):2211–9. https://doi.org/10.1056/NEJMoa1000367.
7. Allison DB, Faith MS, Heo M, Kotler DP. Hypothesis concerning the U-shaped relation between body mass index and mortality. Am J Epidemiol. 1997;146(4):339–49.
8. Whitlock G, Lewington S, Sherliker P, Clarke R, Emberson J, Halsey J, Qizilbash N, Collins R, Peto R. Body-mass index and cause-specific mortality in 900,000 adults: collaborative analyses of 57 prospective studies. Lancet. 2009;373(9669):1083–96. https://doi.org/10.1016/S0140-6736(09)60318-4. 1056/NEJMoa1000367.
9. Calle EE, Thun MJ, Petrelli JM. Rodriguez C, Heath CW Jr. Body-mass index and mortality in a prospective cohort of U.S. adults. N Engl J Med. 1999;341(15):1097–105. https://doi.org/10.1056/NEJM199910073411501.

10. Flegal KM, Kit BK, Orpana H, Graubard BI. Association of all-cause mortality with overweight and obesity using standard body mass index categories: a systematic review and meta-analysis. JAMA. 2013;309(1):71–82. https://doi.org/10.1001/jama.2012.113905.
11. Hubert HB, Feinleib M, McNamara PM, Castelli WP. Obesity as an independent risk factor for cardiovascular disease:a 26-year follow-up of participants in the Framingham heartstudy. Circulation. 1983;67(5):968–77.
12. Wilson PW, D'Agostino RB, Sullivan L, Parise H, Kannel WB. Overweight and obesity as determinants of cardiovascularrisk: the Framingham experience. Arch Intern Med. 2002;162(16):1867–72.
13. Canoy D, Cairns BJ, Balkwill A, Wright FL, Green J, Reeves G, Beral V, Million Women Study Collaborators. Coronary heart disease incidence in women by waist circumference within categories ofbody mass index. Eur J Prevent Cardiol. 2013;20(5):759–62. https://doi.org/10.1177/2047487313492631.
14. Canoy D, Cairns BJ, Balkwill A, Wright FL, Green J, Reeves G, Beral V, Million Women Study Collaborators. Body mass index and incident coronary heart disease in women: a population-based prospective study. BMC Med. 2013;11:87. https://doi.org/10.1186/1741-7015-11-87.
15. Capodaglio P, Faintuch J, Liuzzi A, editors. Disabling obesity. From determinants to health care models. Heidelberg: Springer; 2013. https://doi.org/10.1007/978-3-642-35972-9.
16. Bosello O, Cuzzolaro M. Obesità. Bologna: Mulino; 2013.
17. Bray G, Bouchard C, editors. Handbook of obesity. Clinicalapplications. 3rd ed. Informa Health Care: New York; 2008.
18. Bhaskaran K, Douglas I, Forbes H, Dos-Santos-Silva I, Leon DA, Smeeth L. Body-mass index and risk of 22 specific cancers: a population-based cohort study of 5.24 million UK adults. Lancet. 2014;384(9945):755–65. https://doi.org/10.1016/S0140-6736(14)60892-8.
19. Reaven GM. Banting lecture 1988. Role of insulin resistance in human disease. Diabetes. 1988;37(12):1595–607.
20. Reaven G. Metabolic syndrome: pathophysiology and implications for management of cardiovascular disease. Circulation. 2002;106(3):286–8.
21. National Cholesterol Education Program Expert Panel on Detection Evaluation, Treatment of High Blood Cholesterol in Adults. Third report of the national cholesterol education program (NCEP) expert panel on detection, evaluation, and treatment of high blood cholesterol in adults (adult treatment panel III) final report. Circulation. 2002;106(25):3143–421.
22. Reaven GM. Syndrome x: a short history. Ochsner J. 2001;3(3):124–5.
23. Reaven GM. The metabolic syndrome: requiescat in pace. Clin Chem. 2005;51(6):931–8. https://doi.org/10.1373/clinchem.2005.048611.
24. Grundy SM. Does the metabolic syndrome exist? Diabetes Care. 2006;29(7):1689–92. https://doi.org/10.2337/dc05-2307 (discussion 1693–1686).
25. Eckel RH, Alberti KG, Grundy SM, Zimmet PZ. The metabolic syndrome. Lancet. 2010;375(9710):181–3. https://doi.org/10.1016/S0140-6736(09)61794-3.
26. Reaven GM. The metabolic syndrome: time to get off the merry-go-round? J Intern Med. 2011;269(2):127–36. https://doi.org/10.1111/j.1365-2796.2010.02325.x.
27. Chaput JP, Ferraro ZM, Prud'homme D, Sharma AM. Widespread misconceptions about obesity. Can Fam Physician. 2014;60(11):973–5, 981–974.
28. Lavie CJ, Loberg K. The obesity paradox: when thinner means sicker and heavier means healthier. New York: Hudson Street Press; 2014.
29. Casazza K, Fontaine KR, Astrup A, Birch LL, Brown AW, Bohan Brown MM, Durant N, Dutton G, Foster EM, Heymsfield SB, McIver K, Mehta T, Menachemi N, Newby PK, Pate R, Rolls BJ, Sen B, Smith DL, Thomas DM, Allison DB. Myths, presumptions, and facts about obesity. N Engl J Med. 2013;368(5):446–54. https://doi.org/10.1056/NEJMsa1208051.
30. Capodaglio P, Liuzzi A. Obesity: a disabling disease or a condition favoring disability? Eur J Phys Rehabil Med. 2013;49(3):395–8.

31. American Medical Association House of Delegates. Report of the council on science and public health (CSAPH). Recognition of obesity as a disease. Resolution 420 (A-13). 2013. p. 19. http://www.ama-assn.org/assets/meeting/2013a/a13-adden dum-refcomm-d.pdf. Accessed 11 Nov 2014.
32. American Association of Clinical Endocrinologists (AACE). American association of clinical endocrinologists (AACE) declares obesity a disease state. 2011. http://media.aace.com/press-release/american-association-clinical-endocrinologistsaace-declares-obesity-disease-state. Accessed 11 Nov 2014.
33. Bosello O, Donataccio MP. Obesity paradox. Eat Weight Disord. 2013;18(4):447–8. https://doi.org/10.1007/s40519-013-0080-5.
34. Jensen MD, Ryan DH, Apovian CM, Ard JD, Comuzzie AG, Donato KA, Hu FB, Hubbard VS, Jakicic JM, Kushner RF, Loria CM, Millen BE, Nonas CA, Pi-Sunyer FX, Stevens J, Stevens VJ, Wadden TA, Wolfe BM, Yanovski SZ. 2013 AHA/ACC/TOS guideline for the management of overweight and obesity in adults: a report of the American College of Cardiology/American Heart Association Task Force on Practice Guidelines and the Obesity Society. Circulation. 2014;129(25 Suppl 2):S102–38. https://doi.org/10.1161/01.cir.0000437739.71477.ee.
35. Ravussin E, Ryan DH, The Obesity Society, et al. Expert Panel Report: Guidelines (2013) for the management of eat weight disord 123 overweight and obesity in adults. Obesity. 2014;22(S2):S41–S410. https://doi.org/10.1002/oby.20660.
36. Allison DB, Downey M, Atkinson RL, Billington CJ, Bray GA, Eckel RH, Finkelstein EA, Jensen MD, Tremblay A. Obesity as a disease: a white paper on evidence and arguments commissioned by the Council of the Obesity Society. Obesity. 2008;16(6):1161–77. https://doi.org/10.1038/oby.2008.231.
37. MedPage Today. AMA house votes against council, calls obesity a disease. 18 June 2013. http://www.medpagetoday.com/MeetingCoverage/AMA/39952. Accessed 1 Nov 2015.
38. Fleischmann E, Teal N, Dudley J, May W, Bower JD, Salahudeen K. Influence of excess weight on mortality and hospital stay in 1346 hemodialysis patients. Kidney Int. 1999;4:1560–7. https://doi.org/10.1046/j.1523-1755.1999.00389.x.
39. Kalantar-Zadeh K, Streja E, Kovesdy CP, Oreopoulos A, Noori N, Jing J, Nissenson AR, Krishnan M, Kopple JD, Mehrotra R, Anker SD. The obesity paradox and mortality associated with surrogates of body size and muscle mass in patients receiving hemodialysis. Mayo Clin Proc. 2010;85(11):991–1001. https://doi.org/10.4065/mcp.2010.0336.
40. Kalantar-Zadeh K, Streja E, Molnar MZ, Lukowsky LR, Krishnan M, Kovesdy CP, Greenland S. Mortality prediction by surrogates of body composition: an examination of the obesity paradox in hemodialysis patients using composite ranking score analysis. Am J Epidemiol. 2012;175(8):793–803. https://doi.org/10.1093/aje/kwr384.
41. Allison DB, Zannolli R, Faith MS, Heo M, Pietrobelli A, VanItallie TB, Pi-Sunyer FX, Heymsfield SB. Weight loss increases and fat loss decreases all-cause mortality rate: results from two independent cohort studies. Int J Obes Relat Metab Disord. 1999;23(6):603–11.
42. Gruberg L, Weissman NJ, Waksman R, Fuchs S, Deible R, Pinnow EE, Ahmed LM, Kent KM, Pichard AD, Suddath WO, Satler LF, Lindsay J Jr. The impact of obesity on the short-term and long-term outcomes after percutaneous coronary intervention: the obesity paradox? J Am Coll Cardiol. 2002;39(4):578–84.
43. Stokes A, Preston SH. Smoking and reverse causation create an obesity paradox in cardiovascular disease. Obesity. 2015;23(12):2485–90. https://doi.org/10.1002/oby.21239.
44. Bender R, Jockel KH, Trautner C, Spraul M, Berger M. Effect of age on excess mortality in obesity. JAMA. 1999;281(16):1498–504.
45. Zamboni M, Mazzali G, Zoico E, Harris TB, Meigs JB, Di Francesco V, Fantin F, Bissoli L, Bosello O. Health consequences of obesity in the elderly: a review of four unresolved questions. Int J Obes. 2005;29(9):1011–29. https://doi.org/10.1038/sj.ijo.0803005.

46. McAuley PA, Smith NS, Emerson BT, Myers JN. The obesity paradox and cardiorespiratory fitness. J Obes. 2012;2012:951582. https://doi.org/10.1155/2012/951582.
47. McAuley PA, Kokkinos PF, Oliveira RB, Emerson BT, Myers JN. Obesity paradox and cardiorespiratory fitness in 12,417 male veterans aged 40–70 years. Mayo Clin Proc. 2010;85(2):115–21. https://doi.org/10.4065/mcp.2009.0562.
48. Goel K, Thomas RJ, Squires RW, Coutinho T, Trejo-Gutierrez JF, Somers VK, Miles JM, Lopez-Jimenez F. Combined effect of cardiorespiratory fitness and adiposity on mortality in patients with coronary artery disease. Am Heart J. 2011;161(3):590–7. https://doi.org/10.1016/j.ahj.2010.12.012.
49. Kokkinos P, Faselis C, Myers J, Pittaras A, Sui X, Zhang J, McAuley P, Kokkinos JP. Cardiorespiratory fitness and the paradoxical BMI-mortality risk association inmale veterans. Mayo Clin Proc. 2014;89(6):754–62. https://doi.org/10.1016/j.mayocp.2014.01.029.
50. Sahakyan KR, Somers VK, Rodriguez-Escudero JP, et al. Normal-weight central obesity: implications for total and cardiovascular mortality. Ann Intern Med. 2015;163:827–35. https://doi.org/10.7326/M14-252.
51. McAuley PA, Beavers KM. Contribution of cardiorespiratory fitness to the obesity paradox. Prog Cardiovasc Dis. 2014;56(4):434–40. https://doi.org/10.1016/j.pcad.2013.09.00690.
52. De Schutter A, Lavie CJ, Patel DA, Milani RV. Obesity paradox and the heart: which indicator of obesity best describes this complex relationship? Curr Opin Clin Nutr Metab Care. 2013;16(5):517–24. https://doi.org/10.1097/MCO.0b013e328363bcca.
53. Ekelund U, Ward HA, Norat T, Luan J, et al. Physical activity and all-cause mortality across levels of overall and abdominal adiposity in European men and women: the European prospective investigation into cancer and nutrition study (EPIC). Am J Clin Nutr. 2015;101(3):613–21. https://doi.org/10.3945/ajcn.114.100065.
54. De Schutter A, Lavie CJ, Milani RV. The impact of obesity on risk factors and prevalence and prognosis of coronary heart disease—the obesity paradox. Prog Cardiovasc Dis. 2014;56(4):401–8. https://doi.org/10.1016/j.pcad.2013.08.003.
55. Myers J, McAuley P, Lavie CJ, Despres JP, Arena R, Kokkinos P. Physical activity and cardiorespiratory fitness as major markers of cardiovascular risk: their independent and interwoven importance to health status. Prog Cardiovasc Dis. 2015;57(4):306–14. https://doi.org/10.1016/j.pcad.2014.09.011.
56. Khan UI, Wang D, Karvonen-Gutierrez CA, Khalil N, Ylitalo KR, Santoro N. Progression from metabolically benign to at-risk obesity in perimenopausal women: a longitudinal analysis of study of women across the nation (SWAN). J Clin Endocrinol Metab. 2014;99(7):2516–25. https://doi.org/10.1210/jc.2013-3259.
57. Finelli C, Tarantino G. "Obesity paradox" or "metabolically benign obesity"? Eat Weight Disord. 2013;18(3):337–8. https://doi.org/10.1007/s40519-013-0047-6.
58. Young TK, Gelskey DE. Is noncentral obesity metabolically benign? Implications for prevention from a population survey. JAMA. 1995;274(24):1939–41.
59. Chang Y, Kim BK, Yun KE, Cho J, Zhang Y, Rampal S, Zhao D, Jung HS, Choi Y, Ahn J, Lima JA, Shin H, Guallar E, Ryu S. Metabolically-healthy obesity and coronary artery calcification. J Am Coll Cardiol. 2014;63(24):2679–86. https://doi.org/10.1016/j.jacc.2014.03.042.
60. Wildman RP, Muntner P, Reynolds K, McGinn AP, Rajpathak S, Wylie-Rosett J, Sowers MR. The obese without cardio-metabolic risk factor clustering and the normal-weight with cardio-metabolic risk factor clustering: prevalence and correlates of 2 phenotypes among the US population (NHANES 1999–2004). Arch Intern Med. 2008;168(15):1617–24. https://doi.org/10.1001/archinte.168.15.1617.
61. Bluher M. The distinction of metabolically 'healthy' from 'unhealthy' obese individuals. Curr Opin Lipidol. 2010;21(1):38–43. https://doi.org/10.1097/MOL.0b013e3283346ccc.
62. Boonchaya-anant P, Apovian CM. Metabolically healthy obesity—does it exist? Curr Atheroscler Rep. 2014;16(10):441. https://doi.org/10.1007/s11883-014-0441-1.
63. van Vliet-Ostaptchouk JV, Nuotio ML, Slagter SN, et al. The prevalence of metabolic syndrome and metabolically healthy obesity in Europe: a collaborative analysis of ten large cohort studies. BMC Endocr Disord. 2014;14(1):9. https://doi.org/10.1186/1472-6823-14-9.

64. Gutierrez-Repiso C, et al. Variable patterns of obesity and cardio-metabolic phenotypes and their association with lifestyle factors in the Di@bet.es study. Nutr Metab Cardiovasc Dis. 2014;24:947–55. https://doi.org/10.1016/j.numecd.2014.04.019.
65. Rey-Lopez JP, de Rezende LF, Pastor-Valero M, Tess BH. The prevalence of metabolically healthy obesity: a systematic review and critical evaluation of the definitions used. Obes Rev. 2014;15(10):781–90. https://doi.org/10.1111/obr.12198.
66. Choi MK, Han YA, Roh YK. Utility of obesity indicators for metabolically healthy obesity: an observational study using the Korean National Health and Nutrition Examination Survey (2009–2010). BMC Public Health. 2014;14:1166. https://doi.org/10.1186/1471-2458-14-1166.
67. Peterson MD, et al. Obesity misclassification and the metabolic syndrome in adults with functional mobility impairments: NHANES 2003–2006. Prev Med. 2014;60:71–6. https://doi.org/10.1016/j.ypmed.2013.12.014.
68. Hansen L, Netterstrøm MK, Johansen NB, Rønn PF, Vistisen D, Husemoen LLN, Jørgensen ME, Rod NH, Færch K. Metabolically healthy obesity and ischemic heart disease: a 10-year follow-up of the Inter99 study. J Clin Endocrinol Metab. 2017;102(6):1934–42. https://doi.org/10.1210/jc.2016-3346. ISSN: 1945-7197.
69. Hamer M, Stamatakis E. Metabolically healthy obesity and risk of all-cause and cardiovascular disease mortality. J Clin Endocrinol Metab. 2012;97(7):2482–8. https://doi.org/10.1210/jc.2011-3475.
70. Després JP. Body fat distribution and risk of cardiovascular disease: an update. Circulation. 2012;126(10):1301–13. https://doi.org/10.1161/CIRCULATIONAHA.111.067264.
71. Arnlov J, Ingelsson E, Sundstrom J, Lind L. Impact of body mass index and the metabolic syndrome on the risk of cardiovascular disease and death in middle-aged men. Circulation. 2010;121(2):230–6. https://doi.org/10.1161/CIRCULATIONAHA.109.887521.
72. Arnlov J, Sundstrom J, Ingelsson E, Lind L. Impact of BMI and the metabolic syndrome on the risk of diabetes in middle-aged men. Diabetes Care. 2011;34(1):61–5. https://doi.org/10.2337/dc10-0955.
73. Kuk JL, Ardern CI. Are metabolically normal but obese individuals at lower risk for all-cause mortality? Diabetes Care. 2009;32(12):2297–9. https://doi.org/10.2337/dc09-0574.
74. Lee SK, Kim SH, Cho GY, Baik I, Lim HE, Park CG, Lee JB, Kim YH, Lim SY, Kim H, Shin C. Obesity phenotype and incident hypertension: a prospective community-based cohort study. J Hypertens. 2013;31(1):145–51. https://doi.org/10.1097/HJH.0b013e32835a3637.
75. Lind L, Siegbahn A, Ingelsson E, Sundstrom J, Arnlov J. A detailed cardiovascular characterization of obesity without the metabolic syndrome. Arterioscler Thromb Vasc Biol. 2011;31(8):e27–34. https://doi.org/10.1161/ATVBAHA.110.221572.
76. St-Pierre AC, Cantin B, Mauriege P, Bergeron J, Dagenais GR, Despres JP, Lamarche B. Insulin resistance syndrome, body mass index and the risk of ischemic heart disease. CMAJ. 2005;172(10):1301–5. https://doi.org/10.1503/cmaj.1040834.
77. Aung K, Lorenzo C, Hinojosa MA, Haffner SM. Risk of developing diabetes and cardiovascular disease in metabolically unhealthy normal-weight and metabolically healthy obese individuals. Clin Endocrinol Metab. 2014;99(2):462–8. https://doi.org/10.1210/jc.2013-2832.
78. Häring HU. Novel phenotypes of prediabetes? Diabetologia. 2016;59(9):1806–18. https://doi.org/10.1007/s00125-016-4015-3. Review. PMID:27344314.
79. Heianza Y, Arase Y, Tsuji H, Fujihara K, Saito K, Hsieh SD, Tanaka S, Kodama S, Hara S, Sone H. Metabolically healthy obesity, presence or absence of fatty liver, and risk of type 2 diabetes in Japanese individuals: toranomon hospital health management center study 20 (TOPICS 20). J Clin Endocrinol Metab. 2014;99(8):2952–60. https://doi.org/10.1210/jc.2013-4427.
80. Jung CH, Lee MJ, Hwang JY, Jang JE, Leem J, Yang DH, Kang JW, Kim EH, Park JY, Kim HK, Lee WJ. Association of metabolically healthy obesity with subclinical coronary atherosclerosis in a Korean population. Obesity. 2014;22(12):2613–20. https://doi.org/10.1002/oby.20883.
81. Chang Y, Ryu S, Choi Y, Zhang Y, Cho J, Kwon M-J, Hyun YY, Lee K-B, Kim H, Jung H-S, Yun KE, Ahn J, Rampal S, Zhao D, Suh B-S, Chung EC, Shin H, Pastor-Barriuso R,

Guallar E. Metabolically healthy obesity and development of chronic kidney disease: a cohort study obesity and CKD. Ann Intern Med. 2016;164(5):305–12. https://doi.org/10.7326/M15-1323.
82. Jokela M, Hamer M, Singh-Manoux A, Batty GD, Kivimaki M. Association of metabolically healthy obesity with depressive symptoms: pooled analysis of eight studies. Mol Psychiatry. 2014;19(8):910–4. https://doi.org/10.1038/mp.2013.162.
83. Bluher M. Mechanisms in endocrinology: are metabolically healthy obese individuals really healthy? Eur J Endocrinol. 2014;171(6):R209–19. https://doi.org/10.1530/eje-14-0540.
84. Kramer CK, Zinman B, Retnakaran R. Are metabolically healthy overweight and obesity benign conditions?: a systematic review and meta-analysis. Ann Intern Med. 2013;159(11):758–69. https://doi.org/10.7326/0003-4819-159-11-201312030-00008.
85. Fan J, Song Y, Chen Y, Hui R, Zhang W. Combined effect of obesity and cardio-metabolic abnormality on the risk of cardiovascular disease: a meta-analysis of prospective cohort studies. Int J Cardiol. 2013;168(5):4761–8. https://doi.org/10.1016/j.ijcard.2013.07.230.
86. Heianza Y, Kato K, Kodama S, Suzuki A, Tanaka S, Hanyu O, Sato K, Sone H. Stability and changes in metabolically healthy overweight or obesity and risk of future diabetes: Niigata wellness study. Obesity. 2014;22(11):2420–5. https://doi.org/10.1002/oby.20855.
87. Hwang YC, Hayashi T, Fujimoto WY, Kahn SE, Leonetti DL, McNeely MJ, Boyko EJ. Visceral abdominal fat accumulation predicts the conversion of metabolically healthy obese subjects to an unhealthy phenotype. Int J Obes. 2015;39(9):1365–70. https://doi.org/10.1038/ijo.2015.75.
88. Hamer M, Bell JA, Sabia S, Batty GD, Kivimaki M. Stability of metabolically healthy obesity over 8 years: the English longitudinal study of ageing. Eur J Endocrinol. 2015;173(5):703–8. https://doi.org/10.1530/EJE-15-0449.
89. Hinnouho GM, Czernichow S, Dugravot A, Nabi H, Brunner EJ, Kivimaki M, Singh-Manoux A. Metabolically healthy obesity and the risk of cardiovascular disease and type 2 diabetes: the Whitehall II cohort study. Eur Heart J. 2015;36(9):551–9. https://doi.org/10.1093/eurheartj/ehu123.
90. Bluher S, Schwarz P. Metabolically healthy obesity from childhood to adulthood—does weight status alone matter? Metabolism. 2014;63(9):1084–92. https://doi.org/10.1016/j.metabol.2014.06.009.
91. Rey-Lopez JP, de Rezende LF, de Sa TH, Stamatakis E. Is the metabolically healthy obesity phenotype an irrelevant artifact for public health? Am J Epidemiol. 2015;182(9):737–41. https://doi.org/10.1093/aje/kwv177.
92. Bradshaw PT, Stevens J. Invited commentary: limitations and usefulness of the metabolically healthy obesity phenotype. Am J Epidemiol. 2015;182(9):742–4. https://doi.org/10.1093/aje/kwv178.
93. Muñoz-Garach A, Cornejo-Pareja I, Tinahones FJ. Does metabolically healthy obesity exist? Nutrients. 2016;8:6. https://doi.org/10.3390/nu8060320. pii: E320.
94. Dobson R, Burgess MI, Sprung VS, Irwin A, Hamer M, Jones J, Daousi C, Adams V, Kemp GJ, Shojaee-Moradie F, Umpleby M, Cuthbertson DJ. Metabolically healthy and unhealthy obesity: differential effects on myocardial function according to metabolic syndrome, rather than obesity. Int J Obes. 2016;40(1):153–61. https://doi.org/10.1038/ijo.2015.151.
95. Ortega FB, Lee DC, Katzmarzyk PT, Ruiz JR, Sui X, Church TS, Blair SN. The intriguing metabolically healthy but obese phenotype: cardiovascular prognosis and role of fitness. Eur Heart J. 2013;34(5):389–97. https://doi.org/10.1093/eurheartj/ehs174.
96. Ruderman NB, Schneider SH, Berchtold P. The "metabolically-obese," normal-weight individual. Am J Clin Nutr. 1981;34(8):1617–21.
97. Yoo HJ, Hwang SY, Hong HC, Choi HY, Seo JA, Kim SG, Kim NH, Choi DS, Baik SH, Choi KM. Association of metabolically abnormal but normal-weight (MANW) and metabolically healthy but obese (MHO) individuals with arterial stiffness and carotid atherosclerosis. Atherosclerosis. 2014;234(1):218–23. https://doi.org/10.1016/j.atherosclerosis.2014.02.033.
98. Oliveros E, Somers VK, Sochor O, Goel K, Lopez-Jimenez F. The concept of normal-weight obesity. Prog Cardiovasc Dis. 2014;56(4):426–33. https://doi.org/10.1016/j.pcad.2013.10.003.
99. Lopez-Miranda J, Perez-Martinez P. It is time to define metabolically obese but normal-weight (MONW) individuals. Clin Endocrinol. 2013;79(3):314–5. https://doi.org/10.1111/cen.12181.

100. Hamer M, et al. Waist circumference stronger predictor of death risk than BMI. Ann Intern Med. 2017;166(12):917–8. https://doi.org/10.7326/L17-0022.
101. Grundy SM, Brewer HB Jr, Cleeman JI, Smith SC Jr, Lenfant C, American Heart Association, National Heart, Lung, and Blood Institute. Definition of metabolic syndrome: report of the National Heart, Lung, and Blood Institute/American Heart Association conference on scientific issues related to definition. Circulation. 2004;109(3):433–8. https://doi.org/10.1161/01.CIR.0000111245.75752.C6.
102. St-Onge MP, Janssen I, Heymsfield SB. Metabolic syndrome in normal-weight Americans: new definition of the metabolically obese, normal-weight individual. Diabetes Care. 2004;27(9):2222–8.
103. Romero-Corral A, Somers VK, Sierra-Johnson J, Korenfeld Y, Boarin S, Korinek J, Jensen MD, Parati G, Lopez-Jimenez F. Normal-weight obesity: a risk factor for cardio-metabolic dysregulation and cardiovascular mortality. Eur Heart J. 2010;31(6):737–46. https://doi.org/10.1093/eurheartj/ehp487.
104. Lassale C, Tzoulaki I, Moons KGM, et al. Separate and combined associations of obesity and metabolic health with coronary heart disease: a pan-European case-cohort analysis. Eur Heart J. 2018;39(5):397–406. https://doi.org/10.1093/eurheartj/ehx448.
105. Carnethon MR, De Chavez PJ, Biggs ML, Lewis CE, Pankow JS, Bertoni AG, Golden SH, Liu K, Mukamal KJ, Campbell-Jenkins B, Dyer AR. Association of weight status with mortality in adults with incident diabetes. JAMA. 2012;308(6):581–90. https://doi.org/10.1001/jama.2012.9282.
106. Logue J, Wild S, Sattar N. BMI and mortality among adults with incident type 2 diabetes. N Engl J Med. 2014;370(14):1362. https://doi.org/10.1056/NEJMc1401876#SA3.
107. Badoud F, Perreault M, Zulyniak MA, Mutch DM. Molecular insights into the role of white adipose tissue in metabolically unhealthy normal-weight and metabolically healthy obese individuals. FASEB J. 2015;29(3):748–58. https://doi.org/10.1096/fj.14-263913.
108. Khan UI, Ogorodnikova AD, Xu L, Wang D, Wassertheil-Smoller S, Ho GY, Sowers MF, Rajpathak SN, Allison MA, Mackey RH, Vitolins MZ, Manson JE, Wildman RP. The adipokine profile of metabolically benign obese and at-risk normal-weight postmenopausal women: the women's health initiative observational study. Obesity. 2014;22(3):786–94. https://doi.org/10.1002/oby.20139.
109. Stefan N, Häring HU, Schulze MB. Metabolically healthy obesity: the low-hanging fruit in obesity treatment? Lancet Diabetes Endocrinol. 2018;6(3):249–58. https://doi.org/10.1016/S2213-8587(17)30292-9. pii: S2213-8587(17)30292-9.
110. Banack HR, Kaufman JS. The obesity paradox: understanding the effect of obesity on mortality among individuals with cardiovascular disease. Prev Med. 2014;62:96–102. https://doi.org/10.1016/j.ypmed.2014.02.003
111. Banack HR, Kaufman JS. From bad to worse: collider stratification amplifies confounding bias in the "obesity paradox". Eur J Epidemiol. 2015;30(10):1111–4. https://doi.org/10.1007/s10654-015-0069-7.
112. Greenberg JA. The obesity paradox in the US population. Am J Clin Nutr. 2013;97(6):1195–200. https://doi.org/10.3945/ajcn.112.045815.
113. Sperrin M, Candlish J, Badrick E, Renehan AG, Buchan I. Collider bias is only a partial explanation for the obesity paradox. Epidemiology. 2016;27(4):525–30. http://journals.lww.com/epidem/Pages/comingsoon.aspx.
114. Ahima RS, Lazar MA. The health risk of obesity—better metrics imperative. Science 2013;341(6148):856–8. https://doi.org/10.1126/science.1241244.
115. Blundell JE, Dulloo AG, Salvador J, Fruhbeck G, EASO SAB Working Group on BMI. Beyond BMI—phenotyping the obesities. Obes Facts. 2014;7(5):322–8. https://doi.org/10.1159/000368783.
116. Gray SL, Vidal-Puig AJ. Adipose tissue expandability in the maintenance of metabolic homeostasis. Nutr Rev. 2007;65(5 Pt 2):S7–12.
117. Moreno-Indias I, Tinahones FJ. Impaired adipose tissue expandability and lipogenic capacities as ones of the main causes of metabolic disorders. J Diabetes Res. 2015;2015:970375. https://doi.org/10.1155/2015/970375.

118. Bays H. Adiposopathy, "sick fat," ockham's razor, and resolution of the obesity paradox. Curr Atheroscler Rep. 2014;16:409. https://doi.org/10.1007/s11883-014-0409.
119. Bays H. Adiposopathy. Is "sick fat" a cardiovascular disease. J Am Coll Cardiol. 2011;57:2461–73. https://doi.org/10.1016/j.jacc.2011.02.038.
120. Muller MJ. From BMI to functional body composition. Eur J Clin Nutr. 2013;67(11):1119–21. https://doi.org/10.1038/ejcn.2013.174.
121. Muller MJ, Lagerpusch M, Enderle J, Schautz B, Heller M, Bosy-Westphal A. Beyond the body mass index: tracking body composition in the pathogenesis of obesity and the metabolic syndrome. Obes Rev. 2012;13(Suppl 2):6–13. https://doi.org/10.1111/j.1467-789X.2012.01033.x.
122. Wellen KE, Hotamisligil GS. Obesity-induced inflammatory changes in adipose tissue. J Clin Invest. 2003;112:1785–8. https://doi.org/10.1172/JCI200320514.
123. Fogelholm M. Physical activity, fitness and fatness: relations to mortality, morbidity and disease risk factors. A systematic review. Obes Rev. 2010;11(3):202–21. https://doi.org/10.1111/j.467-789X.2009.00653.x.
124. Global BMI Mortality Collaboration, Di Angelantonio E, et al. Body-mass index and all-cause mortality: individual-participant-data meta-analysis of 239 prospective studies in four continents. Lancet. 2016;388(10046):776–86. https://doi.org/10.1016/S0140-6736(16)30175-1. Epub 2016 Jul 13.
125. Chang Y, Ryu S, Suh BS, Yun KE, Kim CW, Cho SI. Impact of BMI on the incidence of metabolic abnormalities in metabolically healthy men. Int J Obes Lond. 2012;36(9):1187–94. https://doi.org/10.1038/ijo.2011.247.
126. Willett W, et al. Guidelines for healthy weight. N Engl J Med. 1999;341:427–34. https://doi.org/10.1056/NEJM199908053410607.
127. Bangalore S, et al. Body-weight fluctuations and outcomes in coronary disease. N Engl J Med. 2017;376:1332–40. https://doi.org/10.1056/NEJMoa1606148.
128. Roberson LL, Aneni EC, Maziak W, Agatston A, Feldman T, Rouseff M, Tran T, Blaha MJ, Santos RD, Sposito A, Al-Mallah MH, Blankstein R, Budoff MJ, Nasir K. Beyond BMI: the "metabolically healthy obese" phenotype and its association with clinical/subclinical cardiovascular disease and all-cause mortality—a systematic review. BMC Public Health. 2014;14:14. https://doi.org/10.1186/1471-2458-14-14.
129. Phillips CM. Metabolically healthy obesity: definitions, determinants and clinical implications. Rev Endocr Metab Disord. 2013;14(3):219–27. https://doi.org/10.1007/s11154-013-9252-x.
130. Phillips CM, Dillon C, Harrington JM, McCarthy VJ, Kearney PM, Fitzgerald AP, Perry IJ. Defining metabolically healthy obesity: role of dietary and lifestyle factors. PLoS One. 2013;8(10):e76188. https://doi.org/10.1371/journal.pone.0076188.
131. Volkow ND, Wang GJ, Tomasi D, Baler RD. Obesity and addiction: neurobiological overlaps. Obes Rev. 2013;14(1):2–18. https://doi.org/10.1111/j.1467-789X.2012.01031.x.
132. Smith DG, Robbins TW. The neurobiological underpinnings of obesity and binge eating: a rationale for adopting the food addiction model. Biol Psychiatry. 2013;73(9):804–10. https://doi.org/10.1016/j.biopsych.2012.08.026.
133. Harvard Health Publications. Obesity paradox? Just a myth. Harv Heart Lett. 2014;24(8):8.
134. Hill JO, Wyatt HR. The myth of healthy obesity. Ann Intern Med. 2013;159(11):789–90. https://doi.org/10.7326/0003-4819-159-11-201312030-00016.
135. Sharma AM, Kushner RF. A proposed clinical staging system for obesity. Int J Obes. 2009;33(3):289–95.
136. Kuk JL, Ardern CI, Church TS, Sharma AM, Padwal R, Sui X, Blair SN. Edmonton obesity staging system: association with weight history and mortality risk. Appl Physiol Nutr Metab. 2011;36(4):570–6. https://doi.org/10.1139/h11-058.
137. Canning KL, Brown RE, Wharton S, Sharma AM, Kuk JL. Edmonton obesity staging system prevalence and association with weight loss in a publicly funded referral-based obesity clinic. J Obes. 2015;2015:619734. https://doi.org/10.1155/2015/619734.

Studies on Body Image in Children and Adolescents with Overweight/Obesity

14

Caterina Lombardo

14.1 Introduction

Worldwide obesity has doubled since 1980 and the prevalence of overweight and obesity in children under the age of 5 has increased considerably being estimated around 41 million in 2016 (http://www.who.int/dietphysicalactivity/childhood/en/). High BMI has a negative impact on health (e.g., diabetes, cardiovascular problems). Overweight and obesity is also linked to negative psychological outcomes such as negative body image attitudes, low self-esteem, and body image disturbances (e.g., [1, 2]).

This chapter will review evidence related to these psychological outcomes, with a focus on body image attitudes and especially body weight and shape dissatisfaction in overweight and obese children and adolescents taking into account gender and age differences. The chapter will also outline sources and consequences of this weight bias and introduce the concept of positive body image that can help in developing health promotion interventions for improving children's and adolescents' body image.

14.2 Body Dissatisfaction as a Function of Age and Gender in Children and Adolescents with Overweight and Obesity

Previous chapters have outlined that body image is not a realistic perceptual mental representation of one's body but it is the result of a combination of perceptual, attitudinal, and affective characteristics. It develops through interactions with the environment and reflects influences from family, peers, and culture (see Chaps. 1, 8–12,

C. Lombardo
Department of Psychology, Sapienza University of Rome, Rome, Italy
e-mail: caterina.lombardo@uniroma1.it

M. Cuzzolaro, S. Fassino (eds.), *Body Image, Eating, and Weight*,
https://doi.org/10.1007/978-3-319-90817-5_14

22, 24, 28 and 31 of this book). Body dissatisfaction, i.e., negative attitudes towards one's body, is estimated to affect around 50% of the general population (e.g., [3]). Negative body image attitudes, weight concerns, and body dissatisfaction were considered in the past a specific problem for females but nowadays it is evident that an increasing percentage of males also report high body dissatisfaction (e.g., [4]). Concerns about appearance are present in both preschool female and male children but the desire to be thinner is bigger in females than in males at all ages and across countries (e.g., [5]).

Body dissatisfaction is widespread in adolescent girls and adult women of western societies, and it develops early in life: it has been reported by age of 6 (e.g., [5, 6]) and earlier (e.g., [7]). Moreover, it shows a linear increase with age [8] throughout the elementary school years, late elementary school, and early adolescence. Elementary school children express more concern about being overweight and a stronger desire to be thinner than their younger counterparts and body dissatisfaction in late elementary school predicts body esteem and eating problems in early adolescence, and negatively affects the adolescent global self-esteem (e.g., [5]). Negative attitudes and concerns about body weight and size increases in the pre-adolescence and adolescence. It is estimated that, notwithstanding the actual BMI, the percentages of body dissatisfied pre-adolescent girls are about 40–50%, while during adolescence it increases to over 70%, with the 60.4% of males and 80.0% of females being dissatisfied with their bodies [1]. For what attain to transitions from adolescence to adulthood findings are contradictory. There are data indicating that in middle and later adolescence body dissatisfaction stabilizes or sometimes decreases (e.g., [9]) while recent studies (e.g., [10, 11]) report an opposite trend, namely that body dissatisfaction increases between middle school and high school and increases further during the transition to young adulthood. Maybe other variables moderate the age trends, several being socio-cultural while others being personal. Craike et al. [12] found that in non-metropolitan areas, body dissatisfaction decreases with age whereas in metropolitan regions it increases with age. In Craike's et al. [12] study, trends were independent of body perceptions, which were unchanged over time, region, and age. Maybe the stronger predictor of those differences as well as the stronger predictor of increases in body dissatisfaction at increasing age in metropolitan areas is BMI. Data coming from a 10-years longitudinal population-based study (the EAT project) that examined 1902 participants from diverse ethnic/racial and socioeconomic backgrounds in the Minneapolis/St. Paul metropolitan area found that body dissatisfaction increased from early adolescence to young adulthood in both females and males. However, also BMI increased with time and when BMI was controlled, the age trend observed in body dissatisfaction disappeared [10]. As it is consistently reported across studies, when body dissatisfaction appears, it does not go away spontaneously without interventions [13]. Thus, it is relevant for researchers, clinicians, and health providers to increase knowledge about how to prevent not only obesity but also body dissatisfaction which is so strictly related to BMI increases, as evidenced by Bucchianeri and colleagues [10].

14.3 Social Attitudes Towards Obesity

In western societies, there is a strong preference for thinness and leanness (see Chaps. 27–31 of this book). This preference is associated with strong social pressures to be thin for girls and to be muscular for boys. A theory often used for explaining how social preference translates into body dissatisfaction is the social comparison theory (e.g., [14]). According to this theory, individuals compare their own characteristics to the socially prescribed ideals and when discrepancies are detected, negative attitudes are formed; a similar process is used for judging other people and form attitudes towards them (e.g., [15]).

Awareness of the social impact of high body size and of the societal bias against fat people is present in very young children who have internalized this message and are worried about being overweight [5, 16]. Even in early elementary school, children who are overweight or obese report more body dissatisfaction than their average-sized peers, wish they were thinner, chose a thin or average-sized playmate significantly more often than they chose an overweight playmate [17] and are worried about being overweight and thus not having people to play with, being less popular than thin children, having only fat friends or boy/girlfriends [16]. Xanthopoulos and colleagues [18] examined children of fourth to sixth grades finding that, after controlling for both sex and race/ethnicity, body weight was the strongest predictor of body dissatisfaction. However, this association is not consistently reported across studies. Rogers et al. [11], for instance, found that BMI was not strongly associated with varying levels of body dissatisfaction, maybe because not only actual body mass index (BMI) but also perceptions of body weight and size are relevant for explaining negative attitudes towards one's body (e.g., [19]). The internalized prejudice against fat people seems to increase with age [5] and has been reported to be greater in preschool girls than in boys [20].

Usually, with very young children the societal bias against fat people is assessed presenting children with three photographs or silhouettes or dolls and asking them to point to the one who is for instance happy, pretty, sad, has many good friends, has no friends, and so forth. Those instruments have shown that preschool children display a preference for the thin figure compared to both the average-sized and overweight figures [6] and are more likely to attribute negative adjectives towards overweight stimuli and positive adjectives towards thin or average-sized stimuli (e.g., [21]). Similar results have also been reported with 2.5 years old children using two instead of three pictures [22].

14.4 Consequences of Weight Bias

Societal anti-fat attitudes and weight bias have a negative impact on psychological well-being as reported in both cross-sectional and longitudinal studies (e.g., [23, 24]). Griffiths and colleagues [2] in a systematic review evaluating the negative impact of obesity on self-esteem, quality of life, physical competence, physical appearance perceptions, social acceptance, and social functioning showed that obesity was associated to all these negative psychological outcomes with no clear age trend nor differences as a function of gender and ethnicity. Again, it is not obesity per se that may have a negative impact on psychological health, but stigmatization of people whose BMI do not conform to societal standards of beauty. Weight stigmatization is the process that leads to the assignment of people to a category based on their weight and the association to that category of other characteristics that are not necessarily related to weight but considered undesirable as well as the overweight (e.g., stupid, isolated, lazy). See Chap. 28 of this book.

In explaining how anti-fat attitudes are formed, also attributions are important. Attribution theories (e.g., [25, 26]) emphasize causality and controllability of an outcome. Outcomes may be perceived either as the result of internal, controllable causes or as the result of external, uncontrollable causes. In judging individuals belonging to a stigmatized group, people search for the cause of the stigma and if the stigmatized trait is thought to be under personal control, negative attributes are assigned, and discrimination is justified. Research has shown that overweight and obese children are frequently stigmatized and excluded on the bases of their assignment to that weight category (e.g., [6]). Moreover, as reported by Holub [20], internalization of the social anti-fat stereotypes is predicted by children's beliefs about the controllability of weight: those who viewed overweight as uncontrollable held fewer anti-fat attitudes than those who perceived overweight as controllable.

Appearance comparison processes and unfavorable comparisons with others may maintain or increase body dissatisfaction by a feedback loop (e.g., [11]): overweight and obese children and youths as well as their normal-weight peers form their negative attitudes towards fat people through social comparison processes, which in turn give rise to an increase in their level of body dissatisfaction as they do not conform to the social ideals of beauty. Several data indicate that adolescent girls with higher body mass indices are more stigmatized, experience more weight-related teasing and show greater body dissatisfaction than their average weight peers [5, 27, 28] and a study by Puhl and colleagues [29] show that high percentages of weight loss treatment seeking youths report of having been victimized from peers (92%), friends (70%), parents (37%), and teachers (27%).

A second negative feedback loop or vicious cycle has been described for explaining why stigmatized people, instead of losing weight for changing the social category they are included in, are more likely to increase their weight further. The mechanisms of this vicious cycle are described by Brewis [30] as follows:

1. Weight stigma increases eating and reduces exercise behavior: Results of several studies provide evidence that those who feel judged by others because of their body size are less motivated to be physically active (e.g., [31]). Similarly, exposure to stigmatizing materials like videos can trigger higher calorie consumption, especially in those who believe they are overweight [32, 33] and those who report on surveys that they feel stigmatized also report more comfort eating, bingeing, and extreme caloric restriction (e.g., [34]).
2. Weight stigma increases stress: There is a growing body of studies showing that chronic psychosocial stress predicts additional weight gain or greater food intake

especially among those already overweight or obese [35–37]. Research from sexual minority stigma may suggest the pathway that explains negative outcomes also in the case of weight stigmatization: Members of the stigmatized group compare with the other people and make efforts trying to fit it in without succeeding; in turn they receive a constant devaluation which can create chronic stress (e.g., [38]).

3. Weight stigma indirectly affects body weight via changes in social relationships: Adolescent networks influence exercise and eating behavior, but high levels of physical activity also creates and reinforces friendships among people with similar bodies and increases stereotyping and exclusion towards overweight and obese peers (e.g., [39, 40]), thus stigmatized children may become isolated and overeat as a function of that negative affect.
4. Weight stigma indirectly produces structural effects through discrimination: There is evidence that weight bias negatively affects access and opportunity in almost all aspects of everyday life [41]; this negative socioeconomic effect of weight discrimination can lead to additional weight gain [30].

14.5 Sources of Weight Stigmatization

Parents, peers, media, and also health professionals comments may contribute to the internalization of the thin ideal of beauty and thus to develop body dissatisfaction and weight stigmatization (e.g., [11, 27, 41]). See also Chaps. 22 and 27–31 of this book.

14.5.1 Parents

Parents may influence children attitudes towards their bodies through direct and indirect pressures to conform to the societal standards. Parents may directly influence their children attitudes commenting on their appearance and weight or by requiring them to eat or avoid certain foods or encouraging them to slim down (e.g., [42, 43]). The mealtime is often a moment of the day that families spend time together so it is very likely that parents may comment on their children appearance or eating behavior and although parents may or may not explicitly press their overweight/obese children to restrict eating for losing weight, the children perception of this pressure increases the likelihood of being dissatisfied with their bodies [44, 45]. Moreover, parents may indirectly influence their children concerns about body weight and shape through modeling. Dissatisfied children have often parents that remark on the appearance of their own bodies, engage in calorie-restrictive dieting or exercise for losing weight or are concerned about their own and their child's weight (e.g., [46]). Evidence of this relationship in very young children are scarce (e.g., [47]) although Holub and colleagues [42] observed that 3- to 6-year-old children mothers' fear of fatness was associated with children's negative stereotypes about overweight. Studies of older children (pre-adolescents and early adolescents) showed that mothers' negative attitudes towards fat bodies and parents' beliefs about personal control over weight predict high children's weight prejudice (e.g., [48]). More recently, Damiano and colleagues [45] evidenced that mothers' overvaluation of weight and shape predicted use of fat restriction while their internalization of the thin ideal of beauty predicted pushing to eat feeding practices.

Girls may be particularly affected by their mothers' behavior through both direct comments and modeling [47, 49]. The father's influence on their children's, especially sons' attitudes has been investigated only recently. Although Wertheim and colleagues [46] failed in finding an association between fathers' dieting and their adolescent sons' or daughters' body attitudes, more recent findings indicate that fathers' influences are also important in the development of boys' body attitudes. McCabe and Ricciardelli [49] reported that adolescent boys who were pressed by their fathers for losing weight actually tried to lose weight more often than those who did not receive those pressures. Consistently, results of a study conducted by Damiano and colleagues [50] confirm that boys' body size attitudes are associated to fathers' negative attitudes towards obese persons. Moreover, negative comments about weight by fathers predicted binge eating or higher BMI in the sons (e.g., [43]) and Spiel and colleagues [47] reported similar bias in 3-years old children evidencing that fathers' attitudes prospectively predicted boys' weight bias and awareness of weight loss strategies.

The combined influences of both mothers' and peers' were investigated in a study by Lombardo and colleagues [51]. The authors compared two groups of female children practicizing aesthetic and non-aesthetic sports (aesthetic sports are those in which the performance is evaluated by judges, like in gym or dance) [52]. Children in the aesthetic group, despite their lower BMI, desired to be thinner than their peers in the non-aesthetic group. Moreover, their mothers were more dissatisfied with their children's body shape and adopted for themselves more calorie-restrictive dieting than the mothers of the children in the non-aesthetic sports group.

14.5.2 Peers

As children grow up family influences become less relevant while peers influences become stronger (e.g., [53]). Peers directly influence eating and exercise behavior and the closer is a friend the greater is his/her influence (e.g., [54, 55]) with greater effects seen in adolescents as compared to pre-adolescents and boys as compared to girls (e.g., [56]).

Results of the scientific literature are quite consistent in supporting also the influence of peers on body dissatisfaction. As it happens with family members, also peers may impact body dissatisfaction directly through overt comments or indirectly through shaping processes and friends selection. Peers may directly influence body dissatisfaction through negative comments and remarks that may become teasing and bullying (e.g., [23, 24, 57]). Teasing may be defined as a negative appearance-related verbal feedback that informs the recipient that his/her peers have a negative opinion of his/her physical appearance [58]. Verbal feedbacks may be insults or cruel comments and remarks. Results from cross-sectional and longitudinal studies and meta-analysis support the connection between teasing and body dissatisfaction (e.g., [57, 59–63]). Menzel and colleagues [59] suggest that the link between teasing and body dissatisfaction in childhood and adolescence may be causal and predict body dissatisfaction in adulthood. Consistent results also come from the longitudinal study EAT cited above that evidenced that prevalence of weight-related teasing remained longitudinally stable throughout early adolescence, middle adolescence, late adolescence, and young adulthood (e.g., [60]). The association between weight teasing and body dissatisfaction is stronger in children and adolescents than in adults, in female than in male samples [59].

14.5.3 Teachers

The anti-fat attitudes are so widespread that they can also be found at school among teachers (e.g., [49]) and are also within this context a cause of stigmatization and disparity. Several studies (e.g., [64–66]) show that teachers are more likely to have lower expectations for overweight children, across a range of ability areas, and describe them as untidy, emotional, less likely to be successful at work, and more likely to have family problems as compared to their normal-weight peers.

As evidenced by the previously cited study by Puhl and colleagues [29], a high percentage of weight loss treatment seeking youths report of having been victimized not only by peers and friends but also by teachers (27%).

14.5.4 The Media

Media use is widespread in today's western societies. According to a 2013 Nielsen report [67], young people aged 12–24 years spent almost 22 h/week watching traditional TV. A more recent report by the same company confirm that TV is the preferred choice among media users still in 2016 although it is the most heavily consumed platform among adults while children consume multiple types of media and spend many of their waking hours in front of multiple types of screens, often simultaneously. The incidence of TV viewing, however, remains substantial across all age groups. Since 2011 the incidence of TV viewing has decreased slightly: 14–17 aged children show the biggest decrease from 99% in 2011 to 96% in 2014 but part of them is viewing content elsewhere. Given this heavy consumption of media, weight stigmatizing messages can be potentially harmful to young people. Research findings have shown that children's media present positive messages about being thin and negative messages about being overweight; thin characters are associated with desirable characteristics and have central roles, whereas less time is dedicated to overweight characters who usually have minor stereotypical roles, are rarely portrayed in romantic relationships and are more likely to be objects of humor [68].

Eisenberg and colleagues [69] asked 2793 middle and high school children to indicate their favorite television shows. Throughout the 30 episodes analyzed, there were 66 total appearance- or weight-related stigmatizing, weight stigmatizing instances included both male and female characters. Half of the targets were overweight, even though only about one in five characters were overweight across shows. Audience laughter was the response in over 40% of these incidents, thus reinforcing the stigmatization of the characters' weight.

Ata and Thompson [70] surveyed the previous 15 years of research on weight bias and stigmatization in the media and discussed some theoretical models that might help explain the negative effects of such stigmatization. They evidenced that a wide range of media—from television shows to books, newspapers, and the internet—portray overweight and obese individuals in a stigmatizing manner. This is true not only for the adolescents' targeted media programs but also for children's targeted programs. Moreover, results showed that the longer is the time children spend using media the bigger is the impact of the stigmatizing messages on interiorization of those stereotypes. In boys, it was also associated with total time spent watching television. Liking of the obese figures (compared to the non-obese figures) was negatively related to magazine use, which tended to be higher among girls.

14.5.5 Health Providers

Obesity, especially in children and youths, has received significant attention by researchers, professionals, and policy makers due to its relevant consequences on health. As such, health providers often emphasize the need for losing weight or maintain a low BMI and prevention and treatment approaches to obesity address weight loss as the key construct for gaining health (e.g., [71, 72]). Since these negative messages pervade almost every aspect of life (e.g., media, family, work, school) and since also health care providers show high rates of weight bias (e.g., [73]), their messages may strengthen the social negative attitudes towards fat people and indirectly increase stigmatization.

Reviewing the literature on stigma and obesity, Washington [68] evidenced that, as it happens in the general population, also among health providers' stigma towards obesity is highly present and physicians attribute negative characteristics such as "weak-willed" to their obese patients, spend less time with them, and focus more on weight as a cause of their health problems. Negative attitudes about overweight patients have been reported by psychologists, nurses, and physicians [74–76] and also health care professionals treating obesity and eating disorders (e.g., [73, 77]). For instance, Puhl and colleagues [73] assessed through an online survey explicit weight bias, perceived causes of obesity, attitudes towards treating obese patients, perceptions of treatment compliance and success of obese patients, and perceptions of weight bias among their colleagues in 329 professionals treating eating disorders. Participants showed negative weight stereotypes and reported to have colleagues holding negative attitudes towards obese patients. Comparing professionals with less and those with more weight bias, the second were more likely to attribute obesity to behavioral causes, expressed more negative attitudes and frustrations about treating obese patients, and perceived poorer treatment outcomes for these patients.

An improvement (in terms of reduction of stigmatization among health providers) was observed by Budd and colleagues [78] from 1990 to 2007. However, little is known about weight bias in health providers towards children and adolescents obesity, at least at the best of the knowledge of the author of this chapter.

14.6 Positive Body Image and the Health at every Size Movement

Most of the scientific literature summarized above deals with negative body image and its causes and consequences. A change paradigm in the study of body image has been observed a few years ago when the new concept of positive body image was developed. Wood-Barcalow and colleagues [79] defined positive body image as a feeling of love and respect for one's body characterized by appreciation of the unique beauty and functions that it performs, acceptation of the aspects that are inconsistent with idealized images. Those who have this positive image of their bodies are also assumed to be resistant to the external pressure to conform to the socially shared standard of beauty. As for positive psychology, positive body image does not correspond to the absence or low levels of body dissatisfaction but as a sense of full appreciation of the body notwithstanding its imperfections [80].

A complete overview of this position goes beyond the scope of this chapter and a more complete account may be found in Tylka and colleagues [80]. A great impulse to this change paradigm is due to the contribution of feminist scholars (e.g., [81]) who questioned the equation "beautiful bodies equal standard thin bodies." According to this viewpoint, the mass media message that perfect thin bodies are preferable to an individualized concept of health and beauty is probably the most relevant source of body dissatisfaction and weight stigmatization. They proposed to shift the attention from weight to health and gave birth to a trans-disciplinary movement called Health at Every SizeSM (HAES)[2] whose main counter-message is intended to help people understand that it is empowering to resist internalizing media appearance ideals and messages and try to do one's best for gaining health instead of trying to change appearance in order to conform to a standard unrealistic thin body.

The positive body image paradigm be the theoretical framework for designing effective programs that promote the development of a positive image instead of or together with preventing the development of negative attitudes towards children's and adolescents' bodies.

References

1. Griffiths S, Hay P, Mitchison D, Mond JM, McLean SA, Rodgers B, Massey R, Paxton SJ. Sex differences in the relationships between body dissatisfaction, quality of life and psychological distress. Aust N Z J Public Health. 2016;40:518–22. https://doi.org/10.1111/1753-6405.12538.
2. Griffiths LJ, Parsons TJ, Hill AJ. Self-esteem and quality of life in obese children and adolescents: a systematic review. Int J Pediatr Obes. 2010;5:282–304.

3. Fiske L, Fallon EA, Blissmer B, Redding CA. Prevalence of body dissatisfaction among United States adults: review and recommendations for future research. Eating Behav. 2014;15:357–65. https://doi.org/10.1016/j.eatbeh.2014.04.010. Epub 2014 May 14.
4. Blashill AJ. Gender roles, eating pathology, and body dissatisfaction in men: a meta-analysis. Body Image. 2011;8:1–11.
5. Smolak L. Body image development in childhood. In: Cash TF, Smolak L, editors. Body image. A handbook of science, practice, and prevention. 2nd ed. New York: Guilford Press; 2012.
6. Harriger JA, Thompson JK. Psychological consequences of obesity: weight bias and body image in overweight and obese youth. Int Rev Psychiatry. 2012;24(3):247–53. https://doi.org/10.3109/09540261.2012.678817.
7. Tremblay L, Limbos M. Body image disturbance and psychopathology in children: research evidence and implications for prevention and treatment. Curr Psychiatr Rev. 2009;5:62–72.
8. Rohde P, Stice E, Marti CN. Development and predictive effects of eating disorder risk factors during adolescence: implications for prevention efforts. Int J Eat Disord. 2015;48:187–98.
9. Eisenberg ME, Neumark-Sztainer D, Paxton SJ. Five-year change in body satisfaction among adolescents. J Psychosom Res. 2006;61(4):521–7.
10. Bucchianeri MM, Arikian AJ, Hannan PJ, Eisenberg ME, Neumark-Sztainer D. Body dissatisfaction from adolescence to young adulthood: findings from a 10-year longitudinal study. Body Image. 2013;10(1):1–7.
11. Rodgers RF, McLean SA, Marques M, Dunstan CJ, Paxton SJ. Trajectories of body dissatisfaction and dietary restriction in early adolescent girls: a latent class growth analysis. J Youth Adolesc. 2016;45:1664–77. https://doi.org/10.1007/s10964-015-0356-3.
12. Craike M, Young JA, Symons CM, Pain MD, Harvey JT, Eime RM, Payne WR. Trends in body image of adolescent females in metropolitan and nonmetropolitan regions: a longitudinal study. BMC Public Health. 2016;16:1143. https://doi.org/10.1186/s12889-016-3815-1.
13. Wertheim EH, Paxton SJ. Body image development in adolescent girls. In: Cash TF, Smolak L, editors. Body image. A handbook of science, practice, and prevention. 2nd ed. New York: Guilford Press; 2012.
14. Festinger L. A theory of social comparison processes. Hum Relat. 1954;7:117–40.
15. Corcoran K, Jan Crusius J, Mussweiler T. Social comparison: motives, standards, and mechanisms. In: Chadee D, editor. Theories in social psychology. Hoboken: Wiley-Blackwell; 2011. p. 119–39.
16. Rees R, Oliver K, Woodman J, Thomas J. The views of young children in the UK about obesity, body size, shape and weight: a systematic review. BMC Public Health. 2011;11:188.
17. Fraňková S, Chudobová P. Development of body image in preschool girls. Homeost Health Dis. 2000;40:161–9.
18. Xanthopoulos MS, Borradaile KE, Hayes S, Sherman S, Vander Veur S, Grundy KM, Nachmani J, Foster GD. The impact of weight, sex, and race/ethnicity on body dissatisfaction among urban children. Body Image. 2011;8:385–9.
19. Yan F, Johnson AM, Harrell A, Pulver A, Zhang J. Perception or reality of body weight: which matters the most to adolescents' emotional wellbeing? Curr Psychiatr Rev. 2015;11:130–46.
20. Holub SC. Individual differences in the anti-fat attitudes of preschool-children: the importance of perceived body size. Body Image. 2008;5:317–21.
21. Worobey J, Worobey HS. Body-size stigmatization by preschool girls: in a doll's world, it is good to be "Barbie". Body Image. 2014;11:171–4.
22. Turnbull JD, Heaslip S, McLeod HA. Pre-school children's attitudes to fat and normal male and female stimulus figures. Int J Obes. 2000;24:1705–6. https://doi.org/10.1038/sjijo.0801462.
23. Eisenberg ME, Neumark-Sztainer D, Story M. Associations of weight-based teasing and emotional well-being among adolescents. Arch Pediatr Adolesc Med. 2003;157:733–8.
24. Eisenberg ME, Neumark-Sztainer D, Haines J, Wall M. Weight-teasing and emotional well-being in adolescents: longitudinal findings from Project EAT. J Adolesc Health. 2006;38:675–83.

25. Crandall CS. Ideology and lay theories of stigma: the justification of stigmatization. In: Heatherton TF, Kleck RE, Hebl MR, Hull JG, editors. The social psychology of stigma. New York: Guilford Press; 2000. p. 126–52.
26. Crandall CS, D'Anello S, Sakalli N, Lazarus E, Wieczorkowska G, Feather NT. An attribution-value model of prejudice: anti-fat attitudes in six nations. Personal Soc Psychol Bull. 2001;27:30–7.
27. Puhl RM, Latner JD. Stigma, obesity, and the health of the nation's children. Psychol Bull. 2007;133(4):557–80.
28. Neumark-Sztainer D, Falkner N, Story M, Perry C, Hannan PJ, Mulert S. Weight-teasing among adolescents: correlations with weight status and disordered eating behaviors. Int J Obes Relat Metab Disord. 2002;26:123–31.
29. Puhl RM, Peterson JL, Luedicke J. Weight-based victimization: bullying experiences of weight loss treatment–seeking youth. Pediatrics. 2013;131(1):e1–9.
30. Brewis AA. Stigma and the perpetuation of obesity. Soc Sci Med. 2014;118:152–8.
31. Vartanian LR, Novak SA. Internalized societal attitudes moderate the impact of weight stigma on avoidance of exercise. Obesity 2011;19:757–62.
32. Salvy S, Bowker JC, Nitecki LA, Kluczynski MA, Germeroth LJ, Roemmich JN. Impact of simulated ostracism on overweight and normal-weight youths' motivation to eat and food intake. Appetite. 2011;56:39–45.
33. Schvey NA, Puhl RM, Brownell KD. The impact of weight stigma on caloric consumption. Obesity. 2011;19:1957–62.
34. Haines J, Neumark-Sztainer D, Eisenberg ME, Hannan PJ. Weight teasing and disordered eating behaviors in adolescents: longitudinal findings from Project EAT (eating among teens). Pediatrics. 2006;117:209–15.
35. Dallman MF, Pecoraro NC, la Fleur SE. Chronic stress and comfort foods: self-medication and abdominal obesity. Brain Behav Immun. 2005;19:275–80.
36. De Vriendt T, Moreno LA, De Henauw S. Chronic stress and obesity in adolescents: scientific evidence and methodological issues for epidemiological research. Nutr Metab Cardiovasc Dis. 2009;19:511–9.
37. Torres SJ, Nowson CA. Relationship between stress, eating behavior, and obesity. Nutrition. 2007;23:887–94.
38. Sikorski C, Luppa M, Luck T, Riedel-Heller SG. Weight stigma "gets under the skin"-evidence for an adapted psychological mediation framework: a systematic review. Obesity. 2015;23:310–20. https://doi.org/10.1002/oby.20952.
39. Simpkins SD, Schaefer DR, Price CD, Vest AE. Adolescent friendships, BMI, and physical activity: untangling selection and influence through longitudinal social network analysis. J Res Adolesc. 2013;23(3):537–49.
40. Schaefer DR, Simpkins SD. Using social network analysis to clarify the role of obesity in selection of adolescent friends. Am J Public Health. 2014;104:1223–9. https://doi.org/10.2105/AJPH.2013.301768.
41. Puhl RM, Brownell KD. Psychological origins of obesity stigma: toward changing a powerful and pervasive bias. Obes Rev. 2003;4:213–27.
42. Holub SC, Tan CC, Patel SL. Factors associated with mothers' obesity stigma and young children's weight stereotypes. J Appl Dev Psychol. 2011;32:118–26.
43. Berge JM, MacLehose RF, Loth KA, Eisenberg ME, Fulkerson JA, Neumark-Sztainer D. Parent-adolescent conversations about eating, physical activity and weight: prevalence across sociodemographic characteristics and associations with adolescent weight and weight-related behaviors. J Behav Med. 2015;38:122–35. https://doi.org/10.1007/s10865-014-9584-3.
44. Jaffe K, Worobey J. Mothers' attitudes toward fat, weight and dieting in themselves and their children. Body Image. 2006;3:113–20. https://doi.org/10.1016/j.bodyim.2006.03.003.
45. Damiano SR, Hart LM, Paxton SJ. Correlates of parental feeding practices with preschoolers: parental body image and eating knowledge, attitudes, and behaviours. Appetite. 2016;101:192–8.

46. Wertheim EH, Martin G, Prior M, Sanson A, Smart D. Parent influences in the transmission of eating and weight related values and behaviors. Eat Disord. 2002;10:321–34.
47. Spiel EC, Paxton SJ, Yager Z. Weight attitudes in 3- to 5-year-old children: age differences and cross-sectional predictors. Body Image. 2012;9:524–7.
48. Hansson LM, Rasmussen F. Predictors of 10-year-olds' obesity stereotypes: a population-based study. Int J Pediatr Obes. 2010;5:25–33.
49. McCabe MP, Ricciardelli LA. A longitudinal study of body image and strategies to lose weight and increase muscles among children. J Appl Dev Psychol. 2005;26:559–77.
50. Damiano SR, Gregg KJ, Spiel EC, McLean SA, Wertheim EH, Paxton SJ. Relationships between body size attitudes and body image of 4-year-old boys and girls, and attitudes of their fathers and mothers. J Eating Disord. 2015;3:16. https://doi.org/10.1186/s40337-015-0048-0.
51. Lombardo C, Battagliese G, Lucidi F, Frost RO. Body dissatisfaction among pre-adolescent girls is predicted by their involvement in aesthetic sports and by personal characteristics of their mothers. Eat Weight Disord. 2012;17:116–27.
52. Powers P.S. & Johnson C. (1996). Small victories: prevention of eating disorders among athletes, Eating Disord 4:4, 364–377, DOI: https://doi.org/10.1080/10640269608249195.
53. Santrock J. Adolescence. New York: The McGraw-Hill Companies, Inc.; 2007.
54. Barclay KJ, Edling C, Rydgren J. Peer clustering of exercise and eating behaviours among young adults in Sweden: a cross-sectional study of egocentric network data. BMC Public Health. 2013;13(1):1–13.
55. De la Haye K, Robins G, Mohr P, Wilson C. How physical activity shapes, and is shaped by, adolescent friendships. Soc Sci Med. 2011;73:719–28.
56. Sawka KJ, McCormack GR, Nettel-Aguirre A, Hawe P, Doyle-Baker PK. Friendship networks and physical activity and sedentary behavior among youth: a systematized review. Int J Behav Nutr Phys Act. 2013;10(130):1–9.
57. Puhl RM, King KM. Weight discrimination and bullying. Best Pract Res Clin Endocrinol Metab. 2013;27:117–27.
58. Thompson JK, Heinberg LJ. The media's influence on body image disturbance and eating disorders: we've reviled them, now can we rehabilitate them? J Soc Issues. 1999;55:339–53.
59. Menzel JE, Schaefer LM, Burke NL, Mayhew LL, Brannick MT, Thompson JK. Appearance-related teasing, body dissatisfaction, and disordered eating: a meta-analysis. Body Image. 2010;7:261–70.
60. Haines J, Hannan PJ, Van den Berg P, Eisenberg ME, Neumark-Sztainer D. Weight-related teasing from adolescence to young adulthood: longitudinal and secular trends between 1999 and 2010. Obesity (Silver Spring). 2013;21(9):E428–34.
61. Bucchianeri MM, Eisenberg M, Neumark-Sztainer D. Weightism, racism, classism, and sexism: shared forms of harassment in adolescents. J Adolesc Health. 2013;53(1):47–53.
62. Bucchianeri MM, Eisenberg ME, Wall MM, Piran N, Neumark-Sztainer D. Multiple types of harassment: associations with emotional well-being and unhealthy behaviors in adolescents. J Adolesc Health. 2014;54(6):724–9.
63. Haines J, Neumark-Sztainer D, Hannan PJ, Van den Berg P, Eisenberg ME. Longitudinal and secular trends in weight-related teasing during adolescence. Obesity. 2008;16:S18–23.
64. Neumark-Sztainer D, Story M, Harris T. Beliefs and attitudes about obesity among teachers and school health care providers working with adolescents. J Nutr Educ Behav. 1999;31(1):3–9.
65. O'Brien KS, Hunter JA, Banks M. Implicit anti-fat bias in physical educators: physical attributes, ideology and socialization. Int J Obes (Lond). 2007;31(2):308–14.
66. Glock S, Beverborg AOG, Muller BCN. Pre-service teachers' implicit and explicit attitudes toward obesity influence their judgments of students. Soc Psychol Educ. 2016;19:97–115. https://doi.org/10.1007/s11218-015-9315-9.
67. The Nielsen Comparable metrics report 2026. www.nielsen.com.
68. Washington RL. Childhood obesity: issues of weight bias. Prev Chronic Dis. 2011;8:A94.
69. Eisenberg ME, Carlson-McGuire A, Gollust SE, Neumark-Sztainer D. A content analysis of weight stigmatization in popular television programming for adolescents. Int J Eating Disord. 2015;48(6):759–66.

70. Ata R, Thompson JK. Weight bias in the media: a review of recent research. Obes Facts. 2010;3:41–6.
71. Bombak A. Obesity, health at every size, and public health policy. Am J Public Health. 2014;104:e60–7.
72. Saguy A. What's wrong with fat? New York: Oxford University Press; 2013.
73. Puhl RM, Latner JD, King KM, Luedicke J. Weight bias among professionals treating eating disorders: attitudes about treatment and perceived patient outcomes. Int J Eating Disord. 2014;47:65–75.
74. Davis-Coelho K, Waltz J, Davis-Coelho B. Awareness and prevention of bias against fat clients in psychotherapy. Prof Psychol Res Pract. 2000;31:682–4.
75. Maroney D, Golub S. Nurses' attitudes toward obese persons and certain ethnic groups. Percept Mot Skills. 1992;75:387–91.
76. Price JH, Desmond SM, Krol RA, Snyder FF, O'Connell JK. Family practice physicians' beliefs, attitudes, and practices regarding obesity. Am J Prev Med. 1987;3:339–45.
77. Teachman BA, Brownell KD. Implicit anti-fat bias among health professionals: is anyone immune? Int J Obes. 2001;25:1525–31.
78. Budd GM, Mariotti M, Graff D, Falkenstein K. Health care professionals' attitudes about obesity: an integrative review. Appl Nurs Res. 2011;24(3):127–37.
79. Wood-Barcalow NL, Tylka TL, Augustus-Horvath CL. "But I like mybody": positive body image characteristics and a holistic model for young-adult women. Body Image. 2010;7:106–16. https://doi.org/10.1016/j.bodyim.2010.01.001.
80. Tylka TL, Wood-Barcalow NL. What is and what is not positive body image? Conceptual foundations and construct definition. Body Image. 2015;14:118–29.
81. Bacon L, Aphramor L. Weight science: evaluating the evidence for a paradigm shift. Nutr J. 2011;10:9. https://doi.org/10.1186/1475-2891-10-9.

Suggested Reading

Drury CA, Louis M. Exploring the association between body weight, stigma of obesity, and health care avoidance. J Am Acad Nurse Pract. 2002;14(12):554–61.
Eisenberg ME, Neumark-Sztainer D, Perry CL. Peer harassment, school connectedness, and academic achievement. J Sch Health. 2003;73(8):311–6.
Eisenberg ME, Berge JM, Fulkerson JA, Neumark-Sztainer D. Weight comments by family and significant others in young adulthood. Body Image. 2011;8(1):12–9.
Eisenberg ME, Berge JM, Fulkerson JA, Neumark-Sztainer D. Associations between hurtful weight-related comments by family and significant other and the development of disordered eating behaviors in young adults. J Behav Med. 2012;35(5):500–8.
Hussin M, Frazier S, Thompson JK. Fat stigmatization on YouTube: a content analysis. Body Image. 2011;8:90–2.
Lampard AM, MacLehose RF, Eisenberg ME, Neumark-Sztainer D, Davison KK. Weight-related teasing in the school environment: associations with psychosocial health and weight control practices among adolescent boys and girls. J Youth Adolesc. 2014;43(10):1770–80.
Latner JD, Rosewall JK, Simmonds MB. Childhood obesity stigma: association with television, videogame, and magazine exposure. Body Image. 2007;4:147–55.
Neumark-Sztainer D. Obesity and body image in youth. In: Cash TF, Smolak L, editors. Body image. A handbook of science, practice, and prevention. 2nd ed. New York: Guilford Press; 2012.
Tremblay L, Lovsin T, Zecevic C, Larivière M. Perceptions of self in 3–5-year-old children: a preliminary investigation into the early emergence of body dissatisfaction. Body Image. 2011;8:287–92.
Van den Berg P, Neumark-Sztainer D, Eisenberg ME, Haines J. Racial/ethnic differences in weight-related teasing in adolescents. Obesity (Silver Spring). 2008;16(2):S3–S10.

Studies on Body Image in Adults with Non-BED Overweight/Obesity

15

Alessandra Pokrajac-Bulian

15.1 Risk Factors in Negative Body Image Development

There are several research directions in the study of risk factors in negative body image development in higher weight persons: (1) research that focuses on individual characteristics such as gender, age, race, and psychological characteristics of risk (e.g., low self-esteem, depression); (2) research that deals with body weight and its change over time; and (3) research that focuses on interpersonal and social risk factors, such as being teased about weight and appearance, social stigma, and discrimination.

15.1.1 Individual Characteristics. Gender and Ethnic Differences

Compared with overweight men, overweight women are less satisfied with their body and assess themselves to be more overweight even if their BMI is lower. When women and men of similar body weight are compared, women regularly show significantly poorer psychological functioning [1]. Being a woman in our culture is a risk factor in the development of a negative body image [2]. The reasons for these research results most likely come from different socio-cultural ideals regarding the appearance of women and men. Whereas women are expected to be slender, and while they worry about being overweight, men worry about their body image because of the perceived lack of muscles. Numerous studies point out that a lack of muscles is a more significant predictor of a negative body image in men than overweight or excess adipose tissue [3].

A. Pokrajac-Bulian
University of Rijeka, Faculty of Humanities and Social Sciences, Department of Psychology, Rijeka, Croatia
e-mail: pokrajac@ffri.hr

M. Cuzzolaro, S. Fassino (eds.), *Body Image, Eating, and Weight*,
https://doi.org/10.1007/978-3-319-90817-5_15

In their research, Cash and Hicks [4] compared men and women based on their self-assessment of weight as normal or excessive. The results showed that the self-assessment of weight is a more significant predictor of negative body image than actual weight. Overweight women who assessed themselves as such were more dissatisfied with their body than women of normal weight who assessed themselves as overweight. Unlike women, overweight men who assessed themselves as such were less dissatisfied with their body than men of normal weight who assessed themselves as overweight. The authors offer the explanation that corpulent men assess themselves to be bigger and stronger, and not obese. It is possible that this cognitive interpretation protects some men against body image dissatisfaction. In line with this hypothesis is the research carried out on the sample of almost 1900 men and women from Britain [5], in which 3/4 of overweight women perceived themselves as overweight, whereas 2/3 of men did the same. In the interpretation of the results, the authors point out that greater muscularity increases BMI in men, so that their self-assessment of being overweight is not that incorrect. However, it is interesting that women with BMI ranging from 22 to 28 perceive themselves as overweight, whereas men with BMI ranging from 25 to 28 are significantly less likely to be dissatisfied with their body or to perceive themselves as overweight or obese. Although from a psychological standpoint this attitude seems more acceptable and presents a sort of a protective mechanism in negative body image development in men, it does, on the other hand, lead to a conclusion that men are less likely to endeavor to change their body weight by dieting or engaging in physical activity, regardless of the fact that their weight is increased or even at the level of obesity.

Although body image dissatisfaction is rather common in higher weight persons, there are differences between certain ethnic groups. Most studies that link body image with obesity have been carried out on Caucasians, whereas only a few of them look into the effects of race and ethnicity on body image in other races—African Americans, Asians, and Hispanics [6, 7]. Overweight black women generally express more satisfaction with their body than white women with severe obesity; the presumed reason for this is in much more flexible cultural standards of attractiveness, that is, in a much wider range of weight and body shapes that are considered acceptable [7]. Even though very few studies have focused on finding the relationship between obesity and body image in Hispanics and Asians, there are findings that show that women in these groups are approaching the levels of dissatisfaction with their body as expressed by white women, which is happening in parallel with the increase of the former's acculturation to American culture [6].

Franko and Roehrig [8] state that black women show higher levels of accepting obesity and, in contrast to white women, they show moderately less dissatisfaction with their body. A high risk of obesity in black women may point to different forms of oppression that these women were subjected to in the past, or are still being subjected to (e.g., racism, sexual abuse [9]). A more positive body image in black women possibly reflects the need to deny health issues that come with obesity. Some authors believe that a certain level of body image dissatisfaction is necessary as it may motivate higher weight persons, especially in a culture in which obesity is more acceptable, to change their lifestyle by exercising and changing their diet [10].

A meta-analysis of 98 studies published between 1960 and 2004 showed that white and Hispanic women are more dissatisfied with their body compared to black women, but a comparison of mean differences showed that they are relatively small [11]. In some older studies, Hispanic women in comparison to white women assessed themselves to be more attractive even when their weight was significantly higher [12]. A longitudinal research on the sample of young black women showed that 66% of women who were overweight in their 20s became obese in their 30s. However, the relationship between a higher BMI and body satisfaction weakens as they approach higher levels of BMI [13]. Differences in body dissatisfaction between white and black women do not remain constant over time; in the last 25 years, it seems that the difference in body satisfaction has increased, whereas it decreased for body weight. A possible explanation is that white women are becoming less dissatisfied with their body and less concerned with being overweight, whereas in black women their dissatisfaction is increasing, which was shown in longitudinal studies on young adult women [1]. Similar results were obtained in a research carried out on a Pacific island where the prevalence of obesity is very high so that obesity is seen as a more acceptable, positive, and healthier characteristic. Persons with obesity from the Samoan Islands are very satisfied with their body and do not attempt to lose weight [1].

American Asians in comparison with other races (African Americans and Hispanics) are less obese and overweight, but body dissatisfaction, especially in women, is very high—similar to that in white American women [1]. However, an overview of research on Asian women provides contradictory results. In certain cases, they show less body satisfaction, and in other cases, they are significantly more satisfied with their body image than white American women. A third group of studies even shows that they are more like white women in their body satisfaction and weight concern, or that their fear of obesity is even more pronounced [14, 15]. The perception of overweight and obesity, as well as attempts of losing weight, are very common in Asian countries, which points to the significance of cultural factors in shaping attitudes toward weight (e.g., Japanese women have the highest prevalence of perception of overweight, with as much as 63% believing themselves to be overweight) [16].

15.1.2 Low Self-Esteem and Depression

A number of studies found a relationship between an increase in body image dissatisfaction and a higher number of depression symptoms and lower self-esteem in women with obesity seeking weight loss treatment. It seems that this relationship is independent of the degree of obesity [17, 18].

In their research, Matz et al. investigate body image dissatisfaction on the sample of non-binge eating women who applied for weight loss treatment. The most significant predictors of body image dissatisfaction proved to be low self-esteem, being teased about weight in adulthood, and the internalization of cultural appearance standards [19]. There is a significant difference in body image dissatisfaction between genders; women with obesity seeking bariatric surgery are more dissatisfied with their body image compared with men. Self-esteem also proved to be a significant predictor of body image dissatisfaction (BID). In adult persons with severe obesity, it is negatively associated with BID; the less self-esteem a person with obesity has, the greater the body image dissatisfaction [20]. In higher weight persons, preoccupation with own body image does not grow proportionally to the increase of BMI [18].

A study carried out on a group of women with severe obesity, candidates for bariatric surgery, showed that body image dissatisfaction in that group correlates significantly with a high level of depression, and very low self-esteem. What is special in this research is that perfectionism was investigated as well and it, too, proved to be a significant predictor of negative body image [21]—especially those aspects of perfectionism that relate to a tendency to achieve high personal standards and to high criticism in self-assessment. Self-criticism as an indicator of the dimension of maladaptive perfectionism explains the relationship between perfectionism and depression, anxiety, and eating disorder symptoms [22]. Studies are consistent in their conclusions that the indicators of psychological functioning play a very significant role in predicting body image dissatisfaction.

Only a small group of higher weight women is extremely dissatisfied with body image. Research by Sarwer et al. indicates that 8% of women with obesity is extremely dissatisfied with body image, which is in line with the diagnosis of the body dysmorphic disorder [23]. A person with this disorder is worried about one or several non-existent or slight defects in physical appearance. Consequently, a person begins to manifest certain repetitive, compulsive behaviors to reduce concerns about their appearance, e.g., by checking themselves in the mirror, by wearing particular clothes with the aim of covering up a defect, by seeking reassurance and comfort from others (this will be discussed in Chap. 5). However, this diagnosis cannot be applied to women with obesity because by definition the body dysmorphic disorder is associated with concern and discomfort regarding a slight defect in appearance. DSM-V [24] does not have a diagnostic category that includes a significant distress concerning a medical condition that affects physical appearance. In comparison with other higher weight women, those who are extremely dissatisfied with their body image show more symptoms of depression. These research results lead to a conclusion that there is a subgroup of women who experience body image dissatisfaction so intensely that it causes clinically significant psychological disorders [25]. Body image dissatisfaction should be distinguished from body image disorder, which implies more extreme dissatisfaction that causes intense anxiety and severe psychosocial problems. Serious depression, extreme body image dissatisfaction, and significant social anxiety not only prevent individuals in seeking appropriate weight loss treatments, but may also decrease their effectiveness.

It is quite difficult to determine the line between normal and abnormal concern with body image because body image dissatisfaction in higher weight persons is expected and acceptable. Physical deficiency or social prejudice and discrimination to which persons with obesity are subjected to is not something they imagine.

Accepting the attitude that it is normal or desirable for persons with obesity to feel dissatisfied with their body reflects a lack of understanding of the nature of body image disorder and is a form of bias toward obesity that is reflected in the following belief: "Persons with obesity deserve to feel bad about their body." Higher weight persons with body image disorder experience a very disturbing concern with their body image, they believe completely unrealistically that their appearance shows something very negative about their personal worth, they avoid a number of social situations because of their weight, and they are always worried about their bodies being sufficiently hidden or covered [26].

Studies that compare higher weight and normal-weight persons on measures of social anxiety, depression, and self-esteem at times do not confirm the presupposed differences between these two groups. Sarwer et al. compared obese and normal-weight women and found differences in body image satisfaction, but not in the symptoms of depression or self-esteem [23]. Differences between obese and normal-weight persons are sometimes not obtained because studies are carried out on the sample of patients seeking weight loss treatment. Annis et al. also did not find differences in the symptoms of depression and social anxiety between different groups, although the research included women who are currently obese, who were obese, and who were never obese [27]. The researchers found differences only in the self-esteem of currently obese and overweight women and those who never had problems with increased weight, whereas women who were previously obese were not different from other groups; this supports the presumption that self-esteem may partly increase with moderate weight loss. These different research results point to the need for further research on the relationship between body weight, body image dissatisfaction, and psychological symptoms.

15.1.3 Body Weight and Its Changes over Time

On a non-clinical sample of 217 women with obesity, Hill and Williams found that body dissatisfaction significantly worsens with the increase of body weight, that is, that body dissatisfaction is highest in the group with the highest BMI. Similar results were obtained in recent studies [28]. Runfola et al. concluded that body dissatisfaction is present in women throughout the entire range of adulthood and that it is determined by the level of BMI [29]. The conclusion of the authors from a 2016 study on a sample of physically active older women with different BMIs also confirmed that body dissatisfaction is most prominent in women with the highest BMI [30].

The relationship between body dissatisfaction and BMI changes and become less clear when studies are conducted within certain subgroups of higher weight persons. Thus, in the research of Matz et al. [19], no significant correlation between BMI and body dissatisfaction was found in women with non-BED obesity, which led the authors to conclude that the level of nutrition does not have an independent contribution in the importance women attribute to weight and body shape in their self-assessment.

15.1.4 Stigmatization as a Risk Factor

In today's society, obesity is still seen as a problem of the individual. Therefore, it is not uncommon that as a result of stigmatization and discrimination related to obesity, higher weight persons develop a negative body image (see also Chap. 27 of the present book). The experience of weight-based stigmatization is more common in adults with BMI higher than 40 as compared to persons with lower levels of obesity. Persons with the experience of being stigmatized because of overweight have a negative body image [1]. A study by Annis et al. shows that women who are currently obese and overweight and who describe more experiences of weight stigmatization express more body dissatisfaction and distress and exhibit dysfunctional behavior in view of extreme investment in their appearance [27]. In the same study, the authors found that a stigmatizing experience is not related to body image in those women who were previously obese or overweight. Stigmatization significantly correlates with body image distress, which supports the fact that body image is not linked to weight, but is directly related to stigmatization.

Persons with obesity are discriminated both at work and in healthcare, education, and family. Compared to other forms of stigmatization and discrimination, obesity is the only one where an individual cannot hide from others. There are three categories of stigmatization to which higher weight persons may be exposed to: direct stigmatization, in which the person is publicly shamed, stigmatization in the surroundings, which refers, among other things, to occupying a seat in public transportation or in public places, and indirect stigmatization, which refers, for example, to a situation where persons with obesity are critically looked upon while they are shopping for groceries [31]. The stigmatizing experiences of the individuals with obesity are not motivating them to lose weight—on the contrary, they create barriers in regard to change and distance the individual from activities that promote a healthier lifestyle.

An Australian group of authors carried out a qualitative research on body image, self-esteem, and weight stigmatization [32]. The results showed that media depictions continually show that persons with obesity behave in unhealthy ways, are inactive, or eat fast food, which strengthens the social stereotype regarding obesity. The dissatisfaction and shame that persons with obesity feel about their body are constantly reinforced by other people's attitudes and by messages on the need to lose weight coming from family, friends, the media, and public healthcare. Consequently, anxiety and concern arise in situations in which persons with obesity come into contact with other persons, they constantly compare themselves to someone else, and they feel emotional distress due to weight-based stigma [32]. The authors found that persons with obesity choose various ways of dealing with weight-based stigma. Most often, they try to avoid exposing their body to the looks of other people, they avoid mirrors because of the repulsion they feel toward their body, and very often they isolate themselves socially. Some use strategies of diverting attention from their weight and are almost obsessed with grooming and appearance (e.g., women use heavy make-up, do their hair, men try to be immaculately ironed and shaved). They also often use other compensatory behaviors because of their obesity—they work more than others, they try to be exceptional parents and perfect in all that they do, countering thus the usual stereotype that persons with obesity are lazy and inactive. On the other hand, some give up on grooming and invest minimal effort in their appearance, especially those with a BMI higher than 40 and who have been obese all their lives. In order to protect themselves from teasing and weight-based stigma, they try to play the role of extremely cheerful persons; although for them it is often uncomfortable or unnatural, it is easier for them to laugh about themselves than to be constantly upset or mad. This research clearly showed that although there are different personal experiences and coping mechanisms that the persons with obesity use, a negative body image, and a sense of being different regarding their body weight are still dominant [32].

15.2 Assessment of Body Image in Adults with Obesity

Body image dissatisfaction is a multidimensional construct that includes measures of subjective dissatisfaction, cognitive distortion, affective response, avoidance behaviors, and perceptual distortion [33] (see also Chap. 1 of the present book). In the following overview, we look at some of the most commonly used measures that relate to persons with obesity concerns about appearance (see also Chap. 2 of the present book). In selecting measures for the assessment of body image in persons with obesity, special attention is needed as behind similar terms lie different aspects of body image. The most common aspects of body image that are assessed (see review by Sarwer et al. [25]) are classified into several groups: satisfaction with body weight, satisfaction with appearance, investment in body image, and perception of body size.

Body weight satisfaction in persons with obesity is investigated by questionnaires as well as figural ratings. Questionnaires are an expression of an individual's expression of subjective assessment of parts of the body that are related to body weight. An example of such measure is the *Body Shape Questionnaire* [34]. Another way of assessing body image satisfaction is using schematic figures in which, from a number of silhouettes, a person first chooses the one that reflects the person's current figure and then chooses one that reflects the person's ideal figure. The range of figures is from very thin to obese and the discrepancy between these two values is the measure of body image dissatisfaction. Although the use of these measures is quite practical, there are a number of psychometric limitations; difficulties arise because of the impossibility to identify participants with given figures that grow proportionally from the thinnest to the widest figure, which does not necessarily suit all participants or does not provide adequate coverage of obese bodies or bodies with a different somatic weight distribution (e.g., some persons with obesity have less adipose tissue in the lower part of the body, and others have moderate upper body curves). More recent assessment methods that include computer technologies have increased the external validity and accuracy of described measures.

In the assessment of body image dissatisfaction, measures of general satisfaction with appearance may be used. These measures include those aspects of the body that are not related to body weight, such as some parts of the face or muscle mass, and sometimes these assessments relate to appearance in specific clothes (e.g., bathing suit, colorful or loose-fitting clothes) or to other people's assessment. Such measuring instruments are especially useful because they enable the recognition of general concern with appearance or concern with specific parts of the body. Most often in literature we find the *Multidimensional Body-Self Relations Questionnaire* [35], as an especially useful measure because it includes the dimensions of evaluation and focuses on appearance, fitness and health, overweight preoccupation, self-classified weight, and the body areas satisfaction. Cash points out that it is very important to know the extent to which a person invests psychologically into his or her appearance [35]. Appearance investment has two aspects: the extent to which persons pay attention to their appearance and engage in grooming, and the extent to which persons define their worth based on physical appearance. The latter is key in psychological functioning and the quality of life related to body image [25].

The perception of body size has been researched for a long time, but it is only in the last 20 years that studies have shown that perceptual ratings are under the influence of cognitive and affective factors, and not perceptual as previously thought [33]. Apart from being rather impractical and expensive, perceptual measures do not highly correlate with body image satisfaction.

There are cases in which current photographs of an obese person are used for the assessment of body image distortion. However, being photographed is a very stressful situation for overweight and persons with obesity, and this can intensify their concern about body image [1]; anxiety caused in this way may affect the negative assessment of one's body. Studies of body image distortion differ according to the target group that they include, age, origin, socioeconomic status, psychopathology, and type of weight loss program or surgical interventions, which makes it difficult to generalize and to compare obtained results. Nonetheless, regardless of methodological issues, the pattern most often identified indicates that overweight and persons with obesity over-assess their body size compared to persons of normal weight. Previous research on persons with obesity found the tendency to under-assess one's body figure. The explanation provided by Latner and Wilson refers to the idea that over-assessment reflects a sense of self-efficacy [1]. If persons with obesity have the experience of losing weight quickly, there is an increase in the level of personal self-efficacy in relation to weight control. Some studies in which participants assessed their figure before and after treatment showed that the assessments were much more accurate following the treatment.

Studies that investigate body image in persons with obesity should focus on different aspects of body image—from satisfaction to distortion—but they should not disregard personal investment or importance a person attributes to body image. It seems that studies on persons with obesity often disregard the aspect of investment in body image and generally focus on satisfaction. As studies regarding body image assessment most often deal with women, attention should also be directed toward higher weight men to gain a complete picture of the issue at hand.

15.3 Treatment of Body Image in Obese Adults

There are two groups of psychological interventions in the treatment of the negative body image of persons with overweight/obesity; the first one relates to treatments oriented toward weight loss that do not give special attention to body image, and the other one is primarily oriented toward the treatment of body image.

Numerous studies have noted changes in the body image of persons with obesity in weight loss treatment. Cash writes about significant improvement in the body image of women with obesity who reduced their weight 22 kg on average [36]. Foster et al. [17] have similar findings in a group of women with obesity who lost 19 kg on average in mid-treatment and their body image improved significantly. An increase of only a few kilograms led to a mild although significant deterioration of body image. Upon completion of the treatment, in comparison to beginning body image dissatisfaction, the participants showed significant improvement of their body image that was only weakly related to the amount of lost weight. Even a very small loss of weight in persons with obesity may significantly improve body satisfaction. Although high correlation was not found between the amount of weight lost and the degree of improvement of body image, it is very common for persons involved in weight loss treatment to gain weight upon the completion of treatment because they go back to their old, unhealthy diet habits [1]. Gaining weight again means that the body image reverses in the direction of the starting level although some improvements remain.

In a recent review paper and meta-analysis, Chao analyses the effects of improvement of the body image of higher weight individuals who are involved in different weight loss treatments [37]. The results suggest that interventions oriented toward weight loss help in improving body image. This is a very significant finding as body image affects psychological well-being and helps in losing weight and in maintaining it [17]. Chao also finds that various multidimensional aspects of body image, such as body shape concern, body size dissatisfaction, and body satisfaction improve to a significant extent when active interventions are applied [37]. If observed together, these facets include an assessment component and a component of importance to the individual, that is, of investment in body image; this supports the notion that interventions oriented toward weight loss may be effective in improving overall body image—more than in improving only one of its aspects.

Another research direction is moving toward investigating the efficacy of treatments for improving the body image of persons with overweight/obesity without weight loss. Thus, Rosen et al. implement in a group of women with obesity a therapeutic program of cognitive-behavioral orientation with the aim of improving body image [38]. Working in small groups on negative weight-related stereotypes, on modifying intrusive thoughts regarding body dissatisfaction, on appearance-related beliefs, on exposing participants to situations that women with obesity usually avoid, and on removing body checking, the results showed significant improvement in body image. Moreover, there were improvements in self-esteem and regarding shame related to eating, and the participants began to binge less and showed fewer psychological symptoms although there was no weight loss involved.

In a study conducted with a group of women with obesity and men that compared a weight loss treatment with a combination of such treatment and body image therapy, Ramirez and Rosen obtained results that showed improvement in body image and in self-esteem in both groups of patients [39]. Within a year of monitoring, the groups did not differ in view of neither successfulness in maintaining weight nor body image. The authors conclude that body image therapy is very effective with persons with obesity, and that a well-structured cognitive-behavioral weight loss treatment may also be very effective. Sarwer et al. suggest that body image therapy is possibly more effective in that phase of treatment that concerns maintaining weight, as it may enhance the long-term maintenance of achieved results [25].

Heinberg et al. suggest the possibility of a curved relationship between body image dissatisfaction and healthy body weight control through moderate exercise and balanced diet [10]. They believe that a low level of body image dissatisfaction may hamper motivation to get involved in weight control treatment, whereas a very high level of dissatisfaction is a trigger for using extremely unhealthy ways of weight control (e.g., extreme dieting, binging, or bulimic behaviors). Nonetheless, most studies support the view that a greater weight loss can be predicted based on a more positive view of one's body, while an extremely negative body image interferes with positive treatment outcomes.

The studies mentioned above unquestionably show that improving body image is important to persons with obesity and that there are a number of different treatments that have proven effective in resolving the issue. However, it is important to highlight that body image dissatisfaction is only one of the aspects of obesity that are related to satisfaction with life, psychological health, and positive self-esteem. Therefore, it appears it is more important to choose such interventions that along improving negative body image also lead to weight loss—due to health issues. If a person with obesity is satisfied with his or her body image, that is an important achievement, but it is possible that he or she may lose motivation to reduce weight, which is certainly undesirable.

References

1. Latner JD, Wilson RE. Obesity and body image in adulthood. In: Cash TF, Smolak L, editors. Body image: a handbook of science, practice, and prevention. New York: Guilford Press; 2011. p. 189–98.
2. Cash TF, Roy RE. Pounds of flesh: weight, gender, and body images. In: Sobal J, Maurer D, editors. Interpreting weight: the social management of fatness and thinness. Hawthorne: Aldine de Gruyter; 1999. p. 209–28.
3. Cafri G, Thompson JK. Measuring male body image: a review of the current methodology. Psychol Men Masc. 2004;5:18–29.
4. Cash TF, Hicks KF. Being fat versus thinking fat: relationships with body image, eating behaviors, and well-being. Cogn Ther Res. 1990;14:327–41.
5. Wardle J, Johnson F. Weight and dieting: examining levels of weight concern in British adults. Int J Obes. 2002;6:1144–9.
6. Altabe M, O'Garo KN. Hispanic body images. In: Cash TF, Pruzinsky T, editors. Body image: a handbook of theory, research, and clinical practice. New York: Guilford Press; 2002. p. 250–6.

7. Celio AA, Zabinski MF, Wilfley DE. African American body images. In: Cash TF, Pruzinsky T, editors. Body image: a handbook of theory, research, and clinical practice. New York: Guilford Press; 2002. p. 234–42.
8. Franko DL, Roehrig JP. African American body images. In: Cash TF, Smolak L, editors. Body image: a handbook of science, practice, and prevention. New York: Guilford Press; 2011. p. 189–98.
9. Ullman SE, Filipas HH. Ethnicity and child sexual abuse experiences of female college students. J Child Sex Abus. 2005;14 67–89.
10. Heinberg LJ, Thompson JK, Matzon JL. Body image dissatisfaction as a motivator for healthy lifestyle change: is some distress beneficial? In: Striegel-Moore RH, Smolak L, editors. Eating disorders: innovative directions in research and practice. Washington, DC: American Psychological Association; 2001. p. 215–32.
11. Grabe S, Hyde JS. Ethnicity and body dissatisfaction among women in the United States: a meta-analysis. Psychol Bull. 2006;132:622–40.
12. Altabe M. Ethnicity and body image: quantitative and qualitative analysis. Int J Eat Disord. 1998;23:153–9.
13. Roberts A, Cash TF, Feingold A, Johnson BT. Are black–white differences in females' body dissatisfaction decreasing? A meta-analytic review. J Consult Clin Psychol. 2006;74: 1121–31.
14. Cachelin FM, Rebeck RM, Chung GH, Pelayo E. Does ethnicity influence body size preference? A comparison of body image and body size. Obesity. 2002;10(3):158–66.
15. Sanders NM, Heiss CJ. A comparison of body image and eating attitudes in Asian and Caucasian college women. Eat Disord J Treat Prev. 1998;6:15–27.
16. Wardle J, Haase AM, Steptoe A. Body image and weight control in young adults: international comparisons in university students from 22 countries. Int J Obes. 2006;30:644–51.
17. Foster GD, Wadden TA, Vogt RA. Body image before, during, and after weight loss treatment. Health Psychol. 1997;16:226–9.
18. Wadden TA, Sarwer DB, Womble LG, Foster GD, McGuckin BG, Schimmel A. Psychosocial aspects of obesity and obesity surgery. Surg Clin North Am. 2001;8:1001–24.
19. Matz PE, Foster GD, Faith MS, Wadden TA. Correlates of body image dissatisfaction among overweight women seeking weight loss. J Consult Clin Psychol. 2002;70(4):1040–4. https://doi.org/10.1037//0022-006X.70.4.1040.
20. Grilo CM, Masheb RM, Brody M, Burke-Martindale CH, Rothschild BS. Binge eating and self-esteem predict body image dissatisfaction among obese men and women seeking bariatric surgery. Int J Eat Disord. 2005;37:347–51.
21. Rosenberger PH, Henderson KE, Grilo CM. Correlates of body image dissatisfaction in extremely obese female bariatric surgery candidates. Obes Surg. 2006;16:1331–6.
22. Dunkley DM, Blankstein KR, Masheb RM, Grilo CM. Personal standards and evaluative concerns dimensions of "clinical" perfectionism: a reply to Shafran et al. (2002, 2003) and Hewitt et al. (2003). Behav Res Ther. 2006;44:63–84.
23. Sarwer DB, Wadden TA, Foster GD. Assessment of body image dissatisfaction in obese women: specificity, severity and clinical significance. J Consult Clin Psychol. 1998;66(4):651–4.
24. American Psychiatric Association. Diagnostic and statistical manual of mental disorders. 5th ed. Washington, DC: Author; 2013.
25. Sarwer DB, Thompson JK, Cash TF. Body image and obesity in adulthood. Psychiatr Clin N Am. 2005;28:69–87.
26. Rosen JC. Obesity and body image. In: Fairburn CG, Brownell KD, editors. Eating disorders and obesity. New York: Guilford Press; 2002. p. 399–402.
27. Annis NM, Cash TF, Hrabosky JI. Body image and psychosocial differences among stable average-weight, currently overweight, and formerly overweight women: the role of stigmatizing experiences. Body Image. 2004;1:155–67.
28. Hill AJ, Williams J. Psychological health in a non-clinical sample of obese women. Int J Obes. 1998;22:578–83.

29. Runfola CD, Von Holle A, Trace SE, Brownley KA, Hofmeier SM, Gagne DA, Bulik CM. Body dissatisfaction in women across the lifespan: results of the UNC-SELF and gender and body image (GABI) studies. Eur Eat Disord Rev. 2013;21(1):52–9. https://doi.org/10.1002/erv.2201.
30. Raso V, Garber CE, Mancini RB, Matsudo SMM. Body image in a representative sample of overweight, obese and normal weight active older women living in the community: associations with body composition, physical fitness and function. Medical Express (São Paulo, online). 2016;3(4):M160402. https://doi.org/10.5935/MedicalExpress.2016.04.02.
31. Lewis S, Thomas SL, Blood RW, Castle DJ, Hyde J, Komesaroff PA. How do obese individuals perceive and respond to the different types of obesity stigma that they encounter in their daily lives? A qualitative study. Soc Sci Med. 2011;73(9):1349–56.
32. Thomas S, Karunaratne A, Lewis S, Castle D, Knoesen N, Honigman R, Hyde J, Kausman R, Komesaroff P. 'Just bloody fat!': a qualitative study of body image, self-esteem and coping in obese adults. Int J Ment Health Promot. 2010;12(1):39–49. https://doi.org/10.1080/14623730.2010.9721805.
33. Thompson JK, Heinberg LJ, Altabe M, Tanleff-Dunn S. Exacting beauty: theory, assessment, and treatment of body image disturbance. Washington, DC: American Psychological Association; 1999.
34. Cooper PD, Taylor MJ, Cooper Z, Fairburn CG. The development and validation of the body shape questionnaire. Int J Eat Disord. 1987;6:485–94. https://doi.org/10.1002/1098-108X(198707)6:4<485::AID.
35. Cash TF. Cognitive–behavioral perspectives on body image. In: Cash TF, Pruzinsky T, editors. Body image: a handbook of theory, research, and clinical practice. New York: Guilford Press; 2002. p. 38–46.
36. Cash TF. Body image and weight changes in a multisite comprehensive very-low calorie diet program. Behav Ther. 1994;25(2):239–54.
37. Chao H-L. Body image change in obese and overweight persons enrolled in weight loss intervention programs: a systematic review and meta-analysis. PLoS One. 2015;10(5):e0124036. https://doi.org/10.1371/journal.pone.0124036.
38. Rosen JC, Orosan P, Reiter J. Cognitive–behavior therapy for negative body image in obese women. Behav Ther. 1995;26:25–42.
39. Ramirez EM, Rosen JC. A comparison of weight control and body image therapy for obese men and women. J Consult Clin Psychol. 2001;69(3):440–6.

Non-surgical Weight Loss and Body Image Changes in Children, Adolescents, and Adults

16

Federico Amianto

16.1 Overweight and Obesity

Obesity is an increasing problem among adults and children in many developed and developing countries, and it is a major global public health threat [1, 2]. It is a multifactorial disorder characterized by an imbalance between intake and daily requirement of nutrients. The causes of obesity are complex and include genetic, psychological, biochemical, environmental, social, and economic factors. In clinical practice, overweight and obesity are usually defined by the body mass index (BMI, weight in kilograms divided by the square of the height in meters) [3, 4]. According to the World Health Organization (WHO) criteria, overweight is defined as a BMI of 25–29.9 kg/m^2 and obesity as 30 kg/m^2 or greater [5].

Obesity results in significant impairment of health and longevity, increasing individuals' risk of illness and reducing life expectancy. Overweight and obesity are major risk factors for serious chronic diseases, such as type 2 diabetes mellitus, cardiovascular disease, hypertension, stroke, and some forms of cancer [1].

It also has an important impact on individual self-esteem and self-image and limits health-related quality of life [4].

16.2 Assessment

To address correctly and effectively the weight-loss strategies, it's important to make a comprehensive initial assessment and then to use clinical judgement to investigate comorbidities and other factors to an appropriate level of detail [6]. The information should be collected depending on the personal characteristics of the

F. Amianto
Eating Disorders Center for Treatment and Research, Department of Neuroscience, University of Turin, Turin, Italy
e-mail: federico.amianto@unito.it

M. Cuzzolaro, S. Fassino (eds.), *Body Image, Eating, and Weight*,
https://doi.org/10.1007/978-3-319-90817-5_16

individual, the timing of the assessment, the degree of overweight or obesity, and the results of previous assessments. It is necessary to manage comorbidities when they are identified and give the patient information on the benefits of losing weight, healthy eating, and increased physical activity.

To propose a weight-loss treatment, it is fundamental to assess the person's view of the weight and the diagnosis, and possible historical and current psychological reasons for weight gain, to explore eating patterns, physical activity levels, any beliefs about eating, physical activity, and weight gain that are unhelpful if the person wants to lose weight.

It is important to find out what the person has already tried and how successful this has been and to assess the person's readiness to adopt changes. Finally it is very important, from a strategical and psychological point of view, to make a clear distinction between losing weight and maintaining the weight loss [6].

16.3 Treatment and Care of Overweight and Obesity in Adults

Treatment and care of overweight and obesity should take into account the person's preferences, initial fitness, health status, and lifestyle [6].

According to NICE guidelines, therapy should be based on a multi-disciplinary multi-step approach: (1) general advice on healthy weight and lifestyle, (2) diet and physical activity, (3) drugs, (4) surgery. It is fundamental to provide patients and their families and/or carers with information about the options for treatment [6].

Non-pharmacological lifestyle interventions can be combined with psychological interventions to improve adherence to treatment and induce permanent change in the obese or overweight individuals [4, 7].

While many interventions have been shown to have a short-term effect in inducing moderate weight loss, only a minority of people are able to maintain their weight loss. On the other hand, weight loss may improve psychological measures and health-related quality of life and allow for a more active lifestyle and increased physical activity [4].

16.3.1 Lifestyle Interventions

Interventions addressing lifestyle should represent a first-line strategy to induce and maintain weight loss. The greatest part of these interventions are attitudes towards a correct lifestyle that should be common acquisitions among general population. They include behavior change strategies to increase people's physical activity levels or decrease inactivity, improve eating behavior and the quality of the person's diet, and reduce energy intake. Treatments should take into account the social circumstance, the experience and the outcome of previous treatments, the person's level of risk and, where appropriate, any comorbidities. It is important to encourage the family to support any weight management program [4, 6, 8].

16.3.2 Dietary

The main aim of the dietetic intervention is the reduction in fat consumption and increase in healthy food intake [1].

It is important to tailor dietary changes to food preferences and allow for a flexible and individual approach to reducing calorie intake, without unduly restrictive and nutritionally unbalanced diets, because they are ineffective in the long term and can be harmful. Moreover, it is necessary to encourage people to improve their diet even if they do not lose weight because there can be other health benefits. The main requirement of a dietary approach to weight loss is that total energy intake should be less than energy expenditure [6]. Dietary modification is superior to exercise in attaining weight loss in overweight and obese adults: they are a more potent method for creating an energy imbalance than physical activity alone [7].

16.3.3 Physical Activity

Exercise has a positive effect on body weight in people with overweight and obesity. Although exercise alone improved weight loss only marginally compared with no treatment, when combined with dietary interventions, the amount of weight-loss diet resulted greater than diet alone and increasing exercise intensity increased the magnitude of weight loss [7]. Exercise combined with diet, independently by weight loss, also has a positive effect on cardiovascular risk factors, compared with sedentary persons, irrespective of weight [1, 7].

Exercise prescriptions include specific recommendations for the type, intensity, frequency, and duration of any physical activity. Finally, after achieving weight loss, it is important to encourage adults to build up to the recommended activity levels for weight maintenance: a key element of intervention based on physical activity is the reduction of time spent inactive, such as watching television, using a computer or playing video games [6].

16.3.4 Pharmacological Interventions

Non-pharmacological methods of obesity therapy, which include dietary modification, exercise, and behavioral modification, have demonstrated short-term effectiveness. Unfortunately, long-term recidivism rates are high, thus drugs should be used in conjunction with non-pharmacological therapy and with lifestyle modification [5].

Drug treatment is being considered in adults who have a BMI of 28 kg/m^2 or more with associated risk factors, or a BMI of 30 kg/m^2 or more.

The only approved anti-obesity drugs for long-term use belong to the category of the inhibitors of intestinal fat absorption. Orlistat, a drug that inhibits lipases, is the only agent currently available in this class. Side effects are related to malabsorption of fats including steatorrhea, bloating, and malabsorption of fat-soluble vitamins.

Orlistat has positive effects on lipidic profile, reduces blood pressure and diabetes incidence [6, 9].

Less commonly used medications for weight loss are either approved for short-term use (phendimetrazine, diethylpropion, and phentermine), or used off-label (bupropion, metformin, topiramate, and zonisamide) [4–6, 10].

Fluoxetine is currently used in BED treatment with possible clinical benefit in obesity and overweight. It is a selective serotonin reuptake inhibitor (SSRI), enhancing serotonin activity. Its functional consequences include symptoms such as decreased food intake, altered food selection, endocrine changes, and normalization of unusual eating behaviors (such as the frequency and severity of binge eating episodes that may be associated with obesity).

Although not specifically approved for weight loss, it is being prescribed for this indication, but showed higher efficacy in BED than in non-BED obese population [11, 12].

16.3.5 Psychological Interventions

Body image and obesity are related in important ways. Obesity may affect health not only through physical changes but also through psychological distress, which itself is important because it affects quality of life. Body image is one area where distress occurs, and therefore deserves specific attention [13].

Overweight and obese treatment-seekers demonstrate higher rates of psychopathology, including mood disorders (depression, low self-esteem, anxiety) and eating disorders (binge eating disorder, night eating syndrome, body image dissatisfaction), as well as impaired health-related quality of life [14]. Heavier individuals are also at increased risk of discrimination in employment, health care, education, and in interpersonal relationships. Combined, these negative biopsychosocial outcomes result in significant impairments in health-related quality of life [14].

Prominent cognitive processes are involved in the internalization of the slender beauty ideal, development of beliefs that constitute a thinness schema, and a tendency to compare one's weight and shape to the bodies of various other people, such as peers and celebrities [15].

Helping obese individuals to develop a realistic ideal body shape might be helpful in influencing the perceptual component of body image. Perception of one's own body depends on the integration of bodily signals from the outside (exteroception) and the inside (interoception). These signals contribute to self-image, that is, "the picture we have in our minds of the size, shape, and form of our bodies and to our feelings concerning these characteristics and our constituent body parts." Women with higher BMI have greater body image self-discrepancies. Moreover, obese patients usually report the inability to know when to start and stop eating, i.e., to feel the internal signals of hunger and satiety, resulting in an eating behavior led by external signals. Enhancing their interoception, which is impaired by the stress might, eventually, help them to adopt a healthier eating style [16].

Last but not least, body checking and avoidance are behaviors frequently associated with overweight and body image disturbances [17].

The participation in a weight-loss intervention itself has generally been shown to result in improvements in psychological outcomes in the short- to medium-term [14, 15].

A first-line approach to encourage weight loss is represented by psychoeducation, while a wide range of psychological interventions has been used in the treatment of overweight and obesity. The majority of psychological interventions for overweight and obesity are cognitive-behaviorally based, and are typically used in combination with lifestyle interventions [14]. Cognitive-behavior therapy has been proposed that a good time to address them would be following weight loss, in order to enhance weight maintenance [18].

16.3.6 Psychoeducational Interventions

Psychoeducation provides information about core topics like the factors that predispose, trigger, and maintain eating impulsiveness, negative effects of overweight and unbalanced or restrictive diets, and most effective methods of weight regulation [19]. Treatments are focused on plain symptoms explanation, without adopting strategies to influence unconscious or cognitive maintaining factors at a deep level, unlike to what occurs in psychotherapies [19, 20]. These treatments can be structured in weekly group meetings of limited duration [19]. Patients are taught on the pathogenic mechanisms of the disease, to self-monitor food intake, and about correct lifestyles, sustainable in time [19, 20]. Interventions are focused to promote a general improvement of health and quality of life, rather than on weight loss itself. These interventions have showed a preliminary efficacy on binge reduction and eating impulsivity [19, 20].

16.3.7 Psychotherapies

According to literature data, psychotherapies are the most validated and effective treatments for BED [21–23]. Recent studies [21–23] describe binge eating in BED as the possible result of an immediate breakdown of emotion and impulse regulation caused by sudden increases of negative affect and tension, and/or rapid decrease of positive effect. Therapeutic implications of these findings are represented by the development of response-prevention strategies, such as the acceptance of stressful events or the disclosure of mental states.

Cognitive-behavioral therapies (CBT) are the most evaluated and developed psychological intervention for treating BED [21, 22]. The focus is the etiological basis of bingeing and its relation with a self-esteem excessively dependent from body shape [21, 24]. The most widely used CBT models are adaptations of those developed for BN [21, 23]. CBT is a practical and adaptable intervention, with setting and duration that can be tailored on clinical needs and the possibility of being carried out independently or in combination with other pharmacological or BWL approaches [21, 25–27]. A number of researchers, led by Cash and Rosen [28, 29], have devised CBT for improvement of body image. In this process, the experience of the body is shifted from a site of vulnerability and shame to a site of knowledge and agency [15]. Long-term effects of CBT approaches include a gradual normalization of eating patterns and reduced relapse occurrence [30–32]. Unfortunately, evidences about effects on weight reduction are still limited and of unclear clinical significance [22, 33, 34].

Dialectic-behavioral therapy (DBT) is another psychotherapeutic approach that has proved its efficacy in BED; it is more focused on emotion regulation and stress tolerance than CBT [23]. This therapy showed to be effective in binge reduction and in lowering concerns about food and body shape similarly to CBT, but it has not provided clear results on weight loss [35, 36].

Another evidence-based psychological treatment is interpersonal psychotherapy (IPT). This technique focuses on personal relations and role transitions that could have a predisposing and maintaining role in EDs, in order to achieve better social interactions and to cope with interpersonal conflicts [23, 37, 38]. Even if it doesn't focus directly eating symptoms, it can be useful because it targets a specific area of impairment in BED patients [38–40].

Other psychotherapeutic interventions that has been used successfully in the treatment of overweight and obesity include psychodynamic therapy, relaxation therapy, hypnotherapy, eye movement desensitization and reprocessing (EDMR), emotion freedom techniques, and emotion-focused therapy [23].

16.4 Overweight and Obesity in Adolescents and Children

The prevalence of obesity and overweight is increasing in child populations throughout the world, presenting a global public health crisis [2, 41]. In addition to the medical consequences already listed for adults, the condition of obesity can affect the child's mental health and lead to early discrimination, low self-esteem, and depression [2, 41].

Differentiate between obese binge eaters and obese non-binge eaters could be helpful in the assessment and treatment for young obese patients. Obese youngsters who binge tend to have greater psychopathology such as depression, low self-esteem, anxiety, and difficulties in social relationships [42].

16.5 Treatment and Care of Overweight and Obesity in Adolescents and Children

The purposes of interventions in children and adolescents are similar to treatment in adults [2, 41].

However, the primary goal of treatment (i.e., weight reduction or deceleration of weight gain) and the recommended mode of intervention is variable and dependent on the child's age and initial level of overweight, along with other case-specific considerations. The importance of a combined dietary, physical, activity, and behavioral component has been highlighted by several studies [43–56]. Parental involvement has been recognized as an important component of behavioral programs, particularly in pre-adolescent children [2]. Instead at the best of our knowledge, currently there isn't any scientific evidence on the application of psychotherapeutic interventions in the treatment of obesity and overweight during the adolescence or childhood.

16.5.1 Lifestyle Interventions

It is fundamental to create a supportive environment that helps overweight or obese children and their family to make lifestyle changes, tailoring interventions to the needs and preferences of the family system.

The focus may be on either weight maintenance or weight loss, depending on the person's age and stage of growth [6].

16.5.2 Dietary

For overweight and obese children and young people, total energy intake should be below their energy expenditure, but changes should be sustainable. It is recommended not to use unduly restrictive and nutritionally unbalanced diets because they are ineffective in the long term and can be harmful. It is important to encourage young people to improve their diet even if they do not lose weight because there can be other health benefits [6].

16.5.3 Physical Activity

The approach for children is similar to that of adults. Moreover, it is of primary importance to encourage children to reduce inactive behaviors, such as sitting and watching television, using a computer or playing video games.

It has to enlighten the importance of encouraging children and young people to increase their level of physical activity even if they do not lose weight as a result because of the other health benefits exercise can bring [6].

16.5.4 Pharmacological Interventions

Drug treatment is not generally recommended for children younger than 12 years and no drug is approved for this population. Below this age, drug treatment may be used only in exceptional circumstances, if severe comorbidities are present [6, 41].

The only drug approved by the FDA for people over the age of 12 years is Orlistat. However, treatment is only recommended if there are physical comorbidities, and regular review to assess effectiveness, adverse effects, and adherence is recommended [41].

Some off-license drugs used to treat obesity in children and adolescents include fluoxetine and bupropion.

In general, drug interventions can result in a small BMI and weight reduction over the short term. It is unknown whether this is sustainable over the longer term [41].

In any case, it is important to offer support to help maintaining weight loss to people whose drug treatment is being withdrawn; if they did not reach their target weight, in fact, their self-confidence and belief in their ability to make changes may be decreased [6].

16.6 Change in Body Image and Psychological Well-Being During Obesity Treatment

The extent to which someone perceived himself/herself as being overweight was a much better predictor of body dissatisfaction, body esteem, and disordered eating, than the actual BMI [57].

Greater body image dissatisfaction is associated with lower self-esteem, more depressive symptoms, and greater internalization of society's emphasis on the importance of physical appearance. Because of the significant consequences of negative body image in obese individuals, it is important to understand the nature and correlates of body dissatisfaction among individuals who are or who have been overweight. Frequent body checking and avoidance have been documented and shown to be associated with high shape and weight concerns among individuals with obesity or overweight and obese patients with binge eating disorder [18].

Moreover, it has been observed that women with BED suffer from higher levels of body dissatisfaction than women without BED, and they are more exposed to socio-cultural factors that promote the ideal thinness [13, 58].

In a therapeutical and prognostic perspective, body image enhancement should protect against the development of unhealthy behaviors linked to obesity. Therefore, cognitive and affect-related changes that occur during weight management may represent more than positive outcomes and can also influence the effects of an intervention. This is particularly relevant when considering interventions that include regular physical exercise with its well-known positive effects on emotions, self-esteem, depression, and other psychological variables. A recent study conducted by Palmeira and colleagues [59] showed that there might be a predictive role of short-term changes in body size dissatisfaction and self-esteem on long-term weight loss. In fact, individuals who improved self-esteem and body dissatisfaction the most were more likely to obtain long-term weight loss. Therefore, treatments for obesity and overweight should include interventions addressing body image because changes in psychological well-being taking place during weight management programs might independently contribute to long-term success [59].

16.6.1 Body Image, Weight Loss, Dieting, and Qualitative Caloric Intake

Obesity can produce severe psychological consequences. It is sometimes argued that the life dissatisfaction, social abilities, and body image distress produced by obesity are beneficial because they motivate people to lose weight [13].

Instead, body checking and avoidance behavior are major issues in obese patients. The relationship between checking and avoidance behaviors, psychopathology, and weight loss may be particularly important for individuals who are attempting or maintaining behavior change as part of obesity treatment. An overweight person without body dissatisfaction may feel less determined to make health behavior changes than someone with a moderate level of body dissatisfaction. On the other hand, someone with extreme body image distress may be caught in a destructive cycle of negative self-talk that is debilitating and inhibits change [13].

It is often assumed that the key to improving body image is to lose weight. Although a reduction in body weight generally leads to an improvement in body image, the correlation between these variables is not so strong. A possible explanation is that actual changes to the body are less important than perceived changes [60]. In fact, conversely to what is commonly believed, changing body image is more easily achieved by changing the perceptions of one's body and the importance ascribed to that, than by changing body appearance itself. In fact, studies exploring the efficacy of cognitive therapy to body dissatisfaction would indicate that it is possible to improve body image without changing one's appearance [57, 61].

On the other hand, methods based on psychotherapy techniques exist to improve body image and have been applied successfully to obese individuals but these alone do not appear to boost weight loss [13].

More in detail, it has been shown that, when dieting, improvement in body image over treatment is not significantly related to the amount of weight loss. One explanation is that the treatment, rather than weight loss per se, improved body image. Another explanation is that body image improves with relatively small amounts of weight loss, and that further weight loss does not lead to further improvement. Body image, in summary, and other psychological distress such as low self-esteem and binge eating can improve independent of weight loss [13].

When weight loss is obtained through dieting, high levels of dietary restraint and high BMI are associated with low state body image satisfaction after eating. The relationship between dieting, caloric intake, and body image satisfaction appears to be bi-directional: consumption of low calorie foods may induce feelings of body image satisfaction which could support prolonged adherence to a weight-loss diet, whereas consumption of highly caloric food leads to body dissatisfaction. Therefore, body image may be affected also by the way dietary weight-loss is achieved: healthy weight management behaviors, such as a balanced diet with low caloric food intake (and not excessive restrictions or restrictions alternate with high caloric food assumption) improves body image satisfaction and positively reinforce long-term maintenance of weight loss [62].

16.6.2 Body Image and Physical Activity

It has been shown that, like dietary weight-loss interventions, exercise interventions have significant positive effects on body image. In fact, perceived changes to one's body and perceived improvements in one's physical abilities appear to be more consistent correlates of body image change than physique-related changes [60]. It is quite a common finding in studies on body image that body image changes do not always come along with significant changes in body weight, body composition (e.g., fat mass, lean mass), anthropometric variables, or improvement of physical strength (e.g., maximum amount of weight lifted) and endurance (e.g., maximum heart rate, maximum volume of oxygen consumption during exercise) obtained through physical activity. In contrast, body image changes strongly correlate with perceived changes in physical fitness (i.e., body composition, strength, aerobic endurance) and psychological variables such as self-efficacy, conceptualized as confidence in one's abilities to perform activities requiring, aerobic endurance, and muscular strength. Taken together, these findings suggest that how an exerciser perceives changes to her body is a stronger determinant of body image change than the actual magnitude of those changes.

In fact, a review by Martin Ginis et al. [60] demonstrated that perceived change variables emerged as the most consistent unique predictors of body image change. More in detail, perceived body fatness reduction was the most significant predictor of body image improvement. This findings are consistent with the notion that changes in beliefs about one's body, and not actual changes to the body, are the driving force behind body image change in exercise and weight-loss interventions. Even if evidence is scarce, it has been suggested that there is a weight-loss threshold that triggers body image improvements.

Changes in perceived strength also played a significant role in body image change. Strength training may help shift a woman's focus away from her appearance and foster greater awareness of functional aspects of her body. A shift in awareness, coupled with the positive feedback provided by a progressive strength-training regimen may challenge, and ultimately alleviate, negative body image thoughts and feelings. Importantly, these benefits do not seem to diminish over the course of a strength-training intervention, suggesting they play a role in body image change even after the initial period of acute strength increases [60].

About self-efficacy, the finding that aerobic self-efficacy was a stronger predictor of body image than strength self-efficacy likely reflects women placing greater value on aerobic exercise than strength training as a means for losing weight and managing body image concerns. Increased confidence to do aerobic exercise could create the sense that the exerciser is getting closer to the body ideal, thus enhancing body image [60].

Therefore, in treating obese patients, maximizing perceived body changes is more important than obtaining actual body change. Perceived improvements could facilitate patients to develop realistic weight-loss goals that will make them feel good about even relatively small losses. To address body changes perception, it is important to draw patient's attention to improvements in strength and aerobic endurance rather than to weight and body shape modifications and it may be useful to encourage them to record their aerobic and physical-strength achievements [60].

Acknowledgement Dott. Gabriela Dorati contributed to this chapter.

References

1. Mastellos N, Gunn LH, Felix LM, Car J, Majeed A. Transtheoretical model stages of change for dietary and physical exercise modification in weight loss management for overweight and obese adults. Cochrane Database Syst Rev. 2014;(2):CD008066. https://doi.org/10.1002/14651858.CD008066.pub3.
2. Oude Luttikhuis H, Baur L, Jansen H, Shrewsbury VA, O'Malley C, Stolk RP, Summerbell CD. Interventions for treating obesity in children. Cochrane Database Syst Rev. 2009;(1):CD001872.https://doi.org/10.1002/14651858.CD001872.pub2.
3. World Health Organisation (WHO). Obesity: preventing and managing the Global Epidemic—Report of a WHO Consultation on Obesity, 3-5 June 1997. WHO/NUT/ NCD/981; 1998.
4. Roqué i Figuls M, Martínez García L, Martinez-Zapata MJ, Pacheco R, Mauricio D, Bonfill Cosp X. Interventions for treating overweight or obesity in adults: an overview of systematic reviews. Cochrane Database Syst Rev. 2013;(8):CD010665. https://doi.org/10.1002/14651858.CD010665.
5. Rucker D, Padwal R, Li SK, Curioni C, Lau DC. Long term pharmacotherapy for obesity and overweight: updated meta-analysis. BMJ. 2007;335(7631):1194–9. https://doi.org/10.1002/14651858.CD004094.pub2.
6. NICE. Obesity: identification, assessment and management. Clinical guideline. 2014. nice.org.uk/guidance/cg189.
7. Shaw KA, Gennat HC, O'Rourke P, Del Mar C. Exercise for overweight or obesity. Cochrane Database Syst Rev. 2006;(4):CD003817. https://doi.org/10.1002/14651858.CD003817.pub3.
8. NHLBI. Clinical guidelines on the identification, evaluation, and treatment of overweight and obesity in adults: the evidence report. 2000. www.nhlbi.nih.gov/guidelines/obesity/ob gdlns.pdf.
9. NICE. Obesity: guidance on the prevention, identification, assessment and management of overweight and obesity in adults and children. 2006. http://www.nice.org.uk/nicemedia/live/11000/30365/30365.pdf.
10. NIH. National Institute of Diabetes and Digestive and Kidney Diseases (NIDDK). National Institutes of Health. WIN—Publication—Prescription medications for the treatment of obesity. 2010. http://win.niddk.nih.gov/publications/prescription.htm.
11. Melendez G, Serralde-Zúñiga AE, Gonzalez Garay AG, Rodríguez-Carmona Y, Solis Galicia C. Fluoxetine for adult overweight or obese people. Cochrane Database Syst Rev. 2015;(5):CD011688. https://doi.org/10.1002/14651858.CD011688.
12. Amianto F, Ottone L, Abbate Daga G, Fassino S. Binge-eating disorder diagnosis and treatment: a recap in front of DSM-5. BMC Psychiatry. 2015;15:70. https://doi.org/10.1186/s12888-015-0445-6.
13. Schwartz MB, Brownell KD. Obesity and body image. Body Image. 2004;1(1):43–56.
14. Brennan L, Murphy KD, de la Piedad Garcia X, Ellis ME, Metzendorf MI, McKenzie JE. Psychological interventions for adults who are overweight or obese. Cochrane Database Syst Rev. 2016;3. https://doi.org/10.1002/14651858.CD012114.
15. Levine MP, Piran N. The role of body image in the prevention of eating disorders. Body Image. 2004;1(1):57–70. https://doi.org/10.1016/S1740-1445(03)00006-8.
16. Zamariola G, Cardini F, Mian E, Serino A, Tsakiris M. Can you feel the body that you see? On the relationship between interoceptive accuracy and body image. Body Image. 2017;20:130–6.

17. Lewer M, Nasrawi N, Schroeder D, Vocks S. Body image disturbance in binge eating disorder: a comparison of obese patients with and without binge eating disorder regarding the cognitive, behavioral and perceptual component of body image. Eat Weight Disord. 2016;21(1):115–25. https://doi.org/10.1007/s40519-015-0200-5.
18. Latner JD. Body checking and avoidance among behavioral weight-loss participants. Body Image. 2008;5(1):91–8. https://doi.org/10.1016/j.bodyim.2007.08.001.
19. Leombruni P, Ottone L, Lavagnino L, Siccardi S, Nicotra B, Migliore F, et al. Group psychoeducational psychotherapy in binge eating disorder. Minerva Psichiatr. 2010;51(3): 135–44.
20. Balestrieri M, Isola M, Baiano M, Ciano R. Psychoeducation in binge eating disorder and EDNOS: a pilot study on the efficacy of a 10-week and a 1-year continuation treatment. Eat Weight Disord. 2013;18(1):45–51. https://doi.org/10.1007/s40519-013-0014-2.
21. Reas DL, Grilo CM. Review and meta-analysis of pharmacotherapy for binge-eating disorder. Obesity (Silver Spring). 2008;16(9):2024–38. https://doi.org/10.1038/oby.2008.333.
22. Vocks S, Tuschen-Caffier B, Pietrowsky R, Rustenbach SJ, Kersting A, Herpertz S. Meta-analysis of the effectiveness of psychological and pharmacological treatments for binge eating disorder. Int J Eat Disord. 2010;43(3):205–17. https://doi.org/10.1002/eat.20696.
23. Iacovino JM, Gredysa DM, Altman M, Wilfley DE. Psychological treatments for binge eating disorder. Curr Psychiatry Rep. 2012;14(4):432–46. https://doi.org/10.1007/s11920-012-0277-8.
24. Grilo CM, White MA, Gueorguieva R, Wilson GT, Masheb RM. Predictive significance of the overvaluation of shape/weight in obese patients with binge eating disorder: findings from a randomized controlled trial with 12-month follow-up. Psychol Med. 2012;43(6):1335–44. https://doi.org/10.1017/S0033291712002097.
25. Woolhouse H, Knowles A, Crafti N. Adding mindfulness to CBT programs for binge eating: a mixed-methods evaluation. Eat Disord. 2012;20(4):321–39. https://doi.org/10.1080/10640266.2012.691791.
26. Masheb RM, Grilo CM, Rolls BJ. A randomized controlled trial for obesity and binge eating disorder: low-energy-density dietary counseling and cognitive-behavioral therapy. Behav Res Ther. 2011;49(12):821–9. https://doi.org/10.1016/j.brat.2011.09.006.
27. Vancampfort D, Vanderlinden J, De Hert M, Adámkova M, Skjaerven LH, Catalán-Matamoros D, Lundvik-Gyllensten A, Gómez-Conesa A, Ijntema R, Probst M. A systematic review on physical therapy interventions for patients with binge eating disorder. Disabil Rehabil. 2013;35(26):2191–6. https://doi.org/10.3109/09638288.2013.771707.
28. Butters JW, Cash TFJ. Cognitive-behavioral treatment of women's body-image dissatisfaction. Consult Clin Psychol. 1987;55(6):889–97.
29. Rosen JC, Reiter J, Orosan PJ. Cognitive-behavioral body image therapy for body dysmorphic disorder. Consult Clin Psychol. 1995;63(2):263–9.
30. Munsch S, Meyer AH, Biedert E. Efficacy and predictors of long-term treatment success for cognitive-behavioral treatment and behavioral weight-loss-treatment in overweight individuals with binge eating disorder. Behav Res Ther. 2012;50(12):775–85. https://doi.org/10.1016/j.brat.2012.08.009.
31. Vanderlinden J, Adriaensen A, Vancampfort D, Pieters G, Probst M, Vansteelandt K. A cognitive- behavioral therapeutic program for patients with obesity and binge eating disorder: short- and long- term follow-up data of a prospective study. Behav Modif. 2012;36(5):670–86. https://doi.org/10.1177/0145445512439313.
32. Ricca V, Castellini G, Mannucci E, Lo Sauro C, Ravaldi C, Rotella CM, Faravelli C. Comparison of individual and group cognitive behavioral therapy for binge eating disorder. A randomized, three-year follow-up study. Appetite. 2010;55(3):656–65. https://doi.org/10.1016/j.appet.2010.09.019.
33. Castellini G, Lo Sauro C, Mannucci E, Ravaldi C, Rotella CM, Faravelli C, Ricca V. Diagnostic crossover and outcome predictors in eating disorders according to DSM-IV and DSM-V proposed criteria: a 6-year follow-up study. Psychosom Med. 2011;73(3):270–9. https://doi.org/10.1097/PSY.0b013e31820a1838.

34. Grilo CM, Masheb RM, Wilson GT, Gueorguieva R, White MA. Cognitive-behavioral therapy, behavioral weight loss, and sequential treatment for obese patients with binge-eating disorder: a randomized controlled trial. J Consult Clin Psychol. 2011;79(5):675–85. https://doi.org/10.1037/a0025049.
35. Klein AS, Skinner JB, Hawley KM. Adapted group-based dialectical behaviour therapy for binge eating in a practicing clinic: clinical outcomes and attrition. Eur Eat Disord Rev. 2012;20(3):e148–53. https://doi.org/10.1002/erv.2165.
36. Safer DL, Robinson AH, Jo B. Outcome from a randomized controlled trial of group therapy for binge eating disorder: comparing dialectical behavior therapy adapted for binge eating to an active comparison group therapy. Behav Ther. 2010;41(1):106–20. https://doi.org/10.1016/j.beth.2009.01.006.
37. Tasca GA, Balfour L, Presniak MD, Bissada H. Outcomes of specific interpersonal problems for binge eating disorder: comparing group psychodynamic interpersonal psychotherapy and group cognitive behavioral therapy. Int J Group Psychother. 2012;62(2):197–218. https://doi.org/10.1521/ijgp.2012.62.2.197.
38. Wilson GT, Wilfley DE, Agras WS, Bryson SW. Psychological treatments of binge eating disorder. Arch Gen Psychiatry. 2010;67(1):94–101. https://doi.org/10.1001/archgenpsychiatry.2009.170.
39. Kessler RC, Berglund PA, Chiu WT, Deitz AC, Hudson JI, Shahly V, Aguilar-Gaxiola S, Alonso J, Angermeyer MC, Benjet C, Bruffaerts R, de Girolamo G, de Graaf R, Maria Haro J, Kovess-Masfety V, O'Neill S, Posada-Villa J, Sasu C, Scott K, Viana MC, Xavier M. The prevalence and correlates of binge eating disorder in the World Health Organization World Mental Health Surveys. Biol Psychiatry. 2013;73(9):904–14. https://doi.org/10.1016/j.biopsych.2012.11.020.
40. Fassino S, Leombruni P, Pierò A, Abbate-Daga G, Giacomo Rovera G. Mood, eating attitudes, and anger in obese women with and without binge eating disorder. J Psychosom Res. 2003;54(6):559–66.
41. Mead E, Atkinson G, Richter B, Metzendorf MI, Baur L, Finer N, Corpeleijn E, O'Malley C, Ells LJ. Drug interventions for the treatment of obesity in children and adolescents. Cochrane Database Syst Rev. 2016;(11):CD012436.
42. Decaluwé V, Braet C, Fairburn CG. Binge eating in obese children and adolescents. Int J Eat Disord. 2003;33(1):78–84.
43. Epstein LH, Roemmich JN, Stein RI, Paluch RA, Kilanowski CK. The challenge of identifying behavioral alternatives to food: clinic and field studies. Ann Behav Med. 2005;30(3):201–9.
44. Flodmark CE, Ohlsson T, Ryden O, Sveger T. Prevention of progression to severe obesity in a group of obese schoolchildren treated with family therapy. Pediatrics. 1993;91(5):880–4.
45. Golan M, Kaufman V, Shahar DR. Childhood obesity treatment: targeting parents exclusively v. parents and children. Br J Nutr. 2006;95(5):1008–15. https://doi.org/10.1079/BJN20061757.
46. Golley RK, Magarey AM, Baur LA, Steinbeck KS, Daniels LA. Twelve-month effectiveness of a parent-led, family-focused weight-management program for prepubertal children: a randomized, controlled trial. Pediatrics. 2007;119(3):517–25. https://doi.org/10.1542/peds.2006-1746.
47. Hughes AR, Stewart L, Chapple J, McColl JH, Donaldson MD, Kelnar CJ, et al. Randomized, controlled trial of a best-practice individualized behavioral program for treatment of childhood overweight: Scottish Childhood Overweight Treatment Trial (SCOTT). Pediatrics. 2008;121(3):e539–46. https://doi.org/10.1542/peds.2007-1786.
48. Jelalian E, Mehlenbeck R, Lloyd-Richardson EE, Birmaher V, Wing RR. 'Adventure therapy' combined with cognitive-behavioral treatment for overweight adolescents. Int J Obes. 2006;30(1):31–9.
49. Johnston CA, Tyler C, Fullerton G, Poston WSC, Haddock CK, Mcfarlin B, et al. Results of an intensive school-based weight loss program with overweight Mexican American children. Int J Pediatr Obes. 2007;2(3):144–52. https://doi.org/10.1080/17477160701305864.
50. Johnston CA, Tyler C, McFarlin BK, Poston WSC, Haddock CK, Reeves R, et al. Weight loss in overweight Mexican American children: a randomized, controlled trial. Pediatrics. 2007;120(6):e1450–7.

51. Kalavainen MP, Korppi MO, Nuutinen OM. Clinical efficacy of group-based treatment for childhood obesity compared with routinely given individual counseling. Int J Obes. 2007;31(10):1500–8. https://doi.org/10.1038/sj.ijo.0803628.
52. McCallum Z, Wake M, Gerner B, Baur LA, Gibbons K, Gold L, et al. Outcome data from the LEAP (live, eat and play) trial: a randomized controlled trial of a primary care intervention for childhood overweight/mild obesity. Int J Obes. 2007;31(4):630–6.
53. Munsch S, Roth B, Michael T, Meyer AH, Biedert E, Roth S, et al. Randomized controlled comparison of two cognitive behavioral therapies for obese children: mother versus mother-child cognitive behavioral therapy. Psychother Psychosom. 2008;77(4):235–46.
54. Saelens BE, Sallis JF, Wilfley DE, Patrick K, Cella JA, Buchta R. Behavioral weight control for overweight adolescents initiated in primary care. Obes Res. 2002;10(1):22–32.
55. Savoye M, Shaw M, Dziura J, Tamborlane WV, Rose P, Guandalini C, et al. Effects of a weight management program on body composition and metabolic parameters in overweight children: a randomized controlled trial. JAMA. 2007;297(24):2697–704.
56. Williamson DA, Martin PD, White MA, Newton R, Walden H, York-Crowe E, et al. Efficacy of an internet-based behavioral weight loss program for overweight adolescent African-American girls. Eat Weight Disord. 2005;10(3):193–203.
57. Wilson JM, Tripp DA, Boland FJ. The relative contributions of subjective and objective measures of body shape and size to body image and disordered eating in women. Body Image. 2005;2(3):233–47.
58. Bautista-Díaz ML, Franco-Paredes K, Mancilla-Díaz JM, Alvarez-Rayón G, López-Aguilar X, Ocampo Téllez-Girón T, Soto-González Y. Body dissatisfaction and socio-cultural factors in women with and without BED: their relation with eating psychopathology. Eat Weight Disord. 2012;17(2):e86–92.
59. Palmeira AL, Branco TL, Martins SC, Minderico CS, Silva MN, Vieira PN, Barata JT, Serpa SO, Sardinha LB, Teixeira PJ. Change in body image and psychological well-being during behavioral obesity treatment: associations with weight loss and maintenance. Body Image. 2010;7(3):187–93. https://doi.org/10.1016/j.bodyim.2010.03.002.
60. Martin Ginis KA, McEwan D, Josse AR, Phillips SM. Body image change in obese and overweight women enrolled in a weight-loss intervention: the importance of perceived versus actual physical changes. Body Image. 2012;9(3):311–7. https://doi.org/10.1016/j.bodyim.2012.04.002.
61. Menzel JE, Schaefer LM, Burke NL, Mayhew LL, Brannick MT, Thompson JK. Appearance-related teasing, body dissatisfaction, and disordered eating: a meta-analysis. Body Image. 2010;7(4):261–70. https://doi.org/10.1016/j.bodyim.2010.05.004.
62. Lattimore P, Hutchinson R. Perceived calorie intake and state body-image satisfaction in women attempting weight loss: a preliminary investigation. Body Image. 2010;7(1):15–21. https://doi.org/10.1016/j.bodyim.2009.08.002.

17 Studies on Body Image Changes After Bariatric Surgery in Adults

Luca Busetto, Federica Buongiorno, and Sami Schiff

17.1 Introduction

After the failure of various nutritional or dietetic treatments, patients with severe obesity frequently approach bariatric surgery for reasons related to both physical (e.g., weight loss, increased life expectancy) and psychological health (e.g., body image, quality of life, psychological well-being).

After bariatric surgery, the majority of patients show a rapid weight loss, mainly occurring in the first 6–12 months after the procedure, and most of the time the physical health concerns (e.g., type 2 diabetes, hypertension, sleep apnea) improve. In a similar way, also body shape and its functionality undergo extreme changes. These two factors suggest that, after this type of surgical intervention, patients with obesity may improve their quality of life, and reduce the intensity of body image dissatisfaction. However, many factors are able to affect negatively body image and to increase body image dissatisfaction after bariatric surgery.

The ability to cope with life style changes may affect psychological health and body dissatisfaction. After bariatric surgery, the introduction of new healthier habits concerning diet and physical activity are required to maximize long-term goals of weight loss and maintenance. Some patients may decrease or increase their body image dissatisfaction depending on their ability or not to lose weight and/or to maintain weight after loss [1]. Another factor that may affect body image dissatisfaction after weight loss due to bariatric surgery is related to the fact that rapid weight loss can cause excessive skin on the abdomen and other body sites, causing physical or psychological discomfort. For this reason, about 30% of bariatric surgery patients undergo plastic surgery to correct problems with excessive skin [2, 3]. These events may affect negatively body image increasing body image dissatisfaction.

L. Busetto (✉) · F. Buongiorno · S. Schiff
Department of Medicine, University of Padova, Padova, Italy
e-mail: luca.busetto@unipd.it

M. Cuzzolaro, S. Fassino (eds.), *Body Image, Eating, and Weight*,
https://doi.org/10.1007/978-3-319-90817-5_17

In this chapter, we reviewed the existing literature about body image dissatisfaction in patients both before and after bariatric surgery. A short overview about indications to bariatric surgery, its results and the characteristics of the most used types of bariatric procedures have also been included.

17.2 Indication to Bariatric Surgery, Results and Procedures

Bariatric surgery should be considered in the management of adult patients (age range 18–60 years) with severe obesity (BMI > 40 kg/m^2 or BMI > 35 kg/m^2 with comorbid conditions) who failed to lose weight or to maintain long-term weight loss, despite appropriate nonsurgical medical care [4, 5]. Comorbid conditions for which patients with BMI 35–40 kg/m^2 can be considered for bariatric surgery are those that significantly contribute to morbidity and mortality of the obese patient, and in which surgically induced weight loss is expected to improve the disorder (such as metabolic disease, cardio-respiratory disease, and severe joint disease). Bariatric surgery may also be considered, on individual basis, in patients with type 2 diabetes and mild obesity (BMI 30–35 kg/m^2) who do not achieve a substantial weight reduction with nonsurgical methods and in which the diabetes was not adequately controlled by maximal medical therapy [6]. In any cases, patients undergoing bariatric surgery need to be willing to participate in a postoperative long-term follow-up program. Bariatric surgery is contraindicated in patients with absence of a period of identifiable medical management, inability to participate in a long-term medical follow-up, major psychiatric disorders if not otherwise indicated by their caring psychiatrist, alcohol and/or drug abuse, reduced life expectancy, and the inability to care for themselves without adequate family or social support [4, 5].

The weight loss efficacy of bariatric surgery has been confirmed by the results obtained in long-term controlled studies, the main one being the Swedish Obese Subjects (SOS) study, a controlled study that compared the outcome of 2000 patients who underwent bariatric surgery by various techniques with that of a matched control group that received conventional treatment [7]. In the surgery group, after 10 years, the average weight loss from baseline stabilized at 16.1%, whereas in control subjects the average weight during the observation period increased by 1.6%. This substantial difference in weight loss was associated with a higher remission rate of metabolic disease, a highly significant reduction of the incidence of new cases of diabetes, a reduction of cardiovascular events, both fatal and non-fatal, and a reduction of the incidence of new cases of cancer in women. Finally, during a follow-up to 10 years, the cumulative overall mortality in the surgery group was significantly lower than that observed in control subjects (RR: 0.76; 95%CI: 0.59–0.99) [7]. In conclusion, these results provide sufficient evidence that modern bariatric surgery can bring down the increased mortality observed in severely obese patients, provided that the peri-operative mortality is maintained at low levels as reported in various studies (<0.5%). The superiority of bariatric surgery over lifestyle intervention for weight loss and metabolic improvement has been confirmed by some randomized, controlled, clinical trials specifically performed in severely obese patients with type 2 diabetes mellitus [6].

Bariatric surgery is therefore in general safe and effective, but it can cause new clinical problems and is associated with specific diagnostic, preventive and therapeutic needs. Bariatric patients may face new specific multifaceted clinical problems after surgery. Eating habits need to adapt to the new gastro-intestinal physiology, and nutritional deficits may arise according to the type of bariatric procedure. Management of obesity associated disease needs to be modulated according to weight loss taking into account the possibility of changes in drug pharmacokinetics. Specific problems may arise in women during pregnancy, and the patients may experience some psychological difficulties in adapting to the profound changes in eating behavior and body image. Finally, weight regain can occur and should be prevented and managed. Multidisciplinary long-term follow-up is therefore recommended after bariatric surgery, and the provision of an adequate follow-up program is mandatory for bariatric centers [4]. However, giving the accumulating numbers of bariatric patients, follow-up should be at least in part transferred to primary care over time. Moreover, post-bariatric patients may confront obesity specialists, dieticians and nurses not specifically trained in bariatric medicine with thus far unknown problems in their professional activity. Referral to the bariatric center is often necessary and should be possible, but there is a growing need for dissemination of first level knowledge in managing bariatric patients. The basic notions needed to provide first level adequate medical care to post-bariatric patients have been recently summarized [8].

Several bariatric procedures have been introduced in the clinical practice in the last 50 years. Many of them have been abandoned because of insufficient results or severe side effects, and many others remained low in diffusion. According to the most recent survey from the International Federation for the Surgery of Obesity and Metabolic Disorders (IFSO), over 90% of the 579,517 bariatric procedures performed worldwide in 2014 consisted of three type of surgical intervention: sleeve gastrectomy (45.9%), Roux-en-Y gastric bypass (39.6%), and adjustable gastric banding (7.4%) [9].

Sleeve Gastrectomy is a restrictive procedure consisting in the section of the stomach with removal of approximately 2/3 of it. The section takes place parallel to the small curvature in order to create a stomach in a tubular form (Fig. 17.1). The operation reduces drastically the amount of food that can be ingested and causes a feeling of early satiety. However, the removal of a significant part of the stomach and/or modification of the speed of gastric transit also cause changes in the secretion of hormones secreted in the gastro-intestinal tract and having a regulatory action on energy balance and carbohydrate metabolism. Operative mortality is about 0.2% and it is frequently related to leakages at the level of the long gastric suture. Main post-operative specific complications are represented by dilatation of the pouch and gastroesophageal reflux. The results in terms of weight loss can be evaluated at around 60–70% of excess weight. Long-term results are good, but there is a significant number of cases in which patients show at least partial weight regain [10].

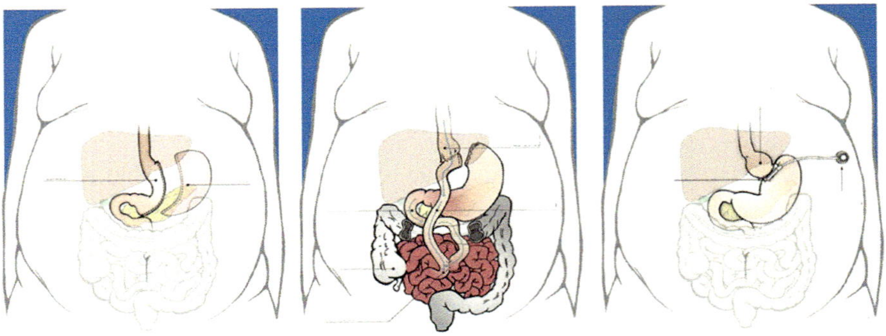

Fig. 17.1 The three major bariatric surgery procedures worldwide. Left: sleeve gastrectomy. Middle: Roux-en-Y gastric bypass. Right: adjustable gastric banding

Gastric bypass consists in the creation of a proximal gastric pouch (15–20 cm^3) which is excluded from the gastric remnant. The small pouch is sutured to the jejunum through a Roux-en-Y intestinal derivation (Fig. 17.1). The stomach and the duodenum are excluded from the transit of the food. Weight loss occurs in part through a restrictive mechanism, but also as the result of the modification of the secretion of entero-acting hormones regulating energy balance and glucose metabolism. The presence of a dumping syndrome following the intake of beverages and/or sweet foods can also participate to the determination of the weight loss. There is not a significant malabsorption of macronutrients (fat, carbohydrates, protein) but there is a certain degree of malabsorption for some micronutrients (Ca, Fe, and Vit. B12). The operative complications are about 2% and the operative mortality is about 0.5%. The main postoperative specific complications are represented by anastomotic leak (1%), anastomotic stenosis (1.5%), anastomotic ulcer (3%), and internal hernias (3%). Possible nutritional complications are represented by multifactorial anemia (more frequently microcytic iron deficiency anemia) and osteoporosis/osteomalacia. Prevention of these complications requires long-life nutritional supplementations. The results in terms of weight loss are evaluated around 55–65% of excess weight with acceptable weight maintenance rates [10].

Gastric banding consists in the placement of a band with a pneumatic internal chamber around the upper part of the stomach. The band is applied under the gastroesophageal junction, and creates a small pouch (25 mL). The chamber is connected to a silicone connecting tube ending with a reservoir placed subcutaneously on the abdominal wall and allows a percutaneous adjustment of the size of the band (Fig. 17.1). Gastric banding has the purpose of slowing down the meal, inducing a feeling of rapid satiety after the introduction of small quantities of food. The patient may be gradually accustomed to the presence of the banding by exploiting the possibility of calibration of the shrinkage. The operative complications are very rare (0.2%) and the operative mortality is very low (<0.1%). The main postoperative complications are represented by migration of the band within the stomach (<1%), gastric pouch dilatation and stomach slippage (3%), disconnection of the port and/

or connecting tube with leakage of the system (3%). Results in terms of weight loss are around 40–50% of excess weight. Long-term results are related to the eating behavior of the patient and there is a significant number of patients with some degree of weight regain [10].

17.3 Body Representation, Body Schema, Body Image and Body Image Dissatisfaction

To better understand the changes of body image and body image dissatisfaction in patients with obesity and after bariatric surgery is necessary to introduce some more general concept about body representation, i.e. the way we represent our own body in its complex physical and psychological components (see also Chap. 1 of the present book). Body representation involves two main aspects: (1) body image and (2) body schema; the first being considered a psychological concept and the second a neuropsychological one. Body schema and body image share the opportunity to represent the totality and complexity of the human body, however it is accepted that the two concepts are different even if interdependent. Indeed, while body schema is a complex perceptual scheme linked to processes related to the spatial localization of the body: body image includes the subjective-cognitive-affective components that integrate body representation.

More specifically, body schema refers to how the brain represents our own body in space and its position in the environment. Neuroscientists located the body schema in the right parietal lobe and attribute to this cortical area most of the disorders of body representation, such as the phantom limb, anosognosia, and unilateral neglect. The neurological model formulated the concept of body schema as a sensorimotor map of the body space mainly based on proprioception, and the body image as a pictorial description of the body based mainly on a visual exteroception [11]. Gallagher [12] advocates a principle distinctions between body schema, considered as a system of postural and sensory–motor capacities that usually functions without perceptual monitoring; and body image, broadly considered as a system of perceptions, attitudes and beliefs pertaining to one's own body. The body schema would be involved in action and interaction with the environment, with the body providing the material perspective on the outside world, whereas the body image would be involved in the sense of body ownership and self-consciousness. According to both Paillard [11] and Gallagher [12], subjective body image is present to consciousness, whereas the body schema is usually not, although inputs from the body schema to the body image can affect spatial perception, the perception of objects and the links with intentional actions.

On the other hand, the cognitive-emotional component is important in the representation of body image [13]. The psychological models conceptualize body image as a complex of inclinations and emotions addressed to our own body, which would result in the way in which we "live" our size, and how we feel our outward appearance in general [14]. From this point of view, body image is the cognitive-emotional-social model of the body, reflecting our subjective experiences, expectations, desires, and emotions. Body image is also affected by the interaction with others in the social context, which, in some cases, may increase discomfort and resulting in an incessant and repeated comparison of our own body image with other people's bodies. Body image encompasses one's body-related self-perceptions and self-attitudes, including thoughts, beliefs, feelings and behaviors [15]. Cash [16] suggested that body image includes at least two components: perceptual body image (i.e., estimation of body size) and attitudinal body image (i.e., affective, cognitive, and behavioral concerns with body size). Body image is therefore a complex multidimensional construct, consisting of cognitive, emotional and behavioral elements, influenced by social and cultural factors.

Most of the research in the field of the relationships between body image and obesity adopted the psychological model. In particular, the problems associated with negative body image are those that have received substantial attention in the research literature and have witnessed a dramatic growth in empirical attention in the last decade [17].

More recently, it was suggested that the emergence of problems with body image and shape in individuals with obesity are related with the link between our body and our mind as described by the Embodied Cognition [18]. Within this theoretical framework, it is assumed that our conceptual system is the result of the interaction between two types of representational systems [19]: schematic (allocentric) and perceptual (egocentric). The egocentric frame of reference is related to the body of the subject and allows the representation of objects location relative to the body center. Within an egocentric frame of reference, we represent objects relative to ourselves. On the other hand, the allocentric frame of reference is related to a space external to the subject. Within the allocentric frame of reference, objects are represented independently of our current relation to them. Following this view, the role of the egocentric representations is "pragmatic": the representation of objects using egocentric coordinates is required for actions like reaching and grasping. Instead, the role of allocentric representations is "semantic": the representation of objects using allocentric coordinates is required for the visual awareness of its size, shape, orientation and meaning [20].

It has been suggested that patients with obesity are prone to be engaged more often in an allocentric view of their body than to represents it considering an egocentric perspective [21, 22]. Individuals with obesity and eating disorders may be locked to an "objectified body" that is no longer or minimally influenced by egocentric representations driven by perception. This phenomenon seems to depend on different factors. Believes and attitudes in considering our own body image, shape and weight, develop along life and is strongly influenced by social context. Subjective body image dissatisfaction in the interaction with the others, in relation to recognized social standard, tends to generate negative emotion and increase shame in obese individuals. Thus, is possible to assume that the contents of the body image is also related to cultural standard, and in the western society is more frequent for individuals with obesity to experience "fat or weight phobia" [23] and body image dissatisfaction [24, 25].

In summary, the dissatisfaction in relation to one's body image is due to the discrepancy between the perceived and desired body shapes, or between our real self and our ideal self, too often influenced by the proposed social models. Therefore, body image dissatisfaction does not depend only on perceptual distortion of the reality, but also on a continuous evaluation of mental images, emotions and thoughts that lead to asssociate body appearance with the personal value in the social context, thus conditining self-esteem.

17.4 Correlates Between Body Weight and Body Image Dissatisfaction in Severe Obesity

Dissatisfaction with its own physical appearance seems to be the rule rather than the exception in patients with severe obesity (see also Chaps. 13 and 14 of this book). The relationship between body image, thoughts, and emotions is a double way, as even our moods can affect the mental representation of our body. Usually, if we feel sad, failed, or disappointed, we will be more likely to consider our body "disappointing" as well, we tend to become hypercritical, as our own body is the cause of our failures ("they reject me because I'm ugly"... "he has not hired myself because I'm obese"). Individuals with obesity generally has a negative body image, which is why they are more easily anxious and embarrassed in various social situations, believes that their appearance reveals their personal inadequacy, contributing to the idea of being persons without willpower and without value.

Body image dissatisfaction is a serious psychosocial problem associated with obesity [26, 27] and certain characteristics and experiences of individuals with obesity appear to be associated with an increased risk of body image dissatisfaction [17, 28]. Research identified several demographic, psychological, and behavioral features associated with body image dissatisfaction, including gender [29, 30], ethnicity [31], body mass index (BMI) [30], binge eating [30, 32], self-esteem [30, 33], and depression [34]. Grilo and colleagues [30] examined a number of correlates of body image dissatisfaction in a series of patients with extreme obesity candidates to bariatric surgery, gastric bypass in particular. Overall, female gender, the presence of binge eating, and a lower self-esteem were confirmed to be significant predictors of body image dissatisfaction. Interestingly, these authors find that binge eating and self-esteem accounted for 56% of the variance of body image dissatisfaction among men, but only 33% of the variance among women. Moreover, they observed higher body image dissatisfaction in women than in men, thus extending this well-known gender difference also to candidates to bariatric surgery. Similarly, Annis and coworkers [35] find that self-esteem in adulthood was significantly and negatively associated with body image dissatisfaction. A positive history for stigmatizing experiences during childhood, adolescence, and adulthood seem also to be significantly associated with poorer body image and psychosocial functioning in women with overweight or obesity. In another study, depression, low self-esteem, and childhood teasing about weight or size jointly acccunted for 28.4% of the variance in body image dissatisfaction in women, while depression, self-esteem, and BMI accounted for 47.4% of the variance in men [36]. These findings confirmed that while there are common components that predict body image dissatisfaction for both sexes, body size might play a more important role in predicting body image dissatisfaction in men. Rosenberger and colleagues [37] investigated correlates of body image dissatisfaction in 131 female candidates to bariatric surgery with extreme obesity and revealed that three indices of psychological functioning (depression, low self-esteem, and perfectionism) accounted for 48% of the variance in body image dissatisfaction. These findings are generally consistent with previous studies investigating body image dissatisfaction in bariatric surgery candidates [30], and in women diagnosed with Binge Eating Disorders [36]. Even if perfectionism was not included as a factor in the previous studies, perfectionism emerged as a strong predictor of body image dissatisfaction in this group of patients. Previous studies also supported that perfectionism is an important feature associated to body image dissatisfaction in diverse groups of females with obesity and/or eating disorders [38–41].

In summary, body image problems should not be considered as universally present in patients with obesity. However, it is clear that body image dissatisfaction is probably the most common factor for psychosocial distress in the population with obesity [33], and especially in women [17, 42]. Poor psychosocial outcomes, such as low self-esteem, depression [43], eating disorders [44], and perfectionism [36] seem to be main variables associated with body image dissatisfaction [45]. Moreover, weight-based teasing [33, 46], childhood onset of obesity [46], internalization of sociocultural appearance standards [33], the presence of binge eating behaviors [47, 48], and shame [37] have also been identified as variables independently associated with body image dissatisfaction in obese candidates to bariatric surgery. Finally, the feeling of distress about its own physical appearance and body weight is the major factor driving the choice of bariatric surgery in about 30% of the obese individuals that candidates themselves to a bariatric procedure [49].

17.5 Body Image Changes Following Bariatric Surgery

Several studies examined the changes of body image dissatisfaction after bariatric surgery. Teufel [50] investigated body image in a longitudinal study 1-year after Laparoscopic Sleeve Gastrectomy. Patients with obesity included in this study had extremely poor body image before bariatric surgery compared to normative samples. However, overall a significant improvement was found after 1 year. Self-evaluation of the body and perception of body dynamics also improved, with individuals reporting a less negative evaluation of its own body and perceived improved body dynamics and vitality. Another study, showed as reductions in body image dissatisfaction associated with concurrent reductions in weight and improvements in weight-related quality of life among adults after gastric bypass surgery patients up to 92 weeks post-surgery [51].

Pecori [1] showed that post-surgical bariatric patients experienced less body image discomfort when compared to a control sample of patients with morbid obesity. The authors suggest that the improvements might reflect changes in attitudinal, affective, and/or cognitive components of body image (i.e., attitudes and beliefs about an individual's body/appearance). Hrabosky [52] also identified significant changes in postoperative body satisfaction after bariatric surgery, with 83% of the patients reporting improvements in body satisfaction after 6 months and 85% reporting improvements after 12 months.

In a longitudinal study in bariatric patients treated with gastric banding, Dixon [53] found significant improvements in patients' appearance evaluation 12 months after surgery, and these improvements maintained out to 4 years. Body image outcomes were also related to excess weight loss, with greater weight loss being associated with higher appearance evaluation. A correlation between excess weight loss and better body image was also found by Sarwer [51], suggesting that weight loss after bariatric surgery is able to reduces body image dissatisfaction in most of the obese individuals. However, despite the above-presented results, it is possible to speculate that while larger weight loss is associated with improvements in multiple quality of life domains, it may not be directly associated with greater improvements in weight and shape concerns. Dixon and colleagues [53] found a discrepancy in changes in body image in persons who underwent laparoscopic adjustable gastric banding. They found improvements in overall body image satisfaction (as assessed by the Appearance Evaluation subscale of the Multidimensional Body-Self Relations Questionnaire, MBSRQ AE) but not changes in body image investment (as assessed by the Appearance Orientation subscale of the measure, MBSRQ AO). No less common are the cases where experience of body image dissatisfaction persists also after bariatric surgery, often associated with excess skin following rapid weight loss that requires body-contouring surgery. As mentioned above, body weight and shape change in a rapid manner and physical and psychological adaptation to the new shape may results in some cases difficult.

About 30% of bariatric surgery patients developed or maintains body image dissatisfaction after surgery and ask for a body-contouring surgery to correct problems with excessive abdominal skin [2, 3]. As reported in a systematic review, residual body image dissatisfaction due to increasing and/or sagging skin has been reported after surgery in as high as 70% of patients, even if 90% were pleased with their overall appearance. Interestingly, patients who reported greater satisfaction after surgery were found to have lost less weight than their dissatisfied counterparts, likely because their "skin problems" were less pronounced. As patients seek out body-contouring surgery to address skin issues, it is important to highlight that also plastic surgeons play an important role in discussing the benefits and costs related with weight loss after bariatric surgery [54].

Song [55] suggested that even if surgery generally improves body image, the profound weight loss following the procedure tend to produce dissatisfaction with other parts of the body. This suggests that as patients become closer to their ideal body image, dissatisfaction may shift to other body parts, being a consequence more of the personality traits and the psychological characteristics of the patients than obesity related [56].

It was finally suggested that body dissatisfaction could become more prominent with time postoperatively, with the occurrence of a disturbance identified as the "phantom fat" syndrome [57]. However, literature examining the "phantom fat" phenomenon is extremely limited. It is relevant to notes that many patients after massive weight loss due to bariatric surgery report some form of body image dysmorphic disorder. For example, they frequently report that they are unable to recognize their own body after the dramatic and fast weight loss. It is possible to speculate that this phenomenon may depend by the fact that, after bariatric surgery, body schema of our own body in the brain persists to be linked with the mental representation of our body before surgery. A well-described similar phenomenon is the "phantom limb syndrome" that affects amputated patients who may persist in perceive the amputated limb and tend to behave as it is still present.

The fact that obese individuals tend to be engaged more in an allocentric view of their body, than to represent it considering an egocentric prospective [21, 22] may be viewed as a factor maintaining the disturbance of body image in obese individuals after bariatric surgery. Recently, virtual reality approaches were developed to manipulate the engagement of obese individuals toward an allocentric frame of reference and to move more often their attention toward egocentric coordinates. In such a way, adaptation of the mental representation of the body schema to the new body shape should be facilitated [58, 59].

Conclusion

In conclusion, body image dissatisfaction is extremely frequent in patients with severe obesity candidates to bariatric surgery, particularly in patients presenting with distinct physical and psychosocial characteristics. Usually, body image dissatisfaction tends to improve after surgery, but not in all the cases and not in a way that is always proportional to weight loss. Rapid and large weight loss, with associated skin excess formation, could worse body image dissatisfaction in some patients.

References

1. Pecori L, Serra Cavalletti GG, Marinari GM, Migliori F, Adami GF. Attitudes of morbidly obese patients to weight loss and body image following bariatric surgery and body contouring. Obes Surg. 2007;17:68–73.
2. Faith MS, Butryn M, Wadden TA, Fabricatore A, Nguyen AM, Heymsfield SB. Evidence for prospective association among depression and obesity in population-based studies. Obes Rev. 2011;12:438–53.
3. Wagenblast AL, Laessoe L, Printzlau A. Self-reported problems and wishes for plastic surgery after bariatric surgery. J Plast Surg Hand Surg. 2014;48:115–21.
4. Yumuk V, Tsigos C, Fried M, Schindler K, Busetto L, Micic D, Toplak H. European guidelines for obesity management in adults. Obes Facts. 2015;8:402–24.
5. De Luca M, Angrisani L, Himpens J, Busetto L, Scopinaro N, Weiner R, Sartori A, Stier C, Lakdawala M, Bhasker AG, Buchwald H, Dixon J, Chiappetta S, Kolberg H-C, Frühbeck G, Sarwer DB, Suter M, Soricelli E, Blüher M, Villalonga R, Sharma A, Shijkora S. Indications for surgery for obesity and weight-related diseases: position statements from the International Federation for the Surgery of Obesity and Metabolic Disorders (IFSO). Obes Surg. 2016;26:1659–96.

6. Rubino F, Nathan DM, Eckel RH, Schauer PR, Alberti KGMM, Zimmet PZ, Del Prato S, Ji L, Sadikot SM, Herman WH, Amiel SA, Kaplan LM, Taroncher-Oldenburg G, Cummings DE, Delegates of the 2nd Diabetes Surgery Summit. Metabolic surgery in the treatment algorithm for type 2 diabetes: a joint statement by international diabetes organizations. Diabetes Care. 2016;39:861–77.
7. Sjöström L. Review of the key results from the Swedish obese subjects (SOS) trial—a prospective controlled intervention study of bariatric surgery. J Intern Med. 2013;273:219–34.
8. Busetto L, Dicker D, Azran C, Batterham RL, Farpour-Lambert N, Fried M, Hjelmesaeth J, Kinzl J, Leitner DR, Makaronidis JM, Schindler K, Toplak H, Yumuk V. Practical recommendations of the Obesity Management Task Force of the European Association for the Study of Obesity for the post-bariatric surgery medical management. Obes Facts. 2017;10:597–632.
9. Angrisani L, Santonicola A, Iovino P, Vitiello A, Zundel N, Buchwald H, Scopinaro N. Bariatric surgery and endoluminal procedures: IFSO worldwide survey 2014. Obes Surg. 2017;27:2279–89.
10. Busetto L, Angrisani L, De Luca M, Forestieri P, Millo P, Santini F. Bariatric surgery. In: Sbraccia P, Nisoli E, Vettor R, editors. Clinical management of overweight and obesity. Recommendations of the Italian Society of Obesity (SIO). Basel: Springer; 2016. p. 53–81.
11. Paillard J. Body schema and body image—a double dissociation in deafferented patients. In: Gantchev GN, Mori S, Massion J, editors. Motor control, today and tomorrow. Sophia: Academic Publishing House; 1999.
12. Gallagher S. How the body shapes the mind. New York: Oxford University Press; 2005.
13. Slade PD. What is body image? Behav Res Ther. 1994;32:497–502.
14. Fisher S. Sexual images of the self: the psychology of erotic sensations and illusions. Hillsdale: L. Erlbaum Associates; 1989.
15. Cash TF. Body image: past, present, and future. Body Image. 2004;1:1–5.
16. Cash TF, Grant JR, Shovlin JM, Lewis RJ. Are inaccuracies in self-reported weight motivated distortions? Percept Mot Skills. 1992;74:209–10.
17. Schwartz MB, Brownell KD. Obesity and body image. Body Image. 2004;1:43–56.
18. Proulx MJ, Todorov OS, Taylor Aiken A, de Sousa AA. Where am I? Who am I? The relation between spatial cognition, social cognition and individual differences in the built environment. Front Psychol. 2016;7:64.
19. Galati G, Pelle G, Berthoz A, Committeri G. Multiple reference frames used by the human brain for spatial perception and memory. Exp Brain Res. 2010;206:109–20.
20. Jeannerod M, Jacob P. Visual cognition: a new look at the two-visual systems model. Neuropsychologia. 2005;43:301–12.
21. Riva G, Gaudio S, Dakanalis A. I'm in a virtual body: a locked allocentric memory may impair the experience of the body in both obesity and anorexia nervosa. Eat Weight Disord. 2013;19:133–4.
22. Riva G. Out of my real body: cognitive neuroscience meets eating disorders. Front Hum Neurosci. 2014;8:236.
23. Lee S. Weight phobia versus fat phobia in anorexia nervosa. Transcult Psychiatr Res Rev. 1995;32:439–40.
24. Pinto-Gouveia J, Matos M. Can shame memories become a key to identity? The centrality of shame memories predicts psychopathology. Appl Cogn Psychol. 2011;25:281–90.
25. Dakanalis A, Riva G. Mass media, body image and eating disturbances: the underline mechanism through the lens of the objectification theory. In: Latzer J, Merrick J, Stein D, editors. Body image: gender differences, sociocultural influences and health implication. New York: Nova Science; 2013. p. 217–36.
26. Friedman M, Brownell KD. Psychological correlates of obesity: moving to the next generation. Psychol Bull. 1995;117:3–20.
27. Thompson JK. Body image, eating disorders, and obesity: an integrative guide for assessment and treatment. Washington, DC: American Psychological Association; 1996.
28. Cash TF, Pruzinsky T. Body image: a handbook of theory, research, and clinical practice. New York: Guilford Press; 2002.

29. Barry D, Grilo CM, Masheb RM. Gender differences in patients with binge eating disorder. Int J Eating Disord. 2002;31:63–70.
30. Grilo CM, Masheb RM, Brody M, Burke-Martindale CH, Rothschild BS. Binge eating and self-esteem predict body image dissatisfaction among obese men and women seeking bariatric surgery. Int J Eating Disord. 2005;37:347–51.
31. Akan G, Grilo CM. Sociocultural influences on eating attitudes and behaviors, body image, and psychological functioning: a comparison of African-American, Asian-American, and Caucasian college women. Int J Eating Disord. 1995;18:181–7.
32. de Zwaan M, Mitchell J, Howell L, Monson N, Swan-Kremeier L, Crosby RD, Seim HC. Characteristics of morbidly obese patients before gastric bypass surgery. Compr Psychiatry. 2003;44:428–34.
33. Matz P, Foster G, Faith M, Wadden TA. Correlate of body image dissatisfaction among overweight women seeking weight loss. J Consult Clin Psychol. 2002;70:1040–4.
34. Wardle J, Waller J, Rapoport L. Body dissatisfaction and binge eating in obese women: the role of restraint and depression. Obes Res. 2001;1:306–24.
35. Annis NM, Cash TF, Hrabosky JI. Body image and psychosocial differences among stable average weight, currently overweight, and formerly overweight women: the role of stigmatizing experiences. Body Image. 2004;1:155–67.
36. Grilo CM, Masheb RM. Correlates of body image dissatisfaction in treatment-seeking men and women with binge eating disorder. Int J Eating Disord. 2005;38:162–6.
37. Rosenberger PH, Henderson KE, Grilo CM. Correlates of body image dissatisfaction in extremely obese female bariatric surgery candidates. Obes Surg. 2006;16:1331–6.
38. Dunkley D, Blankstein K, Masheb RM, Grilo CM. Personal standards and evaluative concerns dimensions of "clinical" perfectionism: a reply to Shafran et al (2002, 2003) and Hewitt et al (2003). Behav Res Ther. 2006;44:63–84.
39. Pratt E, Telch CF, Labouovie EW, Wilson GT, Agras WS. Perfectionism in women with binge eating disorder. Int J Eating Disord. 2001;29:177–86.
40. Joiner TE Jr, Heatherton TF, Rudd MD, Schmidt NB. Perfectionism, perceived weight status, and bulimic symptoms: two studies testing a diathesis-stress model. J Abnorm Psychol. 1997;106:145–53.
41. Bastiani AM, Rao R, Weltzin T, Kaye WH. Perfectionism in anorexia nervosa. Int J Eating Disord. 1995;17:147–52.
42. Sarwer DB, Steffen KJ. Quality of life, body image and sexual functioning in bariatric surgery patients. Eur Eat Disorders Rev. 2015;23:504–8.
43. Nyboe L, Vestergaard CH, Lund H, Møller MK, Videbech P. Metabolic syndrome in first-time hospitalized patients with depression: a 1-year follow-up study. Acta Psychiatr Scand. 2016;133:241–8.
44. Forman M, Davis WN. Characteristics of middle-aged women in inpatient treatment for eating disorders. Eat Disord. 2005;13:231–43.
45. Green AE, Dymek-Valentine M, Pytluk S, Le Grange D, Alverdy J. Psychosocial outcome of gastric bypass surgery for patients with and without binge eating. Obes Surg. 2004;14:975–85.
46. Jackson TD, Grilo CM, Masheb RM. Teasing history, onset of obesity, current eating disorder psychopathology, body dissatisfaction, and psychological functioning in binge eating disorder. Obes Res. 2000;8:451–8.
47. Sarwer DB, Thompson JK, Cash TF. Body image and obesity in adulthood. Psychiatr Clin North Am. 2005;28:68–87.
48. Sarwer DB, Wadden TA, Fabricatore AN. Psychosocial and behavioral aspects of bariatric surgery. Obes Res. 2005;13:639–48.
49. Libeton M, Dixon JB, Laurie C, O'Brien PE. Patient motivation for bariatric surgery: characteristics and impact on outcomes. Obes Surg. 2004;14:392–8.
50. Teufel M, Rieber N, Meile T, Giel KE, Sauer H, Hünnemeyer K, Enck P, Zipfel S. Body image after sleeve gastrectomy: reduced dissatisfaction and increased dynamics. Obes Surg. 2012;22:1232–7.

51. Sarwer DB, Wadden TA, Moore RH, Eisenberg MH, Raper SE, Williams NN. Changes in quality of life and body image after gastric bypass surgery. Surg Obes Relat Dis. 2010;6:608–14.
52. Hrabosky JI, Masheb RM, White MA, Rothschild BS, Burke-Martindale CH, Grilo CM. A prospective study of body dissatisfaction and concerns in extremely obese gastric bypass patients: 6- and 12-month postoperative outcomes. Obes Surg. 2006;16:1615–21.
53. Dixon JB, O'Brien PE. Changes in comorbidities and improvements in quality of life after LAP-BAND placement. Am J Surg. 2002;184:51S–4S.
54. Heitmann C, Germann G. Body contouring surgery after massive weight loss. Part I: abdomen and extremities. Chirurg. 2007;78:273–86.
55. Song AY, Rubin JP, Thomas V, Dudas JR, Marra KG, Fernstrom MH. Body image and quality of life in post massive weight loss body contouring patients. Obesity. 2006;14:1626–36.
56. Pavan C, Marini M, De Antoni E, Scarpa C, Brambullo T, Bassetto F, Mazzotta A, Vindigni V. Psychological and psychiatric traits in post-bariatric patients asking for body-contouring surgery. Aesth Plast Surg. 2017;41:90–7.
57. Cash TF. The psychology of physical appearance: aesthetics, attributes, and images. In: Cash TF, Prunzinsky T, editors. Body images: development, deviance, and change. New York: Guilford Press; 1990. p. 51–79.
58. Riva G, Cárdenas-López G, Duran X, Torres-Villalobos GM, Gaggioli A. Virtual reality in the treatment of body image disturbances after bariatric surgery: a clinical case. Stud Health Technol Inform. 2012;181:278–82.
59. Cárdenas-López G, Torres-Villalobos G, Martinez P, Carreño V, Duran X, Dakanalis A, Gaggioli A, Riva G. Virtual reality for improving body image disorders and weight loss after gastric band surgery: a case series. Stud Health Technol Inform. 2014;196:43–7.

Body Image in Males with Eating and Weight Disorders

18

Emilia Manzato and Giovanni Gravina

18.1 Body Dissatisfaction: Biological, Social, and Cultural Aspects

The Ideal Male Body Image—as well as the Ideal Female Body Image—has remained stable over the centuries inspiring to that typical standard of beauty proposed by the classic Greek sculpture.

The traditional aesthetic canons define as "beautiful" anything which has harmonious proportions capable of satisfying our senses; as for human beings beauty is a real mix of well proportionated shape and good soul [1]. Since the beginning of the last century—particularly in the second half of the last century—the feminine and masculine body ideals have changed due to the spread of new models proposed by media and by the commercial world.

Therefore, the male body ideal has gradually detached from a single model of beauty, for some new models that contributed to increasing the body dissatisfaction in individuals.

So we are now facing different models ranging from an exaggerated sculpted male body to a thin and effeminate male body.

This multiplicity of male body models could be encouraged by a more fluid man/woman dichotomy as well as by commercials and media.

In fact, male body ideals are very far from real male bodies and they could lead men to train compulsively, as well as use beauty treatments, anabolic steroids, and so on, which would account for a considerable income for "beauty industries."

E. Manzato (✉)
University of Ferrara, Ferrara, Italy

G. Gravina
Hospital San Rossore, Pisa, Italy
e-mail: gravina@sanrossorecura.it

M. Cuzzolaro, S. Fassino (eds.), *Body Image, Eating, and Weight*,
https://doi.org/10.1007/978-3-319-90817-5_18

This short foreword underlines how dramatically the changes in ideal male body occurred in the last century have promoted the increase of body dissatisfaction in male exactly as happened in women.

Body dissatisfaction (BD) has been defined as a negative evaluation of weight and shape of one's body. The subject is induced to pursue an ideal body that greatly differs from his/her current body.

Before the late 1980s, BD was often viewed as a specific female problem linked to eating disorders (ED) and other weight-related conditions in women, but recent studies have shown that men also may show body image concerns and BD in particular in Western society [2].

BD is a strong risk factor for the development of an ED in males too [3].

Due to the lower prevalence of Anorexia and Bulimia Nervosa in men, research studies on body image and ED risk among males are more recent than the same ones carried out among females.

However, the newly discovered body image concerns brought along a higher interest in this area as they are considered as a real ED risk factor [4].

Most of the males report a preference for a more muscular physique, which is consistent with the male body ideal frequently portrayed in contemporary Western media.

Despite this, a smaller portion of men desires to lose weight and reduce body mass, as happens in females.

Many factors contributed to body dissatisfaction increase in males, but—up to now—they are not completely clear.

The scientific research focused on the sexual role, due to the initial data suggesting a higher susceptibility to male body ideal proposed by media in gay men. So gay men seemed to be more prone to have a higher body dissatisfaction as well as a greater tendency to leanness [5].

Further surveys did not confirm these data [6].

Now, more recent studies are highlighting the importance of gender role endorsement [7].

The concept of "Gender role endorsement" has been proposed by some sociological trends in the USA in 1970s.

This concept defines the gender (male or female) an individual identifies themselves with. The role endorsement does not necessarily originate from a specific biological gender, and it is not linked to sexual orientation.

Many factors—both social and biological—have been detected as key factors for the development of gender role endorsement.

Social factors include all information linked to "gender" proposed by family, peers, and media. Biological factors include hormonal levels also during the prenatal phase and their genetic regulation.

Masculine and feminine gender role endorsement can play opposing roles in the body image psychopathology amongst males.

Furthermore, gender role endorsement could be responsible for the different ED symptoms in males. That is, both heterosexual and gay men, who tend to endorse a feminine gender role rather than a masculine one, may pursue a thin body image.

On the contrary, those who tend to endorse a more masculine gender role could report a higher tendency to muscularity [8].

The "femininity hypothesis" also suggests that men with typical feminine traits—such as dependence and passivity—have a tendency to lower self-esteem as well.

Furthermore, they tend also to pursue dietary restriction and purging behavior—as well as in females—so as to achieve their personal image of a thinner body.

In the last decades, even the ideal male body images proposed by media such as television, magazines, movies, and social media played a major role [9–11].

Such images tended to depict a more and more muscular male figure, in particular after the discovery of anabolic steroids.

In fact, a key factor in body male image evolution proposed by media was the discovery and the spread of anabolic steroids that have produced, in the last 40 years, an unnatural muscular development which could not be achieved with "regular" exercise.

Considering that the ideal body proposed by media represents a "social rule," many males—who compare themselves to such images—could get more dissatisfaction because of their body and accordingly try to increase their muscles [12].

Some interesting research studies [13] examined the physiques of American action toys (i.e., GI Joe, Superman, Spiderman, and so on), from 1973—when anabolic steroids launched on the market—and 1997.

In fact, before the year 1973, the body shape of action toys had not changed at all.

Conversely, since then, those figures have not simply grown more muscular, but they have even become increasingly defined, with more abdominal definition and plumped pectoral muscles.

Further research confirmed a trend towards an increased muscular shape also in other action toys such as Batman, Hulk, and others [14].

Recent studies also showed that the exposure to videogames emphasizing muscular and powerful heroes could increase BD in male adolescents [15, 16].

The spread of BD in Western society could be linked also to a more frequent use of social media that propose a male model—either leaner or more muscular—over the past few decades [17].

In fact, data research highlighted that those who use Facebook more intensively show higher scores on body image concern measures. They strongly feel they have to lose weight to look thinner or they tend to train strenuously to look more muscular. In both cases, they attempt to achieve an ideal model [18].

Within this scope, an interesting study carried out in Pakistan—a country where the social media have only recently been liberalized—pointed out high rates of "Negative Body Dissatisfaction" (NBID) in university students [19].

In the study, the NBID is defined as a wish to lose weight in males with a BMI under 20 or a wish to gain weight in males with a BMI over 25.

Data showed that individuals more exposed to social media had a higher prevalence of NBID (84.0%) compared to those who were less exposed to social media (16.0%).

Totally unexpected was the higher prevalence of NBID in males (75.3%) than in females (35.0%).

This disparity could be partially ascribed to sociocultural factors. Normally, in those areas, women have to cover their whole body and hair with loose clothes, while men are free to wear what they want and can compare themselves straight to the ideal body image as proposed by social media thus experiencing greater body dissatisfaction.

Another important disturbance in body image is the distortion in Size Perception.

Size Perception defines the ability to identify the body size on a conscious level [20]; it includes sensations detected by the sense organs, individual's beliefs, cultural background, motivation, attitudes, and so on.

Distortion in Size Perception includes either an over-evaluation or an under-evaluation by the subject of their real weight and size.

A disturbed Size Perception could promote BD and consequently facilitate the development of an ED in males as well.

Furthermore, the distortion in Size Perception may become both a predictive factor of overweight and obesity but also an obstacle to weight disorders treatment [21, 22].

Research studies found how the under-evaluation of their weight status in overweight and obese men could be due to cultural influences: in fact, body size underestimation would occur more frequently in cultures where a larger body is considered as desirable and as an ideal body [23].

Within this scope it is interesting to mention a research examining the Ideal Body Size (IBS) in Native Hawaiians, for whom the influence of both their ethnic culture and the American one may lead people to have different opinions about their IBS, depending on the social group they referred to [24].

In fact, Native Hawaiians have always considered a large body as an indicator of health, wealth, and royalty as opposed to the Western ideal body focused on thinness.

This comparison has been carried out within other three different ethnic groups residing in the Hawaii: Filipinos, Japanese, and Whites.

A figures test was administered, and the participants were asked to choose the figure that best represented the Ideal Body Size in the Western culture and the figure that represented the Ideal Body Size typical of their ethnic group as well as their related attitude.

The results showed that Native Hawaiians selected a larger body size than all the other ethnic groups living in Hawai'i.

On the other hand, Filipinos chose a considerably smaller IBS if compared to the Japanese and Whites.

Conversely, a lower level of variability was pinpointed among ethnic groups as for Western IBS.

In any case, males were more likely to select larger body size than females when considering both their typical ethnic IBS model and the one which is typical in the Western world.

Finally, those men who selected a larger ethnic IBS had, in fact, a more negative attitude towards their choice.

This discrepancy between the larger ethnic IBS selected and their related negative attitude in all ethnic groups suggests that individuals could start feeling a real contradiction between their personal size preference and the larger body size proposed by their ethno-cultural canons.

So the ethno-cultural differences in Ideal Body Size could play major role in Size Perception attitude in males too.

18.2 Body Dissatisfaction in Male Adolescents

Adolescence seems to be the riskiest period for developing an ED even in males.

It is widely accepted that body dissatisfaction and other weight and shape concerns have become more prevalent among adolescent boys and adult males [25].

Some studies suggest that boys can experience higher levels of body dissatisfaction than girls, also influencing their psychological wellness and quality of life [26].

An important role is played by their family and peers.

In fact, higher levels of body satisfaction in male adolescents also seem to be highly correlated with positive comments by their mothers and female peers [27]; on the other hand, negative comments by their fathers and male peers could concretely lead them to strategies targeted to modify their body.

Research carried out in the USA basing on data from a large study on adolescents (Growing Up Today Study, GUTS) focused on concerns about body image in male adolescents [28].

Data indicated that 18–21% of kids showed the Muscle-Concerned pattern (great desire for toned and defined muscles and use of muscle-building products) while 19–28% showed the Lean-Concerned pattern (high concern about weight and shape, binge eating together with restrictive dieting behavior).

Additional studies highlighted that body dissatisfaction onsets later in male adolescents than in females [2].

Research data also underlined that late male adolescents—within the healthy Body Mass Index (BMI) percentile range—reported higher weight and shape concern than younger boys within the same BMI range.

A possible reason could be due to their increase in BMI as they grow up, which can be considered as a risk situation for becoming overweight or obese [29].

BMI turned out to be one of the strongest predictors of body dissatisfaction among male adolescents [30].

In fact, overweight and obese boys showed more dissatisfaction with their body than their peers who were underweight or healthy weight [2, 31].

Altered size perception contributes to the development of body dissatisfaction in male adolescents as well.

A recent multicentric research recruited a sample of 250 male adolescents (15–17 years old) who attended their high schools in Ferrara and Pisa and investigated the possible correlations between BMI, body image perception, self-esteem, and muscularity desire.

A comparison between detected and reported measures, showed that only 58.4% reported congruent data with their own BMI (±1 BMI point). Conversely 11.6% underestimated their own BMI (5.6% by more than 2 BMI points) and 20% overestimated their own BMI (7.6% by more than 2 BMI points).

Data showed the highest rates of body dissatisfaction, linked to shape overevaluation, in underweight and overweight boys [32, 33].

18.3 Clinical Picture of Eating Disorders in Males

The clinical symptomatology of ED in males is quite similar to that observed in females [34]. Also in men, as in women, dieting and compensatory behaviors are the typical symptoms and, likewise, the altered eating behavior appears to be related to body dissatisfaction [35], as well as the weight and shape concerns [36].

For males, as for females, the average length of time between onset of illness and treatment is approximately 5 years [37]. However, several studies show some significant differences for AN and BN between males and females.

Physical hyperactivity is more frequent in males with AN while laxative and diuretic use is less common [35, 37]. In men with BN some studies show that the recourse to self-induced vomiting and strict dieting is lower than in females [36, 38–40]. However, other studies indicate a higher number of vomiting episodes in males than females [41]. Furthermore, males with ED are much more likely than females to have been subjected to weight-based victimization, to have a history of being overweight [42], and scored significantly lower than females on harm avoidance and reward dependence [41].

Regarding the comorbidity with other psychiatric disorders, in males and females with AN and BN there are the same high rates of anxiety disorders, major depression, and personality disorders, but in males with BN more elevated rates of substance abuse are found [43, 44].

The studies comparing the Binge Eating Disorder (BED) clinical presentation in males and females show no significant differences concerning the ED symptoms [45]. Men and women with BED show many similarities in current ED features (binge eating, eating concerns, weight and shape concerns), and developmental variables (age at first overweight, age at first diet, age at onset of regular binge eating, or number of weight cycles). However, men have lower BD and drive for thinness, and significantly higher current body mass index (BMI), highest adult BMI, and are significantly more likely to be classified as obese [46]. Men and women with BED do not differ significantly on self-esteem, but men report less emotional eating, a greater frequency of past drug abuse problems, higher rates of current substance abuse and axis-I psychopathology [45, 46].

As to BD, whereas for AN and BN one of the required diagnostic features is a negative body image, the DSM-5 criteria for BED do not include body image disturbance. For the perceptual component, no evidence exists to date that persons with and without BED differ regarding the perception of their body size. However, some studies reveal that individuals with BED-obesity display a higher level of weight and shape concerns than those with non-BED-obesity. Moreover, persons with BED display an enhanced degree of body checking and body avoidance [47], consistently observed to be elevated in people with ED [48–50].

18.4 Body Image Disturbances and Eating Disorders in Males

In recent years, the increasing prevalence of male ED has resulted in a growing number of studies focused on body image disturbances in men [51].

About the body image concerns in a sample of adolescent boys, some studies have shown that both drive for thinness and pursuit of muscularity were related to disordered eating [52]. However, comparing male and female ED, other studies highlighted how, in many cases of male AN and BN, the concerns about the body weight appeared to be linked to the desire of greater muscularity rather than the desire of thinness [53, 54].

Sociocultural differences between males and females about the ideal body shape can be a conditioning factor for different motivations to diet. The search of low body weight—sustained in women also by the current pressure for thinness—does not seem to be the main motivation to diet in many males with ED. For them, the primary goal of dieting seems to be the attempt to reach the ideal male body shape by increasing and defining the muscle mass [55, 56].

Moreover, some authors pointed out that men with ED perceive themselves as fatter than they are, suggesting that distorted body perception, rather than body ideal, may be central to ED in men [57].

However, other Authors, evaluating the male body satisfaction separately from muscularity and body fat, by using two figure tests with different silhouettes of male bodies, have shown the widespread desire for increased muscularity among men and the association between this desire and lower psychological well-being [58].

Finally, there is no conclusive evidence about this matter; both the distorted body perception as well as the pressure for muscular body ideal can play a role in determining body dissatisfaction and ED in males.

18.5 Body Image Perception and Dissatisfaction in Males

In literature, for the higher prevalence of ED in females, most of the body dissatisfaction studies have involved the female gender, and many assessment instruments are more applicable to females than males [59]. The number of assessment tools to study body image has increased substantially over the past 20 years. There is a wide variety of tests to evaluate body image and the multidimensionality of this construct including the measurement of subjective (dis)satisfaction, cognitive distortions, affective reactions, behavioral avoidance, and perceptual inaccuracy [60].

The most investigated aspects of body image have been how accurately body size is perceived (perceptual components) and the dissatisfaction about one's body size and shape (affective components) [61].

The studies focused on body size perception—that involves the processing of information in the brain—have highlighted how different subjective factors can affect the individual judgment on his body image [62].

The evaluation of body size perception is a very controversial area in body image assessment. The early studies of people with ED noted a tendency of subjects with AN to overestimate the size of their bodies.

An extensive review of research studies focused on disturbed size perception by obese men [61] found inconsistent outcomes: nearly the half of the studies showed that individuals with obesity overestimated their body size, while the other half found that obese subjects were relatively accurate. Using the Body Image Assessment Scale (BIAS-BD)—useful to measure both body dissatisfaction and the accuracy of body size estimations—researchers found that men were relatively accurate in estimating their body size, also reporting that men's accuracy was independent of their actual BMI [63]. More recent studies carried out using more sophisticated techniques did not show significant differences between obese and normal-weight men as for size perception although a light trend towards over-evaluation emerged in men with obesity [64]. Moreover, the overvaluation seems to be more frequent also in underweight men. Hence, men resulted as less accurate at evaluating their shape and weight than women.

In recent years, advances in technology permitted new ways of assessing body size perception, by using psychophysical methodologies and digital video-distortion techniques, based on signal detection theory (SDT) analysis and the method of adjustment (MOA). These studies showed no significant difference between obese and normal-weight men in estimating their body size although there was a tendency for individuals with obesity to underestimate their size and weight. The relevance of these works is also to have clarified the respective roles of sensory and non-sensory/affective variables in body size perception, demonstrating that perceptual ratings are affected by sociocultural and other factors [61].

In the same way, the studies on body dissatisfaction showed the role of more factors. Researchers have identified the body mass index (BMI) as the most consistent biological correlate of body dissatisfaction in males [30, 65]. Moreover, some studies found that BMI explained unique variance in body dissatisfaction above and beyond sociocultural variables [66, 67]. Other observations demonstrated the body image improvement in persons with obesity after bariatric surgery and reinforced the role of BMI in body satisfaction [68, 69].

However, although the relationship between BMI and measures of body dissatisfaction is robust across studies, the magnitude of this correlation is variable suggesting, also for body dissatisfaction, a role of other various sociocultural and psychological factors.

18.6 Body Weight and Moderating Factors of Body Dissatisfaction in Males

The 1996 survey in the USA showed that 56% of women and 43% of men were dissatisfied with their overall appearance. Furthermore, two-thirds of women and more than half of men reported dissatisfaction with their body weight [70].

Some of the more commonly used measures to assess weight dissatisfaction are: the Body Dissatisfaction scale of the Eating Disorder Inventory [71], the Body Shape Questionnaire [72], and the Body Uneasiness Test [73]. Other techniques involve the figure rating methodologies (Figure Rating Scale, Contour Rating Scale, and Body Image Assessment Procedure) [74, 75]. To measure the general appearance satisfaction, the most widely used test is the Multi-dimensional Body Self-Relations Questionnaire (MBSRQ) with its subscales [60]. Finally, a test to measure body image specifically in obese patients is the Body Image Assessment for obesity (BIA-O) [76].

On this basis, body dissatisfaction in males can be described as a continuum from none to extreme represented by the Body Dysmorphic Disorder, similar to what is occurring in women [20, 21].

Especially in Western countries, an issue related to body dissatisfaction is the increasing desire for men to have a mesomorphic and muscular V-shaped body [20], including broad shoulders, a flat but muscular stomach, and a narrow waist and hips [77]. Since this ideal is very difficult to attain, the result is an increasing level of body dissatisfaction in men. The simultaneous pursuit of overt musculature and low body fat has led to conceptualize muscle dissatisfaction and body fat dissatisfaction as separate but related constructs that are equally central to male body image [30, 78].

Body dissatisfaction is frequently involved in ED, representing a key diagnostic factor as well as a risk and a maintaining factor, also associated with higher risk of relapse.

More than the simple BD, a feature commonly observed in Western countries and not only in obese people, persons with ED suffer from specific cognitive-perceptive issues linked to body image, with an overvaluation of shape and weight closely related to low self-esteem and other psychological factors.

For these reasons, specific techniques for body image problems in ED are frequently indicated in clinical practice [79].

To understand the role of several variables involved in male body image, researchers have highlighted the role of different factors that can moderate the relation between both BMI and BD as well as ED and BD.

Some studies showed that concurrent and past appearance-related teasing is associated with BD and BD increases in boys and men [10, 66, 80]. Researchers found that appearance-related teasing may be the most powerful predictor of men's BD [81].

Many factors have been found to moderate BD in males with ED are poor impulse control, social anxiety, and internalization of media ideals, as well as emotional dysregulation, body checking, insecure-anxious attachment, and perfectionism [82, 83].

Perfectionism is known as a contributor to eating pathology [84], but rarely it has been investigated about BD [85]. The perfectionistic attitude may include feeling that one cannot meet sociocultural appearance ideals, which could contribute to BD. Moreover, a study has found an association between self-oriented perfectionism and drive for muscularity in men [86].

Other studies, showing that men are negatively affected by exposure to unattainable male body ideals, confirm the role of the media influence on the increased BD and negative mood [9, 10].

Researchers also pointed out the relevance of other moderator factors contributing to body image in men, including male and female peer influences, parent influences, sports involvement and interest, and self-perception of social status [87].

Finally, a recent study proposes a mediator model of disturbed eating and compensatory behavior for men, suggesting that emotion dysregulation and susceptibility to body-related cognitive distortions mediate the relationship between BD and disturbed eating [88].

Conclusions

In the second half of the last century, the masculine body ideal has gradually changed to configure different models and promoting greater body dissatisfaction among males.

Many biological and cultural factors, as well as the gender role endorsement and the role of media and ethnic influences, lead to body image concerns and body dissatisfaction, particularly in adolescent males.

Over the past 30 years, to study body image, many assessment instruments have validated especially for females. Given the increased prevalence of male ED also there was a growing number of studies to evaluate the relationship between body dissatisfaction and eating behavior in males.

Despite a symptomatology quite similar to that observed in females eating disorders, the clinical pictures of ED among males presents, as described, some differences and different moderators who need specific attention and further studies related to the treatment of eating disorders in males.

References

1. Eco U. Storia della Bellezza. Bompiani RCS libri SPA: Bologna; 2004.
2. Mitchison D, Mond J. Epidemiology of eating disorders, eating disordered behaviour, and body image disturbance in males: a narrative review. J Eat Disord. 2015;3:20.
3. Cohane GH, Pope HG Jr. Body image in boys: a review of the literature. Int J Eat Disord. 2001;29:373–9.
4. Manzato E, Zanetti T, Gualandi M, Strumia R. Eating Disorders in males. New York: Nova Science Publishers Inc; 2011.
5. French SA, Story M, Remafedi G, Resnik MD. Sexual orientation and prevalence of body dissatisfaction and eating disordered behaviours: a population-based study of adolescents. Int J Eat Disord. 1996;19:119–26.
6. Strong SM, Williamson DA, Netemeyer RG, Greer JH. Eating disorder symptoms and concerns about body differ as a function of gender and sexual orientation. J Soc Clin Psychol. 2001;19:240–55.
7. Murray SB, Rieger E, Karlov L, Touyz SW. Masculinity and femininity in the divergence of male body image concerns. J Eat Disord. 2013;1:11.
8. Smolak L, Murnen SK. Drive for leanness: assessment and relationship to gender, gender role and objectification. Body Image. 2008;5:251–60.
9. Agliata D, Tantleff-Dunn S. The impact of media exposure on males' body image. J Soc Clin Psychol. 2004;23:7–22.
10. Van den Berg PJ, Paxton SJ, Keery H, Wall M, Guo J, Neumark-Sztainer D. Body dissatisfaction and body comparison with media images in males and females. Body Image. 2007;4:257–68.

11. Duane A, Hargreaves DA, Tiggemann M. Idealized media images and adolescent body image: "comparing" boys and girls. Body Image. 2004;1(4):351–61.
12. Blond A. Impacts of exposure to images of ideal bodies on male body dissatisfaction: a review. Body Image. 2008;5:244–50.
13. Pope HG Jr, Olivardia R, Amanda Gruber A, John Borowiecki J. Evolving ideals of male body image as seen through action toys. Int J Eat Disord. 1999;26:65–72.
14. Baghurst T, Hollander DB, Nardella B, Haff GG. Change in sociocultural ideal male physique: an examination of past and present action figures. Body Image. 2006;3(1):87–91.
15. Mulgrew KE, Volcevski-Kostas D. Short term exposure to attractive and muscular singers in music video clips negatively affects men's body image and mood. Body Image. 2012;9(4):543–6.
16. Barlett CP, Harris JR. The impact of body emphasizing video games on body image concerns in men and women. Sex Role. 2008;59(7):586–60.
17. Pepin Gand Endresz N. Facebook, Instagram, Pinterest and co.: body image and social media. J Eat Disord. 2015;3(Suppl 1):O22.
18. Cohen R, Blaszczynski A. Comparative effects of Facebook and conventional media on body image dissatisfaction. J Eat Disord. 2015;3:23.
19. Khan A, Khalid S, Khan HI, Jabeen M. Impact of today's media on university student's body image in Pakistan: a conservative, developing country's perspective. BMC Public Health. 2011;11:379.
20. Thompson JK, Heinberg LJ, Altabe MN, Tantleff-Dunn S. Exacting beauty: theory, assessment, and treatment of body image disturbance. Washington, DC: American Psychological Association; 2004. p. 290–3.
21. Thompson JK. Body image, eating disorders, and obesity—an emerging synthesis. In: Thompson JK, editor. Body image, eating disorders, and obesity. Washington, DC: American Psychological Association; 1996.
22. Manzato E, Bolognesi A, Simoni M, Cuzzolaro M. Risk factors for weight gain: a longitudinal study in non-weight loss treatment-seeking overweight adults. Eat Weight Disord. 2015;20(3):371–8.
23. Puhl RM, Heuer CA. The stigma of obesity: a review and update. Obesity. 2012;17:941–6.
24. Townsend C, Takishima-Lacasa JY, Latner JD, Grandinetti A, Keawe'aimoku Kaholokula J. Ethnic and gender differences in ideal body size and related attitudes among Asians, Native Hawaiians, and Whites. Hawaii J Med Public Health. 2014;73(8):236–43.
25. Pope HG, Phillips K, Olivardia R. The Adonis complex. How to identify, treat, and prevent body obsession in men and boys. New York: A Touchstone Book; 2000.
26. McCabe MP, Ricciardelli LA. Sociocultural influences on body image and body changes among adolescent boys and girls. J Soc Psychol. 2003;143:5–26.
27. Ricciardelli LA, McCabe MP, Banfield S. Body image and body change methods in adolescent boys. Role of parents, friends, and the media. J Psychosom Res. 2000;49((3):189–97.
28. Calzo JP, Masyn KE, Corliss HL, Scherer EA, Field AE, Austin SB. Patterns of body image concerns and disordered weight- and shape-related behaviors in heterosexual and sexual minority adolescent males. Dev Psychol. 2015;51(9):1216–25.
29. Calzo JP, Sonneville KR, Haines J, Blood EA, Field AE, Austin SB. The development of associations among BMI, body dissatisfaction, and weight and shape concern in adolescent boys and girls. J Adolesc Health. 2012;51(5):517–23.
30. Jones DC, Crawford JK. Adolescent boys and body image: weight and muscularity concerns as dual pathways to body dissatisfaction. J Youth Adolesc. 2005;24:629–36.
31. Manzato E, editor. The different faces of being overweight. Nova Science Publisher: New York; 2015.
32. Manzato E, Gravina G, Giust V, Diloreto G, Piccione C, Nebbiai G, Cuzzolaro M. Body mass index, eating behavior and body image in a sample of male adolescents. Poster 10° International Congress SISDCA 9-11 marzo 2017, Roma.
33. Piccione C, Di Loreto G, Gravina G, Nebbiai G, Giust V, Manzato E, Cuzzolaro M. Body image and muscularity desire in a sample of adolescent males. Poster 10° International Congress SISDCA 9-11 marzo 2017, Roma.

34. Woodside DB, Garfinkel PE, Lin E, Goering P, Kaplan AS, Goldbloom DS, Kennedy SH. Comparison of men with full or partial eating disorders; men without eating disorders, and women with eating disorders in the community. Am J Psychiatry. 2001;158:570–4.
35. Fichter M, Krenn H. Eating disorders in males. In: Treasure J, Schmidt U, van Furth E, editors. Handbook of eating disorders. 2nd ed. Chichester: John Wiley & Sons; 2003.
36. Shu CY, Limburg K, Harris C, McCormack J, Hoiles KJ, Hamilton MJ, Watson HJ. Clinical presentation of eating disorders in young males at a tertiary setting. J Eat Disord. 2015;3:39–45.
37. Braun DL, Sunday SR, Huang A, Halmi KA. More males seek treatment for eating disorders. Int J Eat Disord. 1999;25:415–24.
38. Garfinkel PE, Lin E, Goering P, Spegg C, Goldbloom DS, Kennedy S, Kaplan AS, Woodside DB. Bulimia nervosa in a Canadian community sample: prevalence and comparison of subgroups. Am J Psychiatry. 1995;152:1052–8.
39. Carlat DJ, Camargo CA. Review of bulimia nervosa in males. Am J Psychiatry. 1991;148:831–43.
40. Woodside DB, Kaplan AS. Day hospital treatment in males with eating disorders-response and comparison to females. J Psychosom Res. 1994;38(5):471–5.
41. Núñez-Navarro A, Agüera Z, Krug I, Jiménez-Murcia S, Sánchez I, Araguz N, Gorwood P, Granero R, Penelo E, Karwautz A, Moragas L, Saldaña S, Treasure J, Menchón JM, Fernández-Aranda F. Do men with eating disorders differ from women in clinics, psychopathology and personality? Eur Eat Disord Rev. 2012;20(1):23–31.
42. Gueguen J, Godart N, Chambry J, Brun-Eberentz A, Foulon C, Divac SM, Guelfi JD, Rouillon F, Falissard B, Huas C. Severe anorexia nervosa in men: comparison with severe AN in women and analysis of mortality. Int J Eat Disord. 2012;45:537–45.
43. Carlat DJ, Camargo CA, Herzog DB. Eating disorders in males: a report on 135 patients. Am J Psychiatry. 1997;154:1127–32.
44. Striegel-Moore RH, Garvin V, Dohm FA, Rosenheck RA. Psychiatric comorbidity of eating disorders in men: a national study of hospitalized veterans. Int J Eat Disord. 1999;25:399–404.
45. Tanofsky MB, Wilfley DE, Borman Spurrell E, Welch R, Brownell KD. Comparison of men and women with binge eating disorder. Int J Eat Disord. 1997;21:49–54.
46. Barry DT, Grilo CM, Masheb RM. Gender differences in patients with binge eating disorder. Int J Eat Disord. 2002;31:63–70.
47. Ahrberg M, Trojca D, Nasrawi N, Vocks S. Body image disturbance in binge eating disorder: a review. Eur Eat Disord Rev. 2011;19:375–81.
48. Reas DL, Grilo CM, Masheb RM, Wilson GT. Body checking and avoidance in overweight patients with binge eating disorder. Int J Eat Disord. 2005;37:342–6.
49. Mountford V, Haase A, Waller G. Body checking in the eating disorders: associations between cognitions and behaviors. Int J Eat Disord. 2006;39:708–15.
50. Shafran R, Lee M, Payne F, Fairburn CG. An experimental analysis of body checking. Behav Res Ther. 2007;45:113–21.
51. Jones W, Morgan J. Eating disorders in men: a review of the literature. J Public Ment Health. 2010;9:23–31.
52. Rodgers RF, Ganchou C, Franko DL, Chabrol H. Drive for muscularity and disordered eating among French adolescent boys: a sociocultural model. Body Image. 2012;9:318–23.
53. Olivardia R, Pope HG, Mangweth B, Hudson JI. Eating disorders in college men. Am J Psychiatry. 1995;52:1279–85.
54. Murray SB, Rieger E, Hildebrandt T, Karlov L, Russell J, Boon E, Dawson RT, Touyz SW. A comparison of eating, exercise, shape, and weight related symptomatology in males with muscle dysmorphia and anorexia nervosa. Body Image. 2012;9:193–200.
55. Andersen AE. Eating disorders in males. In: Brownell KD, Fairburn CG, editors. Eating disorders and obesity. New York: Guilford Press; 1995.
56. Griffiths S, Murray SB, Touyz S. Disordered eating and the muscular ideal. J Eat Disord. 2013;1:15.
57. Mangweth B, Hausmann A, Walch T, Hotter A, Rupp CI, Biebl W, Hudson JI, Pope HG Jr. Body fat perception in eating-disordered men. Int J Eat Disord. 2004;35:102–8.

58. Frederick DA, Buchanan GM, Sadehgi-Azar L, Peplau LA, Haselton MG, Berezovskaya A, Lipinski R. Desiring the muscular ideal: Men's body satisfaction in the United States, Ukraine, and Ghana. Psychol Men Masculinity. 2007;8:103–17.
59. McCabe MP, Ricciardelli LA. A longitudinal study of pubertal timing and extreme body change behaviors among adolescent boys and girls. Adolescence. 2004;39:145–66.
60. Sarwer DB, Thompson JK, Cash TF. Body image and obesity in adulthood. Psychiatr Clin N Am. 2005;28:69–87.
61. Gardner RM. Weight status and the perceptual of body image in men. Psychol Res Behav Manag. 2014;7:175–84.
62. Gardner RM, Brown DL. Measurement of the perceptual aspects of body image. In: Greene SB, editor. Body image: perceptions, interpretations and attitudes. New York: Nova Science Publishers; 2011.
63. Gardner RM, Jappe LM, Gardner L. Development and validation of a new figural drawing scale for body-image assessment: the BIAS-BD. J Clin Psychol. 2009;65:113–22.
64. Robinson E, Hogenkamp PS. Visual perceptions of male obesity: a cross-cultural study examining male and female lay perceptions of obesity in Caucasian males. BMC Public Health. 2015;15:492.
65. Jones D. Body image among adolescent girls and boys: a longitudinal study. Dev Psychol. 2004;40:823–35.
66. Paxton SJ, Eisenberg ME, Neumark-Sztainer D. Prospective predictors of body dissatisfaction in adolescent girls and boys: a five-year longitudinal study. Dev Psychol. 2006;42:888–99.
67. Penkal JL, Kurdek LA. Gender and race differences in young adults' body dissatisfaction. Personal Individ Differ. 2007;43:2270–81.
68. Sarwer DB, Wadden TA, Moore RH, Eisenberg MH, Raper SE, Williams NN. Changes in quality of life and body image following gastric bypass surgery. Surg Obes Relat Dis. 2010;6:608–14.
69. Teufel M, Rieber N, Meile T, Giel KE, Sauer H, Hünnemeyer K, Enck P, Zipfel S. Body image after sleeve gastrectomy: reduced dissatisfaction and increased dynamics. Obes Surg. 2012;22:1232–7.
70. Garner DM. The 1997 body image survey results. Psychol Today. 1997;31:30.
71. Garner DM, Olmstead MP, Polivy J. Development and validation of a multidimensional eating disorder inventory for anorexia nervosa and bulimia. Int J Eat Disord. 1983;2:15–34.
72. Cooper PJ, Taylor MJ, Cooper Z, Fairburn CG. The development and validation of the body shape questionnaire. Int J Eat Disord. 1986;6:485–94.
73. Cuzzolaro M, Vetrone G, Marano G, Garfinkel PE. The Body Uneasiness Test (BUT): development and validation of a new body image assessment scale. Eat Weight Disord. 2006;11:1–13.
74. Thompson JK. Assessing body image disturbance: measures, methodology and implementation. In: Thompson JK, editor. Body image, eating disorders, and obesity: an integrative guide for assessment and treatment. Washington, DC: American Psychological Association; 1996. p. 49–81.
75. Stewart TM, Williamson DA. Assessment of body image disturbances. In: Thompson JK, editor. Handbook of eating disorders and obesity. New York: Wiley; 2004. p. 495–514.
76. Williamson DA, Womble LG, Zucker NL, Reas DL, White MA, Blouin DC, Greenway F. Body image assessment for obesity (BIA-O): development of a new procedure. Int J Obes Relat Metab Disord. 2000;24:1326–32.
77. Tiggemann M. Sociocultural perspectives on body image. In: Cash TF, editor. Encyclopedia of body image and human appearance. Burlington: Elsevier Science; 2012.
78. Bergeron D, Tylka TL. Support for the uniqueness of body dissatisfaction from drive for muscularity among men. Body Image. 2007;4:288–95.
79. Paxton SJ, McLean S. Treatment for body image disturbances. In: Grilo C, Mitchell J, editors. The treatment of eating disorders. New York: The Guilford Press; 2009.
80. Eisenberg M, Neumark-Sztainer E, Haines D, Wall JM. Weight-teasing and emotional well-being in adolescents: longitudinal findings from project EAT. J Adolesc Health. 2006;38:675–83.

81. Vartanian LR, Giant CL, Passino RM. Ally McBeal vs. Arnold Schwarzenegger: comparing mass media, interpersonal feedback and gender as predictors of satisfaction with body thinness and muscularity. Soc Behav Pers. 2001;29:711–24.
82. Dakanalis A, Zanetti AM, Riva G, Colmegna F, Volpato C, Madeddu F, Clerici M. Male body dissatisfaction and eating disorder symptomatology: moderating variables among men. J Health Psychol. 2015;20(1):80–90.
83. Dakanalis A, Favagrossa L, Clerici M, Prunas A, Colmegna F, Zanetti MA, Riva G. Body dissatisfaction and eating disorder symptomatology: a latent structural equation modeling analysis of moderating variables in 18-to-28-year-old males. J Psychol. 2015;149:85–112.
84. Stice E. Risk and maintenance factors for eating pathology: a meta-analytic review. Psychol Bull. 2002;128:825–48.
85. Van den Berg PJ, Thompson JK, Obremski-Brandon K, Coovert M. The tripartite influence model of body image and eating disturbance: a covariance structure modeling investigation testing the mediational role of appearance comparison. J Psychosom Res. 2002;53:1007–20.
86. Davis C, Karvinen K, McCreary DR. Personality correlates of a drive for muscularity in young men. Personal Individ Differ. 2005;39:349–59.
87. Bardone-Cone AM, Cass KM, Ford JA. Examining body dissatisfaction in young men within a biopsychosocial framework. Body Image. 2008;5:183–94.
88. Wyssen A, Bryjova J, Meyer AH, Munsch S. A model of disturbed eating behavior in men: the role of body dissatisfaction, emotion dysregulation and cognitive distortions. Psychiatry Res. 2016;246:9–15.

Gender Identity, Sexual Orientation, Body Image, Eating, and Weight

19

Massimo Cuzzolaro and Walter Milano

19.1 Introduction

Physical appearance and internal body image are deeply connected with gender identity. Most people feel as either female or male and consider sex assigned at birth as congruent with their physical appearance and their subjective gender identity. On the contrary, some individuals do not feel at their ease with their natal sex and challenge the socially prescribed gender norms in many different ways.

Several thinkers and scientists have questioned the idea of two opposite sexes and have suggested that gender has various categories or lies on a continuum. However, *gender nonconformities* are not readily accepted, even in Western cultures, and remain a controversial issue. They were considered to be diseases—in particular, mental disorders—until very recent years.

Medicine appropriated homosexuality and classified it as a psychiatric disease in the nineteenth century. In 1968, the second edition of the Diagnostic and Statistical Manual of Mental Disorders (DSM-II) [1] still listed homosexuality in the group of *sexual deviations*, together with pedophilia, transvestitism, etc. (p. 44). In 1980, in DSM-III, *homosexuality* was replaced by the category *ego-dystonic homosexuality*, reserved for people for whom sexual attraction to same sex is a persistent source of distress [2] (p. 281). Some years after, the word *homosexuality* completely disappeared in the DSM-III-R [3], in the tenth edition of the International Classification of Diseases (ICD-10) [4], in the DSM-IV [5], and in the DSM-5 [6]. Therefore, in the major taxonomies, same-sex attraction was no longer considered as a mental

M. Cuzzolaro (✉)
Formerly Medical Pathophysiology Department, Eating Disorders and Obesity Unit, Sapienza University of Rome, Rome, Italy

W. Milano
ASL Napoli 1, Napoli, Italy

Mental Disorders Department, Eating Disorders Unit, Napoli, Italy

M. Cuzzolaro, S. Fassino (eds.), *Body Image, Eating, and Weight*,
https://doi.org/10.1007/978-3-319-90817-5_19

disorder *per se*, and only expressions such as *ego-dystonic sexual orientation* or *persistent and marked distress about sexual orientation* were maintained.

Gender identity disorders first appeared as definite diagnostic categories in 1980, in the DSM-III [2], and included *transsexualism* and *gender identity disorder of childhood* (p. 261).

In 2013, the DSM-5 introduced the new term *gender dysphoria* (GD) to highlight that being gender non-conforming can be considered as a mental disorder only when it is associated with severe suffering.

Two primary conditions are required to fulfill DSM-5 diagnostic criteria for GD:

- Persistent (for at least 6 months) incongruence between the gender that the person feels he/she is, and the biological and legal sex to which he/she was assigned at birth
- Consequent substantial suffering. Body dissatisfaction is the main component of the experienced distress in GD.

The 11th revision of the *International Classification of Diseases and Related Health Problems* (ICD-11) is expected to be approved in 2018. It will most probably retain two diagnoses, to preserve access to health services:

- *Gender incongruence of childhood* that will replace the ICD-10 category *Gender identity disorder of childhood*
- *Gender incongruence of adolescence and adulthood* that will replace the ICD-10 category *Transsexualism*.

However, these categories will be moved out of the ICD-11 chapter on *Mental and Behavioral Disorders* and included in a new section on *Conditions related to sexual health*. This shift is an essential difference from DSM-5. The forthcoming ICD-11 will describe distress and functional impairment as possible associated features—mainly due to disapproving social environments—but they will not be diagnostic requirements [7].

In sum, both DSM-5 and ICD-11 recognize that sexual orientation and transgender identity cannot be considered as mental disorders *per se*.

The modifications mentioned above reflect both advances in research and changes in social attitudes, human rights standards, policies, laws, and clinical practice [8].

In the last few years, many other terms have repeatedly been changed to modify or eliminate expressions that do not appear accurate enough or could offend particular sensibilities. For example, *sex change surg*ery has also been called *gender reassignment surgery, gender confirmation surgery*, and *gender-affirming surgery*. Some individuals who desire or achieve the transition from their natal sex to another, reject being named FtM (female-to-male) or MtF (male-to-female). They claim that they have always been, respectively, males and females, and medical and surgical treatments only make their physical appearance consistent with their true gender identity. Therefore, they ask to be called MtM and FtF.

A list of some current terms and definitions may be helpful to get near this complicate field (Table 19.1).

Table 19.1 Terms and definitions (in alphabetical order)

Agender	People who identify as genderless or gender-neutral
Asexual	People who do not experience sexual attraction
Bisexual	People who are sexually or romantically attracted to both women and men, or to people of various gender identities
Cisgender	A person whose subjective gender identity agrees with the native sex. The term was coined in the 1990s to mean the opposite of transgender. It does not necessarily indicate the sexual orientation
Crossdressing (transvestiting)	Dressing in clothes culturally associated with the opposite sex
Drag kings	Women crossdressers
Drag queens	Men crossdressers
FtM transgender	An individual with female sex assigned at birth who identifies as man (transgender man)
Gender	Either of the two sexes (female and male), with more reference to the social and cultural differences than to the biological ones. It includes physical appearance, beliefs, feelings, and behaviors that a specific culture considers appropriate to women and men. Some authors argue that gender has more than two categories or lies on a continuum
Gender-affirming treatments	Medical and surgical treatments aimed to develop the physical characteristics of the affirmed gender and reduce distress
Gender confirmation surgery (sex change surgery, sex or gender reassignment surgery)	Surgery performed by a multispecialty team to give transgender individuals the physical appearance and functional abilities of the gender they feel themselves to be. Some available procedures for MtF transition: facial feminization, transfeminine top (e.g., breast implants), transfeminine bottom (e.g. vaginoplasty). For FtM transition: facial masculinization, transmasculine top (e.g., mastectomy), transmasculine bottom (e.g., phalloplasty and scrotoplasty)
Gender confusion	The condition of a person who is unclear about his/her gender
Gender diversity	The expression often includes women, men, and non-binary/genderqueer categories
Gender dysphoria	Significant distress caused by a transgender condition
Gender expression	The way a person manifests and communicates his/her gender through body appearance, hairstyle, clothing, voice, behaviors, mannerisms, interests, etc. It may or may not follow the gender-cultural norms linked to the natal sex
Gender identity	The consistent and persistent sense and the concept of being female, male, a blend of both, or neither. It can be the same (cisgender) or different (transgender) from the natal sex
Gender incongruence	A consistent and persistent incongruence between one's experienced/expressed gender and the sex that was assigned at birth
Genderism	Beliefs and practices that discriminate transgender and gender-non-conforming people
Gender non-conformity	To express gender in ways that differ from gender-cultural norms linked to the natal sex. Gender non-conforming individuals may or may not identify as transgender
Genderqueer/non-binary	The non-binary gender of individuals who experience their gender as fluid, changing from time to time: bigender, pangender, genderfluid, or agender

(continued)

Table 19.1 (continued)

Gender role	The social and cultural norms that dictate how females and males should respectively think, feel, speak, dress, behave, interact, etc. The role learned by a person as appropriate to a gender
Gender transition	The process (clothing, behaviors, medical and surgical interventions, etc.) by which transgender persons try to make their physical appearance and functions agree with the gender they feel themselves to be
Homosexuality	Romantic and sexual attraction to same sex. It is not necessarily associated with a transgender condition
Intersex	A person who is born with a mix of male and female biological sex characteristics (chromosomal, gonadal, and anatomical). The old term was hermaphroditism
LGBT	Acronym that stands for lesbian, gay (acronym for good as you), bisexual, and transgender
MtF transgender	An individual with a male sex assigned at birth who identifies as woman (transgender woman)
Natal sex (assigned at birth)	The biological (medical) and legal sex that was assigned at birth
Sexual orientation	Refers to the gender of the people a person is sexually or romantically attracted to
TGNC	Acronym that stands for transgender and gender non-conforming
Transgender	A person whose subjective gender identity or gender expression consistently and persistently differs from the gender the person was assigned at birth. The term may include people genderqueer/non-binary. It does not necessarily indicate the sexual orientation. This condition is not necessarily experienced with significant distress (gender dysphoria). Transgender people may or may not undergo hormone and surgical treatments
Transsexual	Possibly outdated term to indicate a transgender person who desires transition from the natal sex to another and often undergoes hormone treatments and surgery

19.2 Eating Disorders, Gender Identity, and Gender Dysphoria

Janet's patient Nadia refused sexual maturity and after puberty developed severe ED symptoms (see Chap. 1 of the present volume). Should we consider Nadia as a FtM transgender? According to Janet, the answer should be no, and—if we decide to use a current expression—it seems possible to speak of *gender non-conformity* at most.

> "Par tous les moyens possibles elle a cherché à dissimuler son sexe, dont elle a particulièrement honte: ses corsages, ses chapeaux, ses coiffures doivent se rapprocher du costume masculin. Elle coupe ses cheveux à demi longs et les fait boucler et elle voudrait avoir l'aspect d'un jeune étudiant. Il ne faudrait pas croire qu'il y a ici une inversion sexuelle, comme on l'admet beaucoup trop vite dans des cas semblables. Elle serait aussi honteuse d'être un garçon que d'être une fille. Elle voudrait être sans aucun sexe, et même elle voudrait être sans aucun corps, car on voit que toutes les parties du corps déterminent le même sentiment dont le refus d'aliments n'était qu'une manifestation toute partielle" [9] (p. 39–40).

(By all means possible, she has tried to disguise her sex, of which she is especially ashamed: her tops, her hats, her hairstyles should look like the male clothing. She cuts her hair half-long and has it curled, and she would like to have the physical appearance of a young male student. It should not be supposed that this condition is a sexual inversion, as is believed, too quickly, in such cases. She would be as ashamed to be a boy as to be a girl. She would like to be without any sex, and she would even want to be without any body because all parts of the body seem to trigger the same feeling of which the refusal of food is just a very partial manifestation).

The prevalence of GD has probably increased in the past two decades. The figures mirror the growing referral rates to gender identity treatment centers [10–12]. Is it a bona fide increase or only the effect of a greater social and medical acceptance of the phenomenon?

Studies on self-reported transgender identity in children, adolescents, and adults indicate prevalence rates that range from 0.5 to 1.3%, undoubtedly higher than rates observed on clinical samples [13]. Many children with this feeling do not end up being adults with GD. The stability of a transgender identity appears weaker in children, adolescents, and young adults, but this issue has not been sufficiently investigated [13]. As to sex ratio, the prevalence is higher in children and adults born as males. In adolescence, some studies found no significant difference between boys and girls, but other recent surveys found more cases among birth-assigned females [14].

The neurobiological underpinnings of GD are still undefined. Functional magnetic resonance imaging (fMRI) has been used to study functional connections within connectivity networks involved in self-referential processes and own body perception (precuneus, insula, anterior and posterior cingulate, prefrontal, occipital and temporal regions, etc.). Results indicated the presence of some neurofunctional correlates to the subjective incongruence between self-identification and own body perception [15].

A negative body image is a well-known risk factor for eating disordered behaviors [16], and body uneasiness is both a core symptom of several ED and a central component of gender incongruence/dysphoria [17].

Further than genital dissatisfaction, a study found that some body characteristics that influence social gender recognition were remarkably involved in body dissatisfaction in both transgender people: voice and hair in MtF, posture, and muscularity in FtM [18].

Transgender individuals are increasingly seen in ED clinics, and many reports have pointed out the co-occurrence of gender incongruence and ED, in particular in MtF transgender adults [19].

In 2016, a systematic review of the scant literature on these topics suggested that transgender people report high levels of body dissatisfaction and may be particularly vulnerable to disordered eating behaviors. According to this work, GD treatment seems to improve body image [20].

Another review of the literature on GD and mental health indicates that the rates of psychiatric disorders in transgender patients at the time of assessment are higher than in the cisgender population, but they improve after gender-confirming treatment. However, a long-term follow-up study in Sweden suggests that gender confirmation alleviates GD but is not sufficient. Transgender people, after hormonal and surgical gender reassignment, had a significantly higher risk for psychiatric inpatient care, suicide attempts, and overall mortality than the general population [21].

A survey of a random sample of Massachusetts public high schools found that transgendered youth may be at high risk for the development of disordered eating and weight control behaviors [22].

The analysis of an extensive database from 223 US universities showed that rates of past-year self-reported ED diagnosis were highest among transgender students and lowest among cisgender heterosexual men [23].

A Canadian online survey of transgender youth (14–25 years) found a high prevalence of ED symptoms such as fasting, binge eating, and self-induced vomiting. Stigma and violence exposure were significant risk factors. Social support—including family, school, and friends—was a major protective factor [24].

A matched control study explored the association of transgender identity with body dissatisfaction and disordered eating behaviors. The authors compared 200 transgender individuals, 200 persons with ED, and 200 control participants. Transgender people (MtF and FtM) reported greater body dissatisfaction than control participants not only for sex-identifying body parts but also for body weight and shape. MtF transgender individuals appeared to be at particular risk for eating disordered behaviors and unhealthy weight control practices [25]. Some years before also Vocks et al. found that MtF transgender persons reported higher scores than male controls on the drive for thinness, weight and shape concerns, body checking, restrained eating, and bulimia [26].

Hormone treatment can alleviate body uneasiness of persons with gender incongruence. Jones and colleagues studied a large clinical sample of transgender people and found that individuals not on cross-sex hormones reported higher levels of disordered eating behaviors than people in treatment. However, the significant difference between the two groups disappeared after controlling for some well-known risk factors for ED (body dissatisfaction, perfectionism, self-esteem, and anxiety) [27].

Qualitative studies show that transgender persons may internalize the dominant ideals of male and female body image and adopt disordered eating behaviors to accentuate the physical features of their gender identity (e.g., thinness in MtF and muscularity in FtM) and change those pertaining to their natal sex [28, 29].

As to adolescence, the first description of two patients with both ED and GD was published in 2015: a 16-year-old MtF transgender desired to achieve a feminine body and developed a dangerous drive for thinness; conversely, a 13-year-old FtM transgender primarily wanted to arrest breast growth and to increase muscularity [30]. That same year Strandjord described a 16-year-old patient, with natal female sex, who first developed severe AN symptoms (BMI 14.9 kg/m^2) and later disclosed GD (FtM transgender adolescent) [31]. This report was the first to explore the impact—at 19 years of age—of hormone (testosterone cypionate 50 mg/week) and surgical (bilateral mastectomy) treatment. The patient experienced a significant improvement in anxiety and expanded his peer relationships, but 10 months after surgery lost weight (BMI 17.9 kg/m^2) again for restrictive eating and excessive exercise.

19.3 Homosexuality, Bisexuality, Body Image, Eating, and Weight

Four decades ago, from a psychoanalytic point of view, Wilson linked the fear of being fat in males to a female identification and manifest or latent homosexuality [32].

Gay culture emphasizes physical appearance more than lesbian culture. One of the first studies on the influence of sexual orientation on body dissatisfaction in adults found that lesbians and heterosexual women did not differ significantly. On the contrary, gay men reported higher levels of body dissatisfaction than heterosexual men [33].

An old epidemiological research on ED among LGB (lesbian, gay, bisexual) people used the World Health Organization's Composite International Diagnostic Interview and the DSM-IV diagnostic criteria. The ED prevalence was significantly higher among gay and bisexual men compared to heterosexual men. Conversely, there were no differences in ED prevalence between lesbian and bisexual women compared to heterosexual women [34].

Round the turn of the century, other surveys supported the idea that lesbians are not different from heterosexual women in attitudes concerning the appearance, weight, or dieting: homosexual and heterosexual women showed more similarities than differences in eating attitudes and behaviors [35–37]. In particular, a study of a large cohort of adolescents confirmed that gay/bisexual boys were at higher risk of eating disordered behaviors while lesbian/bisexual girls were happier with their bodies than heterosexual girls. However, the same research identified a new group—*mostly heterosexual girls and boys*—at increased risk of ED symptoms [37].

More recently, using pooled data from the 1999 to 2013 Massachusetts Youth Risk Behavior Surveys (N = 26,002) Watson and colleagues found that LGB students reported a higher prevalence of disordered eating behaviors—fasting, purging, assuming diet pills—than heterosexuals [38].

A study mentioned above analyzed data from the American College Health Association's National College Health Assessment II (289,024 students, median age 20 years). Results indicated that cisgender sexual minority young men and women had higher rates of self-reported ED diagnosis and compensatory behaviors (self-induced vomiting, misuse of laxatives, and diet pills) than heterosexual women [23].

Matthews-Ewald et al. used the same data source (2008–2009; N = 110,412) and discovered that dieting to lose weight was more frequent among all sexual minorities (LGB) compared to heterosexual men and women. In particular, gay, unsure, or bisexual men reported higher rates of disordered eating behaviors and ED than heterosexual men [39].

A survey of adolescent males showed that sexual minority males (gay, bisexual) were more likely to be lean-concerned than exclusively heterosexual peers [40].

An American study was recently performed on a representative sample of public high school adolescents [41]. Gay males were more likely to report unhealthy eating and weight control behaviors (fasting, vomiting, taking diet pills, exercising to lose weight) than heterosexual males.

An Italian group studied the influence of gender role orientation (masculinity versus femininity) on eating attitudes in homosexuals, heterosexuals, and transgender. The authors found a positive correlation between femininity and eating problems and a negative correlation between masculinity and eating problems. The authors suggested that these constructs could be more useful than the biological gender to predict possible disordered eating behaviors [42].

Wiseman et al. investigated body image and eating attitudes in a sample of sexual minority men. Results supported the relations assumed in objectification theory among internalization of cultural standards of attractiveness, sexual objectification experiences, body surveillance, body shame, and disordered eating and weight control behaviors [43].

Homosexuality seems to be a risk factor for ED in males also in non-Western countries.

In 2005, Tong et al. described five male ED cases observed in Central China (four with AN and one with BN) [44]. None of these patients reported homosexuality, maybe because it had been decriminalized in China only in 1997 and removed from the official list of mental illnesses some years later. More recently, in 2017, Boon and colleagues studied four males with ED in Singapore. Three of them reported homosexuality [45].

19.4 Some Conclusive Remarks

A 2016 review of the literature indicated that the levels of psychopathology and the rates of psychiatric disorders are higher among transgender persons attending specialized services, at the time of assessment than in cisgender people [46]. A recent case-control study evaluated a sample of Italian GD adolescents with the Body Uneasiness Test [47] (see Chap. 2 of the present volume) and other psychometric instruments. The adolescents with GD reported significantly higher levels of body disparagement and suicidal risk compared to controls [48].

The social costs of gender nonconformities are slowly decreasing, but many LGBT persons still struggle to be accepted by families and social network and to recognize themselves.

A large population-based study found that both health status and care utilization differ between transgender and gender non-conforming (TGNC) adolescents versus cisgender peers. TGNC youth reported significantly poorer physical and mental health but lower rates of health care utilization compared to cisgender individuals [49].

The internalization of social stigma (self-stigma) is a factor that affects self-esteem, mental and physical health, and quality of life. Sometimes multiple stigmas may interact. For example, a survey found that African American sexual minority women reported high rates of obesity and weight-related diseases [50].

Stressful childhood experiences (e.g., sexual, physical, and emotional abuse) are associated with many different psychiatric symptoms, including severe body dissatisfaction and eating disorders. In some studies, LGBT people reported a significantly higher prevalence of such experiences than controls [51].

An Italian study found that, for MtF transgenders, cross-sex hormonal treatment could by itself improve the body uneasiness associated with GD even before genital surgery [52].

Coexisting GD and psychotic symptoms lead to the question of whether the person is experiencing GD or gender delusion, mainly when the feelings of gender incongruence emerged after the psychosis onset. Meijer et al. described four cases (two FtM and two MtF transgender persons, age range 29–57 years) with a schizophrenia-related diagnosis and a coexisting GD [53]. Antipsychotic therapy allowed the stabilization of symptoms. At the same time, gender-affirming interventions were accomplished. The high levels of compliance and satisfaction with the results (minimum follow-up of 3 years) suggest that the presence of mild psychotic symptoms under treatment is not an absolute contraindication to hormone and surgical gender confirmation therapy.

Psychiatric morbidity tends to improve after gender-affirmative treatments, often but not always [46]. Therefore, an expert multi-disciplinary team including mental health professionals should always manage assessment, interventions, and follow-up.

The Endocrine Society guideline, published in November 2017 [54], suggests that most individuals have the mental capacity to give informed consent to these irreversible interventions by age 16 years old, but special attention is required for youths during puberty and older adolescents gender-dysphoric/gender-incongruent. Furthermore, hormone treatment is not recommended before puberty.

As previously mentioned, recent data show that eating pathology risk is increased among sexual minorities, maybe more among MtF transgender and gay individuals. Assessment, treatment, and prevention of eating and weight disorders should include attention to gender identity problems and sexual orientation [55, 56]. There is still a lack of studies in this field and, in particular, the effects of medical and surgical treatments of gender incongruence/dysphoria on eating and weight-related disorders are largely unknown.

References

1. American Psychiatric Association. DSM-II. Diagnostic and statistical manual of mental disorders. 2nd ed. Washington, DC: American Psychiatric Association; 1968.
2. American Psychiatric Association. Diagnostic and statistical manual of mental disorders. DSM III. 3rd ed. Washington, DC: American Psychiatric Association; 1980.
3. American Psychiatric Association. Diagnostic and statistical manual of mental disorders. DSM IIIR. 3rd Revised ed. Washington, DC: American Psychiatric Association; 1987.
4. World Health Organization. The ICD-10 classification of mental and behavioural disorders. Clinical descriptions and diagnostic guidelines. Geneva: World Health Organization; 1992.
5. American Psychiatric Association. Diagnostic and statistical manual of mental disorders, DSM-IV. 4th ed. Washington, DC: American Psychiatric Association; 1994.

6. American Psychiatric Association. Diagnostic and statistical manual of mental disorders, DSM-5. 5th ed. Arlington, VA: American Psychiatric Publishing; 2013.
7. Reed GM, Drescher J, Krueger RB, Atalla E, Cochran SD, First MB, et al. Disorders related to sexuality and gender identity in the ICD-11: revising the ICD-10 classification based on current scientific evidence, best clinical practices, and human rights considerations. World Psychiatry. 2016;15(3):205–21.
8. World Health Organization. Sexual health, human rights and the law. Geneva: World Health Organization; 2015.
9. Janet P. Les obsessions et la psychasthénie (1903). Tome I. Paris: Félix Alcan Éditeur; 1903.
10. Chen M, Fuqua J, Eugster EA. Characteristics of referrals for gender dysphoria over a 13-year period. J Adolesc Health. 2016;58(3):369–71.
11. Fuss J, Auer MK, Briken P. Gender dysphoria in children and adolescents: a review of recent research. Curr Opin Psychiatry. 2015;28(6):430–4.
12. Judge C, O'Donovan C, Callaghan G, Gaoatswe G, O'Shea D. Gender dysphoria—prevalence and co-morbidities in an irish adult population. Front Endocrinol. 2014;5:87.
13. Zucker KJ. Epidemiology of gender dysphoria and transgender identity. Sex Health. 2017;14(5):404–11.
14. Aitken M, Steensma TD, Blanchard R, VanderLaan DP, Wood H, Fuentes A, et al. Evidence for an altered sex ratio in clinic-referred adolescents with gender dysphoria. J Sex Med. 2015;12(3):756–63.
15. Feusner JD, Lidstrom A, Moody TD, Dhejne C, Bookheimer SY, Savic I. Intrinsic network connectivity and own body perception in gender dysphoria. Brain Imaging Behav. 2017;11(4):964–76.
16. Stice E, Ng J, Shaw H. Risk factors and prodromal eating pathology. J Child Psychol Psychiatry. 2010;51(4):518–25.
17. Bandini E, Fisher AD, Castellini G, Lo Sauro C, Lelli L, Meriggiola MC, et al. Gender identity disorder and eating disorders: similarities and differences in terms of body uneasiness. J Sex Med. 2013;10(4):1012–23.
18. van de Grift TC, Cohen-Kettenis PT, Elaut E, De Cuypere G, Richter-Appelt H, Haraldsen IR, et al. A network analysis of body satisfaction of people with gender dysphoria. Body Image. 2016;17:184–90.
19. Beaty L, Trees N, Mehler P. Recurrent persistent hypophosphatemia in a male-to-female transgender patient with anorexia nervosa: case report. Int J Eat Disord. 2017;50(5):606–8.
20. Jones BA, Haycraft E, Murjan S, Arcelus J. Body dissatisfaction and disordered eating in trans people: a systematic review of the literature. Int Rev Psychiatry. 2016;28(1):81–94.
21. Dhejne C, Lichtenstein P, Boman M, Johansson AL, Langstrom N, Landen M. Long-term follow-up of transsexual persons undergoing sex reassignment surgery: cohort study in Sweden. PLoS One. 2011;6(2):e16885.
22. Guss CE, Williams DN, Reisner SL, Austin SB, Katz-Wise SL. Disordered weight management behaviors, nonprescription steroid use, and weight perception in transgender youth. J Adolesc Health. 2017;60(1):17–22.
23. Diemer EW, Grant JD, Munn-Chernoff MA, Patterson DA, Duncan AE. Gender identity, sexual orientation, and eating-related pathology in a national sample of college students. J Adolesc Health. 2015;57(2):144–9.
24. Watson RJ, Veale JF, Saewyc EM. Disordered eating behaviors among transgender youth: probability profiles from risk and protective factors. Int J Eat Disord. 2017;50(5):515–22.
25. Witcomb GL, Bouman WP, Brewin N, Richards C, Fernandez-Aranda F, Arcelus J. Body image dissatisfaction and eating-related psychopathology in trans individuals: a matched control study. Eur Eat Disord Rev. 2015;23(4):287–93.
26. Vocks S, Stahn C, Loenser K, Legenbauer T. Eating and body image disturbances in male-to-female and female-to-male transsexuals. Arch Sex Behav. 2009;38(3):364–77.
27. Jones BA, Haycraft E, Bouman WP, Brewin N, Claes L, Arcelus J. Risk factors for eating disorder psychopathology within the treatment seeking transgender population: the role of cross-sex hormone treatment. Eur Eat Disord Rev. 2018.

28. Algars M, Alanko K, Santtila P, Sandnabba NK. Disordered eating and gender identity disorder: a qualitative study. Eat Disord. 2012;20(4):300–11.
29. Murray SB. Gender identity and eating disorders: the need to delineate novel pathways for eating disorder symptomatology. J Adolesc Health. 2017;60(1):1–2.
30. Couturier J, Pindiprolu B, Findlay S, Johnson N. Anorexia nervosa and gender dysphoria in two adolescents. Int J Eat Disord. 2015;48(1):151–5.
31. Strandjord SE, Ng H, Rome ES. Effects of treating gender dysphoria and anorexia nervosa in a transgender adolescent: lessons learned. Int J Eat Disord. 2015;48(7):942–5.
32. Wilson CP. The fear of being fat and anorexia nervosa. Int J Psychoanal Psychother. 1982;9:233–55.
33. Beren SE, Hayden HA, Wilfley DE, Grilo CM. The influence of sexual orientation on body dissatisfaction in adult men and women. Int J Eat Disord. 1996;20(2):135–41.
34. Feldman MB, Meyer IH. Eating disorders in diverse lesbian, gay, and bisexual populations. Int J Eat Disord. 2007;40(3):218–26.
35. Heffernan K. Eating disorders and weight concern among lesbians. Int J Eat Disord. 1996;19(2):127–38.
36. Moore F, Keel PK. Influence of sexual orientation and age on disordered eating attitudes and behaviors in women. Int J Eat Disord. 2003;34(3):370–4.
37. Austin SB, Ziyadeh N, Kahn JA, Camargo CA Jr, Colditz GA, Field AE. Sexual orientation, weight concerns, and eating-disordered behaviors in adolescent girls and boys. J Am Acad Child Adolesc Psychiatry. 2004;43(9):1115–23.
38. Watson RJ, Adjei J, Saewyc E, Homma Y, Goodenow C. Trends and disparities in disordered eating among heterosexual and sexual minority adolescents. Int J Eat Disord. 2017;50(1): 22–31.
39. Matthews-Ewald MR, Zullig KJ, Ward RM. Sexual orientation and disordered eating behaviors among self-identified male and female college students. Eat Behav. 2014;15(3):441–4.
40. Calzo JP, Masyn KE, Corliss HL, Scherer EA, Field AE, Austin SB. Patterns of body image concerns and disordered weight- and shape-related behaviors in heterosexual and sexual minority adolescent males. Dev Psychol. 2015;51(9):1216–25.
41. Zullig KJ, Matthews-Ewald MR, Valois RF. Relationship between disordered eating and self-identified sexual minority youth in a sample of public high school adolescents. Eat Weight Disord. 2017.
42. Cella S, Iannaccone M, Cotrufo P. Influence of gender role orientation (masculinity versus femininity) on body satisfaction and eating attitudes in homosexuals, heterosexuals and transsexuals. Eat Weight Disord. 2013;18(2):115–24.
43. Wiseman MC, Moradi B. Body image and eating disorder symptoms in sexual minority men: a test and extension of objectification theory. J Counsel Psychol. 2010;57(2):154–66.
44. Tong J, Miao SJ, Wang J, Zhang JJ, Wu HM, Li T, et al. Five cases of male eating disorders in Central China. Int J Eat Disord. 2005;37(1):72–5.
45. Boon E, Zainal KA, Touyz SW. Perceptions of eating disorder diagnoses and body image issues in four male cases in Singapore. J Eat Disord. 2017;5:33.
46. Dhejne C, Van Vlerken R, Heylens G, Arcelus J. Mental health and gender dysphoria: a review of the literature. Int Rev Psychiatry. 2016;28(1):44–57.
47. Cuzzolaro M, Vetrone G, Marano G, Garfinkel PE. The Body Uneasiness Test (BUT): development and validation of a new body image assessment scale. Eat Weight Disord. 2006;11(1):1–13.
48. Fisher AD, Ristori J, Castellini G, Sensi C, Cassioli E, Prunas A, et al. Psychological characteristics of Italian gender dysphoric adolescents: a case-control study. J Endocrinol Invest. 2017;40(9):953–65.
49. Rider GN, McMorris BJ, Gower AL, Coleman E, Eisenberg ME. Health and care utilization of transgender and gender nonconforming youth: a population-based study. Pediatrics. 2018;141(3):e20171683.
50. Matthews AK, Li CC, McConnell E, Aranda F, Smith C. Rates and predictors of obesity among african american sexual minority women. LGBT Health. 2016;3(4):275–82.

51. Schneeberger AR, Dietl MF, Muenzenmaier KH, Huber CG, Lang UE. Stressful childhood experiences and health outcomes in sexual minority populations: a systematic review. Soc Psychiatry Psychiatr Epidemiol. 2014;49(9):1427–45.
52. Fisher AD, Castellini G, Bandini E, Casale H, Fanni E, Benni L, et al. Cross-sex hormonal treatment and body uneasiness in individuals with gender dysphoria. J Sex Med. 2014;11(3):709–19.
53. Meijer JH, Eeckhout GM, van Vlerken RH, de Vries AL. Gender dysphoria and co-existing psychosis: review and four case examples of successful gender affirmative treatment. LGBT Health. 2017;4(2):106–14.
54. Hembree WC, Cohen-Kettenis PT, Gooren L, Hannema SE, Meyer WJ, Murad MH, et al. Endocrine treatment of gender-dysphoric/gender-incongruent persons: an endocrine society* clinical practice guideline. J Clin Endocrinol Metab. 2017;102(11):3869–903.
55. Calzo JP, Blashill AJ, Brown TA, Argenal RL. Eating disorders and disordered weight and shape control behaviors in sexual minority populations. Curr Psychiatry Rep. 2017;19(8):49.
56. Castellini G, Lelli L, Ricca V, Maggi M. Sexuality in eating disorders patients: etiological factors, sexual dysfunction and identity issues. A systematic review. Horm Mol Biol Clin Investig. 2016;25(2):71–90.

20 Sexual Abuse and Body Image in Eating and Weight Disorders

Giovanni Castellini and Valdo Ricca

20.1 Introduction

Sexual abuse defined as unwanted or forced sexual experiences is considered a major public health and medical issue, with community-based samples estimating a lifetime prevalence of 23.3% within men and 37.7% within women in the USA [1] and prevalence increasing up to 43% in sexual minorities [2]. Childhood sexual abuse is defined when the encounter in which touching or penetration of the genitals happened before age 16. Especially when it occurs during adolescence—a crucial period for the development of personality, self-representation, and development of body image—sexual abuse has been associated with several psychopathological conditions, including mood and anxiety disorder [3–5], pathological eating behaviors [6], and body image disturbances [7, 8].

Within the wide range of psychopathological sexual abuse consequences, the onset of pathological eating behaviors has been well demonstrated [9, 10]. It has also been proposed a specific association between eating disorders and sexual abuse, when this occurs during adolescence [10]. As a possible explanation, it has been proposed that pathological eating behaviors come out as primitive and more dysfunctional responses to the tragic event in a period of the life in which brain circuits (i.e., hippocampus and other limbic regions) devoted to the cognitive elaboration of traumatic memories are still immature. In particular, sexual abuse appeared to be clearly associated with onset of bulimic symptoms [11]. Longitudinal studies demonstrated that when the abuse occurs during adolescence, the effect in terms of body image disturbances and pathological eating behaviors are particularly severe [12]. On a different perspective, sexual abuse could also be considered a consequence of the disorder rather than its cause. For example, patients with bulimia nervosa often

G. Castellini · V. Ricca (✉)
Psychiatric Unit, Department of Health Sciences, Florence University School of Medicine, Florence, Italy
e-mail: valdo.ricca@unifi.it

M. Cuzzolaro, S. Fassino (eds.), *Body Image, Eating, and Weight*,
https://doi.org/10.1007/978-3-319-90817-5_20

report impulsivity and the consequent promiscuity in sexual behaviors, which in turn can increase the risk of sexual intercourse [13, 14]. On the other hand, people with anorexia nervosa could be exposed to sexual abuse as a consequence of social withdrawal and relational difficulties, leaving them to the mercy of aggressors [15].

The complex relationship between eating disorders and sexual abuse has been deeply discussed in the last years, in terms of moderators and mediating mechanisms [16]. For example, sexual abuse may act specifically by inducing feelings of poor self-esteem, which could trigger self-starvation, as a reflection of the individual's effort at regaining control on her life [17]. Alternatively, sexual victimization may lead a woman to feel revulsion about her body in a way that may manifest with concerns about body weight, shape, and size. Dissociation defined as "a disruption in the usually integrated functions of consciousness, memory, identity, and perception of the environment" has also been proposed as a psychopathological dimension that can underlie both sexual dysfunction and pathological eating behaviors in victims of sexual assaults [18, 19]. Dissociation plays an important role in binge eating severity for subjects with bulimic symptoms [20], and it is partially involved in the most well-documented theories about binge eating: the "mood modulation" theory [20] and the "escape" theory [21].

Within the all putative mechanism that can mediate the relationship between adverse sexual experiences and development of pathological eating behaviors, this chapter will focus on the role of body image disturbance, which has been reported as a common outcome of sexual abuse, and a core feature of eating disorders. Body image distortion is a core symptom of eating disorders (EDs) [22], and it is defined as "a disturbance in the way in which one's body weight or shape is experienced, undue influence of body weight or shape on self-evaluation, or denial of the seriousness of current low body weight" [23]. Body image disturbance is a key psychological dimensions in persons with eating disorders who typically overvalue their body shape and weight, and mostly define themselves in terms of their shape and weight and their ability to control them. A huge literature support the idea that most of the pathological features of these disorders could be secondary epiphenomena to this more profound pathological core, i.e., an overestimation of the importance of bodily appearance instead of other aspects of existence and personal identity. Indeed, body image disturbance plays a significant role in the persistence of the disorders [24, 25]. Furthermore, shape and weight concerns have been associated with different responses to psychological treatment in several reports [24, 26].

20.2 The Impact of Sexual Abuse on Body Image

Among victims of sexual abuse, the relationship with one's own body may be particularly affected, and the adverse sexual experiences have a long-lasting effect on body image and identity, as well as with self-regulation mechanisms [16]. The traumatic event of sexual abuse during adolescence interferes with the dynamic process of body image development. Each event in this process incorporates into perception of one's own appearance feelings about the body's new information.

As this new information are processed, body image changes. The changes induced by a sexual traumatic experience include body image distortion, sense of shame or guilt associated to the sexual arousal, or avoidance of one's own body image. The impact of sexual abuse can reach an intensity able to challenge the hormonal balance and induce an early menarche [27]. Premature pubertal changes might in turn determine an earlier exposure to negative feelings related to the normal development of adipose tissue and body fat, such as peers commenting about changes in body size and shape.

The impact of sexual abuse on body image should be considered in the light of the a multidimensional pattern, which includes cognitive and affective components (concerns and feelings about the body), perception (estimation of own body size), and behaviors related to the own body perception. Recent observations stressed the greater influence of emotional and somatic factors than the purely perceptual aspect of body size estimation [28–30]. The occurring of sexual abuse during adolescence certainly challenges the process of integration of body image into one's sense of self, a central task of the teenage years. Therefore, sexual violence often disrupts the integrated view of one's own body with consequent hate toward the abused body parts and body mutilation. Furthermore, patients with eating disorders with a history of abuse frequently reported a sense of extraneousness from one's own body and from emotions which can reach the intensity of dissociative experiences. Depersonalization experiences are based on a sense of feeling disconnected from one's body, watching oneself as an observer, or feeling like one's body is unusually large or small. Indeed, some self-harm behaviors such as cutting and burning can be considered as a way to regain control on a compromised interoceptive awareness [31]. In general, dissociation is particularly common in individuals exposed to a traumatic event, with approximately 30% of women with a history of CSA reporting severe daily dissociative symptoms [32]. Individuals who experienced sexual abuse often report experiencing their first dissociative symptoms during or immediately after the abuse, and these symptoms tend to persist in their daily life and throughout adulthood [33].

20.3 Body Image Disturbance as a Mediator of the Sexual Abuse Effects in the Development of Eating Disorder Psychopathology

Several researches focused on the role of body image distortion and body dissatisfaction as potential mediators of the relationship between sexual assault and later development of eating disorder psychopathology [31]. In general, women with history of sexual abuse reported a severe body uneasiness after the traumatic event [34]. In a community sample of women, Preti et al. [15] found that body image dissatisfaction represented a mediator for the effect of sexual abuse intervening during childhood and the degree of distorted eating attitudes and pathological eating behaviors in adulthood. Authors concluded that a possible mechanism leading to psychopathology could be based on the revulsion about the body in ways that may intermix with concerns about body shape, size, and weight [31]. Furthermore, it is possible that the sense of guilt and shame following the abuse was connected with such a revulsion against one's own body; accordingly, body dissatisfaction might be the cause of self-harm behaviors frequently reported among eating disorders patients. As a demonstration to this hypothesis, patients with eating disorders reporting a history of sexual abuse, and they were found to be more likely to engage in auto-mutilation and self-harm more frequently than other patients [35].

The profound uneasiness toward one's own body can be directed toward the whole body representation and dramatically lead to pathological eating behaviors which in many cases are not adequately challenged from the available psychological interventions for eating disorders [7]. The sense of disgust consequent to the abusive experience may deeply affect the cognitive schema of the victim body. In this perspective, dietary restriction represents an attempt to manage discomfort with the body and toward sexuality. It has also suggested that altering the sexual attractive part of the body would make the appearance of the victim less prone to the sexual advances of others [36].

The subjective feeling of loss-of-control following binge eating behaviors has been reported to be particularly severe in victim of sexual abuse [37]. The following attempts to regain control through purging, exercise, or stringent dietary restriction might represent a way to recover a sense of sameness over one's own body. With this regard, several authors focused their researches on the complex phenomenology of sexual abuse, including dissociation, body image distortion, and emotion dysregulation. Authors have explored the processes that to maintain binge eating as being linked to concepts of self-awareness [38]. In survivors of sexual abuse, specific areas of the body (e.g., pubic region and inner thighs) are associated with trauma and linked to highly aversive emotions. Sexual experience, or sensations elicited from this area may act as a trigger for traumatic memories. According to the escape from awareness theory [21], negative feelings associated to traumatic experiences may induce the motivation to escape, which occurs by the patient narrowing his or her awareness from abstract levels (self-evaluation) to the level of the physical surroundings or stimulus (i.e., food, cut, self-harm) [39, 40]. In this context, binge eating results from the temporary loss of inhibition and could be associated with a dissociative experience that "protect" the person from the awareness of traumatic memories.

In this perspective, dissociation represents a defense mechanism to negative affect rising from a body uneasiness or bodily feelings that are experienced as an insult to the self-identity. In particular, it is possible that women with body sensation related to abusive experiences need to "escape" from the awareness of self-evaluation. This may be triggered by sexual experience or confrontation with the thin ideal that makes them feel inadequate, and dissociation may serve as a psychological defense against intolerable emotional states. Finally, the dissociative experience leads to sexual dysfunction and eventually distress, particularly impairing sexual arousal. Laboratory data on cortisol response to sexual stimuli seem to confirm that this process is regulated by affective processes independently from consciousness [41–43].

20.4 Sexual Dysfunction in Patients with Eating Disorders Reporting Sexual Abuse: The Role of Body Image Disturbance

Patients with eating disorder often report sexual dysfunctions including low sexual desire, vaginism, arousal, and orgasm disorders [7, 44, 45]. Sexual functioning in patients with eating disorders has been associated with concerns about body image (e.g., dissatisfaction with body parts, concerns with body size or weight, discomfort with one's body in front of a partner, or others). In general, women who felt more negatively about their bodies reported less sexual desire and arousal, and appeared to be less engaged in sexual activity, as compared with women who had a more positive perception of their bodies [46, 47].

Body image disturbance following a sexual offense has been considered a psychological dimensions underlying both pathological eating behaviors and sexual dysfunction. It is well known that sexual abuse has a significant and lasting effect on a range of different psychological dimensions that can interfere with sexual functioning, including emotional regulation, self-representation of one's body image [42]. Sexual victimization induces feelings of poor self-esteem, which could trigger self-starvation, as a reflection of the individual's effort at regaining control on her life [17], and may lead a woman to feel revulsion about her body in a way that may manifest with concerns about body weight, shape, and size. Also dissociation has been considered a psychological consequence of sexual abuse that can connect trauma, emotion dysregulation, body image disturbance, and sexual dysfunction. Indeed, a disconnection between body and mind might account for individual's subjective experience of sexual arousal inhibition in sexually abused subjects [48]. Sexual abuse survivors experiencing sexual difficulties may have learned to automatically pair sexual stimuli with fear (implicit sexual memories). This condition has been specifically postulated in patients with eating disorders [43].

In a recent study, Castellini et al. [7] demonstrated that patients with eating disorders reporting a history of childhood sexual abuse did not show any significant improvement after cognitive behavioral therapy regarding body shape concerns and sexual functioning. The results of this study showed that among patients with eating disorders, those with a history of sexual abuse represent a subpopulation of persons with a profound uneasiness toward body perception, as well as sexual problems that are not efficaciously challenged during standard psychological interventions. According to other studies, when a clinician meets a person with this traumatic experience in his/her life, he should consider the possibility that these patients would not follow the expected course or improvement. The clinical implication is to specifically target the comorbidities of childhood sexual abuse before useful treatment of an eating disorder can begin. Moreover, it is reasonable to hypothesize that effective treatments specifically targeted on body image perception and cognitive/emotional consequences of sexual abuse would improve sexual activity in this subgroup of patients with eating disorders.

References

1. Chiu GR, Lutfey KE, Litman HJ, Link CL, Hall SA, McKinlay JB. Prevalence and overlap of childhood and adult physical, sexual, and emotional abuse: a descriptive analysis of results from the Boston Area Community Health (BACH) survey. Violence Vict. 2013;28(3):381–402.
2. Rothman EF, Exner D, Baughman AL. The prevalence of sexual assault against people who identify as gay, lesbian, or bisexual in the United States: a systematic review. Trauma Violence Abuse. 2011;12(2):55–66.
3. Maniglio R. The impact of child sexual abuse on health: a systematic review of reviews. Clin Psychol Rev. 2009;29:647–57.
4. Chen LP, Murad MH, Paras ML, Colbenson KM, Sattler AL, Goranson EN, Elamin MB, Seime RJ, Shinozaki G, Prokop LJ, Zirakzadeh A. Sexual abuse and lifetime diagnosis of psychiatric disorders: systematic review and meta-analysis. Mayo Clin Proc. 2010;85:618–29.
5. Carr CP, Martins CM, Stingel AM, Lemgruber VB, Juruena MF. The role of early life stress in adult psychiatric disorders: a systematic review according to childhood trauma subtypes. J Nerv Ment Dis. 2013;201:1007–20.
6. Faravelli C, Giugni A, Salvatori S, Ricca V. Psychopathology after rape. Am J Psychiatry. 2004;161(8):1483–5.
7. Castellini G, Lo Sauro C, Lelli L, Godini L, Vignozzi L, Rellini AH, Faravelli C, Maggi M, Ricca V. Childhood sexual abuse moderates the relationship between sexual functioning and eating disorder psychopathology in anorexia nervosa and bulimia nervosa: a 1-year follow-up study. J Sex Med. 2013;10(9):2190–200.
8. Dyer A, Borgmann E, Kleindienst N, Feldmann RE Jr, Vocks S, Bohus M. Body image in patients with posttraumatic stress disorder after childhood sexual abuse and co-occurring eating disorder. Psychopathology. 2013;46(3):186–91.
9. Thompson KM, Wonderlich SA. Child sexual abuse and eating disorders. In: Thompson KM, editor. Handbook of eating disorders and obesity. Hoboken, NJ: Wiley; 2004. p. 679–94.
10. Johnson JG, Cohen P, Kasen S, Brook JS. Childhood adversities associated with risk for eating disorders or weight problems during adolescence or early adulthood. Am J Psychiatry. 2002;159:394–400.
11. Jacobi C, Hayward C, de Zwaan M, Kraemer HC, Agras WS. Coming to terms with risk factors for eating disorders: application of risk terminology and suggestions for a general taxonomy. Psychol Bull. 2004;130:19–65.
12. Sanci L, Coffey C, Olsson C, Reid S, Carlin JB, Patton G. Childhood sexual abuse and eating disorders in females: findings from the Victorian Adolescent Health Cohort Study. Arch Pediatr Adolesc Med. 2008;162:261–7.
13. Dansky BS, Brewerton TD, Kilpatrick DG, O'Neil PM. The National Women's Study: relationship of victimization and posttraumatic stress disorder to bulimia nervosa. Int J Eat Disord. 1997;21:213–28.
14. Favaro A, Dalle Grave R, Santonastaso P. Impact of a history of physical and sexual abuse in eating disordered and asymptomatic subjects. Acta Psychiatr Scand. 1998;97:358–63.
15. Preti A, Incani E, Camboni MV, Petretto DR, Masala C. Sexual abuse and eating disorder symptoms: the mediator role of bodily dissatisfaction. Compr Psychiatry. 2006;47(6):475–81.
16. Castellini G, Maggi M, Ricca V. Childhood sexual abuse and psychopathology. In: Corona G, Jannini E, Maggi M, editors. Emotional, physical and sexual abuse: impact in children and social minorities. New York: Springer; 2014.
17. Smolak L, Murnen SK. A meta-analytic examination of the relationship between child sexual abuse and eating disorders. Int J Eat Disord. 2002;31:136–150 599.
18. Bird ER, Seehuus M, Clifton J, Rellini AH. Dissociation during sex and sexual arousal in women with and without a history of childhood sexual abuse. Arch Sex Behav. 2014;43(5):953–64.
19. Vanderlinden J, Van Dyck R, Vandereycken W, Vertommen H. Dissociation and traumatic experiences in the general population of the Netherlands. Hosp Community Psychiatry. 1993;44:786–8.

20. McManus F, Waller G. A functional analysis of binge-eating. Clin Psychol Rev. 1995;15:845–63.
21. Heatherton TF, Baumeister RF. Binge eating as escape from selfawareness. Psychol Bull. 1991;110:86–108.
22. Fairburn CG, Harrison PJ. Eating disorders. Lancet. 2003;361(9355):407–16.
23. American Psychiatric Association. Diagnostic and statistical manual for mental disorders. 5th ed. Washington, DC: American Psychiatric Press; 2003.
24. Ricca V, Castellini G, Lo Sauro C, et al. Cognitive-behavioral therapy for threshold and subthreshold anorexia nervosa: a three-year follow-up study. Psychother Psychosom. 2010;79:238–48.
25. Bardone-Cone AM, Harney MB, Maldonado CR, et al. Defining recovery from an eating disorder: conceptualization, validation, and examination of psychosocial functioning and psychiatric comorbidity. Behav Res Ther. 2010;48:194–202.
26. Castellini G, Lo Sauro C, Mannucci E, et al. Diagnostic crossover and outcome predictors in eating disorders according to DSM-IV and DSM-V proposed criteria: a 6-year follow-up study. Psychosom Med. 2011;73:270–9.
27. Chen FR, Rothman EF, Jaffee SR. Early puberty, friendship group characteristics, and dating abuse in US girls. Pediatrics. 2017;8:e20162847.
28. Castellini G, Stanghellini G, Godini L, Lucchese M, Trisolini F, Ricca V. Abnormal bodily experiences mediate the relationship between impulsivity and binge eating in overweight subjects seeking bariatric surgery. Psychother Psychosom. 2015;84(2):124–6.
29. Stanghellini G, Trisolini F, Castellini G, Ambrosini A, Faravelli C, Ricca V. Is feeling extraneous from one's own body a core vulnerability feature in eating disorders? Psychopathology. 2015;48(1):18–24.
30. Stanghellini G, Castellini G, Brogna P, Faravelli C, Ricca V. Identity and eating disorders (IDEA): a questionnaire evaluating identity and embodiment in eating disorder patients. Psychopathology. 2012;45(3):147–58.
31. Preti A, Incani E, Camboni MV, Petretto DR, Masala C, Lockwood R, Lawson R, Waller G. Compulsive features in the eating disorders: a role for trauma? J Nerv Ment Dis. 2004;192:247–9.
32. Van der Kolk BA. The neurobiology of childhood trauma and abuse. Child Adolesc Psychiatr Clin North Am. 2003;12:293–317.
33. Boysan M, Goldsmith RE, Cavuş H, Kayri M, Keskin S. Relations among anxiety, depression, and dissociative symptoms: the influence of abuse subtype. J Trauma Dissociation. 2009;10:83–101.
34. Kearney-Cooke A, Ackard DM. The effects of sexual abuse on body image, self-image, and sexual activity of women. J Gend Specif Med. 2000;3:54–60.
35. Favaro A, Tenconi E, Santonastaso P. The interaction between perinatal factors and childhood abuse in the risk of developing anorexia nervosa. Psychol Med. 2010;40:657–65.
36. Falloon P, Ackard DM. Sexual abuse and body image. In: Cash TF, Pruzinsky T, editors. Body image. Oxford: Guilford Press; 2002. p. 117–8.
37. Reto CS, Dalenberg CJ, Coe MT. Dissociation and physical abuse as predictors of bulimic symptomatology and impulse dysregulation. Eat Disord. 1993;1:226–39.
38. Vanderlinden J, Van Dyck R, Vandereycken W, Vertommen H. Dissociative experiences and trauma in eating disorders. Int J Eat Disord. 1993;13:187–93.
39. Higgins ET. Self-discrepancy: a theory relating self to affect. Psychol Rev. 1987;94:319–40.
40. Vallacher RR, Wegner DM. A theory of action identification. Hillsdale, NJ: Erlbaum; 1985.
41. Castellini G, Lo Sauro C, Ricca V, Rellini AH. Body esteem as a common factor of tendency toward binge eating and sexual dissatisfaction among women: the role of dissociation and stress response during sex. J Sex Med. 2017;14(8):1036–45.
42. Rellini AH, Hamilton LD, Delville Y, Meston CM. The cortisol response during physiological sexual arousal in adult women with a history of childhood sexual abuse. J Trauma Stress. 2009;22(6):557–65.
43. Castellini G, Lelli L, Lo Sauro C, Vignozzi L, Maggi M, Faravelli C, Ricca V. Childhood abuse, sexual function and cortisol levels in eating disorders. Psychother Psychosom. 2012;81(6):380–2.

44. Pinheiro AP, Raney TJ, Thornton LM, Fichter MM, Berrettini WH, Goldman D, et al. Sexual functioning in women with eating disorders. Int J Eat Dis. 2010;43:123–9.
45. Castellini G, Lelli L, Ricca V, Maggi M. Sexuality in eating disorders patients: etiological factors, sexual dysfunction and identity issues. A systematic review. Horm Mol Biol Clin Investig. 2016;25(2):71–90.
46. Reissing ED, Laliberté M, Davis J. Young women's sexual adjustment: the role of sexual self-schema, sexual self-efficacy, sexual aversion and body attitudes. Can J Hum Sex. 2005;14:77–85.
47. La Rocque CI, Cioe J. An evaluation of the relationship between body image and sexual avoidance. J Sex Res 2010;47: 1–12.
48. Chivers M, Seto M, Lalumiere M, Laan E, Grimbos T. Agreement of genital and subjective measures of sexual arousal: preliminary results of a meta-analysis. Paper presented at the annual meeting of the International Academy of Sex Research, Ottawa, Canada, 2005.

Psychoanalysis and Treatment of Body Image Disturbances in Eating and Weight Disorders

21

Secondo Fassino and Federico Amianto

21.1 Introduction: The Body from Phenomenology to the Neurobiology of Intersubjectivity

The lived body (*Leib*, according to Husserl's terminology [1]), compared to the physical body (*Körper* [1]), is at the center of the concepts of self-consciousness and intersubjectivity [2]. Self-conscience does not only consist in knowing an external object, but in getting back it in its own experience. The impression that the body receives from contact with the world produces the feeling of its presence in the world ("*ipseity*") and without this perception no self is possible. Intersubjectivity is based on the direct perception of the emotional nature of others, and the perceptual bond with each other is realized through identification with the body of the other. So intersubjectivity is the intercorporeality, by which we recognize the other as similar to what we are [3].

The model of embodied simulation (ES) [4] is the result of evidences about mirror neurons and constitutes one of the most significant aspects of intersubjectivity understood as "intercorporeality," decisive in recent studies on the factors of change in psychotherapy [5].

The concept of ES is part of the interactionist theory and of the intersubjectivity's theory [6] (importance of social relations) about the significance [7]. The body is the major source of significance since it not only constitutes the experiential aspects of interpersonal relationships but also their linguistic representations.

Reconceptualization of intersubjectivity, as well as resulting from the convergence of recent psychoanalytic developments [8, 9], is also, above all, the result of recent neurobiological acquisitions.

S. Fassino (✉) · F. Amianto
Eating Disorders Center for Treatment and Research, Department of Neuroscience, University of Turin, Turin, Italy
e-mail: secondo.fassino@unito.it; federico.amianto@unito.it

M. Cuzzolaro, S. Fassino (eds.), *Body Image, Eating, and Weight*,
https://doi.org/10.1007/978-3-319-90817-5_21

Brain imaging studies confirm neurodynamics as a basis for psychodynamics [10], useful to redefine the self not just as self-consciousness, but rather as a result of the relationship with the environment and hence with the other.

The intersubjective approach moves psychoanalysis from a mono-personal psychology to a bi-personal psychology, based on the recognition that the most important and efficient aspect of clinical work is the exchange of two subjectivity from which arises "*an unpredictable material co-created*" [10].

The study of the neural bases of our ability to be connected to others' interpersonal relationships gives further empirical value to the model of intersubjectivity. Through the intentional attunement, "*the other*" is much more than a different representation system: it becomes a bodily-self like us. The results of neurobiological research on mirror neurons suggest that "*when we look at the emotion and feelings of others, an important aspect of intersubjectivity is the re-use of the same neural circuits on which our emotional and sensory experiences are based*" [6].

The theoretical assumptions of this development are undoubtedly recognized in Sullivan's interpersonal approach, but even more evident in Adler's Individual Psychology (IP) [11, 12]. In addition to the claim of self-affirmation, the other fundamental element of psychic life, according to the Individual Psychology, is the social sentiment/social interest: the primary affective-social bond that determines a "*necessity*" of cooperation and emotional sharing with peers.

21.2 Disturbance of Body Image in Eating Disorders

21.2.1 Body Dissatisfaction and EDs

Defining Eating Disorders (ED) on purely behavioral issues can not only be reductive, but even misleading as far as therapeutic interventions are concerned. It appears more clinically useful to focus the disturbance on the body image, since patients present a hyper-identification with their own *lived body*.

At the basis of ED symptoms there is a deep distortion of the perception of the size of the own body, which is mistakenly evaluated as too heavy and perceived as uncomfortable [13]. Subjects feel fat in relation to their whole body, even though in many cases a part of the body is perceived in a particularly distorted way: usually the abdomen, the buttocks, the thighs.

Body dissatisfaction (BD) is an important risk and perpetuating factor [14–16] in EDs and is related to the core psychopathological element represented by an overvaluation of body and shape concerns [17]. In the adolescent population, the rate of BD predicts the development of EDs [18]. Heightened BD has also been correlated with an earlier onset in anorexia nervosa (AN) [19]. It also predicts relapse after discharge in AN [20] and can persist altered in recovered anorexic women [21]. Indeed, depressive symptomatology [22] and low self-esteem [23] play an important role in increasing BD, both in EDs [24] and in the healthy population [18].

21.2.2 Body Dissatisfaction in Relationship with ED Symptoms

The tendency to negate the disease complicates the perception of body and of the body image. Subjects with EDs at the initial stages of their disorders often deny the disease and claim to be well in spite of the state of starvation, to the point of not being aware of thinness, hunger, and fatigue. Sometimes the severity and persistence of perceptual distortion can constitute a disorder of body dysmorphism and may take on the features of somatic delirium, requiring targeted treatments.

The fear of gaining weight in subjects with this disorder puts a powerful correlation with internalized body image and dissatisfaction of the own body. Many patients decide to lose weight following comments from friends or schoolmates or as a result of emotional disappointments (life events) or during periods of life where responsibilities increase (fear of maturity). Nevertheless, this is a pathological fear, not justified by the effective weight or attenuated by a weight loss. The rigid diet then becomes a self-maintained behavior and becomes a constant psychophysical commitment throughout the day. At a rational level, there is the conviction of achieving serenity by losing a certain percentage of their weight, but losing weight accentuates the desire for thinness and ascetic non-finalistic tendencies, so the goal is constantly and consistently retrograde downwards as it approaches [25].

The alteration of body image is therefore cognitive-affective and often requires targeted interventions (e.g., mirror exposure therapy). It may also be maintained by both trait alterations (endofenotypic) and state alterations (linked to malnutrition) in neuropsychological functioning (cognitive rigidity, thinking polarization, loss of abstraction, and problem-solving skills) [26].

21.3 Body Dissatisfaction and Its Correlation with the Internal World and the Meanings of Anorexia Nervosa

The disturbance of the body image is accompanied by an altered interoceptive awareness (IA) which represents a deep confusion in discriminating body sensations, feelings, and emotions. It is strictly related to personality immaturity, depressive feelings, and perfectionism [27, 28] and leads to great difficulties in discriminating hunger and satiety.

Eating symptomatology has a sort of adaptive function for those who suffer from AN. The alteration of body perception and consequent eating symptoms represent the attempt of subjects with AN of managing with a deep anguish and struggling emotions that they are not able to copy with, and thus they "move" on eating psychopathology. Few studies to date investigated the relationship between the reported meanings of AN and patients' clinical characteristics [29].

Marzola and coworkers [29] showed that AN may have three main deep meanings. The first is an intrapsychic meaning, intended as a search for a new identity, self-control, and expression of control/power; it appears to be associated with a strong drive for thinness and a personality characterized by a low self-directedness, suggestive of a fragile identity. The second is a relational factor, namely the illness becomes a way to be recognized by others, it is associated with impulse regulation and low self-directedness. The third meaning of AN appears to be the avoidance of negative feelings, emotions, and experiences; it is associated with a higher number of hospitalizations and with an elevated harm avoidance. Given the ego-syntonic nature of AN and the adaptive function of this disorder, the understanding of different perspectives that therapists could refer to, and patients could identify with during the therapeutic process is an indispensable part of treatment to discover the individual meanings of the disorder [30].

Finally, a psychopathologic element that plays a central role in AN is anger. Anger is a powerful emotion that subjects with ED often are not prepared to manage. It represents the reaction to both the sense of confusion, inadequacy and impotence they perceive in their inner world, and the sense of constriction, disengagement, neglect they perceive in the relationships with significant others. Anger is better managed by individuals with greater character strength which is related to better integration of the self [31]. In the treatment of patients with bulimic symptoms, binge-eating is related with Trait Reactive Anger and Anger Expression which are fully mediated by Cooperativeness. Thus relational dynamics and temperament are particularly central in the expression of BN core eating symptoms [32, 33].

21.4 Body Dissatisfaction and Distorted Development of the Self

The relationship between body image disturbance and eating habits is obvious, but more complex than it seems. The eating habit fills the lifestyle, becomes the self, the whole personality of the subject [34]: food and fasting are not just techniques for modifying the own bodily-self, but also ways to change the own state of consciousness, to "feel something," to gain the own perception of self [35].

Recent studies [36] confirm that dysfunctional aspects of the self (Winnicott's "false-self") [37] cause resistance to treatment in patients with EDs [36]. Patients with ED have a particular inner ambivalence towards the illness: eating behaviors produce psychological discomfort but, on the other hand, they dangerously mask the inner conflicts that typically occur during the illness.

It is for this reason that these patients exhibit marked aspects of egosyntonia together with poor awareness of the disease, further contributing to the occurrence of resistance to treatment. Thus, a vicious cycle of resistance to treatment is thus formed and it is reinforced by "contaminant emotions" [38]: conscious and unconscious meanings of body image disturbance, family dynamics, countertransference and therapist's reactions, anger and aggressiveness of the patients and in his/her environment [36, 39].

This vicious circle should be considered when choosing the therapy in patients with EDs. In particular, psychodynamic psychotherapy is not only focused on the symptoms of the disease, but, through the embodied simulation, the intentional attunement, and the central role of the therapist, is centered on the creation of a solid therapeutic relationship, through which a new and mature identity can be acquired, gradually replacing the false-self of the subjects affected with AN. Since resistance can also be considered as a regulator of the therapeutic relationship, therapists should address this issue being aware of transference and countertransference, meanings of symptoms, patients' narcissistic vulnerability, interpersonal dynamics, and resistance to treatments, and carefully managing their own emotions in addition to patients' ones [39, 40].

21.5 Body Dissatisfaction and Attachment Insecurity

A growing body of evidence supports the observation that an insecure attachment plays a central role in the development of mental disorders and that a treatment aimed on enhancing attachment security may improve symptoms and psychopathology [41]. Strong literature data show that an insecure attachment style [15, 42–45] and also affective temperaments [33] are implicated in the pathogenesis of Body Dissatisfaction (BD) in general and in EDs in particular. Although it has been proffered the hypothesis that a constellation of personality traits may explain both attachment insecurity and BD in EDs, it has been shown that attachment insecurity, need for approval in particular, are related to BD in EDs, independent of the patient's personality [46, 47].

Clinicians should focus on attachment concerns in any type of ED presentation because of the primary role played by attachment and need for approval in the therapist–patient relationship [48]. It is crucial to consider the important effects of attachment insecurity on psychotherapy prognosis [49] since it can reduce the ability to form and maintain a trusting relationship with a psychotherapist [50], and this issue may be especially important in the patients with EDs.

Attachment insecurity represents the common root between body image development and the development of the self. The experience of maternal love during childhood is a neurotrophic factor on the GM volume of many brain areas involved both in attachment and in the construction of the self. Non-secure attachment is a core feature of anorexia nervosa both at psychopathological and neurobiological levels while the feeling of anger towards the caregivers has opposite effects on brain areas [51].

21.6 The Self and Anorexia Nervosa

Patients with AN often experience problems of alexithymia, that is difficulties in recognizing and manifesting their inner experiences [52–54] and consequently building and creating a personal narrative [55–57]. This problem can be attributed to a deficit of the self, as Hilde Bruch argues [58]. The self has multiple roles since it coordinates various functions on the affective, cognitive, social, and sensomotor levels in dialectics between the inner and outer world [59]. There are many overlapping areas between self and personality [60], including the identification of predictive factors and responses to treatment [61]. Adler's thought anticipated this observation: in Individual Psychology the Self and Personality are coincident [11, 12].

The self is the connection between intrapsychic and interpersonal activity. It is the foundation of human motivation, knowledge and individual relational ability. This can be defined as " the integrative function of the self," and it seems to be compromised in subjects with a diagnosis of anorexia nervosa.

The self also involves a temporal concept, which goes beyond the synchronic dimension of identity: in fact it describes the ongoing experience of self in the world in relation to the others as it evolves lifelong in each set point of the life cycle (diachronic dimension of self) [62]. It plays a key role in maintaining anorexia nervosa, starting from the troubling experience in adolescence and lasting beyond the food pathology's resolution [63].

Along with Winnicot's conceptualization of the "false-self," Hilde Bruch [58] argues that it is the basis for the difficulty occurring in subjects with AN in discriminating between their own and their caregivers' expectations and needs. This confusion involves body sensations (e.g., hunger) leading to serious difficulties for these subjects to discriminate between physical sensations and emotions (interoceptive awareness) [52].

Also the subjective experience of one's body seems to be not integrated in ED subjects. Their body is often perceived as stranger because it does not refer to their sense of self: it becomes an objectified self-representation ("objectification" of the body) [64–66]. The body assumes the function of a symbolic screen on which subjects with AN display their own suffering as a "concretized metaphor" [52]. At the same time, the perceived body-image represents the only way in which AN subjects perceive their sense of confusion and helplessness denied by the omnipotence of a life without need of food.

Alfred Adler conceives [11] the self as the "lifestyle" expressed by personality traits of the individual. These are the stylistic instruments the individual adopts to reach his/her inner goals. In this sense, the extreme personality traits which are particularly frequent in subjects with AN (high harm avoidance and perfectionism [67, 68]) suggest the construction of rigid frameworks overcompensating the pervasive weakness of the integrative functions of the self (low self-directedness [69]).

21.7 Eating Disorders Treatment: The Self and Psychotherapy

Eating disorders are not just a constellation of eating symptoms, but are underwhelmed by deeper and rooted disorders of the self or the personality. As indicated by a growing number of literature data, psychotherapy, and in particular psychodynamically oriented one, appears to be particularly addressed to the psychopathological core of the disorder [70]. Psychodynamic models consider symptoms on the one hand as an expression of suffering (primary advantage), and on the other hand as an attempt to mitigate their pain (secondary advantage). Therefore, the treatment should not be focused on symptoms, but have to be based on a solid and active therapeutic relationship. Psychodynamic treatment should be directed towards patient's deficits in the formation of the self, including patient's difficulties in understanding and integrating internal states and emotions [40].

21.7.1 The Common Roots of Psychotherapeutic Processes

The understanding of the adaptive value of eating symptomatology to a pervasive anguish due to the deficit in the structure of the self is crucial to help clinicians considering those needs and conflicts underlying the disorder and to plan treatment interventions and goals shared with the patients [39, 40, 71].

To make their self to emerge, patients need to be encouraged and supported to use their own resources to change through psychotherapy. The ability of understanding themselves and a new feeling of self-worthiness felt approaching the progressive construction of the self provides alternative motivations and strategies to give up the disorder [72].

The solid therapeutic relationship based on a specific therapist's awareness of the dynamics related to embodied simulation and intentional attunement is the necessary reparative environment favoring the maturation of a new identity replacing the "ED identity" of the patients [45, 73]. This is in accordance with the early intuition of Alfred Adler:

> *"The treatment involves and transforms both the therapist and the patient"... "the attitude (of the therapist) is essentially empathic, and represented by the late assumption of the maternal function by the therapist...to see with his eyes, hear with his ears... feeling with his hearth..."* [11, 12].

21.7.2 The Role of the Therapist in Dynamic Psychotherapy of AN

As a consequence of their frail self, the patients affected with AN suffer from an overwhelming, globally pervasive sense of inadequacy. Only by becoming partakers of treatment they can achieve differentiation of their self from others, recognize their bodily sensations and emotional states, and go beyond the helpless passivity, submission, and hateful of indiscriminate negativism.

The traditional psychoanalytic setting may represent a despairing re-experience of inadequacy. They can experience that *"someone else knew what they were trying but they themselves do not know it or do not feel (...). Insight for them was just another "thing" had passively accepted by their therapist but then depreciating it as if it meant nothing"* [58].

Approaching to AN patients then, the task of the therapist is not so much interpret the symbolic meaning of symptoms, as to help and encourage the patient to face his/her life, past and present. *"The problem now is to find out their genuine self—what is the truth in them, from a careful consideration of the 'false self'"* [58]. According to the need of an active involvement of the patient, at the beginning of the treatment it is useful a brief explanation on the sense, at the time as the most general meaning of the disease. In order not to further undermine their self-esteem therapist can only hint at the "reparative" function that symptoms of malnutrition exert, and how it interferes with their psychological processes. Being tuned to the more subtle distortion of their sense of reality, the therapist may encourage, without being judgmental, the necessary revaluations. For many patients, the therapy is the first experience to be listened as worthy of attention, instead of receiving an interpretation of their feelings and of the meaning of their communications.

The main therapeutic focus must then move from the content and/or interpretation of deficits and deep conflicts to an emphasis on the relational interaction "here and now" to contain immediately the patients' deep discouragement, even if hidden. The base deficit of the anorexia nervosa, resulting in the deficit of self-concept, is recognized in the lack of encouraging responses to implicit and explicit requests originated from those "good girls" [58]. This formulation promotes a new process of care with an emphasis on encouraging autonomy and initiative in the patient. It is therefore essential to redefine the role of the therapist. The therapist needs to tune to the failure of their intra-psychic experiences, their dysfunctional ways of expressing organize and define their needs, and their emotional confusion in relating to others [47]. The therapeutic relationship is an attempt to correct the defects and cognitive distortions, as well as the sense of dissatisfaction and inadequacy that these patients perceive from their self which is empty and unfinished, and then forced into a general sense of powerlessness, corrected by a grandiose "live without eating or rather die!" [9].

21.7.3 The Process of Encouragement Is the Heart of the Change in Psychodynamic Therapy with AN

The strategies of encouragement configure a set of cognitive-affective processing, attitudes and ways of being, doing, and thinking of the therapist characterized by his trust towards the patient. If the therapeutic relationship is the core engine of clinical intervention on girls with AN, the process of encouragement represents the heart of the therapeutic relationship [9, 58]. In light of the inconsistence of the self in AN patients, therapists' attitude vicariates the deficit function which permits to face and copy with life challenges, otherwise named "courage." Thus for subjects affected with AN the therapeutic work is not so much in the "dig" in the unconscious of mind, but in building a dialogue full of empathic involvement, which crosses the experiential world of both the patient and the therapist and it is able to produce an encouraging co-transference related to the reciprocal organizing activities of both subjects.

The discovery of mirror neurons put the therapeutic process under a totally new light. It is now clear that there is an implicit, unconscious mutual imitation between therapist and patient, and it is responsible for the process of change, in a more substantial way than the verbal intervention itself. The therapeutic relationship is therefore characterized by continuous and reciprocal unaware embodied simulations between patient and therapist. It is likely that the simulation by the patient of the expression modified by the therapist of his/her experience, through intentional attunement, performs regulator therapeutic functions. The model of embodied simulation [4, 5] is important for psychotherapy for several reasons: it provides a unified account of preverbal aspects of interpersonal relationships that probably play an important role in the construction of the self, contributes to new definition of psychopathological processes, and especially reveals the ability to analyze from a different perspective, the specific dynamics that characterize the preverbal interpersonal psychotherapeutic setting. These acquisitions on the development of the self as a neuropsychodynamic process [6, 10] encourage a special revision of psychiatric treatment especially in resistant patients. Many aspects of treatment resistance appear to be related to the therapist's emotional attitudes [39, 48, 74].

21.7.4 Empathetic Comprehension as the Core of the Process of Encouragement

The main goal of the therapy is to build a relationship that will allow security while promoting intimacy, based on an attitude of acceptance towards the patient and trust in his/her ability to change. Special attention is given to the understanding, on the part of the therapist, the quality of the transference. From a relational point of view the aim of transference analysis is to modulate autonomy and dependence, discouraging regressive attachment and idealization. It is therefore in the empathic understanding, resulting in the empathic process, which rank the main drivers of change.

The process of encouragement may be viewed as a progression with different phases: (a) the therapist in the accepting listening attitude consents a controlled contagion driven by embodied simulation from acts, anger emotions, defenses, ambivalences, resistances of the patient; (b) he "metabolizes" the emotions of the patient accepting them empathically as they are; (c) the elaboration of the patient's transference, of the therapist's countertransference, and especially of the metacountertransference [75] induces in him answers (emotions, enactments, content words and prosodic tone, gestures) which are modulated by his/her self, possibly complementary to those of the patient and eventually able to infect her; (d) if the therapist is not discouraged in his empathic firmness the patient, sooner or later, copy and active on these moments his/her embodied simulation; (e) patients may manifest intentional attunements leading to meeting moments bearers of change [9, 76–78]. Empathic understanding—based on embodied simulation and intentional attunement—is therefore the emotional context in which the affective present moments become moments of meeting: these interactions make the experience of being heard which would need above all the AN patients [58]. They will finally represent implicit models, that become part of the implicit procedural memory, which are fundamental agents of development of the self and of change [5]. The willingness to listen in the sense of Bruch [58] allows to perceive and modulate the quantum of closeness/distance that at the moment the patient is able to tolerate without re-activating the regressive defense mechanisms represented by symptoms. Fundamental in this process is the concept of metacountertransference that comes from Michel [75]. It consists that the therapist "*although plagued by despair angry and destructive of the patient is able to recognize and accept these emotions in himself, and suffer, but to use these emotions in favour of the change in the patient... and not in a competition or an aggressive avoidance...*".

In a patient suffering from AN naturally forced to perfectionism, psychotherapy is an opportunity to test new creative self-esteem: the therapist lives here as a person worthy of attention, commitment, concern, and autonomy within an optimal relational involvement amending both. This empathetic transmission of trust in a person affected by suffering, loneliness, and frustration re-activates the *creative self* to take care of herself [12]. Often to the sick AN women this is, after many years, their first experience of receiving listening and attention to "those who are," now and there, instead of receiving an interpretation about their feelings and communications [58, 79].

Anorectic patients, as has been said above, have a profound feeling of being worth nothing [58] and an extraordinary propensity to perfectionism [80].

In the "moments of meeting" therapist and AN patient meet with the regressive deficit, the "secret force" which argues Seidel [81]. "*Only if the patient feels to be not punished for those wrong compensatory goals, only if he is implicitly provided a model of acceptance of his self to forgive himself that he was once so weak from having to orient his life toward perfection, he may give up to those fictitious destinations that require his depression. Forgiven, he can forgive himself*" [81]. In the therapy patient's authentic experience of the deficit along with his therapist gradually corrects the per-version to a con-version of the instances of care of himself, which are so severely compromised as studies on attachment are confirming [44, 82].

The cornerstone of the theory of Bruch for AN was to accept the potential insecurity. All AN patients are eternally concerned about the image they have created in the eyes of others; they have an attitude of basic distrust towards the relationship with others and carry on the conviction that all look at them with contempt and distrust even though the "real" others do not. This is the internalization of a "judging other" and they have to protect against this. Patients need to perceive that focused and alive attention is rewarded with what they have to say and to share. The contact with AN patients involves the therapist in an experience which is quite different from conventional psychotherapy of other diseases because the AN patient is getting away from the contrasts that fuel the possibility of change, the essential focus of the therapy, while the body is consumed further. The AN chronic patients do not accept the treatment as a defining force in their life and fictional adherence to treatment is the most dangerous of resistance reinforcing the fictional self of the patients. The agreement between the therapist and the patient with chronic AN must keep in mind these contrasting perceptions that require a fundamentally different model. Most patients want to free themselves from the tyranny of the disease, but in the end, they will seek constantly to avoid change.

The ability of the psychodynamic therapist is crucial in fostering an attitude of hope in the patient, despite the constant threats of denial and despair. It takes more than a set of technical knowledge, the acquisition of a number of virtues—attitudes of mind and heart—that are embedded in the character and personality of the therapist. Brenner and Khan [83] explore these "psychodynamic virtues": thin and requesting empathy, ability to accept and confirm, curiosity and confidence with the underlying meanings, humility in the face of uncertainties and ambiguity, openness to transference involvement, ability to feel rewards and satisfaction for little things more inherent development of the therapeutic process than its results.

21.7.5 The Counter-Attitude of the Therapist Between Excessive Zeal and Discouragement

The continued efforts of the therapist to understand this strange and perverse disorder in people who want to live without eating, and sometimes rather die can cause over-reactions that depend on the intense emotional activation in the therapist, with alternating excess of zeal or loss of commitment and patience, and even aggression and rejection.

One of the main factors that complicate the psychological treatment of AN is that therapists do often experience negative countertransference stubborn and difficult to manage [47, 80]. Understanding the reasons of the patient is a means to avoid the counter-aggression and discouragement of the therapists which feeds anger and control towards the patient [84]. The alternation between different reactive attitudes of the physician can iatrogenically increase the evil force of AN: accomplishment vs anger and punishment; impotence vs therapeutic fury; affective caregiving vs expulsion; contagion of despair instead of hope; etc. Treasure et al. [74] cautioned therapists that they themselves may play a role in involuntary perpetuating the AN and unwittingly encourage hostility. This may happen when for instance they propose with excessive insistence replenishment and when their pessimism hinders motivation for change. Any attempt to change the food rituals, even if using a gentle and rational approach, will be seen as a request for a leap in the dark a dangerous assault, waiver of inalienable defenses. Fasting, in AN, gives moral force and psychic, while in progressively impairs vital functions. Studies on dopaminergic dysregulation in body emaciation confirm the "doping" effect of fasting. The verbal or implicit pressures of the therapist can make the patient distressed and prone to a further exacerbation of the symptoms: expect the change to a patient who cannot change, from his/her point of view on pain of death, means to reject it and attack him/her. In fact for the patient to encourage eating is not a careful and justifiable demand for a better life. The urgency of the clinician to move quickly with these frighteningly ill patients is understandably difficult to hold, but the risk of iatrogenia is high. The enigma of AN is, in fact, that the symptoms that compromise the life, the body, and the mind can mitigate very well the mental sufferance related to the deficit of the self.

Conclusions

In psychodynamic psychotherapy for ED, a peculiar complexity is encountered in understanding and integrating internal states and emotions. The way patients organize their interiority and relate with the environment is relevant to understand not only the relationship between patients and symptoms, but also the one existing between patient, treatment, and therapist [40]. According to these premises, the treatment should be directed by the patient's personality [36].

Then, how can the therapist exploit for therapeutic purposes what has been evoked in him by the emotion of the patient? It should induce the experienced therapist to implicit virtuous affective participation, instead of leaving the therapist under passive conditions, such as an empty screen placed in front of the patient. Such participation, mediated by the virtues of the therapist, acts implicitly, rather than through verbal expression, generating a movement of care in the patient [85].

The *healer's wound* [86] is in fact the premise-condition of compassionate propensity for therapeutic action.

The change, therefore, is due not to *interpretations that unveil fictitious goals*, but to the deep feeling of being heard, felt, and treated as a deserving person.

Implicit knowledge and system of fictions [9], especially in the therapist, represent a crucial area, a melting pot of empathic imitation, belonging, and cooperation.

The *shared implicit* relationship is the fulcrum of change, representing in the *hic et nunc* a *meaningful intersubjective encounter* of the self with the other, made possible by the developments of the therapist–patient relational history and of the shared coding systems of meaning [85].

References

1. Husserl E. Meditazioni cartesiane, con l'aggiunta dei Discorsi parigini. Bompiani, Milano, 1988; 1931.
2. Schaefer M, Northoff G. Who am I: the conscious and the unconscious self. Front Hum Neurosc. 2017;11:126. https://doi.org/10.3389/fnhum.2017.00126.
3. Stanghellini G, Castellini G, Brogna P, Faravelli C, Ricca V. Identity and eating disorders (IDEA): a questionnaire evaluating identity and embodiment in eating disorder patients. Psychopathology. 2012;45:147–58.
4. Gallese V. Mirror neurons, embodied simulation, and the neural basis of social identification. Psychoanal Dial. 2009;19:519–4536. https://doi.org/10.1080/10481880903231910.
5. Gallese V, Eagle MN, Migone P. Intentional attunement: mirror neurons and the neural underpinnings of interpersonal relations. J Am Psychoanal Assoc. 2007;55(1):131–76.
6. Ammaniti M, Gallese V. La nascita dell'intersoggettività. Milano: Raffaello Cortina Ed; 2014.
7. Gallese V, Lakoff G. The brain's concepts: the role of the sensory-motor system in conceptual knowledge. Cogn Neuropsychol. 2005;22(3):455–79. https://doi.org/10.1080/02643290442000310.
8. Person ES, Cooper AM, Gabbard GO. Psicoanalisi. Teoria, clinica, ricerca. Milano: Raffaello Cortina Ed; 2005.
9. Fassino S. La resistenza ai trattamenti nell'anoressia nervosa: la psicoterapia psicodinamica adleriana ha una specifica indicazione? Riv Psicol Indiv. 2014;76:31–69.
10. Northoff G. Neuropsychoanalysis in practice. Brain, self, objects. Ananke, Torino; 2014/2011.
11. Adler A. The fundamental view of individual psychology. Int J Ind Psych. 1935;1:5–8.
12. Adler A. Preface to *The Diary of Vaslav Nijinsky*. Arch Gen Psychiatry. 1981;38:836–41.
13. Abbate-Daga G, Quaranta M, Marzola E, Amianto F, Fassino S. The relationship between alexithymia and intolerance of uncertainty in anorexia nervosa. Psychopathology. 2015;48(3):202–8. https://doi.org/10.1159/000381587.

14. Stice E, Shaw HE. Role of body dissatisfaction in the onset and maintenance of eating pathology: a synthesis of research findings. J Psychosom Res. 2002;53(5):985–93.
15. Gowers SG, Shore A. Development of weight and shape concerns in the aetiology of eating disorders. Br J Psychiatry. 2001;179:236–42.
16. De Berardis D, Carano A, Gambi F, Campanella D, Giannetti P, Ceci A, Mancini E, La Rovere R, Cicconetti A, Penna L, Di Matteo D, Scorrano B, Cotellessa C, Salerno RM, Serroni N, Ferro FM. Alexithymia and its relationships with body checking and body image in a non-clinical female sample. Eat Behav. 2007;8(3):296–304.
17. Fairburn CG. Cognitive behavior therapy and eating disorders. New York: Guilford Press; 2008.
18. Beato-Fernández L, Rodríguez-Cano T, Belmonte-Llario A, Martínez-Delgado C. Risk factors for eating disorders in adolescents. A Spanish community-based longitudinal study. Eur Child Adolesc Psychiatry. 2004;13(5):287–94.
19. Abbate-Daga G, Pierò A, Rigardetto R, Gandione M, Gramaglia C, Fassino S. Clinical, psychological and personality features related to age of onset of anorexia nervosa. Psychopathology. 2007;40(4):261–8.
20. Carter JC, Blackmore E, Sutandar-Pinnock K, Woodside DB. Relapse in anorexia nervosa: a survival analysis. Psychol Med. 2004:34(4):671–9.
21. Lautenbacher S, Kraehe N, Krieg JC. Perception of body size and body satisfaction in recovered anorexic women: comparison with restrained and unrestrained eaters. Percept Mot Skills. 1997;84(3 Pt 2):1331–42.
22. Wilksch S, Wade TD. Differences between women with anorexia nervosa and restrained eaters on shape and weight concerns, self-esteem, and depression. Int J Eat Dis. 2004;35(4):571–8.
23. McFarlane T, McCabe RE, Jarry J, Olmsted MP, Polivy J. Weight-related and shape-related self-evaluation in eating-disordered and non-eating-disordered women. Int J Eat Dis. 2001;29(3):328–35.
24. Joiner TE Jr, Schmidt NB, Wonderlich SA. Global self-esteem as contingent on body satisfaction among patients with bulimia nervosa: lack of diagnostic specificity. Int J Eat Dis. 1997;21(1):67–76.
25. Fassino S, Pierò A, Gramaglia C, Abbate-Daga G, Gandione M, Rovera GG, Bartocci G. Clinical, psychological, and personality correlates of asceticism in anorexia nervosa: from saint anorexia to pathologic perfectionism. Transcult Psychiatry. 2006;43(4):600–14.
26. Abbate-Daga G, Buzzichelli S, Marzola E, Amianto F, Fassino S. Effectiveness of cognitive remediation therapy (CRT) in anorexia nervosa: a case series. J Clin Exp Neuropsychol. 2012;34(10):1009–15. https://doi.org/10.1080/13803395.2012.704900.
27. Fassino S, Pierò A, Gramaglia C, Abbate-Daga G. Clinical, psychopathological and personality correlates of interoceptive awareness in anorexia nervosa, bulimia nervosa and obesity. Psychopathology. 2004;37(4):168–74.
28. Amianto F, Bertorello A, Migliore F, Abbate-Daga G, Fassino S. Alexithymia in anorexia and bulimia: ubiquitous and primary trait? Cogent Psychology. 2016;3(1). https://doi.org/10.1080/23311908.2016.1185994.
29. Marzola E, Panepinto C, Delsedime N, Amianto F, Fassino S, Abbate-Daga GB. A factor analysis of the meanings of anorexia nervosa: intrapsychic, relational, and avoidant dimensions and their clinical correlates. MC Psychiatry. 2016;16:190. https://doi.org/10.1186/s12888-016-0894-6.
30. Marzola E, Abbate-Daga G, Gramaglia C, Amianto F, Fassino S. A qualitative investigation into anorexia nervosa: The inner perspective. Cogent Psychol. 2015;2(1). https://doi.org/10.1080/23311908.2015.1032493.
31. Fassino S, Abbate-Daga G, Pierò A, Leombruni P, Rovera GG. Anger and personality in eating disorders. J Psychosom Res. 2001;51(6):757–64.
32. Amianto F, Siccardi S, Abbate-Daga G, Marech L, Barosio M, Fassino S. Does anger mediate between personality and eating symptoms in bulimia nervosa? Psychiatry Res. 2012;200(2–3):502–12. https://doi.org/10.1016/j.psychres.2012.07.036.

33. Marzola E, Fassino S, Amianto F, Abbate-Daga G. Affective temperaments in anorexia nervosa: the relevance of depressive and anxious traits. J Affect Disord. 2017;218:23–9. https://doi.org/10.1016/j.jad.2017.04.054.
34. Amianto F, Northoff G, Abbate Daga G, Fassino S, Tasca GA. Is anorexia nervosa a disorder of the self? A psychological approach. Front Psychol. 2016;7:849. https://doi.org/10.3389/fpsyg.2016.00849.
35. Stanghellini G. Corpo (alterazioni del vissuto corporeo). In: Barale F, Bertani M, Gallese V, Mistura S, Zamperina A, editors. Dizionario storico di psicologia, psichiatria, psicoanalisi, neuroscienze. Einaudi, Torino; 2006.
36. Abbate-Daga G, Amianto F, De Bacco C, Delsedime N, Fassino S. Resistance to treatment and change in eating disorders. A review on psychological aspects. BMC Psychiatry. 2013;13:294.
37. Winnicott D. Review of memories, dreams, reflections. Int J Psychoanal. 1964;45:450–5.
38. Strober M. Managing the chronic, treatment-resistant patient with anorexia nervosa. Int J Eat Dis. 2004;36:245–55.
39. Fassino S, Abbate-Daga G. Resistance to treatment in eating disorders: a critical challenge. BMC Psychiatry. 2013;13:282. https://doi.org/10.1186/1471-244X-13-282.
40. Abbate-Daga G, Marzola E, Amianto F, Fassino S. A comprehensive review of psychodynamic treatments for eating disorders. Eat Weight Dis. 2016;21(4):553–80.
41. Mikulincer M, Shaver P. An attachment perspective on psychopathology. World Psychiatry. 2012;11(1):11–5.
42. Troisi A, Di Lorenzo G, Alcini S, Nanni RC, Di Pasquale C, Siracusano A. Body dissatisfaction in women with eating disorders: relationship to early separation anxiety and insecure attachment. Psychosom Med. 2006;68(3):449–53.
43. Eggert J, Levendosky A, Klump K. Relationships among attachment styles, personality characteristics, and disordered eating. Int J Eat Dis. 2007;40(2):149–55.
44. Tasca GA, Balfour L. Eating disorders and attachment: a contemporary psychodynamic perspective. Psychodyn Psychiatry. 2014;42(2):257–76. https://doi.org/10.1521/pdps.2014.42.2.257.
45. Tasca GA, Hilsenroth M, Thompson-Brenner H. Psychoanalytic psychotherapy or cognitive-behavioral therapy for bulimia nervosa. Am J Psychiatry. 2014;171(5):583–4. https://doi.org/10.1176/appi.ajp.2014.13121616.
46. Amianto F, Abbate-Daga G, Morando S, Sobrero C, Fassino S. Personality development characteristics of women with anorexia nervosa, their healthy siblings and healthy controls: What prevents and what relates to psychopathology? Psychiatry Res. 2011;187(3):401–8. https://doi.org/10.1016/j.psychres.2010.10.028.
47. Abbate-Daga G, Gramaglia C, Amianto F, Marzola E, Fassino S. Attachment insecurity, personality, and body dissatisfaction in eating disorders. J Nerv Ment Dis. 2010;198(7):520–4. https://doi.org/10.1097/NMD.0b013e3181e4c6f7.
48. Tereno S, Soares I, Martins C, Celani M, Sampaio D. Attachment styles, memories of parental rearing and therapeutic bond: a study with eating disordered patients, their parents and therapists. Eur Eat Dis Rev. 2008;16(1):49–58.
49. Goodwin RD, Fitzgibbon ML. Social anxiety as a barrier to treatment for eating disorders. Int J Eat Dis. 2002;32(1):103–6.
50. Mahon J, Bradley SN, Harvey PK, Winston AP, Palmer RL. Childhood trauma has dose-effect relationship with dropping out from psychotherapeutic treatment for bulimia nervosa: a replication. Int J Eat Dis. 2001;30(2):138–48.
51. Cicerale A, Settanta C, D'Agata F, Caglio M, Caroppo P, Coriasco M, Spalatro A, Mortara P, Fassino S, Ardito RDB, Amianto F. Neuroanatomical correlates of state of mind with respect to attachment in patients with anorexia nervosa. Clin Neuropsychiatry. 2013;5:217–55.
52. Skårderud F. Eating one's words, part I: 'Concretised metaphors' and reflective function in anorexia nervosa—an interview study. Eur Eat Dis Rev. 2007;15(3):163–74.
53. Rothschild-Yakar L, Waniel A, Stein D. Mentalizing in self vs. parent representations and working models of parents as risk and protective factors from distress and eating disorders. J Nerv Ment Dis. 2013;201(6):510–518.6.

54. Tapajóz Pereira de Sampaio F, Soneira S, Aulicino A, Allegri RF. Theory of mind in eating disorders and their relationship to clinical profile. Eur Eat Dis Rev. 2013;21(6):479–87. https://doi.org/10.1002/erv.2247.
55. Lang K, Treasure J, Tchanturia K. Acceptability and feasibility of self-help cognitive remediation therapy for anorexia nervosa delivered in collaboration with carers: a qualitative preliminary evaluation study. Psychiatry Res. 2015;225(3):387–94. https://doi.org/10.1016/j.psychres.2014.12.008.
56. Oldershaw A, Hambrook D, Stahl D, Tchanturia K, Treasure J, Schmidt U. The socio-emotional processing stream in anorexia nervosa. Neurosc Biobehav Rev. 2011;35(3):970–88. https://doi.org/10.1016/j.neubiorev.2010.11.001.
57. Treasure J, Schmidt U. The cognitive-interpersonal maintenance model of anorexia nervosa revisited: a summary of the evidence for cognitive, socio-emotional and interpersonal predisposing and perpetuating factors. J Eat Dis. 2013;1:13. https://doi.org/10.1186/2050-2974-1-13.
58. Bruch H. Anorexia nervosa: therapy and theory. Am J Psychiatry. 1982;139(12):1531–8.
59. Northoff G. Brain and self—a neurophilosophical account. Child Adolesc Psychiatry Ment Health. 2013;7(1):28. https://doi.org/10.1186/1753-2000-7-28.
60. Fassino S, Abbate-Daga G, Amianto F, Leombruni P, Boggio S, Rovera GG. Temperament and character profile of eating disorders: a controlled study with the Temperament and Character Inventory. Int J Eat Dis. 2002;32(4):412–25.
61. Fassino S, Abbate-Daga G, Pierò A, Rovera GG. Dropout from brief psychotherapy in anorexia nervosa. Psychother Psychosom. 2002;71:200–6.
62. Doering S, Enzi B, Faber C, Hinrichs J, Bahmer J, Northoff G. Personality functioning and the cortical midline structures—an exploratory FMRI study. PLoS One. 2012;7(11):e49956. https://doi.org/10.1371/journal.pone.0049956.
63. Wagner S, Barbarich-Marsteller NC, Frank GK, Bailer UF, Wonderlich SA, Crosby RD, Henry SE, Vogel V, Plotnicov K, McConaha C, Kaye WH. Personality traits after recovery from eating disorders: do subtypes differ? Int J Eat Dis. 2006;39(4):276–84.
64. Eshkevari E, Rieger E, Longo MR, Haggard P, Treasure J. Persistent body image disturbance following recovery from eating disorders. Int J Eat Dis. 2014;47(4):400–9. https://doi.org/10.1002/eat.22219.
65. Fitzsimmons-Craft EE, Bardone-Cone AM, Kelly KA. Objectified body consciousness in relation to recovery from an eating disorder. Eat Behav. 2011;12(4):302–8. https://doi.org/10.1016/j.eatbeh.2011.09.001.
66. Greenleaf C, McGreer R. Disordered eating attitudes and self-objectification among physically active and sedentary female college students. J Psychol. 2006;140(3):187–98.
67. Hurst K, Zimmer-Gembeck M. Focus on perfectionism in female adolescent anorexia nervosa. Int J Eat Dis. 2015;48(7):936–41. https://doi.org/10.1002/eat.22417.
68. Wilksch SM, Durbridge MR, Wade TD. A preliminary controlled comparison of programs designed to reduce risk of eating disorders targeting perfectionism and media literacy. J Am Acad Child Adolesc Psychiatry. 2008;47(8):937–47. https://doi.org/10.1097/CHI.0b013e3181799f4a.
69. Fassino S, Amianto F, Sobrero C, Abbate-Daga G. Does it exist a personality core of mental illness? A systematic review on core psychobiological personality traits in mental disorders. Panminerva Med. 2013;55(4):397–413.
70. Zipfel S, Wild B, Groß G, Friederich HC, Teufel M, Schellberg D, Giel KE, de Zwaan M, Dinkel A, Herpertz S, Burgmer M, Löwe B, Tagay S, von Wietersheim J, Zeeck A, Schade-Brittinger C, Schauenburg H, Herzog W, ANTOP Study Group. Focal psychodynamic therapy, cognitive behaviour therapy, and optimised treatment as usual in outpatients with anorexia nervosa (ANTOP study): randomised controlled trial. Lancet. 2014;383(9912):127–37. https://doi.org/10.1016/S0140-6736(13)61746-8.
71. Skårderud F. Bruch revisited and revised. Eur Eat Dis Rev. 2009;17(2):83–8. https://doi.org/10.1002/erv.923.

72. Thompson-Brenner H. Discussion of "Eating disorders and attachment: a contemporary psychodynamic perspective:" does the attachment model of eating disorders indicate the need for psychodynamic treatment? Psychodyn Psychiatry. 2014;42(2):277–84. https://doi.org/10.1521/pdps.2014.42.2.277.
73. Poulsen S, Lunn S, Daniel SIF, Folke S, Mathiesen BB, Katznelson H, Fairburn CG. A randomized controlled trial of psychoanalytic psychotherapy or cognitive-behavioral therapy for bulimia nervosa. Am J Psychiatry. 2014;171(1):109–16. https://doi.org/10.1176/appi.ajp.2013.12121511.
74. Treasure J, Crane A, McKnight R, Buchanan E, Wolfe M. First do no harm: iatrogenic maintaining factors in anorexia nervosa. Eur Eat Dis Rev. 2011;19(4):296–302. https://doi.org/10.1002/erv.1056.
75. Michel L. Des stereotypes culturels au transfert-contre-transfert dans la relation psychothérapique Interculturelle. Psychothérapies. 1999;19(4):247–55.
76. Stern D. The present moment in psychotherapy and everyday life. New York: WW Norton; 2004.
77. Rovera GG. Le strategie dell'incoraggiamento. Riv Psicol Indiv. 2009;66:139–60.
78. Stern D, Boston Change Process Study Group. The foundational level of psychodynamic meaning: implicit process in relation to conflict, defense and the dynamic unconscius. Int J Psychoanal. 2007;88:843–60. https://doi.org/10.1516/ijpa.2007.843.
79. Thompson-Brenner H, Satir D, Franko D, Herzog D. Clinician reactions to patients with eating disorders: a review of the literature. Psych Serv. 2012;63(1):73–8. https://doi.org/10.1176/appi.ps.201100050.
80. Vitousek K, Watson S, Wilson GT. Enhancing motivation for change in treatment-resistant eating disorders. Clin Psychol Rev. 1998;18(4):391–420.
81. Seidel V. Regression als therapeutisches Agens in der individualpsychologische Therapie. Beiträge zur Individualpsichologie. 1985;6:90.
82. Tasca GA, Balfour L. Attachment and eating disorders: a review of current research. Int J Eat Dis. 2014;47:710–7. https://doi.org/10.1002/eat.22302.
83. Brenner A, Khan F. The training of psychodynamic psychiatrists: the concept of "psychodynamic virtue". Psychodyn Psychiatry. 2013;41(1):57–74.
84. Rovera GG. Patient-therapist matching. Riv Psicol Indiv. 2015;78:3–19.
85. Fassino S. Finzioni e processo di cambiamento. Riv Psicol Indiv. 2010;68:59–79.
86. Guggenbuhl-Craig A. Al di sopra del malato e della malattia. Raffaello Cortina, Milano, 1987; 1983.

Family Functioning and Body Image

22

Federico Amianto and Secondo Fassino

22.1 Introduction

Body image dissatisfaction, the negative subjective evaluation of one's physical or outward appearance (figure, weight, specific body parts) is an important risk and perpetuating factor for eating disorders, being related to their central psychopathological elements, and a prospective factor for low self-esteem, depression, and unhealthy behaviors [1].

Body image and its subjective evaluation is a core aspect of the self as developing in childhood, adolescence, and adulthood [2]. Since the development of the self is heavily driven by the attachment patterns which arise from family functioning, this may represent a crucial issue in the development of body satisfaction and dissatisfaction.

22.2 Methodological Considerations

Approaching the research on this crucial issue, some considerations on methodological limitations in the research on family functioning and body image should be made. First, only longitudinal research can explore causality, confirming or not the chronological precedence of risk factors and mediating variables. Instead many of the studies on family functioning and body image are of a cross-sectional nature, so they capture associations from which causality cannot be inferred. The use of scales that are based on self-report assessment and recollection of interactions within the family can result in well-known biases like the under-report of negative behaviors or the differential recollection based on current status (the so-called Effort after

F. Amianto (✉) · S. Fassino
Eating Disorders Center for Treatment and Research, Department of Neuroscience, University of Turin, Turin, Italy
e-mail: federico.amianto@unito.it; secondo.fassino@unito.it

M. Cuzzolaro, S. Fassino (eds.), *Body Image, Eating, and Weight*,
https://doi.org/10.1007/978-3-319-90817-5_22

meaning bias) [3, 4]. Another particularly important issue in body image research is that instruments suitable for girls, which are mainly centered on the body image perception from a female point of view (e.g., those used in research on eating disorders), may not be transferable to boys, thus accounting for substantial differences in the literature. Moreover, the parallel investigation of parents and the offspring should utilize comparable measures. Different methods of assessing recollection of childhood memories and the inclusion or absence of instruments for the evaluation of mediation variables can lead to different findings across studies.

Finally, research should focus not only on body dissatisfaction but also on aspects like positive body image, which has emerged to be a different construct with different psychological correlates from the simple opposite of negative body image.

22.3 Parental Modeling and Attitudes Towards Eating

As analyzed in the review by Rodgers and Chabrol (2009) [4] the research on parent–child interactions and body image has classically explored two main modalities of influence. A first theory suggests that parents serve as a model for the development of the children's body image and eating behaviors. While a negative modeling effect (e.g., negative body image and eating behaviors in daughters shaped after those of the mothers) has been more studied, there is also evidence for a positive model effect, as emerging from the study of Fulkerson and coworkers (2006) that evidenced the regularity of family meals seems to be related to less disordered eating in the offspring [5, 6].

A second theory emphasizes the role of parental verbal messages (in the form of critics, teasing, and encouragement to control weight) directed towards the offspring and concerning the body size and shape, weight and eating behaviors of daughters and sons. Both of these modalities find support in the literature, but there seem to be a stronger relationship between body image dissatisfaction and parental attitudes than with parental modeling, for which longitudinal studies don't come to consistent findings [4, 7].

Concerning the active influences from parents, it would be important not to consider only the explicit and negatively connotated messages, but also more subtle and indirect messages as well as comments directed to other individuals. Furthermore, while parental teasing might be a rare event, appearance-related messages from parents are often intended as encouraging but can nevertheless harm the offspring's body esteem. Helfert and Warschburger (2011) found parental encouragement to control weight and shape as the most prevalent aspect of parental pressure perceived by girls and boys [8]. Kluck (2010) identified parental encouragement to control weight and size as the strongest predictor of body dissatisfaction in a retrospective study on young women [9]. The perception of the frequency of messages by the offspring can be different from that reported by the parents and can also be influenced by already present body concerns. Individuals that already have body image concerns can be more sensitive to messages that wouldn't be considered relevant and remembered by others.

22.4 Parents, Peers, and Media: Internalization and Social Comparison

The biopsychosocial model take into account biological characteristics, psychological variables and sociocultural influences and their interactions in the individual development of health and disease. Research on body image based on this model has identified two further main sources of environmental pressure along with family, namely peers and media. Concerning peers, Menzel and coworkers (2010) in their review found a well-established positive association between teasing and body dissatisfaction [10]. The role of family in managing peers pressures on young family member may be reduced in current society because of the role of social cyber communication which is mainly of control and sometimes may evolve in acts of cyberbullism [11].

As regards the media, these are responsible for the spread diffusion among general population of the thin ideal (the unattainable and unhealthy ideal of slenderness) which has become a cultural standard of beauty to which particularly western women are subjected. The possibility that family introjects and interprets towards offspring the implicit requests of this thin ideal was claimed by Gendall and coworkers (1982) at the beginning of the world ED epidemic as a major risk factor concerning family functioning [12, 13].

In addition, these three sources of influences can interact with each other and are actually considered to be stronger predictors of body dissatisfaction when combined together than any one of them taken singularly. The tripartite model which incorporates influences from family, peers and media proposes a way for them to have an impact on body image and eating disturbances that includes internalization of social norms and social comparison as mediating factors. While Keery and coworkers (2004) found influences from parents to be fully mediated by internalization and social comparison, a replication of the model by Shroff and Thompson (2006) found support for a direct effect of parental influences [14, 15]. Comments from parents can have an effect not directly related to their content but to the facilitation of other influences. Parents and peers can contribute to the development of an appearance-focused environment in which the adolescents are more easily subjected to beauty ideals and appearance-related behaviors, thus growing more concerned with their appearance. For example, Nathanson and Botta (2003) evidenced that the focus on appearance rather than the complimentary or critical nature of the comments that parents directed to TV characters was related to disordered eating in the offspring [16].

22.5 The Role of Attachment

Since social pressures and ideals around body size and shape are ubiquitous at least in western societies, but not every individual exposed to unattainable ideals of beauty internalizes these models or develops body dissatisfaction, research has focused on what makes some individuals and not others incorporate them into a self-concept.

Recent research points to attachment as a key factor for this mediation in the development of body satisfaction and dissatisfaction.

Getting along with peers and parental nurturance are core social connections that influence body image. Loving and supportive relationships with parents are prospective contributors to body image satisfaction for adolescent boys and girls, while distant relationships are linked to negative evaluation of self from the children. There are studies that tend to conclude for a greater impact of parental support than peer support on adolescent body image [17, 18].

Attachment theory (Bowlby, 1969) posits that the quality of early relational experiences with parental figures is fundamental for developing internal working models about the self and the others that are maintained stable throughout the lifetime [19]. These internal models influence the individual's adult relationships and the degree of discomfort in handling separation and intimacy. Attachment can be secure or insecure. Securely attached individuals hold a positive view of the self while having trust in others. On the other hand, an early insufficient respondence between children needs and parental availability may lead to insecure attachment styles. Insecure attachment can be further subtyped in avoidant or anxious [20]. Individuals characterized as avoidantly attached have a positive model of the self but a negative model of others and are uncomfortable with intimacy. Anxiously attached individuals have a positive model of others but a negative model of the self and have anxiety about separation. The high need for approval and negative view of the self of this style of attachment, by making the individual more "other" oriented, may confer vulnerability to external negative influences. Some research on body dissatisfaction seems to lead in the direction of a more evident role for anxious attachment than for the avoidant type [21].

Hardit and Hannum (2012) examined a sample of undergraduate women in the framework of the tripartite model [22]. They found the relationship between environmental influences and body dissatisfaction in these sample to be moderated by anxious attachment; young women who reported anxiety about relationships were also more concerned about their bodies. In this view, body size and shape would be a concrete way for valuate or devaluate the self. Lower anxious attachment may function as a buffer and protecting factor against environmental pressures. Thus, the authors suggest that the cultural and social influences highlighted in the tripartite model might be promoted by attachment insecurity.

Cheng and Mallinkcrodt (2009) found that the effect of anxious attachment on body dissatisfaction in a sample on college women was mediated by media internalization [23]. They developed a model to test how the quality of parental bonds and the security of attachment could help women resisting the internalization of media images, leading them to experience body satisfaction. They did not find a direct relationship between either of the parents' care and media internalization, but they found mother's and father's care related to attachment anxiety which in turn was linked to body dissatisfaction through the mediation of media internalization. The examination of the paths of influence for fathers and mothers separately evidence their differing contributions to body dissatisfaction.

Insecure attachment is also recognized to be implicated in the genesis of eating disorders [24]. The description of fathers as distant made by individuals with eating disorders is associated with body dissatisfaction [25]. In general, lower mother and father care are associated with greater rate of psychiatric disorders and psychological disturbances. Some researchers have suggested that anorexia nervosa is associated with avoidant attachment, while bulimia nervosa with preoccupied attachment style [26]. However, other research has found no difference in attachment insecurity subtype across the different eating disorders subgroups (pointing to a greater importance of the severity rather than the type of the disorder) [27].

Grenon and coworkers (2016) recently replicated the model of Cheng and Mallinkcrodt (2009) in a clinical sample of girls with eating disorders [28]. While the recollection of mothers as less caring was directly related to body dissatisfaction, the recollection of fathers as less caring was related to attachment anxiety and higher media internalization that mediated the relation with body dissatisfaction. They suggest that the fostering of a secure attachment by fathers can potentially protect the daughters from the internalization of media images. Memories of poorer emotional bonding with mothers (the retrospective account made by the individual of the parents' contribution to the parent–child relationship in terms of mother and father overprotection and care, a concept similar to parents' emotional availability) seem to be directly related to daughters' self-evaluation and body esteem. Again attachment anxiety seems to be central to body dissatisfaction development, due to negative view of self, positive view of others, and a high need of approval.

Along this line of research relating the inter- and intrapersonal factors of body dissatisfaction, Abbate Daga and coworkers (2010) questioned if personality traits could explain both attachment insecurity and body dissatisfaction in eating disorders patients [29]. This was previously shown in studies on healthy population that suggested that attachment insecurity could be totally dependent on personality traits [30]. Using the TCI (Temperament and Character Inventory), a widely used and validated personality assessment questionnaire that allows to identify innate (temperament) and acquired (character) personality dimensions, the authors obtained the portrait of a patient with eating disorders as a person with low Self Directedness and Cooperativity (only partially developed character), high Harm Avoidance (fearful, likely to use behavior inhibition strategies), and high Reward Dependence (strong dependence on external reinforcement). They also found evidence for high attachment insecurity in this population. However, their results refuted the hypothesis of attachment as a variation in personality: the need for approval scale (measuring a dimension of insecure attachment) was the only variable that independently predicted ED subjects' body concern after the confounding variables and personality traits were considered together. Thus, the influences of personality and attachment on body image disturbances cannot be considered overlapped. The interpretation given by the authors was that in these patients thinness might be a way to maintain connections with others, avoiding to be dismissed (interestingly, personality factors appeared to play a greater role when the symptomatology was less severely anorectic). Alternatively, these data support the hypothesis that the lacking approval (e.g., psychological validation) from attachment figures may impair subjects affected with AN in accepting their body image and introjecting it into their developing self-image [2].

22.6 Evidence Across the Life Span

An important priority for research on body image is to investigate the development of body image across the life span and identify the factors that contribute to it.

So far the few studies that examined the relationships between family functioning and body image satisfaction and dissatisfaction provided mixed results. For example, Presnell and coworkers (2004) didn't find prospective evidence for links between parental support and body dissatisfaction [31], whereas in a later study Bearman and coworkers (2006) found support from parents to predict body dissatisfaction in boys and girls [17].

Holsen and coworkers (2012) analyzed body satisfaction in a Norwegian sample beginning at age 13 and ending at age 30, thus capturing the years of adolescence and early adulthood [32]. Their goal was to examine the impact of early relationships with parents on the development of body image. First they found, as predicted, a clear evidence for gender difference in body image satisfaction, with males having a more positive body image than females in a way that did not diminish with age. They also confirmed the role of BMI across adolescence and early adulthood. In contrast with some previous research, they documented a relatively stable growth in body image satisfaction during adolescence and a stabilization in adulthood. They also found that the quality of parent–child interactions represented a significant predictor of initial level of body satisfaction, after controlling for BMI. Again this finding highlights the relevance of the relationships with others for the evaluation of the physical self. However, the negative effect of initial negative relationships seemed to diminish entering early adulthood. In this period, individuals who reported less positive relationships at the beginning recovered with a steeper growth in body image satisfaction. Concerning relationships with peers, these emerged less relevant than the quality of the relationships with parents, which seemed to continue to exert an effect even when the growing adolescents spent less time with parents and more with peers.

The systemic perspective on family underscore the interdependence of individuals as elements of a system, suggesting that children and parents can influence each other in a dynamic way.

Family connectedness, the sense of belonging and psychological closeness of the family, has been linked to several positive outcome for adolescents.

Boutelle and coworkers (2009) found that parent–child connectedness predicted body satisfaction for girls 5 years later, while body satisfaction predicted parent–child connectedness for boys [33].

Crespo and coworkers (2010) took on this perspective and focusing on body satisfaction examined its relation with family connectedness [34]. They found that for girls the perceived family connectedness across time predicted body satisfaction, which was in turn a predictor of family connectedness.

Yu (2016) examined longitudinal data from a sample of young boys and girls in South Korea, which is the country with the highest rate of cosmetic surgery per capita [35]. Adolescents in this country seem to be particularly burdened by cultural pressures and unrealistic standards of beauty. The author found different trajectories of body dissatisfaction. The different growth trajectories had different antecedents and girls who reported lower parent–child connectedness at baseline were likely to be in a development class characterized by high body dissatisfaction. The stability of body dissatisfaction pointed to a lasting role of early influences. Again connectedness to parents emerged as a protective factor for body dissatisfaction for boys and girls. It is noteworthy that also the feeling of low autonomy predicted greater body dissatisfaction in the growing adolescents.

Helfert and Warschburger (2011) found longitudinal evidence for the link between parental encouragement to control weight and shape and body dissatisfaction 1 year later [36]. As shown in cross-sectional research, this points the attention to encouraging parental comments regarding weight and shape meant to be supportive but with negative effects. As in previously cited reports also in this case teasing from peers and parents did not result as relevant for the development of body concerns.

22.7 Gender, Age, and Parental Influences

As evidenced before, there are gender similarities and differences in the contributions of relationships with parents to body image. Some studies suggest a greater impact of parental interactions for girls [34, 37]. Girls are also supposed to be more likely to perceive and act on their body dissatisfaction at more precocious levels than boys [38, 39].

It is widely recognized that in westernalized society body ideals are gender specific, thus girls appear to be more likely to engage in behaviors to lose weight and boys in strategies to increase muscles. Boys and girls are thought to share body ideals with same gender adults. In this direction, there are studies supporting the relation between mothers' and daughters' levels of body dissatisfaction [5, 40, 41]. Regarding gender differences in parental messages, it appears that they are more strongly linked to behaviors in girls. Instead, it seems that daughters receive more messages related to appearance from fathers than from mothers [5].

Research on children has proposed that body image dissatisfaction can emerge since 5 years of age, particularly for girls [42, 43]. Although generally considered to increase in the challenging time of adolescence, literature findings may range from those showing a worsening of body image to those showing an improvement in the adolescence years.

As reviewed by Tatangelo and coworkers (2016), some studies seem to indicate that a growing number of children from the age of 6 are not satisfied with their appearance, while others suggest children to be generally satisfied with their bodies [44–46]. However, it's clear that even younger children have a preference for thin bodies, indicating an early adhesion to the thin ideal in western culture. So it is relevant to determine the role of parents in shaping this preference and more importantly if it's related to the evaluations that the children might perform of their own bodies [47].

Wong and coworkers (2013) showed that the primary caregiver's satisfaction of the body size of their preschool children was related to the satisfaction of the children [48]. As for adolescents' verbal messages from parents about the appearance of the child seems to exert a relevant influence on preschool children's body image. Research in this area has mainly considered mothers influences. As said before for adolescents, it would be useful to investigate the differential pathways by which mothers and fathers influence body image development.

Along with fathers it could be relevant to study also the impact of relationships with siblings. Sinton and Birch (2006) showed older siblings to be particularly influent on preschool children body image [49].

Finally, some research supports the hypothesis that the family versus peer influences on the development of subject's body image may exert different weights depending on each development phase. Some authors suggest that connectedness to parents would play a major role in developing offspring's body image during childhood, while peer pressure would exert greater influence during the adolescence. In adulthood, the relationship with romantic partners or other attachment experiences might grow in relevance as source of influences for body image. Avalos and Tylka (2006) found that the acceptance from the person (for example, the romantic partner) that adult subjects considered the most influential in their life as object of attachment was related to greater perceived acceptance of their body by others (and to intuitive eating) [50].

22.8 Interventions on the Family Functioning

The role of attachment dynamics in the management of individuals with body image disturbances has been strongly evidenced by the study of Tereno and colleagues (2008) [51]. The parent–child attachment memories of patients were strictly related to the current quality of therapeutic relationship with a heavy potential influence on the outcome of the treatment.

Moreover, a more precise knowledge of the family-related predictors of body dissatisfaction can guide more informed strategies for prevention through individual and family targeted intervention. The evidence of different trajectories of development of body dissatisfaction related to family functioning that comes from longitudinal studies may help the design of specific preventive interventions for subgroups of population. For instance, a great attention should be paid to the attachment dynamics with parents and also to parental criticism on body image and weight during early childhood since this period is crucial for the early development of body image. Instead, more attention should be paid to the criticism of peers during adolescence.

Attachment-based models suggest specific areas of preventive intervention since early childhood, for example, addressing the attachment insecurity which has been demonstrated as a typical risk factor for body dissatisfaction in eating disorders patients. Primary preventive interventions should focus on supporting parents to reduce attachment anxiety in their offspring fostering the development of secure attachment. This could counteract the negative influences on body image evaluation by preventing their internalization.

Secondary preventive interventions may be carried on parents in the therapeutic settings, e.g., during family therapies or family counseling interventions [52]. Therapists should assess attachment style and family recollection when treating patients characterized by body image disturbances.

On the other hand, specific psycho-educational programs should be developed to help parents in preventing the negative influence of media on their relationship with children. Parents should be discouraged to pursue the thin ideals in the education of their offspring. Instead, they should be warned that to maintain an adequate body weight and image in their children they should maintain a warm and supportive relation that fosters secure attachment, thus helping and developing a positive view of self and others [53].

If preschool were confirmed to be the time when body image concerns begin to form, the delivery of positive body image messages for children and parents could be particularly efficacious since the birth of the child. Mental healthcare should consider that only programs for parent education during this early period of child life could really prevent the emergence of body image disturbances in the offspring. McCabe and coworkers (2014) implemented a program in which the parents of 3–6 years old boys participated at two educational workshops and found after such intervention a greater awareness in the parents of how they may impact on their sons and daughters body image [54].

Finally, it must be accounted for that the knowledge coming from the systemic perspective on family that any member can influence the others is dense of practical implications that should be considered when developing prevention programs, for instance including all family members or being present at a population level.

Acknowledgement Dr. Matteo Martini contributed to this chapter.

References

1. Stice E, Shaw HE. Role of body dissatisfaction in the onset and maintenance of eating pathology—a synthesis of research findings. J Psychosom Res. 2002;53:985–93. https://doi.org/10.1016/S0022-3999(02)00488-9.
2. Amianto F, Northoff G, Abbate Daga G, Fassino S, Tasca GA. Is anorexia nervosa a disorder of the self? A psychological approach. Front Psychol. 2016;7:849. https://doi.org/10.3389/fpsyg.2016.00849.
3. Fassino S1, Amianto F, Rocca G, Daga GA. Parental bonding and eating psychopathology in bulimia nervosa: personality traits as possible mediators. Epidemiol Psichiatr Soc. 2010;19(3):214–22.
4. Rodgers R, Chabrol H. Parental attitudes, body image disturbance and disordered eating amongst adolescents and young adults: a review. Eur Eat Disord Rev. 2009;17:137–51. https://doi.org/10.1002/erv.907.
5. Elfhag K, Linne Y. Gender differences in associations of eating pathology between mothers and their adolescent offspring. Obes Res. 2005;13:1070–6. https://doi.org/10.1038/oby.2005.125.
6. Fulkerson JA, Story M, Mellin A, Leffert N, Neumark-Sztainer D, French SA. Family dinner meal frequency and adolescent development: relationships with developmental assets and high-risk behaviors. J Adolesc Health. 2006;39:337–45. https://doi.org/10.1016/j.jadohealth.2005.12.026.

7. Paxton SJ, Eisenberg ME, Neumark-Sztainer D. Prospective predictors of body dissatisfaction in adolescent girls and boys: a five-year longitudinal study. Dev Psychol. 2006;42:888–99.
8. Helfert S, Waschburger P. The face of appearance-related social pressure: gender, age and body mass variations in peer and parental pressure during adolescence. Child Adolesc Psychiatry Ment Health. 2011;17:7–16. https://doi.org/10.1186/1753-2000-7-16.
9. Kluck AS. Family influence on disordered eating: the role of body image dissatisfaction. Body Image. 2010;7:8–14. https://doi.org/10.1016/j.bodyim.2009.09.009.
10. Menzel JE, Schaefer LM, Burke NL, Mayhew LL, Brannick MT, Thompson JK. Appearance-related teasing, body dissatisfaction, and disordered eating: a meta-analysis. Body Image. 2010;7:261–70. https://doi.org/10.1016/j.bodyim.2010.05.004.
11. Amianto F, Fassino S. Psychiatric problems emerging in teens: the situation for the design of future interventions. Acta Psychopathol. 2017;3:1. https://doi.org/10.4172/2469-6676.100073.
12. Gendall KA, Joyce PR, Sullivan PF, Bulik CM. Personality and dimensions of dietary restraint. Int J Eat Disord. 1998;24:371–9.
13. Fassino S, Svrakic D, Abbate-Daga G, Leombruni P, Amianto F, Stanic S, Rovera GG. Anorectic family dynamics: temperament and character data. Compr Psychiatry. 2002;43(2):114–20. https://doi.org/10.1053/comp.2002.30806.
14. Keery H, Berg PV, Thompson JK. An evaluation of the tripartite influence model of body dissatisfaction and eating disturbance with adolescent girls. Body Image. 2004;1:237–51. https://doi.org/10.1016/j.bodyim.2004.03.001.
15. Shroff H, Thompson KJ. The tripartite influence model of body image and eating disturbance: a replication with adolescent girls. Body Image. 2006;3:17–23. https://doi.org/10.1016/j.bodyim.2005.10.004.
16. Nathanson AI, Botta RA. Shaping the effects of television on adolescents' body image disturbance: the role of parental mediation. Commun Res. 2003;30:304–31.
17. Bearman SK, Presnell K, Martinez E, Stice E. The skinny on body dissatisfaction. A longitudinal study of adolescent girls and boys. J Youth Adolesc. 2006;35:229–41. https://doi.org/10.1007/s10964-005-9010-9.
18. Leung N, Thomas G, Waller G. The relationship between parental bonding and core beliefs in anorexic and bulimic women. Br J Clin Psychol. 2000;39(2):205–13. https://doi.org/10.1023/A:1024515519160.
19. Bowlby J. Attachment and loss: attachment. New York: Basic Books; 1969.
20. Mikulincer M, Shaver PR, Pereg D. Attachment theory and affect regulation: the dynamics, development, and cognitive consequences of attachment-related strategies. Motiv Emotion. 2003;27(2):77–102. https://doi.org/10.1023/A:1024515519160.
21. Cash TF, Theriault J, Annis NW. Body image in an interpersonal context: adult attachment, fear of intimacy, and social anxiety. J Soc Clin Psychol. 2004;23:89–103. https://doi.org/10.1521/jscp.23.1.89.26987.
22. Hardit SK, Hannum JW. Attachment, the tripartite model, and the development of body dissatisfaction. Body Image. 2012;4:469–75. https://doi.org/10.1016/j.bodyim.2012.06.003.
23. Cheng HL, Mallinckrodt B. Parental bonds, anxious attachment, media internalization, and body image dissatisfaction: exploring a mediation model. J Couns Psychol. 2009;56:365–75. https://doi.org/10.1037/a0015067.
24. Troisi A, Di Lorenzo G, Alcini S, Nanni R, Di Pasquale C, Siracusano A. Body dissatisfaction in women with eating disorders: relationship to early separation anxiety and insecure attachment. Psychosom Med. 2006;68:449–53. https://doi.org/10.1097/01.psy.0000204923.09390.5b.
25. Pace U, Cacioppo M, Schimmenti A. The moderating role of father's care on the onset of binge eating symptoms among female late adolescents with insecure attachment. Child Psychiatry Hum D. 2012;43:282–92. https://doi.org/10.1007/s10578-011-0269-7.
26. Candelori C, Ciocca A. Attachment and eating disorders. In: Bria P, Ciocca A, De Risio S, editors. Psychotherapeutic issues in eating disorders: models, methods and results. Rome: Universo; 1998. p. 139–53.
27. O'Shaughnessy R, Dallos R. Attachment research and eating disorders: a review of the literature. Clin Child Psychol Psychiatry. 2009;14:559–74. https://doi.org/10.1177/1359104509339082.

28. Grenon R, Tasca GA, Maxwell H, Balfour L, Proulx G, Bissada H. Parental bonds and body dissatisfaction in a clinical sample: the mediating roles of attachment anxiety and media internalization. Body Image. 2016;19:49–56. https://doi.org/10.1016/j.bodyim.2016.08.005.
29. Abbate-Daga G, Gramaglia C, Amianto F, Marzola E, Fassino S. Attachment insecurity, personality and body dissatisfaction in eating disorders. J Nerv Ment Dis. 2010;198(7):520–4. https://doi.org/10.1097/NMD.0b013e3181e4c6f7.
30. Eggert J, Levendosky A, Klump K. Relationships among attachment styles, personality characteristics and disordered eating. Int J Eat Disord. 2007;40:149–55. https://doi.org/10.1002/eat.20351.
31. Presnell K, Bearman SK, Stice E. Risk factors for body dissatisfaction in adolescent boys and girls: a prospective study. Int J Eat Disord. 2004;36:389–401.
32. Holsen I, Jones DC, Birkeland MS. Body image satisfaction among Norwegian adolescents and young adults. A longitudinal study of the influence of interpersonal relationships and BMI. Body Image. 2012;9(2):201–8. https://doi.org/10.1016/j.bodyim.2012.01.006.
33. Boutelle K, Eisenberg ME, Gregory ML, Neumark-Sztainer D. The reciprocal relationship between parent–child connectedness and adolescent emotional functioning over 5 years. J Psychom Res. 2009;66:309–16.
34. Crespo C, Kielpikowski M, Jose PE, Pryor J. Relationships between family connectedness and body satisfaction: a longitudinal study of adolescent boys and girls. J Youth Adolesc. 2010;39:1392–401. https://doi.org/10.1007/s10964-009-9433-9.
35. Yu JJ. Trajectories of body dissatisfaction among South Korean youth: findings from a nationally representative sample. Body Image. 2016;19:186–94. https://doi.org/10.1016/j.bodyim.2016.10.002.
36. Helfert S, Warschburger P. A prospective study on the impact of peer and parental pressure on body dissatisfaction in adolescent girls and boys. Body Image. 2011;8:101–9. https://doi.org/10.1016/j.bodyim.2011.01.004.
37. Barker ET, Galambos NL. Body dissatisfaction of adolescent girls and boys: risk and resource factors. J Early Adolesc. 2003;23:141–65. https://doi.org/10.1177/0272431603023002002.
38. Jones DC. Body image among adolescent girls and boys: a longitudinal study. Dev Psychol. 2004;40:823–35. https://doi.org/10.1037/0012-1649.40.5.823.
39. Smolak L. Body image in children and adolescents: where do we go from here? Body Image. 2004;1:15–28. https://doi.org/10.1016/S1740-1445(03)00008-1.
40. Fulkerson JA, McGuire MT, Neumark-Sztainer D, Story M, French SA, Peery CL. Weight related attitudes and behaviors of adolescent girls and boys who are encouraged to diet by their mothers. Int J Obesity. 2002;26:1579–87. https://doi.org/10.1038/sj.ijo.0802157.
41. Keery H, Eisenberg ME, Boutelle K, Neumark-Sztainer D, Story M. Relationships between maternal and adolescent weight-related behaviors and concerns: the role of perception. J Psychosom Res. 2006;61:105–11. https://doi.org/10.1016/j.jpsychores.2006.01.011.
42. Davison KK, Markey CN, Birch LL. Etiology of body dissatisfaction and weight concerns among 5-year-old girls. Appetite. 2000;35:143–51. https://doi.org/10.1006/appe.2000.0349.
43. Lowes J, Tiggemann M. Body dissatisfaction, dieting awareness, and the impact of parental influence on young children. Br J Health Psych. 2003;8:135–47. https://doi.org/10.1348/135910703321649123.
44. Tatangelo G, McCabe M, Mellor D, Mealey A. A systematic review of body dissatisfaction and sociocultural messages related to the body among preschool children. Body Image. 2016;18:86–95. https://doi.org/10.1016/j.bodyim.2016.06.003.
45. Harriger JA, Calogero RM, Witherington DC, Smith JE. Body size stereotyping and internalisation of the thin ideal in preschool girls. Sex Roles. 2010;63:609–20. https://doi.org/10.1007/s11199-010-9868-1.
46. Musher-Eizenman DR, Holub SC, Edwards-Leeper L, Persson AV, Goldstein SE. The narrow range of acceptable body types of pre-schoolers and their mothers. App Dev Psychol. 2003;24:259–72. https://doi.org/10.1016/S0193-3973(03)00047-9.
47. Tremblay L, Lovsin T, Zecevic C, Larivière M. Perceptions of self in 3–5-year-old children a preliminary investigation into the early emergence of body dissatisfaction. Body Image. 2011;8:287–92. https://doi.org/10.1016/j.bodyim.2011.04.004.

48. Wong Y, Chang YMS, Lin CMS. The influence of primary caregivers on body size and self-body image of preschool children in Taiwan. Asia Pac J Clin Nutr. 2013;22:283. https://doi.org/10.6133/apjcn.2013.22.2.05.
49. Sinton MM, Birch LL. Individual and sociocultural influences on pre-adolescent girls' appearance schemas and body dissatisfaction. J Youth Adolesc. 2006;35:157–67. https://doi.org/10.1007/s10964-005-9007-4.
50. Avalos LC, Tylka TL. Exploring a model of intuitive eating with college women. J Couns Psychol. 2006;53:486–97. https://doi.org/10.1037/0022-0167.53.4.486.
51. Tereno S, Soares I, Martins C, Celani M, Sampaio D. Attachment styles, memories of parental rearing and therapeutic bond: a study with eating disordered patients, their parents and therapists. Eur Eat Disord Rev. 2008;16:49–58. https://doi.org/10.1002/erv.801.
52. Amianto F, Bertorello A, Spalatro A, Milazzo M, Signa C, Cavarero S, Abbate Daga G, Fassino S. Adlerian parental counseling in eating disorders: preliminary data of a controlled clinical trial. Eat Weight Disord. 2013;19(3):303–14. https://doi.org/10.1007/s40519-013-0079-y.
53. Amianto F, Ercole R, Abbate Daga G, Fassino S. Exploring parental bonding in BED and non-BED obesity compared with healthy controls: clinical, personality and psychopathology correlates. Eur Eat Disord Rev. 2015;24:187–96. https://doi.org/10.1002/erv.2419.
54. McCabe MP, Mellor D, Mealey A. An educational programme for parents on the body image of preschool-aged boys. J Health Psychol. 2014;21(7):1241–8. https://doi.org/10.1177/1359105314551078.

Transdiagnostic Cognitive Behavioural Theory and Treatment of Body Image Disturbance in Eating Disorders

23

Riccardo Dalle Grave and Simona Calugi

23.1 Introduction

According to the Diagnostic and Statistical Manual of Mental Disorders (DSM-5) [1], body image disturbance is one of the diagnostic criteria for anorexia nervosa and bulimia nervosa, but not for binge-eating disorder [1]. It is associated with a greater severity of eating-related psychopathology and psychological distress [2], and is also a predictor of eating disturbance in adolescence [3]. In fact, body image disturbance is one of the most important prognostic factors in the treatment of bulimia nervosa [4], anorexia nervosa [5], and binge-eating disorder [6].

Body image is a multidimensional construct that includes cognitive, behavioural, affective, and perceptual components [7, 8]. However, interest in the perceptual component, measured with body size estimation techniques, has gradually diminished in recent years due to uncertainty over its specificity [9, 10], and the unresolved methodological and theoretical confusion over its measurement [11]. Instead, the recently proposed and empirically supported transdiagnostic cognitive behavioural theory of eating disorders places more emphasis on a specific cognitive component of body image disturbance, the overvaluation of shape and weight, as their distinctive "core psychopathology" [12, 13].

23.2 The Overvaluation of Shape and Weight

Patients with eating disorders tend to overvalue or focus entirely on shape and weight control as a means of judging their own self-worth. This psychopathological feature is common to anorexia nervosa and bulimia nervosa, and occurs in more than 50% of patients with binge-eating disorder [14], as well as a large subgroup of

R. Dalle Grave (✉) · S. Calugi
Department of Eating and Weight Disorders, Villa Garda Hospital, Garda (VR), Italy

M. Cuzzolaro, S. Fassino (eds.), *Body Image, Eating, and Weight*,
https://doi.org/10.1007/978-3-319-90817-5_23

other specified eating disorders. Observed in both female and male patients, it is unique to the eating disorders, and is rarely seen in the general population, as people without eating disorders generally evaluate themselves on the basis of their perceived performance in a variety of life domains, e.g. relationships, work, sport, and parenting. Individuals with eating disorders, however, by placing excessive value on their shape and weight, become single-mindedly focused on control of the same, actively pursuing weight loss and an assiduously avoidance of "fatness" and weight gain [15].

Overvaluation of shape and weight should be differentiated from body dissatisfaction, as studies have shown that the former is more closely associated to self-esteem than the latter [16], and better differentiates individuals with eating disorders from those without [17, 18].

23.3 The Transdiagnostic Perspective

Unlike the DSM-5, which seeks to distinguish between different eating disorder categories, transdiagnostic cognitive behavioural theory instead focuses on their common maintaining mechanisms. This theory, developed by Fairburn, Cooper, and Shafran [12, 13], is supported by the fact that eating disorders share the same clinical features (e.g. preoccupation with thoughts about shape, weight, and eating control, strict dieting, binge-eating episodes, purging behaviours, excessive exercising, body checking, body avoidance, and feeling fat) [13], and that studies assessing the course of the various eating disorders show that a large subgroup tend to transition between the various DSM categories [19, 20]. Hence, the transdiagnostic theory suggests that shared processes may be instrumental in maintaining eating disorders, that the overvaluation of shape and weight control is the core psychopathology distinguishing eating disorders from other psychiatric disorders, and is of central importance in maintaining eating disorder psychopathology.

23.4 Overvaluation of Shape and Weight as a Central Eating Disorder Maintenance Mechanism

The majority of clinical features of eating disorders apparently stem from patients' overvaluation of shape and weight and their control, and this core feature is of primary importance in maintaining eating disorder psychopathology (Fig. 23.1). This manifests via extreme weight-control behaviours (e.g. dietary restraint and restriction, self-induced vomiting, misuse of laxatives and diuretics, and excessive exercising), various forms of body checking and avoidance, feeling fat, and preoccupation with thoughts about eating, shape and weight. In some patients, efforts to maintain prolonged undereating are "successful", causing them to become severely underweight, while others fall prey to the one eating disorder feature that is not obviously a direct consequence of the core psychopathology, namely binge eating. That being said, the transdiagnostic theory suggests that binge eating is largely the consequence

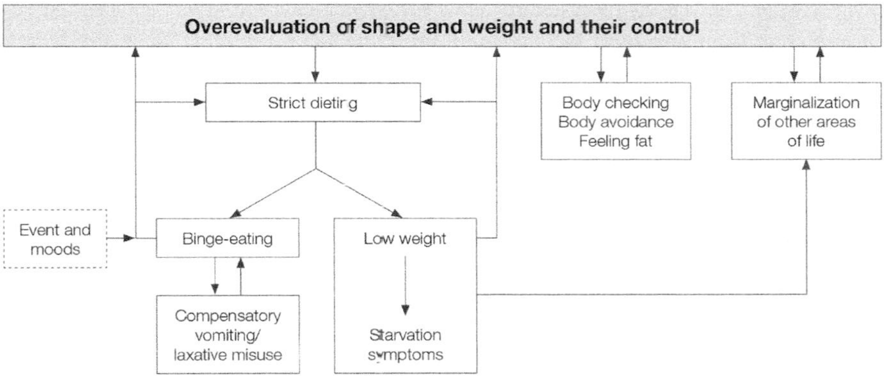

Fig. 23.1 The central role of the overvaluation of shape and weight and their control in maintaining the principal eating disorder features

of a breakdown in self-imposed extreme and rigid dietary rules, and/or used to modulate events and associated mood changes.

The central role of the overvaluation of shape and weight in the maintenance of eating disorder psychopathology is supported by the following evidence:

- Among patients with bulimia nervosa who showed a full response to treatment, those with the highest residual level of overvaluation of shape and weight were most prone to relapse [4].
- Trials of two psychological treatments for bulimia nervosa have shown that behavioural approaches that did not address the overvaluation of shape and weight were associated with a greater risk of relapse than those that did [21, 22].
- A prospective study of the natural course of bulimia nervosa found that baseline levels of shape and weight overvaluation predicted the persistence of binge eating (over 15 months), and that the degree of dietary restraint partially mediated this relationship [23].
- In a transdiagnostic sample (comprising patients with bulimia nervosa and those with anorexia nervosa), a reciprocal relationship has been discovered between the weight and shape overvaluation and moderate-to-extreme dietary restraint and exercising [24].

23.5 An Overview of CBT-E

Based on the transdiagnostic theory of eating disorders, enhanced cognitive behavioural therapy (CBT-E) (described in detail in the main treatment guide of Fairburn [15]) has four major goals:

1. To actively engage the patients in the treatment and change—CBT-E is designed to make patients feel in control of their own treatment, and to participate actively in all procedures adopted to help them overcome their eating problem.

2. To remove the eating disorder psychopathology behind features such as disturbed eating, low weight, extreme weight-control behaviours, and/or preoccupation with thoughts about body shape, weight, and eating control.
3. To correct the mechanisms maintaining the patient's psychopathology with a personalized, flexible and transdiagnostic treatment, based on their individual needs.
4. To ensure the changes are lasting, by providing patients with effective strategies to promptly respond to any setbacks.

The key strategy is to create a personalized formulation, which describes the main maintenance mechanisms to be targeted by the treatment. The eating disorder psychopathology is then addressed by means of a flexible series of sequential and well-specified strategies and procedures, integrated with progressive patient education. The aim is to modify thinking and implement changes in behaviour via strategies such as ongoing self-monitoring and targeted homework tasks between sessions. Hence, in the first phase of treatment, patients are encouraged to observe themselves enacting their formulation in real time, and to engage in an attempt to change their behaviour by considering the effect it is having. Once change is underway, i.e. when the main maintenance processes have been disrupted, patients then learn to de-centre from their eating problems, and eventually to identify their eating disorder mindset and learn to control it.

Transdiagnostic CBT-E may be administered via one of two versions, a "focused" form, which exclusively addresses the processes maintaining the individual's eating disorder psychopathology, or a "broad" form, which also addresses one or more of the three adjunctive maintenance mechanisms. According to the transdiagnostic theory, these are *clinical perfectionism*, *core low self-esteem*, and *interpersonal difficulties*. Mood intolerance has recently been incorporated into the focused version of the treatment.

For patients who are not significantly underweight, generally with a BMI of 18.5 kg/m^2 or above, CBT-E can be administered in an outpatient setting. A typical programme comprises 20 weekly individual sessions and is divided into four stages. *Outpatient CBT-E* may also be adapted for underweight patients, generally by prolonging the treatment (usually up to 40 weeks), and conducting twice-weekly sessions to address the typical low motivation to change and the need for a healthy weight, until the patient is consistently gaining weight. Outpatient CBT-E programmes for adolescents are similar to those designed for adults, but tend to be shorter, as change often occurs more quickly (e.g. with underweight patients 30 sessions may well be sufficient) [25]. Where possible, such programmes also feature parental involvement, generally in a single assessment session with the parents alone within the first 2 weeks, and then a series of brief (15–20 min) sessions together with the patient, scheduled immediately after an individual session, and continued throughout the course of treatment [26].

If patients are having difficulty modifying their eating habits in response to conventional outpatient CBT-E, but do not require hospitalization, they could benefit from *intensive outpatient CBT-E*. This contains additional CBT-E strategies and procedures, some developed specifically for this group of patients. For instance, patients may be offered three supervised daily meals on weekdays, twice-weekly individual CBT-E sessions, consultations with a CBT-E-trained dietician to plan and review weekend meals, and regular reviews with a CBT-E-trained physician [27, 28]. If patients cannot be managed safely on an outpatient basis, however, *inpatient CBT-E* may be more suitable. Described in detail elsewhere [27, 29], this adopts the main strategies and procedures of CBT-E, but with three main differences. First and foremost, the treatment is delivered by a specifically trained multidisciplinary team of physicians, psychologists, dieticians, and nurses. Assistance with eating is also provided during the initial weeks of treatment, and, although treatment is based on individual CBT-E sessions, some elements are administered in a group format. The inpatient CBT-E programme lasts 20 weeks, comprising 13 weeks of inpatient treatment and 7 weeks of day-hospital, followed by 20 weeks of post-inpatient outpatient CBT-E.

23.6 CBT-E Clinical Services

The adaptability of this treatment to different levels and settings of care, and the fact that it is suitable for treating adults and adolescents from all eating disorder diagnostic categories, has led to the establishment of "umbrella" clinical services based entirely on CBT-E. This approach, called "multistep CBT-E" [28], was pioneered by Villa Garda Hospital (Italy) and adopted soon after in the Netherlands, Norway, Sweden, and the USA. Similar strategies and procedures are administered at different levels of care, and the only difference between the various "steps" is the *intensiveness* of treatment, with less unwell patients being treated using outpatient CBT-E procedures, the more severely affected being channelled directly to inpatient CBT-E, and intensive outpatient CBT-E being used as third option for those unsuited to either.

In comparison with the traditional clinical services available (often eclectic, rather than evidence-based), a clinical service designed entirely around CBT-E offers two major advantages. First, patients are treated with a well-delivered, scientifically valid treatment; and, second, problems associated with transitions from outpatient to intensive treatment and vice versa (which may be confusing and disruptive) are minimized.

23.7 The CBT-E Body Image Module

CBT-E places great emphasis on addressing overvaluation of shape and weight and its expressions through a specific "body image module" featuring specific integrated multimodal strategies and procedures [15] (Table 23.1). The module, which is described in the main Fairburn's CBT-E guide [15], usually forms part of Stage Three of the 20-session version of the treatment, or Step Two of 40-session version, i.e. when underweight patients reach a BMI of 17.5 kg/m^2.

Table 23.1 Main strategies and procedures of the CBT-E body image module

1. Identifying overvaluation and its consequences
2. Enhancing the importance of other self-evaluation domains
3. Reducing the importance of shape and weight
(a) Addressing body checking
(b) Addressing body avoidance
(c) Addressing feeling fat
4. Exploring the origins of overvaluation of shape and weight

23.7.1 Identifying Overvaluation and Its Consequences

Patients first need to be educated on the concept of self-evaluation. In order for them to draw up their personal self-evaluation schema, the therapist helps the patient generate a list of life areas that are important to their self-worth. Once the list has been drawn up, the therapist should then go on to explore with the patient the relative importance of each of the identified self-evaluation domains, ranking them and sketching out a provisional pie chart. Each slice of the pie is used to represent the relative importance that the patient attaches to that area of life in their self-evaluation schema (Fig. 23.2), which can be discerned from the intensity and duration of the patients' response to things going badly in each area.

This schema provides the patient with a visual representation of the excessive importance they give to shape, weight and eating control, and can be used by the therapist to elicit the advantages and disadvantages of using a system of self-evaluation based predominantly on that domain. Through this type of analysis, the patient is led to the conclusion that, although having one predominant self-evaluation domain may have short-term advantages—it is simpler to gauge self-worth via a single, controllable, and measurable domain, it is in fact a dysfunctional

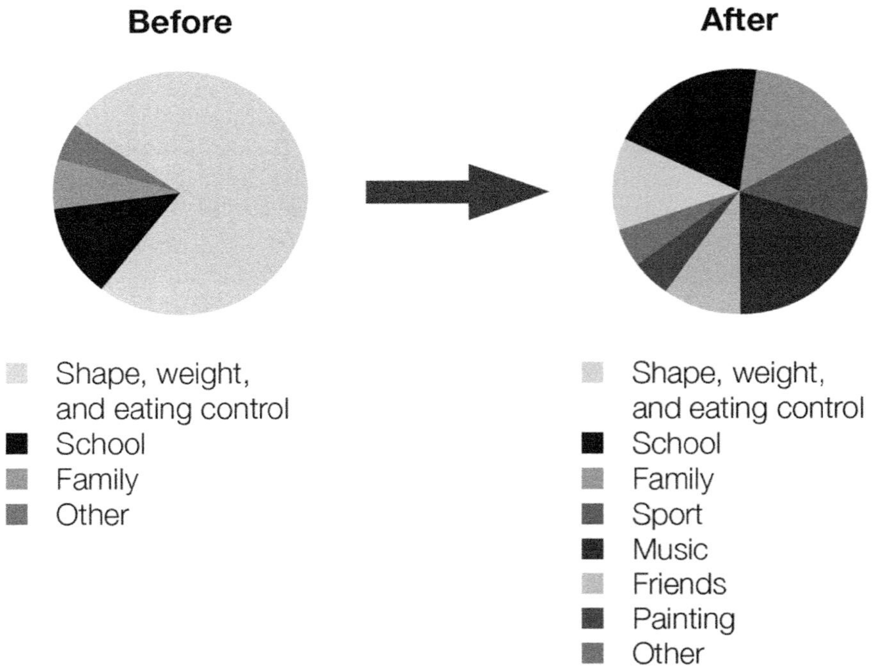

Fig. 23.2 The self-evaluation schema of a young woman with an eating disorder before and after the body image module

form of self-evaluation in the long term. Indeed, while multiple means of judging self-worth (e.g. school marks, relationships, sports performance, personal qualities) may be less easy to control, the single-minded pursuit of "thinness" severely marginalizes other important aspects of life (e.g. relationships, school, work, hobbies). It can also be linked directly or indirectly to behaviours that characterize and maintain eating problems (e.g. strict dieting, binge-eating episodes), and produces severe physical and psychosocial complications. Furthermore, although a single criterion may improve mood when things are going well, if something goes wrong (e.g. weight gain or a binge-eating episode) it inevitably leads to a collapse of self-worth.

Having thus illustrated to the patient that a stable, balanced self-evaluation system is preferable, the therapist then helps them to create an "extended" personal formulation, which includes the main expressions of shape and weight overvaluation that are fuelling their preoccupation, namely *body checking*, *body avoidance*, *feeling fat*, and marginalization of other areas of life, to be addressed by the treatment (see Fig. 23.1). Based on this formulation, the therapist helps the patient to devise a plan for tackling their concerns about shape and weight control through two complementary strategies: (1) enhancing the personal significance of other self-evaluation domains and (2) reducing the emphasis placed on shape and weight.

23.7.2 Enhancing the Importance of Other Self-Evaluation Domains

This involves helping patients to identify any activities or areas of life that they would like to work on, and assisting them to do so. The aim is for patients to increase the number and significance of other self-evaluation domains, particularly in the interpersonal sphere, and indirectly to reduce their overvaluation of shape and weight.

23.7.3 Reducing the Importance of Shape and Weight

A second direct strategy is to target the behavioural expressions of the patient's overvaluation of shape and weight. This is applied at the same time as enhancing the importance of other self-evaluation domains, and involves tackling behaviours linked to body checking, body avoidance, and feeling fat.

23.7.3.1 Addressing Body Checking

Body checking is common among healthy individuals, but in those who tend to overvalue shape and weight it manifests far more frequently and in very unusual ways, for example standing naked in front of the mirror for long periods of time and looking at the body from different angles [30]. Body checking maintains overvaluation of shape and weight through several mechanisms: (1) repeated scrutiny of "unsatisfactory" parts of the body tends to magnify apparent defects; (2) focusing on specific parts of the body in isolation rather than the body as a whole increases body dissatisfaction because it maintains the "problem" continually under the eyes; (3) paying superficial attention to the body parts of atypical persons (e.g. models or actresses), thin people, or those with idealized features (e.g. a flat stomach) confirms the patients' belief that their body is the wrong size and/or shape; and (4) frequently checking body weight may lead to erroneous interpretation of minimal changes (generally due to hydration status) as a sign of "getting fat", thereby promoting an increase in dietary restraint.

Patients are often not aware that they are engaging in these behaviours, and therefore need to be educated about the adverse effects of anomalous body checking. Likewise, patients should be asked to monitor for any episodes occurring over a two-day period in order that they can assess their frequency and implications. Typical body checking behaviours to address are dysfunctional mirror use, focusing on certain body parts (which magnify apparent defects), and comparison with thin, attractive people (a behaviour that can only lead to the conclusion that one is fat and unattractive). In cases where this type of unhealthy comparison is focused on celebrities shown in magazines, one useful strategy may be to point out to patients that such images are not representative of realistic body models (there are numerous examples of "The Photoshop Effect" on the internet which may be helpful in this regard). The importance of such strategies for addressing body checking should not be overlooked, particularly as one recent study has shown that CBT-E procedures to improve body image are associated with a reduction of shape and weight concerns in patients with anorexia nervosa [31].

23.7.3.2 Addressing Body Avoidance

Body avoidance is another typical expression of the overvaluation of shape and weight [30]. It acts to maintain body dissatisfaction and therefore the overvaluation of shape and weight itself. This is because not having a clear idea of one's appearance tends to foster concerns and fears about shape and weight. Body avoidance is also a huge obstacle to healthy socialization, intimacy with a partner, and everyday activities such as clothes shopping or swimming.

Typical body avoidance behaviours include avoiding: (1) checking body weight; (2) looking at one's own body; (3) touching one's own body; and (4) exposing one's body to others. In CBT-E, such behaviours are addressed via a "gradual exposure" strategy, in which the therapist helps patients to identify their own main manifestations of body avoidance. Thus enlightened, they can be assisted to plan and progressively enact exposure of specific body parts, beginning with those that cause less discomfort. In this way, patients gradually become accustomed to the sight and feel of their own body, and ultimately feel comfortable exposing it in the presence of others. Generally speaking, this process does not require many sessions, and leads to a marked reduction in the damaging behaviours, and attendant secondary benefits.

23.7.3.3 Addressing Feeling Fat

Many people report feeling fat, but the experience is extremely intense and frequent among those with eating disorders. This may be a consequence of their mislabelling certain emotions (like anxiety or depression), unpleasant physical states (e.g. feeling full, bloated, or sluggish), or body awareness (fuelled by body checking, wearing tight clothes and/or receiving comments on the body). CBT-E theorists suggest that excessive feeling fat could be a consequence of patients' longstanding and prolonged preoccupation with body shape [15], and as patients often equate feeling fat with being fat (even if they are of normal or low weight) it requires urgent attention. Feeling fat is addressed by encouraging patients to ask themselves what *else* they are feeling when they feel fat, and teaching them to address that emotion or circumstance directly.

23.8 Exploring the Origins of Overvaluation of Shape and Weight

Towards the end of treatment, patients should re-draw their self-evaluation schema to highlight any changes that they have been able to make. If good progress has been made, the pie chart will feature new slices, and that representing shape and weight will be smaller (Fig. 23.2). At this point it may also be helpful to explore with the patient how their overvaluation of shape and weight developed and evolved, enabling them to become consciously aware of how their eating problem arose, see how its early positive function (e.g. the feeling of being in control) may no longer be applicable, and distance themselves further from the eating disorder mindset.

23.9 Empirical Status of CBT-E for Eating Disorders

CBT-E has shown promise as a treatment for eating disorders in several samples of adult and adolescent outpatients and inpatients. For example, one controlled trial of CBT-E compared the broad and focused forms of the treatment with a delayed treatment group in a transdiagnostic sample (BMI >17.5 and <40.0 kg/m^2) from two treatment centres [32]. This study showed that patients treated using the two versions of CBT-E experienced substantial and equivalent change, with about two-thirds achieving remission by the end of treatment. These results were consistent with findings at 1-year follow-up, and the improvement noted was significantly greater than that achieved by those whose treatment was delayed. Interestingly, the broad version of CBT-E, which also addresses adjunctive maintenance mechanisms, was found to be superior to the focused form in patients in whom at least two of the four additional mechanisms were clinically significant at the beginning of treatment Stage Two, while the focused form was found to be more effective in the remainder.

Studies have compared the focused version of CBT-E with psychoanalytic psychotherapy [33] and integrative-affective therapy (ICAT) in adult patients with bulimia nervosa [34], with focal psychodynamic treatment in adult patients with anorexia [35], and with interpersonal psychotherapy (IPT) in a transdiagnostic sample (BMI >17.5 and <40.0 kg/m^2) [36]. These found that CBT-E was significantly more efficacious than psychoanalytic psychotherapy in bulimia nervosa and IPT in the transdiagnostic sample, but no significant difference was found between CBT-E and ICAT for bulimia nervosa or CBT-E and focal psychodynamic therapy for anorexia nervosa. However, it should be noted that the version of CBT-E compared with ICAT did not include the body image module (a central component of CBT-E), and the CBT-E compared with focal psychodynamic treatment comprised a fusion of the focused and broad forms of CBT-E with some general CBT procedures like social skills training and cognitive restructuring (not features of the standard outpatient CBT-E). This was combined with the option of hospitalization, which was shown to have played an important role in promoting weight gain in about one-third of patients. Moreover, in neither of these studies did the therapist receive supervision by an expert in CBT-E. However, in the most recent psychological treatment comparison study (the SWAN Study), CBT-E was found to be superior than both Maudsley Anorexia Nervosa Treatment for Adults (MANTRA) and Specialist Supportive Clinical Management (SSCM) in its ability to help patients achieve a physically healthy weight (59% at 12 month follow-up compared to 47.5% in SSCM and 44% in MANTRA) [37].

CBT-E has also shown promise in case series studies assessing its effects on adults [38], adolescents with anorexia nervosa [39], and not-underweight adolescents [40]. In these samples, about 40% of adults and almost 60% of adolescents with anorexia nervosa reached and/or maintained a normal weight range, while about 67.6% of not-underweight adolescents had reached minimal residual eating disorder psychopathology by the end of treatment. Very promising results have been also reported for patients with anorexia nervosa treated using inpatient CBT-E [41, 42], with about 40% of adults and 80% of adolescents having reached a healthy BMI 12 months after discharge, even those with anorexia nervosa classed as severe and enduring [43]. Finally, two uncontrolled studies in standard clinical settings indicate that the outcome for completers treated with CBT-E is similar to that reported in research trials, although treatment completion rates were lower [44, 45].

Conclusions

Adopting an individualized transdiagnostic approach to address patients' overvaluation of shape and weight and the other psychopathological maintenance mechanisms, irrespective of their initial DSM diagnosis, CBT-E has led to great advances in the treatment of eating disorders. However, many issues remain to be resolved. In order to identify who would benefit from treatment and under what conditions, it will be essential to uncover treatment response predictors and moderators, and treatment mediators need to be identified in order to provide better understanding of how CBT-E works. In particular, we need to ascertain how it manages to reduce the core overvaluation of shape and weight control. This should enable us to enhance the active components of treatment and discard redundant ones, thereby improving its efficacy even further. Last but not least, there is an urgent need to develop new strategies and procedures for disseminating CBT-E, since few patients with eating disorders are receiving it, despite the promising results achieved so far.

References

1. American Psychiatric Association. Diagnostic and statistical manual of mental disorders (DSM-5). Washington, DC: American Psychiatric Association; 2013.
2. Grilo CM. Why no cognitive body image feature such as overvaluation of shape/weight in the binge eating disorder diagnosis? Int J Eat Disord. 2013;46(3):208–11. https://doi.org/10.1002/eat.22082.
3. Thompson JK, Coovert MD, Richards KJ, Johnson S, Cattarin J. Development of body image, eating disturbance, and general psychological functioning in female adolescents: covariance structure modeling and longitudinal investigations. Int J Eat Disord. 1995;18(3):221–36.
4. Fairburn CG, Peveler RC, Jones R, Hope RA, Doll HA. Predictors of 12-month outcome in bulimia nervosa and the influence of attitudes to shape and weight. J Consult Clin Psychol. 1993;61(4):696–8.
5. Ricca V, Castellini G, Lo Sauro C, Mannucci E, Ravaldi C, Rotella F, et al. Cognitive-behavioral therapy for threshold and subthreshold anorexia nervosa: a three-year follow-up study. Psychother Psychosom. 2010;79(4):238–48. https://doi.org/10.1159/000315129.
6. Grilo CM, Masheb RM, Crosby RD. Predictors and moderators of response to cognitive behavioral therapy and medication for the treatment of binge eating disorder. J Consult Clin Psychol. 2012;80(5):897–906. https://doi.org/10.1037/a0027001.
7. Slade PD. What is body image? Behav Res Ther. 1994;32(5):497–502.
8. Thompson JK, Heinberg LJ, Altabe M, Tantleff-Dunn S. Exacting beauty. Washington, DC: American Psychological Association; 1999.
9. Farrell C, Shafran R, Fairburn CG. Body size estimation: testing a new mirror-based assessment method. Int J Eat Disord. 2003;34(1):162–71. https://doi.org/10.1002/eat.10174.
10. Cornelissen PL, Johns A, Tovee MJ. Body size over-estimation in women with anorexia nervosa is not qualitatively different from female controls. Body Image. 2013;10(1):103–11. https://doi.org/10.1016/j.bodyim.2012.09.003.
11. Smeets MAM. The rise and fall of body size estimation research in anorexia nervosa: a review and reconceptualization. Eur Eat Disord Rev. 1997;5:75–95.
12. Cooper PJ, Fairburn CG. Confusion over the core psychopathology of bulimia nervosa. Int J Eat Disord. 1993;13(4):385–9.
13. Fairburn CG, Cooper Z, Shafran R. Cognitive behaviour therapy for eating disorders: a "transdiagnostic" theory and treatment. Behav Res Ther. 2003;41(5):509–28.
14. Grilo CM, White MA, Gueorguieva R, Wilson GT, Masheb RM. Predictive significance of the overvaluation of shape/weight in obese patients with binge eating disorder: findings from a randomized controlled trial with 12-month follow-up. Psychol Med. 2013;43(6):1335–44. https://doi.org/10.1017/s0033291712002097.
15. Fairburn CG. Cognitive behavior therapy and eating disorders. New York: Guilford Press; 2008.
16. Masheb RM, Grilo CM. The nature of body image disturbance in patients with binge eating disorder. Int J Eat Disord. 2003;33(3):333–41. https://doi.org/10.1002/eat.10139.
17. Goldfein JA, Walsh BT, Midlarsky E. Influence of shape and weight on self-evaluation in bulimia nervosa. Int J Eat Disord. 2000;27(4):435–45.
18. Grilo CM, Hrabosky JI, White MA, Allison KC, Stunkard AJ, Masheb RM. Overvaluation of shape and weight in binge eating disorder and overweight controls: refinement of a diagnostic construct. J Abnorm Psychol. 2008;117(2):414–9. https://doi.org/10.1037/0021-843x.117.2.414.
19. Milos G, Spindler A, Schnyder U, Fairburn CG. Instability of eating disorder diagnoses: prospective study. Br J Psychiatry. 2005;187:573–8. https://doi.org/10.1192/bjp.187.6.573.

20. Smink FR, van Hoeken D, Hoek HW. Epidemiology, course, and outcome of eating disorders. Curr Opin Psychiatry. 2013;26(6):543–8. https://doi.org/10.1097/YCO.0b013e328365a24f.
21. Cooper PJ, Steere J. A comparison of two psychological treatments for bulimia nervosa: implications for models of maintenance. Behav Res Ther. 1995;33(8):875–85.
22. Fairburn CG, Jones R, Peveler RC, Hope RA, O'Connor M. Psychotherapy and bulimia nervosa. Longer-term effects of interpersonal psychotherapy, behavior therapy, and cognitive behavior therapy. Arch Gen Psychiatry. 1993;50(6):419–28.
23. Fairburn CG, Stice E, Cooper Z, Doll HA, Norman PA, O'Connor ME. Understanding persistence in bulimia nervosa: a 5-year naturalistic study. J Consult Clin Psychol. 2003;71(1):103–9.
24. Tabri N, Murray HB, Thomas JJ, Franko DL, Herzog DB, Eddy KT. Overvaluation of body shape/weight and engagement in non-compensatory weight-control behaviors in eating disorders: is there a reciprocal relationship? Psychol Med. 2015;45(14):2951–8. https://doi.org/10.1017/s0033291715000896.
25. Calugi S, Dalle Grave R, Sartirana M, Fairburn CG. Time to restore body weight in adults and adolescents receiving cognitive behaviour therapy for anorexia nervosa. J Eat Disord. 2015;3:21. https://doi.org/10.1186/s40337-015-0057-z.
26. Dalle Grave R, Cooper Z. Enhanced cognitive behaviour treatment adapted for younger patients. In: Wade T, editor. Encyclopedia of feeding and eating disorders. Singapore: Springer; 2016.
27. Dalle Grave R. Intensive cognitive behavior therapy for eating disorders. Hauppauge, NY: Nova; 2012.
28. Dalle Grave R. Multistep cognitive behavioral therapy for eating disorders: theory, practice, and clinical cases. New York: Jason Aronson; 2013.
29. Dalle Grave R, Bohn K, Hawker D, Fairburn CG. Inpatient, day patient and two forms of outpatient CBT-E. In: Fairburn CG, editor. Cognitive behavior therapy and eating disorders. New York: Guilford Press; 2008. p. 231–44.
30. Shafran R, Fairburn CG, Robinson P, Lask B. Body checking and its avoidance in eating disorders. Int J Eat Disord. 2004;35(1):93–101. https://doi.org/10.1002/eat.10228.
31. Calugi S, El Ghoch M, Dalle Grave R. Body-checking behaviours and treatment outcomes in anorexia nervosa. Int J Eat Disord. 2017;50(4):437–41. https://doi.org/10.1002/eat.22677.
32. Fairburn CG, Cooper Z, Doll HA, O'Connor ME, Bohn K, Hawker DM, et al. Transdiagnostic cognitive-behavioral therapy for patients with eating disorders: a two-site trial with 60-week follow-up. Am J Psychiatry. 2009;166(3):311–9. https://doi.org/10.1176/appi.ajp.2008.08040608.
33. Poulsen S, Lunn S, Daniel SI, Folke S, Mathiesen BB, Katznelson H, et al. A randomized controlled trial of psychoanalytic psychotherapy or cognitive-behavioral therapy for bulimia nervosa. Am J Psychiatry. 2014;171(1):109–16. https://doi.org/10.1176/appi.ajp.2013.12121511.
34. Wonderlich SA, Peterson CB, Crosby RD, Smith TL, Klein MH, Mitchell JE, et al. A randomized controlled comparison of integrative cognitive-affective therapy (ICAT) and enhanced cognitive-behavioral therapy (CBT-E) for bulimia nervosa. Psychol Med. 2014;44(3):543–53. https://doi.org/10.1017/s0033291713001098.
35. Zipfel S, Wild B, Gross G, Friederich HC, Teufel M, Schellberg D, et al. Focal psychodynamic therapy, cognitive behaviour therapy, and optimised treatment as usual in outpatients with anorexia nervosa (ANTOP study): randomised controlled trial. Lancet. 2014;383(9912):127–37. https://doi.org/10.1016/s0140-6736(13)61746-8.
36. Fairburn CG, Bailey-Straebler S, Basden S, Doll HA, Jones R, Murphy R, et al. A transdiagnostic comparison of enhanced cognitive behaviour therapy (CBT-E) and interpersonal psychotherapy in the treatment of eating disorders. Behav Res Ther. 2015;70:64–71. https://doi.org/10.1016/j.brat.2015.04.010.
37. Byrne S, Wade T, Hay P, Touyz S, Fairburn CG, Treasure J, et al. A randomised controlled trial of three psychological treatments for anorexia nervosa. Psychol Med. 2017:1–11. https://doi.org/10.1017/s0033291717001349.
38. Fairburn CG, Cooper Z, Doll HA, O'Connor ME, Palmer RL, Dalle Grave R. Enhanced cognitive behaviour therapy for adults with anorexia nervosa: a UK-Italy study. Behav Res Ther. 2013;51(1):R2–8. https://doi.org/10.1016/j.brat.2012.09.010.

39. Dalle Grave R, Calugi S, Doll HA, Fairburn CG. Enhanced cognitive behaviour therapy for adolescents with anorexia nervosa: an alternative to family therapy? Behav Res Ther. 2013;51(1):R9–R12. https://doi.org/10.1016/j.brat.2012.09.008.
40. Dalle Grave R, Calugi S, Sartirana M, Fairburn CG. Transdiagnostic cognitive behaviour therapy for adolescents with an eating disorder who are not underweight. Behav Res Ther. 2015;73:79–82. https://doi.org/10.1016/j.brat.2015.07.014.
41. Dalle Grave R, Calugi S, El Ghoch M, Conti M, Fairburn CG. Inpatient cognitive behavior therapy for adolescents with anorexia nervosa: immediate and longer-term effects. Front Psychiatry. 2014;5:14. https://doi.org/10.3389/fpsyt.2014.00014.
42. Dalle Grave R, Calugi S, Conti M, Doll H, Fairburn CG. Inpatient cognitive behaviour therapy for anorexia nervosa: a randomized controlled trial. Psychother Psychosom. 2013;82(6): 390–8. https://doi.org/10.1159/000350058.
43. Calugi S, El Ghoch M, Dalle Grave R. Intensive enhanced cognitive behavioural therapy for severe and enduring anorexia nervosa: a longitudinal outcome study. Behav Res Ther. 2016;89:41–8. https://doi.org/10.1016/j.brat.2016.11.006.
44. Byrne SM, Fursland A, Allen KL, Watson H. The effectiveness of enhanced cognitive behavioural therapy for eating disorders: an open trial. Behav Res Ther. 2011;49(4):219–26. https://doi.org/10.1016/j.brat.2011.01.006.
45. Knott S, Woodward D, Hoefkens A, Limbert C. Cognitive behaviour therapy for bulimia nervosa and eating disorders not otherwise specified: translation from randomized controlled trial to a clinical setting. Behav Cogn Psychother. 2015;43(6):641–54. https://doi.org/10.1017/s1352465814000393.

Feminist Perspectives on the Etiology and Treatment of Body Dissatisfaction, Eating, and Weight-Related Disorders

24

Melinda A. Green

24.1 A Feminist Conceptualization of Etiology

A feminist conceptualization of the etiology of body dissatisfaction, eating, and weight-related disorders rests upon a greater understanding of the sociocultural forces which dictate appearance-related ideals and how these culturally prescribed ideals differ as a function of gender [1, 2]. It also necessitates a cultural analysis of the changing body ideals across place and time and their relation to changing gender roles [1, 2].

First and foremost, it is essential to recognize over 90% of patients with eating disorders are women and girls [3]. Men and boys are also affected by eating disorders but at a far lower rate. Men comprise approximately 10% of the patient population, with isolated subsets of men showing greater risk [3, 4]. Existing research indicates sexual minority men are at particular risk; eating disorder symptoms are as common among gay and bisexual men as they are among heterosexual, bisexual, and lesbian women [4]. That said, eating disorder diagnoses display among the largest discrepant gender ratio of any form of mental illness and affect women and girls at a much higher rate compared to men and boys.

This lopsided gender ratio may be explained in several ways. There may be unique genetic and other biological risk factors which predispose women and girls to struggle at an increased rate with body dissatisfaction and eating disorders compared to men and boys. Alternately, socialization forces could significantly predispose women and girls to greater risk. These fundamental etiological questions reflect the historic nature versus nurture debate. Existing science dictates any reasonable solution to this debate assumes both forces play a role. The question then becomes which force is exerting a greater impact and via what mechanisms.

M. A. Green
Body Dissatisfaction and Eating Disorder Research Laboratory, Department of Psychology, Cornell College, Mt Vernon, IA, USA
e-mail: mgreen@cornellcollege.edu

M. Cuzzolaro, S. Fassino (eds.), *Body Image, Eating, and Weight*,
https://doi.org/10.1007/978-3-319-90817-5_24

A feminist analysis has historically focused on sociocultural forces which predispose increased risk for eating disorders and body dissatisfaction among girls and women; therefore, sociocultural etiological factors and their interaction with biological vulnerabilities reflect the focus of this chapter.

Volumes of research support the importance of sociocultural forces in the development and maintenance of eating disorders. In order to begin understand the relevant forces at play, a historical perspective is required.

24.2 Historical Perspectives

In earlier eras, and still in some non-Westernized countries today, the ideal feminine form was robust. Ample body weight was an indicator of wealth, reflecting the plentiful food sources and leisurely lifestyles of those with abundant financial resources. Eager to herald and model indicators of wealth, women and girls aspired to attain fuller figures. Thinness was viewed with an attitude of disdain and the prevalence of eating disorders was relatively low [1].

This largely derogatory view of thinness dramatically changed in Westernized cultures in the latter half of the twentieth century. Food-related resources, labor saving devices, and sedentary lifestyles became increasingly commonplace. The ability to store excess energy as fat was no longer a luxury reserved for the wealthy. Levels of obesity and overweight increased significantly and the feminine appearance ideal shifted. The fashion industry, the mass media, and other influential socialization forces began to model and promote a much thinner ideal female body type [5]. In a matter of a few short decades, the ideal feminine body type morphed significantly and socialization forces of the modern era dictated a level of thinness that could not be attained by the majority of women via healthy means.

During this era, the bodyweights of sociocultural icons of feminine beauty plunged. The majority of models, actresses, and centerfolds displayed bodies which placed them in the underweight or severely underweight categories according to World Health Organization guidelines. Katzmarzyk and Davis [6] examined the body mass indices (BMIs) of Playboy centerfolds for two consecutive decades (1978–1998). Their examination revealed 70% of the centerfolds were underweight and 77.5% were less than 85% of their ideal body weight. Many Western female beauty icons of this modern era operated at the margins of health in pursuit of extreme thinness. As weights of beauty icons decreased, disordered eating, eating disorders, and body dissatisfaction became widespread among women and girls exposed to these thin images [7].

Many researchers have examined the relationship between the changing bodyweights of female beauty icons of this modern era and the risk of eating disorders among women and girls. Results indicate the lay public, habitually exposed to thin images, and repeatedly seeing those thin images linked to positive outcomes, developed a great liking for thinness and the social rewards associated with it [7].

24.3 Consequences of the Thin-Ideal

The cultural acceptance of thinness as the ideal feminine body type carries many consequences. Several empirical studies have established the link between exposure to the media thin-ideal [7], body dissatisfaction, and an increased risk for eating disorders. Meta-analytic findings indicate body dissatisfaction is significantly higher among women, especially young women, after viewing images of thin models compared to average size models, plus size models, or neutral objects [8].

Becker and colleagues [9] examined the impact of the media thin-ideal via a novel study. The researchers evaluated the disordered eating attitudes and behaviors of two samples of Fijian girls before and after the introduction of Westernized television into the culture. Nadroga, Fiji was selected for the study because, prior to the introduction of Westernized television, the ideal feminine body type was robust, measures to induce thinness were discouraged, and the prevalence of eating disorders was very low. After the introduction of Westernized television, rates of disordered eating among Fijian schoolgirls dramatically increased. During interviews, the schoolgirls revealed they were seeking thinness in order to attain thin bodies similar to those possessed by the actresses on their favorite Westernized television shows.

As the thin-ideal became all-pervasive during this modern era, body dissatisfaction among women became so widespread that researchers referred to it as "normative discontent" since it now reflected the norm, rather than the exception, for the majority of women [10]. As the ideal spread, women and girls in Westernized cultures were bombarded by socialization forces which heralded and rewarded a thin body-type. These influences persist today and continue to largely define the worth of women and girls across socialization contexts in Westernized cultures.

24.4 Rewarding Thin Bodies

Conformity to the thin-ideal is associated with rewards in the educational, occupational, and relational realms. Deviations from the thin-ideal are associated with a host of punishments and lost opportunities. Women are much more likely than men to be punished for failing to conform to the thin-ideal [11]. This punishment occurs across socialization contexts and occurs at a lower level of excess weight compared to weight-related punishments experienced by men.

Data from the occupational realm indicate women are 16 times more likely than men to report experiencing discrimination attributable to excess weight in the occupational realm [12] and verified punishments occur at a much lower level of excess weight for women compared to men. Cawley [13] indicated significantly overweight women were paid less than their average weight counterparts. Baum and Ford [14] reported women experienced a wage penalty tied to excess weight that was significantly higher than the weight penalty experienced by men and it occurred at a lower weight level. Findings were replicated by Fonda et al. [15] who demonstrated obese and overweight women showed significantly decreased net worth at retirement-age compared to thin women. The trend was reversed for men; findings indicated overweight and obese men showed higher net worth at retirement-age.

Taken together, results suggest women who are overweight or obese experience significant discrimination in the occupational realm and therefore, experience considerable pressure to obtain and maintain a thin body-type in order to preserve financial and occupational success. See Fikkan and Rothblum [11] for a comprehensive review of data examining wage discrimination as a function of gender and weight. Occupational and economic weight-related pressures represent one socialization realm in which women get a clear message that a thin body is necessary for reward and success.

Data from the educational realm further reiterate the ubiquitous nature of socialization forces which emphasize the thin-ideal. Many educational studies reflect the consequences women and girls face when they deviate from this cultural ideal. Crosnoe [16] reported young obese women were significantly less likely to pursue postsecondary education even after controlling for academic ability, socioeconomic status, and other relevant indicators which traditionally predict educational aspirations. Obesity was not a significant predictor of pursuit of postsecondary education among young men. Data from the relational realm further elucidate pressures women and girls receive regarding weight. Data indicate men in romantic relationships are significantly more likely than women to rank their preferences for romantic partners based on weight [17]. Therefore, overweight and obese heterosexual women and sexual minority men encounter greater expectations for low bodyweight due, in part, to the fact that their preferred sexual audience preferences thin romantic partners.

Weight-based discrimination also punishes women and girls in other socialization realms. Within the political arena, perceptions of larger women are disparaging. Miller and Lundgren [18] found obese female political candidates were evaluated negatively compared to non-obese candidates. This trend was reversed for obese male candidates, who were rated more highly than non-obese male candidates. Amy and colleagues [19] demonstrated obese women were less likely to receive screening tests for gynecological cancer because of perceived barriers related to their weight. Reluctance to seek pelvic exams and breast exams has been linked directly to excess weight and body dissatisfaction among obese women [20].

Powerful socialization forces across multiple realms provide sustained, habitual reinforcements and punishments which keep women and girls preoccupied with weight and thinness. Failure to conform to the cultural thin-ideal exerts a negative impact on the lives of women and girls across these many facets of everyday life. The influence of the cultural thin-ideal is particularly noteworthy in Westernized cultures which herald appearance as a key indicator of social worth. To the extent that a culture defines one's social worth in terms of appearance, overweight and obese women and girls are viewed to be "less worthy" than their thin counterparts.

24.5 The Cultural Objectification of Women and Girls

The effects of this toxic body environment are exacerbated by the pervasiveness of the objectification of women and girls in Westernized cultures. Cultural objectification refers to the tendency to reduce the social worth of women and girls to their sexual appeal. The frequency with which women and girls are objectified in Western cultures is increasing, as reflected in mass media portrayals and consumer products which promote women and girls as sexual objects whose appearances are used for the gratification of others [21].

The objectification of women and girls occurs across most socialization contexts. It is ubiquitous in nearly every form of media communication, including television, video games, movies, social media, music, commercials, and other forms of marketing. Objectification is apparent even in socialization contexts traditionally associated with the advancement of women and girls, including competitive sports. The passage of Title IX and the development and advancement of women's professional sports teams represented an extension of the rights and opportunities of women into areas that were previously off limits. Participation in sports confers many psychological and physical health benefits for participants; this pertinent legislation and its associated opportunities allowed women and girls a greater opportunity to experience the many benefits of participating in organized sports.

Objectification has become increasingly commonplace in this traditionally progressive domain of competitive sports. Fink and Kensicki [22] conducted a content analysis of sports media coverage of female and male athletes in *Sports Illustrated (SI)* from 1997 to 1999 and found only 10% of the photographs portrayed female athletes. Of this 10%, half the photos featured sexually objectified female athletes; only 2% of the photographs of male athletes were sexually objectified. There is additional evidence that this situation has worsened in subsequent years, with female athletes being revered as sexual objects rather than talented athletes [21]. This is a missed opportunity for many girls and women. Instead of finding strength and body competence through increased participation in sports, female athletes are again met with messages which reduce their bodies to sexual objects for the gratification of others.

The widespread promotion of this thin, objectified ideal contributes to marked body dissatisfaction and disordered eating among women and girls who internalize this ideal [23]. This process is referred to as trait self-objectification and is linked to a host of negative psychological outcomes. Girls and women exhibiting high levels of trait self-objectification exhibit habitual body monitoring, maladaptive appearance-based social comparison, body shame, depression, anxiety, and an increased risk for eating disorders.

24.6 Relation to Gender Roles

The timing of the introduction of the thin-ideal into Westernized cultures is often of considerable interest to feminist theorists who explore the sociocultural etiology of eating disorders. Promotion of this thin-ideal occurred during an era in many Westernized countries when women's gender roles were shifting decidedly. The second World War required dramatic shifts in the labor force to support war efforts in many developed countries and women began entering the workforce in unprecedented numbers while men fought on the battlefields of Europe. When the war ended, many women chose to remain in the labor force and traditional gender roles started to shift precipitously. The civil rights movement followed shortly thereafter, and advocacy efforts and key advances in the second wave of the women's movement occurred in the United States. During the same time period, the ideal feminine body shifted from one that was ample and robust to one that was thin and objectified [1].

Thinness and objectification became key determinants of social worth for women and girls and started to be widely promoted in fashion and mass media outlets in the 1960s and 1970s. It is curious that this ubiquitous sociocultural pressure which equated thinness with feminine social worth temporally coincided with key advances in the women's movement. Many feminist analyses do not view this to be coincidental. In a time period in which women were entering the workforce in unprecedented numbers, sociocultural forces were encouraging them to shrink in physical form—to literally "take up less space." Some theorists view the cultural thin-ideal as a concerted effort to oppress women, hypothesizing that keeping women weight-obsessed effectively distracted them from other ambitious endeavors, such as striving for educational or occupational achievements [1]. Others view these as two separate cultural phenomenon which are temporally, but not causally, related.

This debate is not easily resolved, but relevant research does exist. Nasser and colleagues [24] note in their edited book many examples of the relationship between rapidly shifting cultural norms, including gender-related norms in many cultures, and a concomitant increase in the pervasiveness of the thin-ideal and the prevalence of eating disorders. If, as these data suggest, eating disorder represents a syndrome precipitated by shifting gender-related norms and cultural ideals, then prescriptions for social change may be fostered by social advocacy efforts.

24.7 Prescriptions for Social Change

Research indicates exposure to a wide variety of body types in mass media portrayals of women and girls is critical to reducing body dissatisfaction and disordered eating behaviors among women and girls [25]. Results suggest reducing risk for eating disorders and body dissatisfaction may be as simple as ensuring that average size models and larger models are represented in the media in positive ways. In other words, media representations of women and girls should include diverse body types.

Alternative feminine body ideals have been largely absent in media representation during the modern era. When an alternative feminine body type is portrayed in the media, it is most often linked with hostility and negativity. For this reason, persons in Westernized cultures have been conditioned to show a cognitive bias toward underweight bodies and this tendency is especially ingrained among women with eating disorders [26].

There are many different approaches to curbing the negative impact of the media thin-ideal and encouraging the introduction of diverse body types into mainstream Westernized media. The first is via regulation and policy. Several countries have now developed public policies which require public disclosure when media images are photo edited to make models and actresses appear thinner. Because such disclosures detract from the quality of the image, these policies have the net effect of discouraging the use of photo editing which promotes extreme thinness.

While a notable approach, many of the models and actresses recruited for media portrayals are very thin prior to photo editing. Therefore, the discouragement of photo editing alone, though an important step, is not sufficient to promote the proliferation of larger and average sized images. This can occur via several methods. First, models and actresses may be required to maintain a certain body mass index to continue to appear in high profile media roles. Several countries have implemented such policies. The potential downside of such policies is that these practices may discriminate against the small percentage of women who possess underweight body types via genetic means alone (even when engaged in healthy eating and weight-related behaviors).

A second alternative is to introduce policy which requires corporations to integrate models and actresses with diverse body types into their marketing campaigns, movies, videogames, and other media products. For example, of all female targets appearing in a certain product, there could be a required percentage of diverse body types represented.

If policymakers are not sufficiently progressive on such issues, change could also be initiated at the level of the consumer. Intentionality on the part of companies and corporations is often driven by market forces motivated by changes in consumer behavior. In that regard, it may be important for advocacy efforts to begin with the consumer.

Media literacy campaigns represent one effective way to educate the consumer regarding the health risks associated with the objectified media thin-ideal [27]. Prevention and treatment programs which incorporate media literacy components which discourage the objectified thin-ideal may be particularly helpful in combatting body dissatisfaction and disordered eating among women and girls. Dissonance-based programs have been shown to be particularly effective in this regard [7].

24.8 Implications for Treatment and Prevention

Based on Festinger's [28] theory of cognitive dissonance, dissonance-based eating disorder interventions instruct symptomatic participants to voluntarily adopt verbal, written, and behavioral exercises designed to denounce the thin-ideal [29]. These counterattitudinal exercises evoke psychological tension (i.e., cognitive dissonance). Participants are motivated to reduce this tension via the adoption of consistent attitudes and behaviors which denounce thin-ideal internalization and reduce body dissatisfaction and eating disorder symptomatology [29, 30].

The *Body Project* is a dissonance-based eating disorder prevention program which has received significant empirical support across multiple trials (see [29, 31]). The *Body Project* consists of four 60-min group sessions (led by a trained facilitator) and nine homework assignments which incorporate verbal, written, and behavioral exercises designed to induce dissonance and reduce thin-ideal internalization. The *Body Project* has demonstrated greater reductions in eating disorder risk factors (thin-ideal internalization, body dissatisfaction, dietary restriction, and negative affect) and eating disorder symptoms (binge behaviors, purge behaviors, maladaptive exercise, and dietary restriction) compared to assessment-only control conditions or alternative interventions among women with subclinical symptoms [32]. The efficacy of the program has also been demonstrated recently within the treatment realm [33]. The program has online version available for ease of administration, cost-effectiveness, and more widespread availability [32].

Conclusion

Effective treatment and prevention efforts which reduce thin-ideal internalization, decrease self-objectification, and decrease maladaptive social comparison are essential to address sociocultural risk factors for disordered eating. Feminist theorists dedicated to the successful treatment and prevention of body dissatisfaction and eating disorders should continue to develop, test, and refine such interventions in order to continue to improve their efficacy. Practitioners of feminist techniques should continue to implement these empirically supported interventions to effectively assist clients struggling with these disorders.

References

1. Fallon P, Katzman MA, Wooley SC. Feminist perspectives on eating disorders. New York: Guilford Press; 1994.
2. Malson H, Burns M. Critical feminist approaches to eating disorders. New York: Routledge; 2009.
3. American Psychiatric Association. Diagnostic and statistical manual of mental disorders. 5th ed. Arlington, VA: American Psychiatric Publishing; 2013.
4. Davids CM, Green MA. A preliminary investigation of body dissatisfaction and eating disorder symptomatology with bisexual individuals. Sex Roles. 2011;65:533–47. https://doi.org/10.1007/s11199-011-9963-y.
5. Morris AM, Katzman DK. The impact of media on eating disorders in children and adolescents. Pediatr Child Health. 2003;8:287–9.
6. Katzmarzyk PT, Davis C. Thinness and body shape of Playboy centerfolds from 1978 to 1998. Int J Obes Relat Metab Disord. 2001;25:590–2.
7. Stice E, Shaw H. Adverse effects of the media portrayed thin-ideal on women and linkages to bulimic symptomatology. J Soc Clin Psychol. 1994;13:288–308. https://doi.org/10.1521/jscp.1994.13.3.288.
8. Groesz LM, Levine MP, Murnen SK. The effect of experimental presentation of thin media images on body satisfaction: a meta-analytic review. Int J Eat Disord. 2002;31:1–16.
9. Becker AE, Burwell RA, Gilman SE, Herzog DB, Hamburg P. Eating behaviours and attitudes following exposure to television among ethnic Fijian adolescent girls. Br J Psychiatry. 2002;180:509–14.
10. Rodin J, Silberstein L, Striegel-Moore R. Women and weight: A normative discontent. Nebr Symp Motiv. 1984;32:267–307.
11. Fikkan J, Rothblum E. Is fat a feminist issue? Exploring the gendered nature of weight bias. Sex Roles. 2012;66:575–97.
12. Roehling MV, Roehling PV, Pichler S. The relationship between body weight and perceived weight-related employment discrimination: the role or sex and race. J Vocat Behav. 2007;71:300–18. https://doi.org/10.1016/j.jvb.2007.04.008.

13. Cawley J. The impact of obesity on wages. J Hum Resour. 2004;39:451–74. https://doi.org/10.2307/3559022.
14. Baum CL, Ford WF. The wage effects of obesity: a longitudinal study. Health Econ. 2004;13:885–99. https://doi.org/10.1002/hec.881.
15. Fonda SJ, Fultz NH, Jenkins KR, Wheeler LM, Wray LA. Relationship of body mass and net worth for retirement-aged men and women. Res Aging. 2004;26:153–76. https://doi.org/10.1177/0164027503258739.
16. Crosnoe R. Gender, obesity, and education. Sociol Educ. 2007;80:241–60. https://doi.org/10.1177/003804070708000303.
17. Chen EY, Brown M. Obesity stigma in sexual relationships. Obes Res. 2005;13:1393–7.
18. Miller BJ, Lundgren JD. An experimental study of the role of weight bias in candidate evaluation. Obesity. 2010;18:712–8. https://doi.org/10.1038/oby.2009.492.
19. Amy NK, Aalborg A, Lyons P, Keranen L. Barriers to routine gynecological cancer screening for White and African-American obese women. Int J Obes. 2006;30:147–55. https://doi.org/10.1038/sj.ijo.0803105.
20. Puhl R, Brownell KD. Bias, discrimination, and obesity. Obes Res. 2001;9:788–805.
21. American Psychological Association Task Force on the Sexualization of Girls. Report of the APA task force on the sexualization of girls. 2007. http://www.apa.org/pi/women/programs/girls/report-full.pdf
22. Fink JS, Kensicki LJ. An imperceptible difference: visual and textual constructions of femininity in Sports Illustrated and Sports Illustrated for Women. Mass Commun Soc. 2002;5:317–39.
23. Fredrickson BL, Roberts T, Noll SM, Quinn DM, Twenge JM. That swimsuit becomes you: sex differences in self-objectification, restrained eating, and math performance. J Pers Soc Psychol. 1998;75:269–84.
24. Nasser M, Katzman M, Gordon R. Eating disorders and cultures in transition. New York: Taylor & Francis; 2001.
25. Want SC. Meta-analytic moderators of experimental exposure to media portrayals of women on female appearance satisfaction: social comparisons as automatic processes. Body Image. 2009;6:257–69. https://doi.org/10.1016/j.bodyim.2009.07.008.
26. Green MA, Rogers J, Ohrt T, Nguyen C, Blasko K, Martin A. Attentional bias to weight-related stimuli in disordered eating: cardiac and affective indicators. J Soc Clin Psychol. 2016;*35*(1):21–44. https://doi.org/10.1521/jscp.2016.35.1.21.
27. Brown JD, Witherspoon EM. The mass media and American adolescents' health. J Adolesc Health. 2002;31:153–70.
28. Festinger L. A theory of cognitive dissonance. Stanford, CT: Stanford University Press; 1957.
29. Stice E, Chase A, Stormer S, Appel A. A randomized trial of dissonance-based eating disorder prevention program. Int J Eat Disord. 2001;29:247–62.
30. Green M, Scott N, Diyankova I, Gasser C, Pederson E. Eating disorder prevention: an experimental comparison of high level dissonance, low level dissonance, and no-treatment control. Eat Disord. 2005;13:157–69. https://doi.org/10.1080/10640260590918955.
31. Stice E, Rohde P, Shaw H, Gau J. An effectiveness trail of a selected dissonance-based eating disorder prevention program for female high school students: long-term effects. J Consult Clin Psychol. 2011;79(4):500–8. https://doi.org/10.1037/a0024351.
32. Stice E, Rohde P, Durant S, Shaw H. A preliminary trial of a prototype internet dissonance-based eating disorder prevention program for young women with body image concerns. J Consult Clin Psychol. 2012;80:907–16. https://doi.org/10.1037/a0028016.
33. Green MA, Willis M, Fernandez-Kong K, Reyes S, Linkhart R, Johnson M, Thorne T, Kroska E, Woodward H, Lindberg J. Effect of a dissonance-based eating disorder program on cardiac risk. Health Psychol. 2016. Advance online publication.

Virtual Reality for the Treatment of Body Image Disturbances in Eating and Weight Disorders

25

Giuseppe Riva, Santino Gaudio, Silvia Serino, Antonios Dakanalis, Marta Ferrer-García, and José Gutiérrez-Maldonado

25.1 Introduction

25.1.1 Virtual Reality: A Definition

What is Virtual Reality (VR)? If we follow the Oxford English Dictionary, the meaning of VR is: "A computer-generated simulation of a lifelike environment that can be interacted with in a seemingly real or physical way by a person, esp. by means of responsive hardware such as a visor with screen or gloves with sensors." (online: http://www.oed.com/view/Entry/328583?redirectedFrom=virtual+reality).

G. Riva (✉) · S. Serino
Centro Studi e Ricerche di Psicologia della Comunicazione, Università Cattolica del Sacro Cuore, Milan, Italy

Applied Technology for Neuro-Psychology Lab, Istituto Auxologico Italiano, Milan, Italy
e-mail: giuseppe.riva@unicatt.it

S. Gaudio
Department of Neuroscience, Functional Pharmacology, Uppsala University, Uppsala, Sweden

Centre for Integrated Research (CIR), Area of Diagnostic Imaging, Università "Campus Bio-Medico di Roma", Rome, Italy

A. Dakanalis
Department of Medicine and Surgery, University of Milano Bicocca, Milan, Italy

Department of Brain and Behavioral Sciences, University of Pavia, Pavia, Italy

Department of Clinical Psychology and Psychobiology, University of Barcelona, Barcelona, Spain

Applied Technology for Neuro-Psychology Lab, Istituto Auxologico Italiano, Milan, Italy

M. Ferrer-García · J. Gutiérrez-Maldonado
Department of Clinical Psychology and Psychobiology, University of Barcelona, Barcelona, Spain

M. Cuzzolaro, S. Fassino (eds.), *Body Image, Eating, and Weight*,
https://doi.org/10.1007/978-3-319-90817-5_25

In this definition VR is described as a set of fancy technologies [1–3]: an interactive *3D visualization system* (a computer, a game console, or a smartphone) supported by *input tools* (trackers, gloves, joystick, mice, etc.) that continually report the position and movements of the users; and ***output tools*** (visual, aural, haptic, etc.) that immerse the user in the virtual environment.

On the basis of the hardware and software included in a VR system, it is possible to distinguish between:

- **Desktop VR**: It uses as main output tool a standard PC screen. The feeling of immersion can be improved through stereoscopic vision. Input tools usually include a mouse, joystick, or typical VR peripherals such as a data glove.
- **Fully Immersive VR**: It uses advanced output devices (head-mounted display, force feedback robotic arms, etc.) and a system of head/body tracking to guarantee the exact correspondence and co-ordination of users' movements with the feedback of the environment. In immersive VR, the user appears to be fully inserted in the computer-generated environment.
- **CAVE**: This is a small room where a computer-generated world is projected on the walls. The projection is made on both front and side walls. This solution is particularly suitable for collective VR experiences because it allows different people to share the same experience at the same time.

NASA recently provided a less technical definition of VR: "the use of computer technology to create the effect of an interactive three-dimensional world in which the objects have a sense of spatial presence. In this definition, 'spatial presence' means that the objects in the environment effectively have a location in three-dimensional space relative to and independent of your position. Note that this is an effect, not an illusion. The basic idea is to present the correct cues to your perceptual and cognitive system so that your brain interprets those cues as objects" out there "in the three-dimensional world". (Online: https://www.nas.nasa.gov/Software/VWT/vr.html).

In this view, what distinguishes VR from other media is the sense of "presence," i.e., the feeling of "being there," in the synthetic experience produced by the technology [4, 5]. While there is still no general consensus about what presence actually *is* from a psychological viewpoint (for an introduction to the subject, see [6]), it is fair to say that most investigators agree about what it is *not* [7, 8]. As underlined by Riva and colleagues [9–25] "presence is not the degree of technological immersion, it is not the same thing as emotional engagement, it is not absorption or attention or action; but all of these have a potential role in understanding the experience of presence in interaction – the experience of interacting with presence" (p. 1).

25.1.2 The Clinical Use of VR

The sense of presence and emotional engagement offered by VR can be a powerful tool for personal change because it provides a high level of personal efficacy and self-reflectiveness [26]. As underlined by Glantz and colleagues [27]: "One reason it is so difficult to get people to update their assumptions is that change often requires a prior step – recognizing the distinction between an assumption and a perception. Until revealed to be fallacious, assumptions constitute the world; they seem like perceptions, and as long as they do, they are resistant to change" (p. 96). On one side, VR offers synthetic worlds in which an individual can be placed and live a particular experience [28]. More, VR allows a higher level of self-reflectiveness than that provided by memory and imagination, and a higher level of control than that offered by direct "real" experience [29]. In fact, VR has also been described as an experiential form of imagery that is as effective as reality in inducing emotional responses [30].

These features clearly explain the increasing use of VR in clinical psychology. In a recent publication, Riva et al. [29] reported the available reviews and meta-analyses about the use of VR in clinical and health psychology. They were related to addictions (2 reviews, 1 meta-analysis; 53 studies), pain (4 reviews; 48 studies), anxiety disorders (3 reviews, 4 meta-analyses; 175 studies), stress-related disorders (4 reviews; 41 studies), depression (1 review and meta-analysis; 19 studies), EDs (3 reviews; 33 studies), schizophrenia and other psychotic disorders (2 reviews, 1 meta-analysis; 23 studies), and autism (2 reviews; 39 studies). The highest number of studies has been conducted in anxiety disorders and stress-related disorders, supporting the efficacy of VR in the treatment of phobias, stress management, post-traumatic stress disorder, panic disorder, and agoraphobia. The evidence for the treatment of social phobia is not definitive. The reviews related to addictions show that VR is effective in inducing craving to substances such as cocaine, alcohol, and tobacco, allowing its use in cue exposure treatments and to develop coping skills. In autism, the reviews support the use of VR to train social skills. This kind of training has also been used in patients with schizophrenia, and preliminary results are promising, but there is still no strong evidence for the efficacy of VR in the treatment of this disorder and other psychotic disorders. Similarly, there is only evidence for a moderate effect of the VR interventions on depression. As a pain reduction technique, VR has shown strong efficacy in short-term interventions, but little evidence exists for longer-term benefits. In EDs, the reviews performed to date show that VR cue exposure to food stimuli and VR body image treatments are effective [31]. We will discuss more in detail these results in the next paragraphs.

25.1.3 Virtual Reality Technology

The implementation of VR-based applications for clinical use has always depended heavily on the development of advanced technology. Consequently, for a long time the research in this area was limited by the cost of the technology required. Furthermore, the field was largely restricted to academic research and very few technology companies sought to transfer the results of this research into clinical VR applications.

Today, however, VR technology is advancing quickly. Both Oculus Rift (http://www.oculus.com) and HTC (https://www.htcvive.com/) are showcasing high-quality VR experiences at reasonable price points—less than $2000 for a fully configured system—which are now widely available to consumers [32]. Thus, the first major obstacle to the widespread use of the VR seems to have been overcome. The second one, the presence of technological difficulties, remains, but probably not for very long. The use of VR systems involves the management of complex devices that require a certain level of technological knowledge and the assistance of technical staff. Therefore, it is not surprising that some therapists and clinicians, especially veteran practitioners, are reluctant to introduce VR systems into their daily practice. However, this scenario is about to change largely due to the expansion of VR in the field of consumer electronics; the commercialization of VR systems among the general population will bring down costs and enhance the development of user-friendly devices. Furthermore, for younger generations the use of VR technology will be part of their everyday routine and the technical difficulties will disappear.

25.2 Virtual Reality Applications in Eating and Weight Disorders

As discussed widely in other chapters of this book, body image disturbance is a central feature of eating and weight disorders (EWDs) and plays an important role in the development, maintenance, and risk of relapse of these conditions [6, 29, 33, 34]. However, the study of body disturbances is not easy. In fact, our experience of the body is not direct (Fig. 25.1), but it is [35–37]:

- Mediated by perceptual information.
- Influenced by internal information.
- Recalibrated through stored implicit and explicit body representation (body memory).

More, body image distortion can be seen as a multidimensional construct (Fig. 25.1) that, according to neuroimaging studies [38–45], includes three different components: cognitive, affective, and perceptive. The cognitive and affective components of body image distortion are widely accepted and related both:

- *To brain dysfunctions* [37, 40, 46]: alterations of the prefrontal cortex, the amygdala, and the insula [47], and
- *To sociocultural issues* [41, 46, 48]: internalization of an ideal body figure [43], social body comparison [49–51], and self-objectification [52].

Recent different functional magnetic resonance imaging (fMRI) [53] also suggest a perceptual component of body image distortion. According to Gaudio and colleagues "several brain regions could be involved body image disturbances and may sustain an impaired integration between real and perceived internal/external state of one's own body in AN patients" (p. 582).

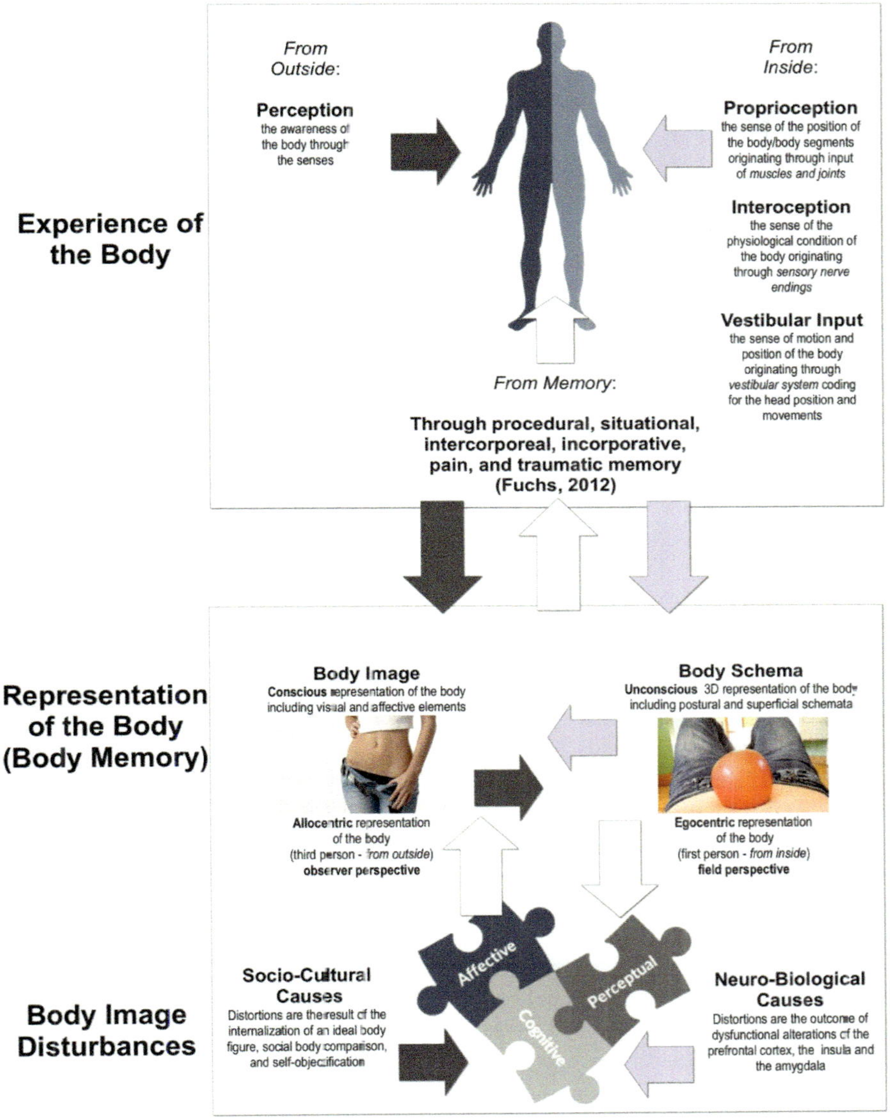

Fig. 25.1 From the experience of the body to body image disturbances

Given the complexity of body image, researchers usually target only one of the different components of body image disturbances [54–56]:

- *The perceptual distortion of body image*: the inability to perceive the size of the body accurately, and
- *The cognitive/affective body dissatisfaction*: the degree to which a person likes or dislikes the size and shape of his/her body and values it.

This complexity can also explain why body image disturbance is often overlooked in EWDs treatments, despite being considered a core feature of these disorders.

In this context, the development of VR has provided researchers and clinicians with a new technology that seems to be particularly well suited to the study, assessment, and treatment of body image disturbances for its ability of targeting all these dimensions. The use of immersive VR systems brings patients face to face with their virtual body in its actual size. More, VR simulates real-life situations in which different aspects of body image disturbances can be studied, assessed, and even treated in a secure, private, and controlled setting [57, 58]. Moreover, the possibility of developing three-dimensional figures that represent the body of the participants and whose size and shape can be modified enables patients to embody their mental representations of the different components of body image (e.g., perceived vs. ideal body image). Finally, VR allows bodily illusions [59–62]—the controlled illusory generation of unusual bodily feelings, such as the feeling of ownership over a virtual limb, that affect the experience of a body part or the entire body (i.e., body-swap illusion)—whose results have been presented in three recent reviews [63–65] and will be further discussed in the next paragraphs.

25.3 Virtual Reality for the Treatment of Body Image in EWDs: The Rationale

Most women are dissatisfied with their body [66]: one adolescent girl out of two reports body dissatisfaction [42]. For this reason, the "objectification theory" suggests a significant role of culture and society in the etiology of these disorders. Introduced by Fredrickson and Roberts [67], this theory suggests that our culture imposes a specific self-evaluation model—self-objectification—that defines women's behavioral and emotional responses [68].

At its simplest, the objectification theory holds that [69]:

1. There exists an objectified societal ideal of beauty (within a particular culture).
2. This is transmitted via a variety of sociocultural channels.
3. This ideal is then internalized by individuals.
4. Satisfaction (or dissatisfaction) with appearance will be a function of the extent to which individuals do (or do not) meet the ideal prescription.

According to Fredrickson and colleagues [70, 71], repeated experiences of sexual objectification—when women are treated as bodies that exist for the use and pleasure of others—cause them to gradually adopt an observer's perspective of their physical self; that is, they begin to treat themselves as an object to be looked at and evaluated on the basis of physical appearance. The self is so defined in terms of how the body appears to others.

The internalization of an observer's perspective on one's own body is labeled as "self-objectification" [72] and reduces a woman's worth to her perception of her body's semblance to cultural standards of attractiveness [69]. Self-objectification is typically manifested as persistent body surveillance or habitual monitoring of the body's outward appearance and is believed to lead to different negative experiential consequences such as body shame, social physique anxiety, lack of awareness of internal bodily states, and decreased peak motivational states/flow experiences [73, 74], and is recognized as the most robust risk factor for clinical and subclinical EWDs [43, 75].

There are two possible criticisms of this view. The first is that males, who apparently are less prone to self-objectification, also experience EWDs. Second, only a small subset of all the female and male subjects exposed to idealized body models develop clinically diagnosable EWDs [76].

Nevertheless, different recent studies have underlined the possible role of self-objectification in the etiology of male EWDs [43, 71, 76–78]. Specifically in males, self-objectification is manifested as body surveillance [79].

A possible response to the second criticism is offered by a new etiological model, i.e., the "*Allocentric Lock (AL) Theory*" [20, 52, 80–82]. This theory suggests that EWDs, including anorexia nervosa, are the outcome of a deficit in the processing and integration of multisensory bodily representations and signals [40, 83, 84] that alters the way the body is "experienced" and "remembered." Specifically, individuals with (or developing) this disorder may be locked to an allocentric (third person) disturbed memory of their body that, independently of its causes, is not more updated by experiential data, even after a successful diet and/or a significant weight reduction (Fig. 25.2).

Differently from other physical objects, our body is experienced both as object (third person)—we perceive our body as a physical object in the external world—and as subject (first person)—we experience our body through different neural representations that are not related to its physical appearance [85].

These frames influence also the way memories are stored and retrieved [86, 87]: the rememberer may "see" the event from his or her perspective as in normal perception (field mode), or "see" the self engaged in the event as an observer would (observer mode). More, they influence the ability of representing and recalling our body: an egocentric representation of how our body looks is matched by an allocentric one, used by our brain in different situations [88]: from spatial cognition to social perception.

But what are the differences between field and observer modes of remembering? As Eich and colleagues clearly underline [87]: "...adopting an observer perspective is tantamount to a literal disembodiment at the neural level." (p. 177). In simpler words, remembering our body in the observer mode overrides the actual contents of our bodily self-consciousness. If this process is impaired for either exogenous (i.e., high level of stress) or endogenous causes (i.e., alteration of neurotransmitters and/or brain areas), the experience of the body is locked to an old memory.

From a cognitive viewpoint, this situation can be explained as the effect of a functional disconnection between top-down, premorbidly learned predictions regarding the experience of the body and the processing of bottom-up perceptual information regarding its current state [20, 74].

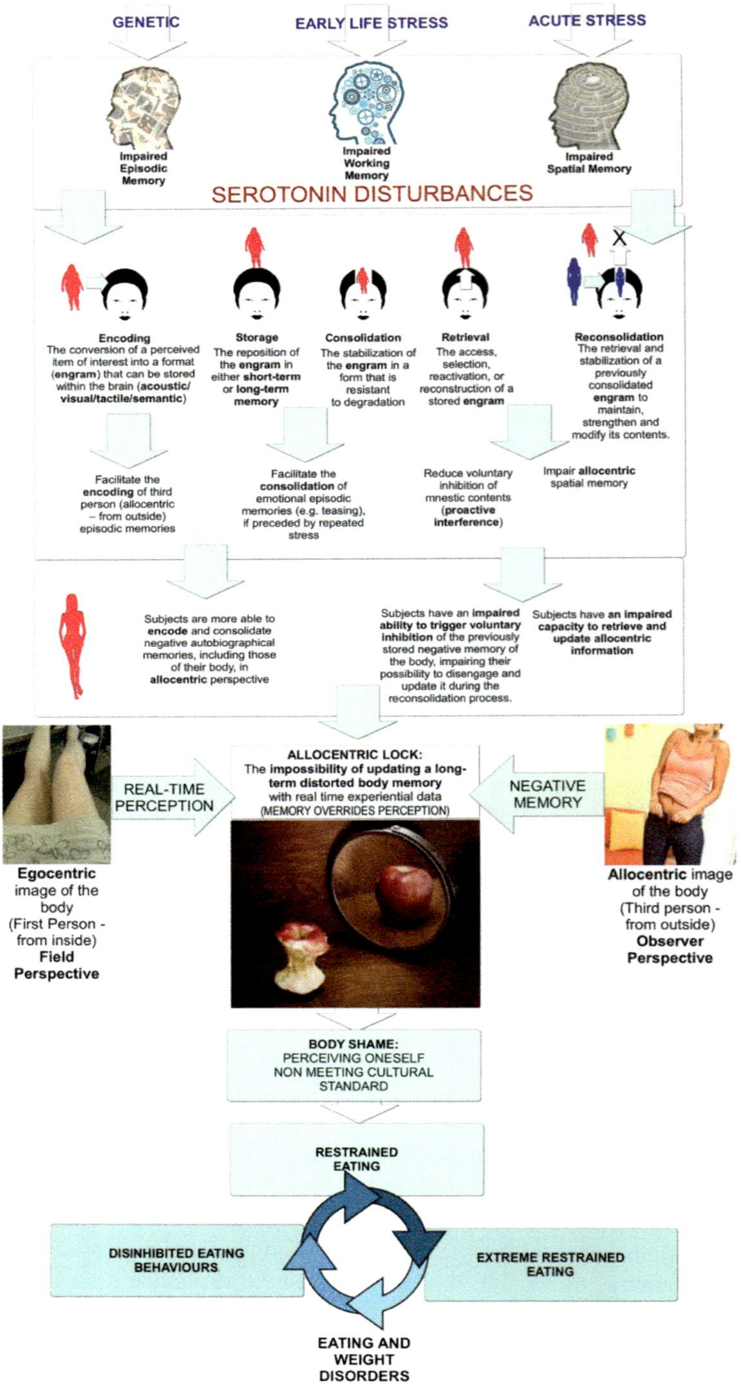

Fig. 25.2 The allocentric lock theory

More, this theory also fits well with the recent neurobiological model developed by Kaye and colleagues [89, 90] suggesting that AN patients are characterized by a dysregulation in the anterior ventral striatal pathway that may create a vulnerability for dysregulated appetitive behaviors. One of the effects of this dysregulation is an altered serotoninergic activity [91–94] related to the impairment of serotonin (5-HT) neurotransmitters. As discussed in a recent review [40], serotonin disturbances may (see Fig. 25.2):

- Facilitate the encoding of allocentric (from outside) episodic memories.
- Facilitate the consolidation of emotional episodic memories (e.g., teasing), if preceded by repeated stress.
- Reduce voluntary inhibition of mnestic contents.
- Impair allocentric spatial memory.

If we discuss these data within the interpretative frame suggested by the allocentric lock hypothesis, it is possible to hypothesize that these patients [40]:

(a) *Are more able to store and consolidate negative autobiographical memories, including those of their body, in allocentric perspective.*
(b) *Have an impaired ability to trigger voluntary inhibition of the previously stored negative memory of the body, impairing their possibility to disengage and update it during the reconsolidation process.*
(c) *Have an impaired capacity to retrieve and update allocentric information.*

In conclusion, there is a possible link between serotonin dysfunctions and body image disturbances in AN: the impossibility of updating a disturbed body memory using real-time experiential data—I'm locked to an old negative body stored in long-term memory—pushes patients to control body weight and shape even when underweight. Moreover, if even successful dieting attempts are unable to balance body image disturbance, people may either start more radical dieting attempts or, at the opposite end, all their attempts to control eating are abandoned and they engage in disinhibited eating behaviors that can be followed by compensatory behaviors, which can turn into a vicious cycle (for a broader review, see [95, 96]).

25.4 Virtual Reality for the Treatment of Body Image in EWDs: Protocols and Studies

To modify this situation, the use of VR, a synthetic egocentric experience, is an emerging and promising approach [97–100]. In particular, the two research groups mentioned above (Riva's group in Milan and Perpiñá's group in Castellón and Valencia) are using VR to improve CBT, and have also developed VR-based software for the assessment and treatment of body image disturbances [101].

The first approach is offered by VR-enhanced cognitive behavior therapy called Experiential Cognitive Therapy (ECT) developed by Giuseppe Riva and his group inside the VREPAR and VEPSY Updated European funded projects. It is a relatively short-term, patient-oriented approach that focuses on individual discovery [102]. ECT shares with CBT the use of a combination of cognitive and behavioral procedures to help the patient identify and change the maintaining mechanisms. However, it differs from CBT in the following ways:

- *Use of VR*: There are 15 VR sessions. The first session is used to assess any stimuli that could elicit abnormal eating behavior. Specifically, attention is focused on the patient's concerns about food, eating, shape, and weight. At the end of the first VR session the therapist uses the *miracle question*, a typical approach used by the solution-focused brief therapy [103–106]. Using VR to experience the effects of the miracle [34, 107–110] individuals are more likely not only to gain an awareness of their need to do something to create change but also to experience a greater sense of personal efficacy.
- *Focus on the negative emotions related to the body (a major reason patients want to lose weight) and on supporting the empowerment process.* In eight VR sessions, the therapist helps patients to recognize why they eat and what they need to either avoid or cope with specific emotional/behavioral triggers. Cue exposure techniques are also used [111, 112]. During exposure, patients face high-risk situations for reducing or extinguishing the conditioned response of anxiety when exposed to food-related cues [113, 114]. Exposure ends after a significant reduction in the level of anxiety.
- *Focus of the experience of the body:* VR is used in a sensory training to unlock the body memory (body image rescripting protocol) by increasing the contribution of new egocentric/internal somatosensory information directly related to the existing allocentric memory [31, 115]. In the protocol (see Fig. 25.3), involving six VR sessions, different body-related situations are experienced from both first-person (the patient does not see his/her body in the scene) and third-person perspectives (the patient sees his/her body in the scene) integrating the therapeutic methods used by Butter and Cash [116] and Wooley and Wooley [117].

This approach was validated by various case studies [3, 118] and trials [107, 119–122].

The most recent controlled trial (ISRCTN59019572) included 211 obese (BMI>40 female patients and 90 obese (BMI>40) female patients with BED [109, 110]. In the trial ECT was compared with CBT and an integrated treatment (IT) including nutritional groups, a low-calorie diet (1200 kcal/day) and physical training.

In both studies [109, 110], only ECT was effective at improving weight loss at 1-year follow-up. Conversely, control participants regained most of the weight they had lost during the inpatient program.

Furthermore, in the BED study [109] binge eating episodes decreased to zero during the inpatient program but were reported again in all the groups at 1-year follow-up. However, a substantial regain was observed only in the group who received the integrated treatment alone, while both ECT and CBT were successful in maintaining a low rate of monthly binge eating episodes.

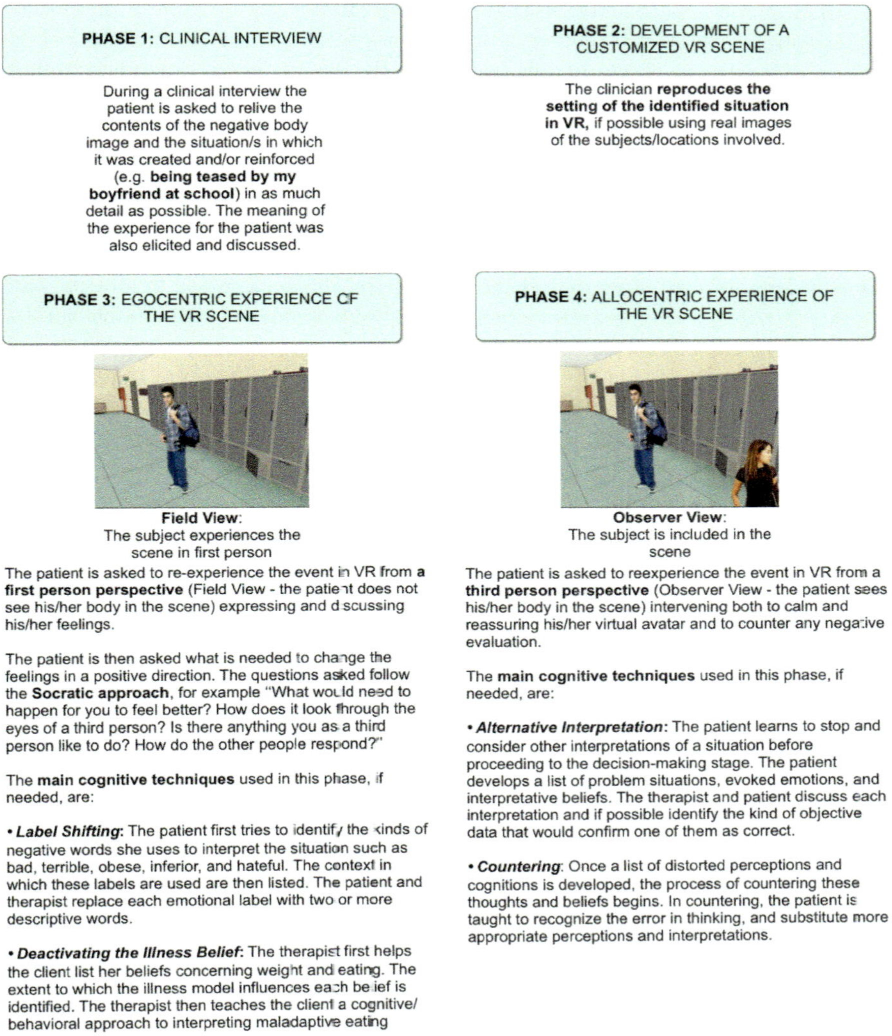

Fig. 25.3 The VR body image rescripting protocol (Adapted from Riva et al. 2006, Riva, 2011)

To further improve the efficacy of ECT, Riva and colleagues recently started to explore the possibility of integrating the emerging field of bodily illusions in the protocol [115, 123]. A first study [97] showed that the body-swap illusion was able to update the negative stored representation of the body. It has been found that after embodying a virtual body with a skinny belly, women updated their "remembered body," reporting a significant (post-illusion) decrease in their body-size distortion. A similar result was obtained recently by Keizer and colleagues [124] using body swapping with a sample of 30 anorectic subjects: they decreased the overestimation of their shoulders, abdomen, and hips both after the illusion was induced and after a short follow-up (2 h and 45 min after the illusions).

Support for the use of bodily illusions to alter the dysfunctional experience of the bodily self also came from a recent published study [125] showing that a (VR) body-swap illusion, which generates the (converse) illusion that a fat person is thin, was able to increase body satisfaction and reduce body-size distortion in a non-operable super-super obese patient (i.e., with body mass index >60 kg/m^2). In addition to the improvement in the bodily experience, the illusion was able to increase the patient's motivation to maintain healthy eating behaviors. While no studies to date have directly exploited the potential of bodily illusions in ED treatment, the evidence deriving from the extant experimental studies may suggest clinical applications for these methods [65, 126, 127].

Preston and Ehrsson [128] also used these illusions to explore the relation between body satisfaction and body perception. The body swapping was induced over a mannequin body digitally manipulated to be both wider and slimmer than the participants' actual body size. The results showed that the illusion of ownership over a slimmer body significantly decreases perceived body width and increases body satisfaction. Preston and colleagues [129] also used multisensory full-body illusions to modulate feelings of ownership over a mannequin body. The third-person mirror perspective elicited strong feelings of ownership over the mannequin and increased physiological responses to the mannequin being threatened. This result suggests that mirrors are special for viewing the self by providing a unique first-person perspective of our body from the outside. In a later study, Preston and Ehrsson [130] used multisensory illusions to elicit illusory ownership of obese and slim bodies during functional magnetic resonance imaging. Their results suggest the involvement of the anterior insula and the anterior cingulate cortex in the development of negative feelings toward the body through functional interactions with the posterior parietal cortex, which mediates perceived obesity.

Perpiñá's group compared the effectiveness of VR with that of CBT for body image improvement. Specifically, they developed six different virtual environments, including a 3D figure whose body parts (arms, thighs, legs, breasts, stomach, buttocks, etc.) could be enlarged or reduced. The proposed approach addressed several body image dimensions: the body could be evaluated wholly or in parts; the body could be placed in different contexts (for instance, in the kitchen, before eating, after eating, facing attractive persons, etc.); behavioral tests could be performed in these contexts, and several discrepancy indices related to weight and figure could be combined (actual weight, subjective weight, desired weight, healthy weight, how the person thinks others see her/him, etc.).

In the published trial, 18 outpatients who had been diagnosed as suffering from EDs disorders (AN or BN) were randomly assigned to one of the two treatment conditions: the VR condition (CBT plus VR) and the standard body image treatment condition (CBT plus relaxation). The results showed that all patients improved significantly following treatment. However, those who had been treated with the VR component showed a significantly greater improvement in general psychopathology,

ED psychopathology, and specific body image variables. What is more, these results were maintained at 1-year follow-up [131].

This group's most recent controlled trial included 34 patients diagnosed with ED [42]. Seventeen patients underwent VR-enhanced CBT and 17 classical CBT. The CBT program for EDs enhanced by a body image-specific component using VR techniques was shown to be more efficient than CBT alone. Furthermore, improvement was maintained in post-treatment and at 1-year follow-up.

Conclusions

VR has proven to be a useful technology in the study, assessment, and treatment of a variety of psychological disorders. Studies on the application of this technology in the treatment of EDs were some of the first ones conducted in the early 1990s. Since then, several VR applications have been developed to be used in conjunction with traditional treatments, and their effectiveness has been tested in case studies, as well as in non-controlled and controlled trials. VR-based interventions in EDs usually combine exposure to VR environments with components based on CBT.

Although various longitudinal studies highlight the unhealthy weight-control behaviors used to counter body dissatisfaction as the common antecedents of eating and weight disorders, trans-disciplinary efforts for further elucidating this mechanism and improving the effectiveness of the available evidence-based interventions are imperative at this time.

To achieve a better explanation of these mechanisms, Riva proposed the "Allocentric Lock Hypothesis" [20, 43, 52, 74, 82, 83]. The key hypothesis of this framework is that both OB and EDs [i.e., Anorexia Nervosa (AN) and Bulimia Nervosa (BN)] are the outcome of a deficit in the processing and integration of multisensory bodily representations and signals [40, 83, 84] that alters the way the body is "experienced" and "remembered": EWDs patients may be locked to an allocentric disembodied negative memory of the body that is not updated even after a demanding diet and a significant weight loss. They cannot win: whatever they will do to modify their real body, they will be always present in a virtual body that they hate (e.g., "My body is fat").

As presented and discussed in this chapter, virtual reality can have a key role in the process of updating and improving the experience of the body [5]. So, it is likely that some of the new interventions on EWDs that derive from the allocentric lock theory and from the findings related to multisensory bodily illusions may be enhanced by the use of virtual reality, as recently demonstrated by different pioneering studies [65, 124, 125].

In conclusion, the two factors that are currently holding back the widespread use of VR technology in this field are the high cost and complexity of its use and maintenance [28]. The first of these barriers is about to disappear. As noted above, high-quality, highly immersive HMD devices are now available at a remarkably low cost [32]. Support should now be provided for the testing of new devices as they become available in order to assess the value of VR in clinical and health psychology as a whole, and more specifically in the field of EWDs.

Acknowledgments This chapter was supported by the research project: "Unlocking the memory of the body: Virtual Reality in Anorexia Nervosa" (201597WTTM) by the Italian Ministry of Education, Universities and Research.

References

1. Riva G, editor. Virtual reality in neuro-psycho-physiology: cognitive, clinical and methodological issues in assessment and rehabilitation. Amsterdam: IOS Press; 1997.
2. Riva G, Melis L, Bolzoni M. Treating body image disturbances. Commun ACM. 1997;40(8):69–71.
3. Riva G. Modifications of body image induced by virtual reality. Percept Mot Skills. 1998;86:163–70.
4. Wiederhold BK, Riva G, Gutiérrez-Maldonado J. Virtual reality in the assessment and treatment of weight-related disorders. Cyberpsychol Behav Soc Netw. 2016;19(2):67–73.
5. Gutierrez-Maldonado J, Wiederhold BK, Riva G. Future directions: how virtual reality can further improve the assessment and treatment of eating disorders and obesity. Cyberpsychol Behav Soc Netw. 2016;19(2):148–53.
6. Riva G, et al. Presence-inducing media for mental health applications. In: Lombard M, et al., editors. Immersed in media. New York: Springer; 2015. p. 283–332.
7. Riva G, Waterworth JA. Presence and the self: a cognitive neuroscience approach. Presence-Connect. 2003;3(1). http://presence.cs.ucl.ac.uk/presenceconnect/articles/Apr2003/jwworthApr72003114532/jwworthApr72003114532.html.
8. Gorini A, et al. The role of immersion and narrative in mediated presence: the virtual hospital experience. Cyberpsychol Behav Soc Netw. 2011;14(3):99–105.
9. Zahoric P, Jenison RL. Presence as being-in-the-world. Presence Teleoperators Virtual Environ. 1998;7(1):78–89.
10. Riva G, Waterworth JA, Murray D, editors. Interacting with presence: HCI and the sense of presence in computer-mediated environments. Berlin: De Gruyter Open; 2014. http://www.presence-research.com/.
11. Riva G, Davide F, IJsselsteijn WA, editors. Being there: concepts, effects and measurements of user presence in synthetic environments. In: Riva G, Davide F, editors. Emerging communication: studies on new technologies and practices in communication. Amsterdam: Ios Press; 2003. http://www.emergingcommunication.com/volume5.html.
12. Lee KM. Presence, explicated. Commun Theory. 2004;14(1):27–50.
13. Lombard M, et al., editors. Immersed in media. Telepresence theory, measurement & technology. Heidelberg: Springer; 2015.
14. Waterworth JA, Riva G. Feeling present in the physical world and in computer-mediated environments. Basingstoke: Palgrave Macmillan; 2014.
15. Banos RM, et al. Immersion and emotion: their impact on the sense of presence. Cyberpsychol Behav. 2004;7(6):734–41.
16. Banos RM, et al. Presence and emotions in virtual environments: the influence of stereoscopy. Cyberpsychol Behav. 2008;11(1):1–8.
17. Pillai JS, Schmidt C, Richir S. Achieving presence through evoked reality. Front Psychol. 2013;4:86.
18. Di Lernia D, Serino S, Pezzulo G, Pedroli E, Cipresso P, Riva G. Feel the time. Time perception as a function of interoceptive processing. Front Hum Neurosci. 2018;12:74. https://doi.org/10.3389/fnhum.2018.00074.
19. Seth AK, Suzuki K, Critchley HD. An interoceptive predictive coding model of conscious presence. Front Psychol. 2011;2:395.
20. Riva G. Neuroscience and eating disorders: the allocentric lock hypothesis. Med Hypotheses. 2012;78:254–7.
21. Riva G. Is presence a technology issue? Some insights from cognitive sciences. Virtual Real. 2009;13(3):59–69.

22. Ling Y, et al. A meta-analysis on the relationship between self-reported presence and anxiety in virtual reality exposure therapy for anxiety disorders. PLoS One. 2014;9(5):e96144.
23. Sanchez-Vives MV, Slater M. From presence to consciousness through virtual reality. Nat Rev Neurosci. 2005;6(4):332–9.
24. Slater M, Wilbur S. A framework for immersive virtual environments (FIVE): Speculations on the role of presence in virtual environments. Presence Teleoperators Virtual Environ. 1997;6(6):603–16.
25. Slater M. Presence and the sixth sense. Presence Teleoperators Virtual Environ. 2002;11(4):435–9.
26. Riva G, Gaggioli A, Villani D, Preziosa A, Morganti F, Corsi R, et al. NeuroVR: an open source virtual reality platform for clinical psychology and behavioral neurosciences. Stud Health Technol Inform. 2007;125:394–9.
27. Glantz K, et al. Virtual reality (VR) and psychotherapy: opportunities and challenges. Presence Teleoperators Virtual Environ. 1997;6(1):87–105.
28. Riva G, Gamberini L. Virtual reality in telemedicine. Telemed J E Health. 2004;6(3):327–40. https://doi.org/10.1089/153056200750040183.
29. Riva G, Baños RM, Botella C, Mantovani F, Gaggioli A. Transforming experience: the potential of augmented reality and virtual reality for enhancing personal and clinical change. Front Psych. 2016;7:164.
30. Vincelli F. From imagination to virtual reality: the future of clinical psychology. Cyberpsychol Behav. 1999;2(3):241–8.
31. Riva G. Letter to the Editor: virtual reality in the treatment of eating and weight disorders. Psychol Med. 2017;47(14):2567–8.
32. Zanier ER, Zoerle T, Di Lernia D, Riva G. Virtual reality for traumatic brain injury. Front Neurol. 2018;9:345.
33. Dakanalis A, Timko A, Serino S, Riva G, Clerici M, Carrà G. Prospective psychosocial predictors of onset and cessation of eating pathology amongst college women. Eur Eat Disord Rev. 2016;24(3):251–6.
34. Dakanalis A, Gaudio S, Serino S, Clerici M, Carrà G, Riva G. Body-image distortion in anorexia nervosa. Nat Rev Dis Primers. 2016;2:16026.
35. Riva G. The neuroscience of body memory: From the self through the space to the others. Cortex. 2018;104:241–60.
36. Blanke O, Slater M, Serino A. Behavioral, neural, and computational principles of bodily self-consciousness. Neuron. 2015;88(1):145–66.
37. Pazzaglia M, Zantedeschi M. Plasticity and awareness of bodily distortion. Neural Plast. 2016;2016:9834340.
38. Cash TF, Deagle EA. The nature and extent of body-image disturbances in anorexia nervosa and bulimia nervosa: a meta-analysis. Int J Eat Disord. 1997;22(2):107–26.
39. Gaudio S, Nocchi F, Franchin T, Genovese E, Cannatà V, Longo D, Fariello G. Gray matter decrease distribution in the early stages of Anorexia Nervosa restrictive type in adolescents. Psychiatry Res. 2011;191(1):24–30.
40. Riva G. Neurobiology of anorexia nervosa: serotonin dysfunctions link self-starvation with body image disturbances through an impaired body memory. Front Hum Neurosci. 2016;10:600.
41. Esposito R, et al. The role of body image and self-perception in anorexia nervosa: the neuroimaging perspective. J Neuropsychol. 2018;12(1):41–52.
42. Marco JH, Perpiñá C, Botella C. The treatment of the body image disturbances in eating disorders and clinically significant change. Ann Psychol. 2014;30(2):422–30.
43. Dakanalis A, Riva G. Mass media, body image and eating disturbances: the underline mechanism through the lens of the objectification theory. In: Latzer J, Merrick J, Stein D, editors. Body image: gender differences, sociocultural influences and health implication. New York: Nova Science; 2013. p. 217–36.
44. Eshkevari E, et al. Persistent body image disturbance following recovery from eating disorders. Int J Eat Disord. 2014;47(4):400–9.
45. Thompson JK, Smolak L. Body image, eating disorders, and obesity in youth: assessment, prevention, and treatment. New York: Taylor & Francis; 2001.

46. Sato Y, et al. Neural basis of impaired cognitive flexibility in patients with anorexia nervosa. PLoS One. 2013;8(5):e61108.
47. Gaudio S, Quattrocchi CC. Neural basis of a multidimensional model of body image distortion in anorexia nervosa. Neurosci Biobehav Rev. 2012;36(8):1839–47.
48. Suchan B, Vocks S, Waldorf M. Alterations in activity, volume, and connectivity of body-processing brain areas in anorexia nervosa. Eur Psychol. 2015;20(1):27–33.
49. van den Berg P, et al. The Tripartite Influence model of body image and eating disturbance: a covariance structure modeling investigation testing the mediational role of appearance comparison. J Psychosom Res. 2002;53(5):1007–20.
50. Tylka TL. Refinement of the tripartite influence model for men: dual body image pathways to body change behaviors. Body Image. 2011;8(3):199–207.
51. Swami V. Cultural influences on body size ideals unpacking the impact of westernization and modernization. Eur Psychol. 2015;20(1):44–51.
52. Riva G, Gaudio S, Dakanalis A. The neuropsychology of self-objectification. Eur Psychologist. 2015;20(1):34–43.
53. Gaudio S, Wiemerslage L, Brooks SJ, Schiöth HB. A systematic review of resting-state functional-MRI studies in anorexia nervosa: evidence for functional connectivity impairment in cognitive control and visuospatial and body-signal integration. Neurosci Biobehav Rev. 2016;71:578–89.
54. Cash TF. Body image: past, present, and future. Body Image. 2004;1(1):1–5.
55. Grogan S. Body image: understanding body dissatisfaction in men, women and children. 3rd ed. New York: Routledge; 2016.
56. Halliwell E. Future directions for positive body image research. Body Image. 2015;14:177–89.
57. Gutierrez-Maldonado J, Ferrer-Garcia M, Dakanalis A, Riva G. Virtual reality: applications to eating disorders. In: Agras SW, Robinson A, editors. The Oxford handbook of eating disorders. 2nd ed. Oxford: Oxford University Press; 2017. p. 146–61.
58. Riva G, Gutiérrez-Maldonado J, Wiederhold BK. Virtual worlds versus real body: virtual reality meets eating and weight disorders. Cyberpsychol Behav Soc Netw. 2016;19(2):63–6.
59. Serino S, Dakanalis A. Bodily illusions and weight-related disorders: clinical insights from experimental research. Ann Phys Rehabil Med. 2017;60(3):217–9.
60. Olive I, Berthoz A. Combined induction of rubber-hand illusion and out-of-body experiences. Front Psychol. 2012;3:128.
61. Pomes A, Slater M. Drift and ownership toward a distant virtual body. Front Hum Neurosci. 2013;7:908.
62. Maselli A, Slater M. Sliding perspectives: dissociating ownership from self-location during full body illusions in virtual reality. Front Hum Neurosci. 2014;8:693.
63. Costantini M. Body perception, awareness, and illusions. Wiley Interdiscip Rev Cogn Sci. 2014;5(5):551–60.
64. Gallace A, Spence C. Outside the boundaries of our bodies: the relationship between touch and the representation of the body in our mind. In: Gallace A, Spence C, editors. In touch with the future: the sense of touch from cognitive neuroscience to virtual reality. Oxford: Oxford University Press; 2014. p. 102–24.
65. Serino S, Scarpina F, Dakanalis A, Keizer A, Pedroli E, Castelnuovo G, et al. The role of age on multisensory bodily experience: an experimental study with a virtual reality full-body illusion. Cyberpsychol Behav Soc Netw. 2018;21(5):304–10. https://doi.org/10.1089/cyber.2017.0674.
66. Riva G. Virtual environment for body-image modification: virtual reality system for the treatment of body image disturbances. Comput Hum Behav. 1998;14(3):477–90.
67. Fredrickson BL, Roberts T. Objectification theory: toward understanding women's lived experiences and mental health risks. Psychol Women Q. 1997;21:173–206.
68. Calogero RM, Tantleff-Dunn S, Thompson JK. Self-objectification in women: causes, consequences, and counteractions. Washington, DC: American Psychological Association; 2010.
69. Dakanalis A, Carra G, Calogero R, Fida R, Clerici M, Zanetti MA, Riva G. The developmental effects of media-ideal internalization and self-objectification processes on adolescents'

negative body-feelings, dietary restraint, and binge eating. Eur Child Adolesc Psychiatry. 2015;28(8):997–1010. https://doi.org/10.1007/s00787-014-0649-1.
70. Fredrickson BL, Roberts TA, Noll SM, Quinn DM, Twenge JM. That swimsuit becomes you: sex differences in selfobjectification, restrained eating, and math performance. J Pers Soc Psychol. 1998;75(1):269–84.
71. Nell SM, Fredrickson BL. A mediational model linking self-objectification, body shame and disordered eating. Psychol Women Q. 1998;22:623–36.
72. Tiggemann M, Lynch D. Body image across the life span in adult women: The role of self-objectification. Dev Psychol. 2001;37(2):243–53.
73. Dakanalis A, et al. Objectified body consciousness (OBC) in eating psychopathology. Assessment. 2017;24(2):252–74.
74. Riva G. Out of my real body: cognitive neuroscience meets eating disorders. Front Hum Neurosci. 2014;8:236.
75. Dakanalis A, et al. Psychosocial moderators of the relationship between body dissatisfaction and symptoms of eating disorders: a look at a sample of young Italian women. Eur Rev Appl Psychol. 2013;63(5):323–34.
76. Dakanalis A, et al. Internalization of sociocultural standards of beauty and eating disordered behaviours: the role of body surveillance, shame, and social anxiety. J Psychopathol. 2013;20:33–7.
77. Calogero RM. Objectification processes and disordered eating in British women and men. J Health Psychol. 2009;14(3):394–402.
78. Dakanalis A, Clerici M, Bartoli F, Caslini M, Crocamo C, Riva G, Carra G. Risk and maintenance factors for young women's DSM-5 eating disorders. Arch Womens Ment Health. 2017;11 https://doi.org/10.1007/s00737-017-0761-6.
79. Dakanalis A, et al. body dissatisfaction and eating disorder symptomatology: a latent structural equation modeling analysis of moderating variables in 18-to-28-year-old males. J Psychol. 2015;149(1):85–112.
80. Riva G, Gaudio S, Dakanalis A. I'm in a virtual body: a locked allocentric memory may impair the experience of the body in both obesity and anorexia nervosa. Eat Weight Disord. 2013;19(1):133–4.
81. Gaudio S, Riva G. Body image disturbances in anorexia: the link between functional connectivity alterations and reference frames. Biol Psychiatry. 2013;73(9):e25–6.
82. Riva G, Gaudio S. Allocentric lock in anorexia nervosa: new evidences from neuroimaging studies. Med Hypotheses. 2012;79(1):113–7.
83. Riva G, Dakanalis A. Altered processing and integration of multisensory bodily representations and signals in eating disorders: a possible path toward the understanding of their underlying causes. Front Hum Neurosci. 2018;12:49.
84. Riva G, Gaudio S. Locked to a wrong body: eating disorders as the outcome of a primary disturbance in multisensory body integration. Conscious Cogn. 2018;59:57–9. https://doi.org/10.1016/j.concog.2017.08.006.
85. Luongo MA, Pazzaglia M. Commentary: body image distortion and exposure to extreme body types: contingent adaptation and cross adaptation for self and other. Front Hum Neurosci. 2016;10:526.
86. Eich E, et al. Neural systems mediating field and observer memories. Neuropsychologia. 2009;47(11):2239–51.
87. Eich E, et al. Field and observer perspectives in autobiographical memory. In: Forgas JP, Fiedler K, Sedikides C, editors. Social thinking and interpersonal behavior. New York: Taylor & Francis; 2012. p. 163–81.
88. Juurmaa J, Lehtinen-Railo S. Visual experience and access to spatial knowledge. J Vis Impair Blind. 1994;88:157–70.
89. Kaye WH, Fudge JL, Paulus M. New insights into symptoms and neurocircuit function of anorexia nervosa. Nat Rev Neurosci. 2009;10(8):573–84.
90. Kaye WH, et al. Nothing tastes as good as skinny feels: the neurobiology of anorexia nervosa. Trends Neurosci. 2013;36(2):110–20.

91. Jean A, et al. The nucleus accumbens 5-HTR4-CART pathway ties anorexia to hyperactivity. Transl Psychiatry. 2012;2:e203.
92. Kumar KK, Tung S, Iqbal J. Bone loss in anorexia nervosa: leptin, serotonin, and the sympathetic nervous system. Ann N Y Acad Sci. 2010;1211:51–65.
93. Calati R, et al. The 5-HTTLPR polymorphism and eating disorders: a meta-analysis. Int J Eat Disord. 2011;44(3):191–9.
94. Chen J, et al. The 5-HTTLPR confers susceptibility to anorexia nervosa in Han Chinese: evidence from a case-control and family-based study. PLoS One. 2015;10(3):e0119378.
95. Murray SB, et al. A comparison of eating, exercise, shape, and weight related symptomatology in males with muscle dysmorphia and anorexia nervosa. Body Image. 2012;9(2):193–200.
96. Cafri G, Olivardia R, Thompson JK. Symptom characteristics and psychiatric comorbidity among males with muscle dysmorphia. Compr Psychiatry. 2008;49(4):374–9.
97. Serino S, et al. Virtual reality body-swapping: a tool for modifying the allocentric memory of the body. Cyberpsychol Behav Soc Netw. 2016;19(2):127–33.
98. Serino S, et al. Out of body, out of space: impaired reference frame processing in eating disorders. Psychiatry Res. 2015;230(2):732–4.
99. Riva G. Embodied medicine: what human-computer confluence can offer to health care. In: Gaggioli A, et al., editors. Human computer confluence: transforming human experience through symbiotic technologies. Warsaw: De Gruyter Open; 2016. p. 55–79.
100. Perpiña C, Botella C, Baños RM. Virtual reality in eating disorders. Eur Eat Disord Rev. 2003;11(3):261–78.
101. Ferrer-Garcia M, Gutiérrez-Maldonado J, Riva G. Virtual reality based treatments in eating disorders and obesity: a review. J Contemp Psychol. 2013;43(4):207–21.
102. Riva G. The key to unlocking the virtual body: virtual reality in the treatment of obesity and eating disorders. J Diabetes Sci Technol. 2011;5(2):283–92.
103. Riva G. Medical clinical uses of virtual worlds. In: Grimshaw M, editor. The Oxford handbook of virtuality. New York: Oxford University Press; 2014. p. 649–65.
104. deShazer S. Keys to solutions in brief therapy. New York: W.W. Norton; 1985.
105. Riva G, et al. e-health in eating disorders: virtual reality and telemedicine in assessment and treatment. Stud Health Technol Inform. 2002;85:402–8.
106. Riva G, et al. The use of VR in the treatment of eating disorders. Stud Health Technol Inform. 2004;99:121–63.
107. Riva G, et al. Virtual reality-based multidimensional therapy for the treatment of body image disturbances in obesity: a controlled study. Cyberpsychol Behav. 2001;4(4):511–26.
108. Riva G, et al. Virtual-reality-based multidimensional therapy for the treatment of body image disturbances in binge eating disorders: a preliminary controlled study. IEEE Trans Inf Technol Biomed. 2002;6(3):224–34.
109. Cesa GL, et al. Virtual reality for enhancing the cognitive behavioral treatment of obesity with binge eating disorder: randomized controlled study with one-year follow-up. J Med Internet Res. 2013;15(6):e113.
110. Manzoni GM, et al. Virtual reality-enhanced cognitive-behavioral therapy for morbid obesity: a randomized controlled study with 1 year follow-up. Cyberpsychol Behav Soc Netw. 2016;19(2):134–40.
111. Ferrer-Garcia M, Gutierrez-Maldonado J, Pla-Sanjuanelo J, Vilalta-Abella F, Riva G, Clerici M, et al. A randomised controlled comparison of second-level treatment approaches for treatment-resistant adults with bulimia nervosa and binge eating disorder: assessing the benefits of virtual reality cue exposure therapy. Eur Eat Disord Rev. 2017;25(6):479–90. https://doi.org/10.1002/erv.2538.
112. Pla-Sanjuanelo J, Ferrer-García M, Vilalta-Abella F, Riva G, Dakanalis A, Ribas-Sabaté J, et al. Testing virtual reality-based cue-exposure software: which cue-elicited responses best discriminate between patients with eating disorders and healthy controls? Eat Weight Disord. 2017; https://doi.org/10.1007/s40519-017-0419-4.
113. Ferrer-Garcia M, et al. The validity of virtual environments for eliciting emotional responses in patients with eating disorders and in controls. Behav Modif. 2009;33(6):830–54.

114. Pla-Sanjuanelo J, et al. Identifying specific cues and contexts related to bingeing behavior for the development of effective virtual environments. Appetite. 2015;87:81–9.
115. Dakanalis A, et al. Towards novel paradigms for treating dysfunctional bodily experience in eating disorders. Eat Weight Disord. 2017;22:373–5.
116. Butters JW, Cash TF. Cognitive-behavioral treatment of women's body image satisfaction: a controlled outcome-study. J Consult Clin Psychol. 1987;55:889–97.
117. Wooley SC, Wooley OW. Intensive out-patient and residential treatment for bulimia. In: Garner DM, Garfinkel PE, editors. Handbook of psychotherapy for anorexia and bulimia. New York: Guilford Press; 1985. p. 120–32.
118. Riva G, et al. Virtual reality based experiential cognitive treatment of anorexia nervosa. J Behav Ther Exp Psychiatry. 1999;30(3):221–30.
119. Rinaldi S, et al. La terapia cognitivo-esperienziale: un approccio integrato per la valutazione e il trattamento dei disturbi del comportamento alimentare. Quaderni di Psicoterapia Cognitiva. 1999;4(2):6–21.
120. Cesa GL, et al. Integrated experiential therapy for the treatment of obesity and binge eating disorder: a clinical trial. Cyberpsychol Behav. 2005;8(4):310–1.
121. Riva G, et al. Virtual reality environment for body image modification: a multidimensional therapy for the treatment of body image in obesity and related pathologies. Cyberpsychol Behav. 2000;3(3):421–31.
122. Riva G, et al. Virtual reality based experiential cognitive treatment of obesity and binge-eating disorders. Clin Psychol Psychother. 2000;7(3):209–19.
123. Serino S, Chirico A, Pedroli E, Polli N, Cacciatore C, Riva G. Two-phases innovative treatment for anorexia nervosa: the potential of virtual reality body-swap. Annu Rev Cybertherapy Telemed. 2017;15:111–5.
124. Keizer A, et al. A virtual reality full body illusion improves body image disturbance in anorexia nervosa. PLoS One. 2016;11(10):e0163921.
125. Serino S, Scarpina F, Keizer A, Pedroli E, Dakanalis A, Castelnuovo G, Chirico A, Novelli M, Gaudio S, Riva G. A novel technique for improving bodily experience in a non-operable super-super obesity case. Front Psychol. 2016;7:83.
126. Gutierrez-Maldonado J, et al. Virtual reality: applications to eating disorders. In: Agras SW, Robinson A, editors. The Oxford handbook of eating disorders. 2nd ed. Oxford: Oxford University Press; 2017. p. 146–61.
127. Riva G, et al. Embodied medicine: mens sana in corpore virtuale sano. Front Hum Neurosci. 2017;11:120.
128. Preston C, Ehrsson HH. Illusory changes in body size modulate body satisfaction in a way that is related to non-clinical eating disorder psychopathology. PLoS One. 2014;9(1):e85773.
129. Preston C, Kuper-Smith BJ, Henrik Ehrsson H. Owning the body in the mirror: the effect of visual perspective and mirror view on the fullbody illusion. Sci Rep. 2015;5:18345.
130. Preston C, Ehrsson HH. Illusory obesity triggers body dissatisfaction responses in the insula and anterior cingulate cortex. Cereb Cortex. 2016;26(12):4450–60.
131. Marco JH, Perpina C, Botella C. Effectiveness of cognitive behavioral therapy supported by virtual reality in the treatment of body image in eating disorders: One year follow-up. Psychiatry Res. 2013;209(3):619–25.

Drug Treatment of Body Image Disturbance in Mental Disorders

26

Matteo Balestrieri

26.1 Drug Treatment for Eating Disorders

Body image disturbance is a cognitive misperception of self-appearance in the context of different mental health disorders, but in particular of eating disorders (ED) (see also Chaps. 1–12 of this book). If we intend to use drug treatments for such disturbance, we must first analyze how much such treatments are appropriate for ED. In fact, we know that, apart from the exception of fluoxetine in the treatment of bulimia, no other psychotropic drug has an approved indication for ED. As such, the pieces of evidence of each study on different drugs must be taken with caution, even if this represents the essential basis for a treatment founded on the state-of-art knowledge.

26.1.1 Anorexia Nervosa

Studies on the effectiveness of *antidepressants* (AD) in anorexia nervosa (AN) are limited. As for tricyclics, preliminary studies with amitriptyline and clomipramine showed modest or no benefit of these drugs in comparison with placebo [1, 2]. This trend was also confirmed with selective serotonin reuptake inhibitors (SSRI). Most studies with fluoxetine showed that it was poorly useful in the treatment of AN. Even if a small, open study reported positive results on depressive symptoms and a significant weight gain [3], other studies failed to demonstrate the efficacy of fluoxetine over placebo [4, 5]. Two studies explored if fluoxetine was able to maintain over time the weight that had been previously restored. Kaye et al. [6] reported a reduced relapse with fluoxetine in comparison with placebo and a reduction of depressive and anxiety symptoms. However, negative results were found in a

M. Balestrieri
DAME, University of Udine, Udine, Italy
e-mail: matteo.balestrieri@uniud.it

M. Cuzzolaro, S. Fassino (eds.), *Body Image, Eating, and Weight*,
https://doi.org/10.1007/978-3-319-90817-5_26

subsequent larger clinical trial funded by the NIMH [7], which showed that CBT alone was equivalent to CBT plus medication with respect to time to relapse.

Two studies with citalopram showed that also this SSRI was of limited usefulness in AN. In the trial of Bergh et al. [8], patients on citalopram and psychotherapy lost much more weight than patients treated with psychotherapy alone. Moreover, Fassino et al. [9] did not report differences in weight gain between citalopram and a waiting-list condition, even though depression, obsessive–compulsive symptoms, and impulsiveness were better with the drug.

Santonastaso et al. [10] conducted an open trial on the effects of sertraline in a sample of 11 AN patients treated in an outpatient setting. The SSRI did not attain beneficial effects on body weight while it was efficacious on depressive symptoms.

Lastly, two case reports by Safer et al. [11, 12] showed that mirtazapine and duloxetine could be useful in some cases of AN, in particular for the control of affective symptoms.

In conclusion, available data demonstrated that AD are of limited efficacy in the control of weight, but may be useful for affective and anxiety symptoms that are present in the course of AN.

As far as *first-generation antipsychotics* are concerned, we have some evidence on the efficacy of haloperidol on delusional body image alteration in AN. In limited series of patients, Cassano et al. [13] and Mauri et al. [14] showed that haloperidol might be effective as an adjunctive treatment for patients with severe restrictive-type AN. Moreover, in a single-blind comparison of amisulpride, fluoxetine, and clomipramine in the treatment of hospitalized patients with AN, those treated with amisulpride showed a greater increase in mean body weight. In spite of this, no significant difference was found for weight phobia, body image disturbance, and amenorrhea [15].

More evidence is available for *second-generation antipsychotics* [16–18]. With a meta-analytic approach, Kishi et al. [16] identified four studies with olanzapine, and one each with risperidone, quetiapine, and sulpiride. Both individually and pooled together, antipsychotics did not differ from placebo or usual care concerning effects on weight gain, scores on questionnaires related to AN (with some exceptions for quetiapine, which did better), or affective symptoms. Lebow et al. [19] published a similar meta-analysis adding a further study with olanzapine and obtaining the same results.

As far as quetiapine is concerned, there are three open-label studies with controversial results (see also further on). Bosanac et al. [20] demonstrated an efficacy of the drug on weight restoration, while Powers et al. [21] and Court et al. [22] did not.

Finally, Trunko et al. [23] reported some case reports showing that adding aripiprazole to antidepressants triggered a reduction in eating-specific anxiety and obsessive thoughts.

In conclusion, the available evidence does not permit an optimistic approach to the treatment of AN with antipsychotics. These drugs might be used in specific cases where a psychotic dimension is clearly evident, while an unselective use of them in AN is questionable. Moreover, it is well known that trials with drugs are difficult to carry out in AN patients because of their lack of insight and fear of weight gain. Thus, patients included in the trials may represent only a subset of AN patients potentially eligible. This fact implies that in the context of a real-world AN, antipsychotics are even less useful than what clinical trials demonstrate. The efficacy of antipsychotics on weight restoration seems anyway doubtful, while that on anxiety or depression symptoms is more promising.

26.1.2 Bulimia Nervosa

The World Federation of Societies of Bipolar Disorder (WFSBP) published in 2011 a review of 36 studies demonstrating that there was evidence for the efficacy of tricyclics and some SSRI for reducing binge eating and purging in bulimia (BN), while lithium was not efficacious [24]. As for tricyclics, five studies showed that desipramine and imipramine were superior to placebo, while in two studies the efficacy over placebo was unproven. Moreover, three other studies demonstrated that CBT treatment was superior to tricyclics, and thus combined treatment was recommended. Fluoxetine was the best-studied SSRI and is the only medication approved for BN (at a dosage of 60 mg/day) by the United States Food and Drug Administration (U.S. FDA) and by the European Medicines Agency (EMA). In many controlled studies, fluoxetine demonstrated a greater efficacy vs. placebo. Where CBT treatment was included, combined treatment was superior to fluoxetine alone. In two studies, citalopram demonstrated to be effective. The data on fluvoxamine are not unequivocal, with some evidence of efficacy in a few studies. Sertraline is another SSRI that has been shown to be effective, as demonstrated in a small, RCT. Trazodone showed as well a good efficacy in an RCT, and the same happened with bupropion, even if four subjects experienced grand mal seizures during treatment. Topiramate has also shown to be effective. However, it should be used with caution since adverse reactions are common.

In conclusion, the role of psychotropic drug treatment in bulimia seems promising. However, the bulk of evidence regards tricyclics and fluoxetine, which mostly were able to demonstrate their efficacy. For other drugs, it is necessary to replicate the results so far obtained to corroborate the few positive outcomes obtained. In general, there is a need for more robust studies, information on the long-term efficacy of these treatments, and benefit for weight and shape overconcern.

26.1.3 Binge Eating Disorder

The WFSBP [24] reported that, according to an analysis of 26 randomized controlled trials (RCTs), many psychotropic drugs proved to be efficacious in the treatment of binge eating disorder (BED). In particular, the best grade of evidence of efficacy was obtained by tricyclics (imipramine and desipramine), citalopram, escitalopram, sertraline, and topiramate. Instead, other well-known serotonergic agents (fluoxetine, fluvoxamine, venlafaxine) reached worse results. Since then, McElroy et al. [25] found two other RCTs with duloxetine and bupropion. The first was superior to placebo in reducing binge eating episodes, global severity of BED symptoms, global severity of depressive symptoms, and body weight. The latter was similar to placebo in reducing binge eating frequency, but produced greater weight loss.

Some other substances that have been tried in BED: anti-obesity agents (orlistat, sibutramine, rimonabant), an opioid antagonist (naloxone), a GABAergic agent (baclofen), and a psychostimulant (lisdexamfetamine). All these drugs, including anti-obesity medications, were able to reduce binge eating episodes or time spent binge eating. Lisdexamfetamine is the only medication approved for BED by the U.S. FDA.

In conclusion, different drugs, not necessarily belonging to the classic psychotropic substances, were able to control binge eating behavior. The choice of what to use is related to the strategy of treatment. Several studies were carried out in combination with psychotherapy, mostly CBT. This approach showed quite often to be superior in obtaining weight loss when compared with drug treatment alone.

26.2 Drug Treatment for Body Image Disturbances in Eating Disorders

The drug treatment for each of the three major ED has specific outcome measures. As for AN, the primary measure is the weight restoration, for BN the first goal is the reduction of binge eating and purging, while for BED is the reduction of binge eating and weight loss.

In some studies, also other psychological dimensions are considered as secondary measures of the results. Body image disturbance/dissatisfaction is one of these issues and is particularly relevant for the characterization of the outcome in AN patients. This happens because body image disturbance—namely "Disturbance in the way in which one's body weight or shape is experienced, undue influence of body weight or shape on self-evaluation, or denial of the seriousness of the current low body weight"—is one of the three DSM-5 criteria for AN [26]. As a matter of fact, the evaluation of body image disturbance is seldom considered in RCT, and when it happens, it is usually assessed only with an Eating Disorder Inventory (EDI) subscale and very rarely with a specific instrument.

The DSM-5 diagnosis of BN requires five criteria, one of which is "self-evaluation unduly influenced by body shape and weight." Strictly speaking, this symptom may not be interpreted as a body image disturbance. Thus, the results on body image dissatisfaction reported in the drug trials on BN (as well as on BED) have a different meaning as compared with those obtained in AN, but the psychometric scale used is often the same.

26.2.1 Anorexia Nervosa

I tried to review all the studies which explicitly reported body image disturbance or body image dissatisfaction as primary or secondary measures of outcome (Table 26.1). In most cases, this dimension was studied taking into consideration the body image dissatisfaction subscale of EDI-2 (EDI-2 BD). I considered only the

Table 26.1 Drug treatment of anorexia considering response on body image dissatisfaction

	Treatments	Resp on EDI	Resp on other scales of bid
Mauri et al. [14]	Haloperidol	Yes on delusional bid	
Mondraty et al. [28]	Olanzapine, chlorpromazine	Equal	
Brambilla et al. [29]	CBT+olanzapine, CBT+placebo	Equal	
Attia et al. [30]	Olanzapine, placebo	–	BSQ: equal in two groups
Kafantaris et al. [31]	Olanzapine in add-on	–	Bid assessment: no effect
Powers et al. [21]	Quetiapine, placebo	Equal	
Bosanac et al. [20]	Quetiapine	No	
Court et al. [22]	Quetiapine, TAU	Equal	
Hagman et al. [32]	Risperidone, placebo	Equal	BIS, CAPT: equal
Misra et al. [35]	Estradiol, progesterone, placebo	Equal	
Fassino et al. [9]	Citalopram, waiting list	Equal	

Note: *bid* body image dissatisfaction; *BIS*, Body Image Software Program; *CAPT*, Color-A-Person-Test; *EDI*, Eating Disorder Inventory.

studies that reported the results on this specific subscale, excluding those that analyzed only the total score of EDI-2. Moreover, I selected also all studies that used specific measures of body concern, such as the Body Shape Questionnaire (BSQ), released by Cooper et al. [27], a 34-item instrument designed to measure concerns about body shape among young women.

Mauri et al. [14] reported on a chart review conducted on nine severe and treatment-resistant patients with AN restricted type, BMI <13, and a delusional body image disturbance. Patients received low doses (0.5–3.3 mg/day) of *haloperidol* during hospitalization in a median period of 42 days. Three patients also assumed antidepressants. No specific scales for insight or the assessment of clinical response were administered, and no matched controls were compared. BMI increased from the initial mean value 12.2–16.0. All patients improved: the delusional body image disturbance and the desire for thinness were subjectively perceived as less intense. The authors suggested that haloperidol might act both on delusional thinking and on severe body image distortion. The small sample size, the absence of a control group, and of validated scales limit the generalizability of these findings anyway.

In 2005, Mondraty et al. [28] assessed 26 AN patients and recruited 15 of them (57.7%) to carry out an RCT that compared *olanzapine* with *chlorpromazine*. The principal outcome was the reduction of anorectic rumination. The study showed that olanzapine significantly reduced the level of rumination as compared with the chlorpromazine group. On the other hand, the authors did not find significant difference in the degree of weight gain between the two groups. As for the subscale EDI-2 BD, the differences only approached statistical significance, with olanzapine doing better than chlorpromazine. A limitation of these results was that nearly two-thirds of the patients on olanzapine were also taking antidepressants.

In a double-blind RCT, Brambilla et al. [29] compared 30 women with AN treated with a 3-month course of CBT plus at random *olanzapine* or placebo. The original study sample included 35 patients, but five of them dropped out (14.28%). The authors found greater improvement in depression, anxiety, obsessive–compulsiveness, and aggressiveness in the olanzapine group. Weight generally improved but without significant group difference. Moreover, the analysis for repeated measures regarding the EDI-2 total score and the subscales (including body image dissatisfaction) revealed no significant differences between the two treatments (CBT plus olanzapine vs. CBT plus placebo), even when the patients were split according to AN type.

In 2011, Attia et al. [30] published the results of an RCT where 603 patients with AN were first evaluated through a telephone screening, and then 49 subjects proceeded to in-person evaluation. The 23 outpatients suffering from AN who accepted to participate in the trial were randomly assigned to receive either *olanzapine* or placebo for 8 weeks. Seventeen patients completed the study with a dropout rate of 27% in the olanzapine group and 25% in the placebo group. The patients were free of other psychotropic medication for at least 4 weeks before the study enrollment, except for SSRI or SNRI that were permitted. At the end of treatment, BMI was greater in the group receiving olanzapine, but the authors did not detect any psychological improvement associated with olanzapine when compared with placebo. This result was true also for the assessment with the BSQ, showing that no differences on body shape concerns were uncovered between treatments.

In the same year, Kafantaris et al. [31] carried out a placebo-controlled trial on a young population with AN who used *olanzapine* as adjunctive treatment. Of the 94 eligible participants, 74 (78%) refused to participate in the study, mostly because of fear to gain weight using medications. Fifteen of the twenty AN patients enrolled completed the 10-week trial successively with a dropout rate of 30% in the treatment group and 20% in the placebo group. A body image assessment was carried out asking the patients their opinion about nine silhouettes. No differences were found in BMI between the groups. Moreover, the addition of olanzapine did not improve general psychopathology and yielded no effect on body image assessment.

Powers et al. [12] compared in a small group of 15 patients *quetiapine* vs. placebo. Only 10.4% of the 207 patients initially screened signed informed consensus. There was no difference in outcome for any of the measures between the group of participants who received quetiapine and the group who received placebo, including EDI-2 total scores or scores on any of the subscales.

Bosanac et al. [20] in an 8-week open trial reported on a small group of adult AN patients treated with *quetiapine*. Of the eight patients enrolled, only five completed the study (37% dropout rate). Over 4 weeks there was no significant difference in BMI and in the EDE-12 shape concern score.

A naturalistic open-label randomized trial compared 10 AN patients treated with *quetiapine* (100–400 mg/day) with 11 AN patients receiving treatment as usual [22]. The dropout rate was 33.3% for the quetiapine group and 38.9% for the control group. No differences in BMI and in ED symptoms (including scores on EDI-2 BD) were found between the two groups.

Hagman et al. [32] published an RCT of *risperidone* for the treatment of AN for 9 weeks. Two hundred and sixty young patients were assessed for eligibility. One hundred and seventy-four did not meet inclusion criteria, and 45 refused to participate, 41 female subjects with AN were randomized to receive risperidone or placebo. The dropout rates were 15.8% in the treatment group and 0% in the placebo group. The main adopted measures were the EDI-2, the Body Image Software Program (BIS), a computer program that measures body size distortion and body image dissatisfaction [33] and the Color-A-Person-Test (CAPT), a tool used to assess body image dissatisfaction [34]. No significant differences between the two groups were found in BMI variation, while scores on EDI-2 subscale of interpersonal distrust significantly decreased with risperidone. On the contrary, there were no significant differences between risperidone and placebo in change over time for measures of body image dissatisfaction or body image distortion on any of the specific scales (EDI-2 BD, BIS, or CAPT).

In 2002, Fassino et al. [9] conducted a prospective RCT to examine the efficacy of *citalopram*, as compared with a waiting-list condition, in the treatment of outpatients suffering from AN restricting-type. Twenty-six AN patients treated with citalopram showed significant differences in reducing depression, obsessive–compulsive symptoms, impulsiveness, and trait anger compared with the control group but not in BMI improvement. Seven patients in the citalopram group (29.6%) and six patients in the control group (30%) did not complete the study. No differences were found in EDI-2 body image dissatisfaction scale.

More recently, Misra et al. [35] randomized young girls with AN to transdermal *estradiol* (100 μg twice weekly) with cyclic progesterone or placebo patches and pills for 18 months. Measures of psychopathology included the EDI-2, the BSQ and a tool for measuring trait and state anxiety. Seventy-two girls completed these measures at baseline and 37 at 18 months (dropout of 48.6%). The two groups did not differ for changes in weight or BMI (secondary measures) over 18 months. As far as the primary measures are concerned, physiologic estrogen replacement improved trait but not state anxiety, eating attitudes, or body shape perception (both EDI-2 BD and BSQ).

In conclusion, the efficacy of different psychotropic drugs in AN seems so far questionable. No single drug has proven to be efficacious in body image disturbances, apart the single study which demonstrated an efficacy of haloperidol over body image disturbances of delusional nature.

26.2.2 Bulimia Nervosa

The comprehensive review of WFSBP [24] included 36 studies that assessed the efficacy of psychotropic drugs on bulimia. Most of these studies adopted as a primary outcome measure the reduction of binge eating and/or purging. However, 12 of these studies included also inventories (mostly EDI-2) measuring eating attitudes, and in just a few cases it was possible to enucleate the specific effect on body image dissatisfaction (Table 26.2).

Table 26.2 Drug treatment of bulimia nervosa considering response on body image dissatisfaction

	Treatments	Resp on EDI	Resp on other scales of bid
Barlow et al. [36]	Desipramine, placebo	No	
Blouin et al. [42]	Desipramine, fenfluramina	Yes	
Leitenberg et al. [37]	Desipramine, CBT		BSQ No
Fichter et al. [38]	Fluoxetine 60 mg, placebo	Equal	
Goldbloom et al. [39]	Fluoxetine, CBT		EDE No
Leombruni et al. [43]	Citalopram, fluoxetine	Equal	BSQ equal
Brambilla et al. [40]	CBT, amineptine, fluvoxamine	No	
Fichter et al., 1996 [45]	Fluvoxamine, placebo	EDI bulimia Yes	
Carruba et al., 2001 [41]	Moclobemide, placebo	Equal	
Fassino et al. [44]	Reboxetine	Yes	BSQ Yes
Hedges et al. [46]	Topiramate, placebo	Yes	

The results of this review are somewhat contradictory. Negative results on eating attitudes were obtained with *desipramine* [36, 37], *fluoxetine* [38, 39], *fluvoxamine* [40], and *moclobemide* [41]. On the other hand, in other studies a positive outcome was reported with *desipramine* [42], with both *citalopram* and *fluoxetine* using both EDI and BSQ [43] and with *fluvoxamine* even if only on the bulimia subscale of EDI [44]. More specifically, besides a positive effect on eating attitudes, in a trial on 28 patients lasting 3 months, Fassino et al. [44] reported with *reboxetine* a specific effect on the EDI-2 body image dissatisfaction scale and BSQ. Furthermore, Hedges et al. [46] in a 10-week trial obtained in 96 patients a positive outcome with *topiramate*, including the reduction of scores of EDI-2 body image dissatisfaction scale.

In conclusion, a still limited literature seems to show that in BN a few psychotropic drugs, in particular antidepressants (desipramine, citalopram, fluoxetine, reboxetine), may be helpful not only in the control of bingeing and purging, but also in the amelioration of eating attitudes, including body image dissatisfaction. Fluoxetine is the only FDA and EMA approved drug for BN, but does not seem to produce a relevant effect on eating attitudes. Other studies addressed to expand these findings are evidently needed.

26.2.3 Binge Eating Disorder

The literature on drug treatment of body image dissatisfaction in BED is even more scanty (Table 26.3). Marcus et al. [47] assigned 45 obese subjects (half with binge-eating problems) to *fluoxetine* (60 mg/day) or placebo in a 52-week double-blind trial. Patients treated with fluoxetine plus behavior modification lost significantly more weight than those treated with placebo plus behavior modification. However, the drug did not appear to have a differential benefit for binge-eaters and did not modify the EDI-2 BD score. Ricca et al. [48] found no advantage on eating attitudes

Table 26.3 Drug treatment of binge eating disorder considering response on body image dissatisfaction

	Treatments	Resp on EDI	Resp on other scales of BD
Marcus et al. [47]	Fluoxetine, placebo	No	
Ricca et al. [48]	Fluoxetine, fluvoxamine added to CBT		EDE No
Leombruni et al. [43]	Sertraline, placebo	No	
Golay et al. [49]	Orlistat, placebo	Yes (BD No)	

when adding *fluoxetine* and *fluvoxamine* to CBT. Leombruni et al. [43], who analyzed the efficacy of *sertraline* vs. placebo in BED patients, found a significant improvement in weight and a reduction in the frequency of binges, but no differences on the EDI-2 BD. Golay et al. [49] randomized 89 BED patients in a double-blind fashion to 24 weeks of treatment with 120 mg of *orlistat* or placebo three times daily. The authors found that the mean weight loss from baseline for orlistat-treated patients was significantly greater than for patients receiving placebo and that the overall EDI-2 score, but not the EDI-2 BD score, was lower in patients treated with orlistat than in those in the placebo group.

In conclusion, no benefit on body image dissatisfaction was evidenced with the use of different drugs in BED.

26.3 Drug Treatment for Body Dysmorphic Disorder

26.3.1 Body Dysmorphic Disorder

Body image disturbances also occur in other disorders, such as in Body Dysmorphic Disorder (BDD), where the presence of appearance concerns is the core criterion for the diagnosis. It is estimated that the point prevalence of BDD ranges from 1.7 to 2.4% of representative samples [50]. BDD differs from normal appearance concerns because it is associated with significant distress and can lead to significant functional impairment in interpersonal relationships and occupational status. When physical defects are present, people with BDD manifest excessive worries about the severity of the defect, as revealed by a high frequency and intensity of preoccupation. These individuals show ritualistic patterns of thoughts and behaviors associated with hiding, correcting, or fixing the perceived defect, such as intrusive thoughts about appearance, mirror checking, and camouflaging.

The analogies and differences between AN and BDD have repeatedly been investigated. While individuals with BDD may have appearance concerns about their face, skin, or other specific body areas, persons with AN typically think that they or parts of their body are too fat despite being dangerously underweight. In any case, a recent review suggests that the two disorders are highly comorbid, and show similar ages of onset, illness courses, and comparable clinical and personality characteristics, even though may respond differently to psychosocial and psychotropic treatments [51].

Even the nature of body concern has been analyzed. While these appearance-related beliefs have been considered of obsessive nature [52–54], recent research indicates that they are often delusional as well [50, 55, 56]. This fact has important consequences for the treatment, both because the insight has a key role in the adherence to the medication and because different classes of drugs may be implicated.

26.3.2 Clinical Trials

The literature on psychotropic drug treatment of BDD is scarce and predominantly concentrated on SSRI antidepressants, which are currently considered the medication of choice for BDD, even if no drug has been approved by FDA and EMA for BDD.

The main outcome measure used in drug trials on BDD is the Yale-Brown Obsessive Compulsive Scale, modified for body dysmorphic disorder (BDD-YBOCS) [57], even if other measures have been used, such as the Body Dysmorphic Disorder Examination (BDDE) [58].

So far, in the literature on drug and psychosocial treatments of BDD we can find only a trial which compared different drugs [59]. In this double-blind cross-over trial, two tricyclics—*clomipramine* and *desipramine*—were tested on 29 subjects per drug, randomized to 8 weeks of treatment. Clomipramine, which is characterized by a more definite serotonergic profile as compared with desipramine, proved to be more efficacious, independently from comorbid OCD, depression, or social phobia.

In a study comparing the efficacy on 67 BDD participants of 12 weeks of placebo-controlled *fluoxetine* treatment, 53% of subjects responded to fluoxetine and 18% to placebo [60]. Trials without a control group included one each with *citalopram* [61], *escitalopram* [62], *fluvoxamine* [63, 64], and *venlafaxine* [65], all showing an efficacy over BDD symptoms with a response rate varying from 53 to 73%. Patients usually experienced improvement on all items of the BDD-YBOCS, including urges to perform compulsive/safety behaviors, and control over BDD obsessions and compulsions. However, higher dosages than those used for anxiety and affective disorders were usually recommended [66, 67].

Sometimes BDD is characterized by body image misperceptions of delusional nature, and it is debated if SSRI can control also these symptoms. For example, in the study comparing *clomipramine* and *desipramine*, the superior efficacy of clomipramine was present regardless of whether or not the patients were delusional [58]. Similarly, a placebo-controlled study with *fluoxetine* showed that this drug was just as efficacious for individuals with delusional BDD as it was for those with non-delusional BDD [59].

Conversely, anecdotal studies report that antipsychotic augmentation of SSRI therapy is scarcely efficacious in delusional BDD. For example, a retrospective chart-review study of 90 patients with DSM-IV BDD, treated for up to 8 years, showed that second-generation antipsychotics augmentation of SSRI determined a response in only 2 out of 13 cases [68]. *Pimozide* augmentation was not efficacious in a subsequent trial [69] and the same happened with *olanzapine* augmentation [70]. On the contrary, Nakaaki et al. [71] were able to demonstrate in one SSRI-resistant patient the efficacy of 5 mg/day *olanzapine* augmentation. Furthermore, Uzun and Ozdemir [72] presented a case of a patient with treatment-resistant BDD who responded to the addition of *aripiprazole* to fluvoxamine treatment. Finally, Loréa and Van Wijnendaele [73] reported weak responses with *risperidone* and *clozapine* augmentation in psychotic patients with BDD features.

In conclusion, the literature seems to show that SSRI, mostly at a higher dosage than those used for depression, and other serotonergic agents may be useful for the treatment of BDD. To note, delusional BDD patients respond to SSRI just as likely as non-delusional BDD patients, and the use of antipsychotics should be considered as an add-on therapy only in selected, particularly resistant and delusional patients.

Conclusions

Nowadays, the management of ED with drugs can be based on an increasing number of studies. Not all drugs are efficacious and not all ED can benefit from drug treatment, but many substances showed to be efficacious in clearly definite eating disturbances.

The anorexia is particularly difficult to approach with psychotropic drugs. In particular, the antidepressants may be useful for comorbid affective and anxiety symptoms and antipsychotics may be used in cases where a psychotic dimension is clearly evident. On the contrary, an indiscriminate drug approach in AN is not recommended.

The efficacy of psychotropic drug treatment in BN seems promising, and this is confirmed in particular with classic psychotropic drugs, such as tricyclics and fluoxetine. Instead, in BED different drugs, not necessarily typical, can control binge eating behavior. For bulimia as well as for BED, the combination with CBT showed to be superior in reducing binge eating and weight.

When considering the specific dimensions of *body image disturbance* and *body image dissatisfaction*, we must first understand the different meaning of the two dimensions in the various ED, and in the BDD. Taking this into account, we must admit that the efficacy of psychotropic drugs in AN seems questionable: no single drug proved to be efficacious on body image disturbance, apart one single study with haloperidol. On the other hand, literature seems to show that in BN a few psychotropic drugs, in particular antidepressants, may be helpful not only in the control of bingeing end purging but also in the amelioration of body image dissatisfaction. These positive results should be counterbalanced by other negative data, which limit the evidence of efficacy. Furthermore, in BED no benefit on body image dissatisfaction was demonstrated by the use of different drugs.

Finally, we may use a different clinical condition to implement our knowledge on how to treat body image disturbance. The body dysmorphic disorder offers a good model to compare. In fact, in BDD the SSRI, mostly at a higher dosage than those used for depression, as well as other serotonergic agents, showed to be efficacious also in the presence of delusional patients. Moreover, an add-on therapy with antipsychotics could be started in selected, particularly resistant and delusional patients.

To conclude, the clinical target of ameliorating body image disturbance with drugs may be realistically reached in bulimia nervosa and BDD, while is less convincing in AN, where drugs are hardly useful, and in BED. The model of BDD may suggest that higher dosages of SSRI than those usually recommended may be helpful. In any case, we know that body image disturbance is particularly resistant to therapy, and thus it can probably be faced with a combined treatment where psychotherapy has an essential role. See Chaps. 21–25 of this book.

References

1. Halmi KA, Eckert E, LaDu TJ, Cohen J. Anorexia nervosa. Treatment efficacy of cyproheptadine and amitriptyline. Arch Gen Psychiatry. 1986;43:177–81.
2. Lacey JH, Crisp AH. Hunger, food intake and weight: the impact of clomipramine on a refeeding anorexia nervosa population. Postgrad Med J. 1980;56(Suppl 1):79–85.
3. Gwirtsman HE, Guze BH, Yager J, Gainsley B. Fluoxetine treatment of anorexia nervosa: an open clinical trial. J Clin Psychiatry. 1990;51:378–82.
4. Attia E, Haiman C, Walsh BT, Flater SR. Does fluoxetine augment the inpatient treatment of anorexia nervosa? Am J Psychiatry. 1998;155:548–51.
5. Barbarich NC, McConaha CW, Gaskill J, La Via M, Frank GK, Achenbach S, et al. An open-trial of olanzapine in anorexia nervosa. J Clin Psychiatry. 2004;65:1480–2.
6. Kaye WH, Nagata T, Weltzin TE, Hsu LK, Sokol MS, McConaha C, et al. Double-blind placebo-controlled administration of fluoxetine in restricting- and restricting-purging-type anorexia nervosa. Biol Psychiatry. 2001;49:644–52.
7. Walsh BT, Kaplan AS, Attia E, Olmsted M, Parides M, Carter JC, et al. Fluoxetine after weight restoration in anorexia nervosa: a randomized controlled trial. JAMA. 2006;295:2605–12.
8. Bergh C, Eriksson M, Lindberg G, Södersten P. Selective serotonin reuptake inhibitors in anorexia. Lancet. 1996;348(9039):1459–60.
9. Fassino S, Leombruni P, Daga G, Brustolin A, Migliaretti G, Cavallo F, Rovera G. Efficacy of citalopram in anorexia nervosa: a pilot study. Eur Neuropsychopharmacol. 2002;12:453–9.
10. Santonastaso P, Friederici S, Favaro A. Sertraline in the treatment of restricting anorexia nervosa: an open controlled trial. J Child Adolesc Psychopharmacol. 2001;11:143–50.
11. Safer DL, Darcy AM, Lock J. Use of mirtazapine in an adult with refractory anorexia nervosa and comorbid depression: a case report. Int J Eat Disord. 2011;44:178–81.
12. Safer DL, Arnow KD. Suprathreshold duloxetine for treatment-resistant depression, anorexia nervosa binge-purging type, and obsessive-compulsive disorder: a case report. Innov Clin Neurosci. 2012;9(3):13–6.
13. Cassano GB, Miniati M, Pini S, Rotondo A, Banti S, Borri C, et al. Six-month open trial of haloperidol as an adjunctive treatment for anorexia nervosa: a preliminary report. Int J Eat Disord. 2003;33:172–7.
14. Mauri M, Miniati M, Mariani MG, Ciberti A, Dell'Osso L. Haloperidol for severe anorexia nervosa restricting type with delusional body image disturbance: a nine-case chart review. Eat Weight Disord. 2013;18(3):329–32.
15. Ruggiero GM, Laini V, Mauri MC, Ferrari VM, Clemente A, Lugo F, Mantero M, Redaelli G, Zappulli D, Cavagnini F. A single blind comparison of amisulpride, fluoxetine and clomipramine in the treatment of restricting anorectics. Prog Neuro-Psychopharmacol Biol Psychiatry. 2001;25:1049–59.
16. Kishi T, Kafantaris V, Sunday S, Sheridan EM, Correll CU. Are antipsychotics effective for the treatment of anorexia nervosa? Results from a systematic review and meta-analysis. J Clin Psychiatry. 2012;73(6):e757–66.

17. Balestrieri M, Oriani MG, Simoncini A, Bellantuono C. Psychotropic drug treatment in anorexia nervosa. Search for differences in efficacy/tolerability between adolescent and mixed-age population. Eur Eat Disord Rev. 2013;21(5):361–73.
18. Miniati M, Mauri M, Ciberti A, Mariani MG, Marazziti D, Dell'Osso L. Psychopharmacological options for adult patients with anorexia nervosa. CNS Spectr. 2016;21(2):134–42.
19. Lebow J, Sim LA, Erwin PJ, Murad MH. The effect of atypical antipsychotic medications in individuals with anorexia nervosa: a systematic review and meta-analysis. Int J Eat Disord. 2013;46(4):332–9.
20. Bosanac P, Kurlender S, Norman T, Hallam K, Wesnes K, Manktelow T, Burrows G. An open-label study of quetiapine in anorexia nervosa. Hum Psychopharmacol. 2007;22:223–30.
21. Powers PS, Klabunde M, Kaye W. Double-blind placebo-controlled trial of quetiapine in anorexia nervosa. Eur Eat Disord Rev 2012;20(4):331–4.
22. Court A, Mulder C, Kerr M, Yuen HP, Boasman M, Goldstone S, Fleming J, Weigall S, Derham H, Huang C, McGorry P, Berger G. Investigating the effectiveness, safety and tolerability of quetiapine in the treatment of anorexia nervosa in young people: a pilot study. J Psychiatr Res. 2010;44:1027–34.
23. Trunko ME, Schwartz TA, Duvvuri V, Kaye WH. Aripiprazole in anorexia nervosa and low-weight bulimia nervosa: case reports. Int J Eat Disord. 2011;44(3):269–75.
24. Aigner M, Treasure J, Kaye W, Kasper S, WFSBP Task Force On Eating Disorders. World Federation of Societies of Biological Psychiatry (WFSBP) guidelines for the pharmacological treatment of eating disorders. World J Biol Psychiatry. 2011;12(6):400–43.
25. McElroy SL, Guerdjikova AI, Mori N, Keck PE Jr. Psychopharmacologic treatment of eating disorders: emerging findings. Curr Psychiatry Rep. 2015;17(5):35.
26. American Psychiatric Association. Diagnostic and statistical manual of mental disorders. 5th ed. Arlington, VA: American Psychiatric Publishing; 2013.
27. Cooper PJ, Taylor MJ, Cooper Z, Fairburn CG. The development and validation of the body shape questionnaire. Int J Eat Disord. 1987;6:485–94.
28. Mondraty N, Birmingham CL, Touyz S, Sundakov V, Chapman L, Beumont P. Randomized controlled trial of olanzapine in the treatment of cognitions in anorexia nervosa. Australas Psychiatry. 2005;13:72–5.
29. Brambilla F, Garcia CS, Fassino S, Daga GA, Favaro A, Santonastaso P. Olanzapine therapy in anorexia nervosa: psychobiological effects. Int Clin Psychopharmacol. 2007;22: 197–204.
30. Attia E, Kaplan AS, Walsh BT, Gershkovich M, Yilmaz Y, Musante D, et al. Olanzapine versus placebo for out-patients with anorexia nervosa. Psychol Med. 2011;41(10):2177–82.
31. Kafantaris V, Leigh E, Hertz S, Berest A, Schebendach J, Sterling WM, et al. A placebo-controlled pilot study of adjunctive olanzapine for adolescents with anorexia nervosa. J Child Adolesc Psychopharmacol. 2011;21(3):207–12.
32. Hagman J, Gralla J, Sigel E, Ellert S, Dodge M, Gardner R, et al. A double-blind, placebo-controlled study of risperidone for the treatment of adoles- cents and young adults with anorexia nervosa: a pilot study. J Am Acad Child Adolesc Psychiatry. 2011;50(9): 915–24.
33. Gardner RM, Boice R. A computer program for measuring body size distortion and body dissatisfaction. Behav Res Methods Instrum Comput. 2004;36(1):89–95.
34. Wooley OW, Roll S. The Color-A-Person Body Dissatisfaction Test: stability, internal consistency, validity, and factor structure. J Pers Assess. 1991;56(3):395–413.
35. Misra M, Katzman DK, Estella NM, Eddy KT, Weigel T, Goldstein MA, Miller KK, Klibanski A. Impact of physiologic estrogen replacement on anxiety symptoms, body shape perception, and eating attitudes in adolescent girls with anorexia nervosa: data from a randomized controlled trial. J Clin Psychiatry 2013;74(8):e765–71.
36. Barlow J, Blouin J, Blouin A, Perez E. Treatment of bulimia with desipramine: a double-blind crossover study. Can J Psychiatry. 1988;33:129–33.
37. Leitenberg H, Rosen JC, Wolf J, Vara LS, Detzer MJ, Srebenik D. Comparison of cognitive-behaviour therapy and desipramine in the treatment of builimia nervosa. Behav Res Ther. 1994;32:37–45.

38. Fichter MM, Leibl K, Rief W, Brunner E, Schmidt-Auberger S, Engel RR. Fluoxetine versus placebo: a double blind study with bulimic in patients undergoing intensive psychotherapy. Pharmacopsychiatry. 1991;24:1–7.
39. Goldbloom DS, Olmsted M, Davis R, Clewes J, Heinmaa M, Rockert W, Shaw B. A randomised controlled trial of fluoxetine and cognitive behavioural therapy for bulimia nervosa: short-term outcome. Behav Res Ther. 1997;35:803–11.
40. Brambilla F, Draisci A, Peirone A, Brunetta M. Combined cognitive-behavioral, psychopharmacological and nutritional therapy in bulimia nervosa. Neuropsychobiology. 1995;32:68–71.
41. Carruba MO, Cuzzolaro M, Riva L, Bosello O, Liberti S, Castra R, et al. Efficacy and tolerability of moclobemide in bulimia nervosa: a placebo-controlled trial. Int Clin Psychopharmacol. 2001;16:27–32.
42. Blouin AG, Blouin JH, Perez EL, Bushnik T, Zuro C, Mulder E. Treatment of bulimia with fenfluramine and desipramine. J Clin Psychopharmacol. 1988;8(4):261–9.
43. Leombruni P, Amianto F, Delsedime N, Gramaglia C, Abbate-Daga G, Fassino S. Citalopram versus fluoxetine for the treatment of patients with bulimia nervosa: a single-blind randomized controlled trial. Adv Ther. 2006;23:481–94.
44. Fassino S, Amianto F, Gramaglia C, Facchini F, Abbate Daga G. Temperament and character in eating disorders: ten years of studies. Eat Weight Disord. 2004;9(2):81–90.
45. Fichter MM, Krüger R, Rief W, Holland R, Döhne J. Fluvoxamine in prevention of relapse in bulimia nervosa: effects on eating-specefic psychopathology. J Clin Psychopharmacol. 1996;16:9–18.
46. Hedges DW, Reimherr FW, Hoopes SP, Rosenthal NR, Kamin M, Karim R, Capece JA. Treatment of bulimia nervosa with topiramate in a randomized, double-blind, placebo-controlled trial, part 2: improvement in psychiatric measures. J Clin Psychiatry. 2003; 64(12):1449–54.
47. Marcus MD, Wing RR, Ewing L, Kern E, McDermott M, Gooding W. A double-blind, placebo-controlled trial of fluoxetine plus behavior modification in the treatment of obese binge-eaters and non-binge-eaters. Am J Psychiatry. 1990;147:876–81.
48. Ricca V, Mannucci E, Mezzani B, Moretti S, Di Bernardo M, Bertelli M, et al. Fluoxetine and fluvoxamine combined with individual cognitive-behaviour therapy in binge eating disorder: a one-year follow-up study. Psychother Psychosom. 2001;70:298–306.
49. Golay A, Laurent-Jaccard A, Habicht F, Gachoud JP, Chabloz M, Kammer A, et al. Effect of orlistat in obese patients with binge eating disorder. Obes Res. 2005;13:1701–8.
50. Buhlmann U, Glaesmer H, Mewes R, Fama JM, Wilhelm S, Brähler E. Updates on the prevalence of body dysmorphic disorder: a population-based survey. Psychiatry Res. 2010;178(1):171–5.
51. Hartmann AS, Greenberg JL, Wilhelm S. The relationship between anorexia nervosa and body dysmorphic disorder. Clin Psychol Rev. 2013;33(5):675–85.
52. Hollander E, Wong CM. Body dysmorphic disorder, pathological gambling, and sexual compulsions. J Clin Psychiatry. 1995;56(Suppl 4):7–12.
53. Jolanta JRJ, Tomasz MS. The links between body dysmorphic disorder and eating disorders. Eur Psychiatry. 2000;15:302–5.
54. Phillips KA, Kaye WH. The relationship of body dysmorphic disorder and eating disorders to obsessive-compulsive disorder. CNS Spectr. 2007;12(5):347–58.
55. Phillips KA, Hollander E. Treating body dysmorphic disorder with medication: evidence, misconceptions, and a suggested approach. Body Image. 2008;5(1):13–27.
56. Mancuso SG, Knoesen NP, Castle DJ. Delusional versus nondelusional body dysmorphic disorder. Compr Psychiatry. 2010;51(2):177–82.
57. Phillips KA, Hollander E, Rasmussen SA, Aronowitz BR, DeCaria C, Goodman WK. A severity rating scale for body dysmorphic disorder: development, reliability, and validity of a modified version of the Yale-Brown Obsessive Compulsive Scale. Psychopharmacol Bull. 1997;33(1):17–22.
58. Rosen JC, Reiter J. Development of the body dysmorphic disorder examination. Behav Res Ther. 1996;34(9):755–66.

59. Hollander E, Allen A, Kwon J, Aronowitz B, Schmeidler J, Wong C, et al. Clomipramine vs desipramine crossover trial in body dysmorphic disorder: Selective efficacy of a serotonin reuptake inhibitor in imagined ugliness. Arch Gen Psychiatry. 1999;56(11):1033–9.
60. Phillips KA, Albertini RS, Rasmussen SA. A randomized placebo-controlled trial of fluoxetine in body dysmorphic disorder. Arch Gen Psychiatry. 2002;59(4):381–8.
61. Phillips KA, Najjar F. An open-label study of citalopram in body dysmorphic disorder. J Clin Psychiatry. 2003;64(6):715–20.
62. Phillips KA. An open-label study of escitalopram in body dysmorphic disorder. Int Clin Psychopharmacol. 2006;21(3):177–9.
63. Perugi G, Giannotti D, Di Vaio S, Frare F, Saettoni M, Cassano GB. Fluvoxamine in the treatment of body dysmorphic disorder (dysmorphophobia). Int Clin Psychopharmacol. 1996;11(4):247–54.
64. Phillips KA, Dwight MM, McElroy SL. Efficacy and safety of fluvoxamine in body dysmorphic disorder. J Clin Psychiatry. 1998:59(4):165–71.
65. Allen A, Hadley SJ, Kaplan A, Simeon D, Friedberg J, Priday L, Baker BR, Greenberg JL, Hollander E. An open-label trial of venlafaxine in body dysmorphic disorder. CNS Spectr. 2008;13(2):138–44.
66. Ipser JC, Sander C, Stein DJ. Pharmacotherapy and psychotherapy for body dysmorphic disorder. Cochrane Database Syst Rev. 2009;1:CD005332.
67. Fang A, Matheny NL, Wilhelm S. Body dysmorphic disorder. Psychiatr Clin North Am. 2014;37(3):287–300.
68. Phillips KA, Albertini RS, Siniscalchi JM, Khan A, Robinson M. Effectiveness of pharmacotherapy for body dysmorphic disorder: a chart-review study. J Clin Psychiatry. 2001;62(9):721–7.
69. Phillips KA. Olanzapine augmentation of fluoxetine in body dysmorphic dis-order. Am J Psychiatry. 2005;162(5):1022–3
70. Phillips KA. Placebo-controlled study of pimozide augmentation of fluoxetine in body dysmorphic disorder. Am J Psychiatry. 2005;162(2):377–9.
71. Nakaaki S, Murata Y, Furukawa TA. Efficacy of olanzapine augmentation of paroxetine therapy in patients with severe body dysmorphic disorder. Psychiatry Clin Neurosci. 2008;62(3):370.
72. Uzun O, Ozdemir B. Aripiprazole as an augmentation agent in treatment-resistant body dysmorphic disorder. Clin Drug Investig. 2010;30(10):707–10.
73. Loréa N, Van Wijnendaele R. Body dysmorphic disorder and psychosis. Case reports and discussion. Encéphale. 2012;38(1):37–41.

Studies on Body Shame in Eating and Weight Disorders

27

Giada Pietrabissa, Giorgia Varallo, Cesare Cavalera, Gian Mauro Manzoni, Roberto Cattivelli, Alessandro Rossi, Margherita Novelli, Federica Scarpina, Valentina Villa, Enrico Molinari, and Gianluca Castelnuovo

27.1 Introduction

Shame is a painful emotion comprising cognitive, behavioral, affective, social, and physiological components. It can be seen as resulting from comparison of the self's action with the self's standards [1] and its expression goes from disgust and anger to anxiety, including social confrontation [2]. Shame is, in fact, strictly related with significant negative affect deriving from adverse external evaluations, such as being perceived inadequate, inferior, unattractive, or defective by others [3–5].

G. Pietrabissa · R. Cattivelli · E. Molinari · G. Castelnuovo (✉)
Istituto Auxologico Italiano IRCCS, Psychology Research Laboratory, Ospedale San Giuseppe, Verbania, Italy

Department of Psychology, Catholic University of Milan, Milan, Italy
e-mail: gianluca.castelnuovo@auxologico.it; gianluca.castelnuovo@unicatt.it

G. Varallo · A. Rossi · M. Novelli · V. Villa
Istituto Auxologico Italiano IRCCS, Psychology Research Laboratory, Ospedale San Giuseppe, Verbania, Italy

C. Cavalera
Department of Psychology, Catholic University of Milan, Milan, Italy

G. M. Manzoni
Istituto Auxologico Italiano IRCCS, Psychology Research Laboratory, Ospedale San Giuseppe, Verbania, Italy

Faculty of Psychology, eCampus University, Novedrate (Como), Italy

F. Scarpina
Istituto Auxologico Italiano IRCCS, Psychology Research Laboratory, Ospedale San Giuseppe, Verbania, Italy

"Rita Levi Montalcini" Department of Neuroscience, University of Turin, Turin, Italy

M. Cuzzolaro, S. Fassino (eds.), *Body Image, Eating, and Weight*,
https://doi.org/10.1007/978-3-319-90817-5_27

27.2 Body Shame in Eating and Weight Disorders

Shame has been significantly associated with mental disorders [5], or dangerous eating attitudes and body image difficulties [6–8]. Particularly, studies have established a significant link between body shame and eating disorders [9–16], and "attention has recently turned towards examining the effect of body shame (as opposed to general shame) on eating pathology [17–19]. Though some studies have used a composite measure that includes body shame, behavioral shame and characterological shame (e.g., [20–22]), those that measure body shame separately generally find that it is a stronger predictor of eating pathology than is general shame [23] or that it is independently predictive [24]" ([9], p. 375). Troop (2016) also noted that "… if we experience shame, we may change our behaviour in order to escape this aversive state, we may also modify our behaviour in order to avoid feeling shame in the first place. One may, for example, attempt to lose weight if one feels ashamed of one's current body size while, if one feels that to gain weight would be shameful, then one may engage in preventive dieting rather than weight loss dieting ([25])" ([9], p. 365–366). In fact, "It has been suggested that disordered eating behaviours, such as dieting, may emerge as maladaptive strategies adopted to avoid this threatening emotion (shame) and to strive for approval and acceptance by others (e.g., through reaching a socially valued thin physical appearance [2, 26, 27]). Binge eating may also be conceptualized as a maladaptive strategy to avoid or escape from disturbing thoughts or negative emotions [28–31]. However, binge eating paradoxically increase negative affect and negative self-evaluations, being associated with increased shame, guilt and criticism [9, 21, 25, 30]" ([3], p. 196).

"Shame activates therefore a series of automatic defensive behavioural outputs (e.g., concealment, avoidance, control and excessive self-monitoring) in order to protect the self from such perceived threats" ([3], p. 196). However, the consequences of shame are still not clear, and further research is needed in order to better understand the impact of shame, body image, weight, shape, and eating concerns on disordered eating attitudes, particularly Binge Eating Disorder (BED) [3]. In this regard, a recent research by Duarte et al. [3] demonstrated that the greater is the binge eating symptomatology, the higher are the severity of eating concerns, the level of depression, and the shame experienced by the person [6], as well as the cognitive fusion concerning body image [3].

A significant role in this process is, in fact, played by the individuals' Cognitive Fusion (CF) which is "the degree to which one's internal experiences are perceived as trustworthy presentations of reality and acted upon, instead of experienced as transitory and subjective mental events" ([3], p. 196). CF may provoke avoidance-driven actions that lead to negative consequences, such as increased suffering and anxiety [32–36]. Also, it seems to be related to difficulties in modifying behaviors, even if change anticipates a state of well-being [37, 38]. Therefore, when negative thoughts refer to body image dissatisfaction, CF may increase the risk of developing eating disorder symptomatology [18, 39, 40].

In addition, Troop (2016) [9] found that "those who feel more body shame eat more, not less, over the following week" (p. 380), whereas, according to the Miller's theories [41], if feelings of shame have a punishing-aversive effect, consuming less calories may reduce this negative emotional state [9]. Allan and Goss [2] described the shame-shame cycle [2] as the possibility that eating more may represent an attempt to limit or avoid negative feelings connected with shame. In case of anticipation of body shame due to weight gain, instead, another possible reaction is to: "eat less over the following week, which supports Miller's proposition [41] that shame is prohibiting. In fact, the strength of the association between anticipated body shame and subsequent caloric intake is stronger than that between current body shame and intake." ([9], p. 380).

27.3 Assessment

Body shame typically relates with Eating Disorders (EDs) and Body Dysmorphic Disorders (BDD) [42] (see also Chaps. 4, 5, 8–10 of this book). Scales more related to eating concerns than BDD are here below specifically considered. In fact, according to Weingarden et al. [42], "although there are existing self-report measures of body shame (e.g., Body Image Guilt and Shame Scale, BIGSS [19]), these measures tend to capture weight- and eating-based shame, which is more likely to occur in individuals with eating disorders. Unlike eating disorders, primary concerns in BDD are not weight or eating based; rather, they tend to focus on the skin, facial features, or other specific body parts ..." ([42], p. 10).

27.3.1 The Experience of Shame Scale

The Experience of Shame Scale—Body subscale (ESS [43]) is a measure of body shame focused on assessing BDD criteria rather than shame (exemplifying items are "Have you worried about what other people think of your appearance?"; "Have you avoided looking at yourself in the mirror?"). This tool is not the most accurate to capture the typical features of body shame in a possible context of BDD [42].

27.3.2 The Body Image Guilt and Shame Scale

The Body Image Guilt and Shame Scale (BIGSS) was developed by Thompson, Dinnel, and Dill in 2003 [19], in order to detect weight- and eating-based shame typically occurring in patients with eating problems. The BIGSS scale reports a significant level of reliability and validity focusing primarily on shame related to weight- and eating-concerns.

27.3.3 The Body-Focused Shame and Guilt Scale

Inspired by both the Test of Self-Conscious Affect (TOSCA) scale, which induces shame, guilt or externalizing responses toward a given set of scenarios [20], and the BIGSS [27], the Body-Focused Shame and Guilt Scale (BF-SGS) [42] "presents scenarios that are likely to evoke self-conscious emotions regarding one's body parts (e.g., "You go to the mall, and everybody seems better looking than you")" ([42], p. 11). Authors created "not only shame-driven response options (e.g., "You would feel so awful that you'd want to hide"), but also guilt-driven (e.g., "You would think, "I should spend more time trying to improve my appearance") and externalization-of-blame (e.g., "You would think, 'They don't lead busy lives, so they are able to spend more time on their appearance'") response options" ([42], p. 11).

27.3.4 The Bodily Shame Scale

In 2006, Troop and colleagues developed the Bodily Shame Scale (BSS) [23], an 11-item self-report questionnaire focused on the measurement of feelings, thoughts, and behaviors related to the experience of shame in association with the individuals' actual body. In fact "the BSS included scales measuring current body shame (the shame that is experienced in relation to one's current body size) and anticipated body shame (shame that is anticipated if one were to gain weight)" ([9], p. 376). Still, to assess current and anticipated body shame in different populations (clinical and not clinical ones) may lead to different outputs: "... in a non-clinical sample of women, current and anticipated body shame predicted fear of weight gain and restrictive efforts to reduce weight. This was also true in women with a history of EDs although current body shame also predicted bulimic behaviours (specifically binge eating and laxative abuse)" ([9], p. 376). When looking at a clinical sample (females with a history of EDs), instead, it is possible to note that "while current body shame predicted an increase in the degree of underweight and misperception of body size, anticipated body shame predicted an increase in fear of weight gain" ([9], p. 376).

27.3.5 The Body Pride and Shame Scale

The Body Pride and Shame Scale (BPSS) is composed by 30 items deriving from the Bodily Shame Scale (BSS [23]). In fact, while the BSS questionnaire is focused on assessing thoughts, feelings, and behaviors related to the experience of shame in strict relationship with the body, the BPSS scale overcomes the limitations of the BSS scale measuring the psychological constructs of pride and the associations between shame and pride with weight-related variables (weight loss, weight gain, and current weight). A detailed description of the BPSS scale is reported in Troop (2016), who stated: "Thus, five shame items and five pride items measuring behavioural, affective and attitudinal aspects were included to which participants indicated the degree to which they experienced (or anticipated they would experience) these emotions in relation to current body weight, imagined weight gain and imagined weight loss. The 10 items in each of these three sections were identical except insofar as they reflected different temporal perspectives (current versus anticipated). There are 30 items in total and each is scored on a 10-point Likert scale with response options ranging from "not at all true of me" to "completely true of me"" ([9], p. 376).

27.3.6 The Other as Shamer Scale

According to Gilbert [24], there are two distinct elements of the shame experience: internal and external shame. Internal shame involves negative self-evaluation and self-criticism, whereas external shame originates from how a person experiences him/herself in the minds of others, and it involves the belief that others view the self negatively [44]. Since strongly associated with social difficulties, such as ostracism and social criticism, which adversely affect the representation of the self, a growing body of studies underlines the need to measure and address external shame [45]. In fact, the perception of being seen negatively by others too often leads the individual to inhibit the activation of positive affect. This process will then reinforce external shame and give rise to a vicious circle maintained by the application of maladaptive coping strategies for managing shame [46].

External shame is measured by the Other as Shamer Scale (OAS [5, 47]), and a detailed description of the OAS is provided by Duarte (2017): "this scale includes 18 items measuring external shame. Participants are asked to rate the items on a 5-point Likert scale (0 = 'Never' to 4 = 'Almost always') according to the frequency with which they make certain evaluations about how others negatively judge, look down or criticize them. In the original study the scale showed good reliability, with a Cronbach's alpha of 0.92" ([47], p. 197).

27.3.7 The Cognitive Fusion Questionnaire-Body Image

Due to the impact of cognitive fusion related to body image on eating psychopathology, an adequate operationalization of this construct may be of great utility in clinical practice. As underlined by Duarte et al. (2017) [3], the Cognitive Fusion Questionnaire-Body Image (CFQ-BI [39]) "was based on the original Cognitive Fusion Questionnaire [32] and includes 10 items measuring cognitive fusion related to body image. Participants are asked to rate the extent to which each statement (e.g., 'My thoughts relating to my body image cause me great distress or emotional pain') is true regarding their own experience, using a 7-point Likert scale (1 = 'Never true' to 7 = 'Always true'). This scale presents good internal consistency, retest reliability, as well as discriminant, convergent and divergent validities [39]..." ([3], p. 197).

27.4 Treatment

Cognitive Behavioral Therapy (CBT) is the gold standard treatment for obesity and BED [48]. However, according to Duarte et al. (2017) "although the comprehensiveness and the practical nature of CBT approach are positive, this psychotherapy does not necessarily produce a successful weight loss" ([3], p. 167). Working on "body shame" and "shame" would, therefore, help people to reduce or modify negative self-evaluations and to promote acceptance of internal experiences, also limiting individuals' engagement in avoidance behaviors that may trigger a dangerous vicious circle of maintenance of the problem [28, 29, 37, 49, 50].

In fact, according to Goss and colleagues (2009), it is very useful in a clinical context to assess shame prior to and during EDs treatments [2]. However, healthcare professionals are not always prepared to identify and manage shame-related issues that may, therefore, remain unsolved. Still, "an empathic, collaborative and empowering stance is likely to be crucial in treatment, as shame is likely to be triggered relatively easily, particularly at the beginning of therapy. In general, safety behaviours (i.e., behaviours that help patients manage difficult affect) are functional and clients resist giving them up. However, for most other disorders, safety behaviours are not a source of internal or external pride. In EDs, safety behaviours (such as weight control) are sometimes an initial source of external pride and frequently a source of internal pride; indeed, they may be the sole source of self-esteem and central to self-identity. Therapists will need to explore this and be empathic to the intense fear of change and the painful dilemmas this involves" ([2], p. 312–313).

In order to better cope with shame concerns, a multi-context intervention including individual psychotherapy, psychoeducation for patients and caregivers, promotion of a functional not-shaming attitude in the individual's wider social network, group-based interventions based on CBT [51] or Compassion Focused Therapy approach (CFT) is required [2, 52].

Specifically, as suggested by Troop (2016) [9], psychotherapeutic interventions should focus more on emotions rather than cognitions. The self-compassion approach, for example, is aimed to modulate negative feelings using self-kindness and common humanity [53]. Also, Hayaki et al. underlined that shame can be significantly and quickly reduced in EDs patients by improving self-compassion [54]. Goss and colleagues also corroborated the utility of treatments improving self-compassion in the EDs management [49, 55].

27.5 Prevention

Studies demonstrated that body shame and appearance anxiety may lead to dysfunctional eating behaviors. "The most consistent support has been found for body shame, which is not very surprising as recurrent opportunities for women to experience body shame in both public and private contexts are powerful motivators to engage in disordered eating. In contrast, mixed or no support has been shown for the role of interoceptive awareness or flow experience in the context of self-objectification and disordered eating" ([56], p. 578).

A theory that is interesting in both primary and secondary prevention settings is the Fredrickson and Roberts's Objectification Theory [57]. The authors "identified self-objectification as the first psychological consequence to emerge among girls and women as a result of living in a sexually objectifying cultural milieu. Self-objectification is defined as the adoption of a third-person perspective on the self as opposed to a first-person perspective such that girls and women come to place greater value on how they look to others rather than on how they feel or what they can do. An objectified body is a malleable, measureable, and controllable body. By viewing and treating themselves as sexual objects, it is argued that girls and women act as their own first surveyors in anticipation of being evaluated by others. Thus, the body becomes the site of reparative action and vigilant monitoring to manage the sexual objectification. When girls and women view themselves through this self-objectified lens, they take a peculiar stance on their own bodies that is fundamentally disruptive to the self–body relationship" ([56], p. 575). Preventing the development of such a dangerous self-objectification among girls and women may avoid or reduce several psychopathological consequences, including high level of body shame and appearance, as well as safety anxiety [56].

A preventive approach may be to work more on shame proneness. In fact, findings from a recent research carried out by Cavalera et al. [8] "provide support for the view that shame proneness is related to eating disorder symptomatology because of a strong correlation with psychological variables. Therefore, shame proneness not only correlates with body shame or drive for thinness … but is also associated with many psychological aspects related to very different domains of eating disorders" (p. 379).

27.6 Body Shaming: A New Phenomenon in the Social Media Era

While traditional media consumption has been widely linked to Body Image Dissatisfaction (BID) and disordered eating behaviors, few studies suggest that nowadays one of the biggest source of self-objectification and body image concerns comes from Social networking websites (SNSs) [58–62]. Specifically, a recent investigation confirmed that Internet exposure and Facebook (FB) usage are associated with internalization of the thin ideal, body surveillance, and drive for thinness [58]. Moreover, Fardouly et al. showed that FB and fashion magazine usage were positively correlated with self-objectification and that these relationships were mediated by appearance comparisons [63]. SNSs are commonly used to build social relationships and search for information about others [64]. This process is defined "social grooming" [64] and it is characterized by checking friends' profiles, leaving messages, and commenting on them [65]. These social behaviors may increase occasions for users to view the images that social media friends post on their profiles, thus leading to compare their appearance to others.

Increased exposure to FB has been also recognized as factor that further raises the risk of negative social comparison [66], negative self-evaluations, and rumination about not being "good enough" [67]. However, a detailed study observed that the time spent on FB is less significant than the degree of exposure to body appearance-activity such as FB photo sharing, and that FB usage is positively associated with body image concerns [68].

Notably, the effects that FB can have on body image may depend on how it is used: people who post images and statuses to compete with or compare themselves to others may experience negative consequences, such as low self-esteem or body image concerns, but the risk of experiencing a higher rate of BID is minimal for those who use FB to connect and share with friends [69, 70].

Still, recent research has observed that SNSs users are more inclined to expose their body in an online public space where it can be freely accessed (Online body display) in order to attract mates, express dominance, and project positive self-image. Also, a study conducted by Nadkarni and Hofmann concluded FB use to be primarily driven by two human needs: belongingness and self-presentation [71]; and Toma and Hancock [72] further found that FB profiles help satisfy individuals' needs for self-worth and self-integrity.

Also, SNSs may promote authentic self-expression; but the sense of anonymity that they also drive, may foster inappropriate and hostile communications, including cyberbullying [73]. Cyberbullying occurs when individuals use technology (i.e., e-mail, cellphones, text messages, webpages) to write aggressive, embarrassing, or hateful messages to/about peers in order to intimidate, harass, shame, and control, and being a growing phenomenon, its impact is often underestimated [74].

Together with FB, Twitter represents another popular social media platform, and appearance-related issue seems to be a recurrent tweet topic. In October 2013, a group of users dedicated an entire week to "fat shaming" posting negative comments about others' body weight and shape followed by "#FatShamingWeek." Almost 1500 Tweets were posted with this hashtag and many of these were weight-stigmatizing. Tweets might be encouraged by the belief that "hurting people's feelings is the quickest way to get them to change," as on the page accountable for #FatShamingWeek. This belief has also been sustained in traditional media as a motivating strategy [75]. However, research suggests that shaming has negative effects on health-related behavior change [75].

Teasing regarding body weight has been associated to body image dissatisfaction, eating disordered behaviors, low self-esteem, and negative psychological consequences such as depression and suicide ideation [76–78]. Since BID plays a pivotal role in the development of EDs [79], it is necessary to identify factors that contribute to increase body dissatisfaction in order to improve prevention and reforming targeted earlier intervention programs, such as developing "Twitter chats," or FB pages promoting information, acceptance of body sizes, and positive messages.

References

1. Lewis M. Shame: the exposed self. New York: Free Press; 1992.
2. Goss K, Allan S. Shame, pride and eating disorders. Clin Psychol Psychother. 2009;16(4):303–16.
3. Duarte C, Pinto-Gouveia J, Ferreira C. Ashamed and fused with body image and eating: binge eating as an avoidance strategy. Clin Psychol Psychother. 2017;24(1):195–202.
4. Pinto-Gouveia J, Ferreira C, Duarte C. Thinness in the pursuit for social safeness: an integrative model of social rank mentality to explain eating psychopathology. Clin Psychol Psychother. 2014;21(2):154–65.
5. Matos M, Pinto-Gouveia J, Duarte C. Above and beyond emotional valence: the unique contribution of central and traumatic shame memories to psychopathology vulnerability. Memory. 2012;20(5):461–77.

6. Duarte C, Pinto-Gouveia J, Ferreira C. Escaping from body image shame and harsh self-criticism: exploration of underlying mechanisms of binge eating. Eat Behav. 2014;15(4):638–43.
7. Manasse SM, et al. Slowing down and taking a second look: inhibitory deficits associated with binge eating are not food-specific. Appetite. 2016;96:555–9.
8. Cavalera C, et al. Erratum to: Shame proneness and eating disorders: a comparison between clinical and non-clinical samples. Eat Weight Disord. 2017;22(2):379.
9. Troop NA. The effect of current and anticipated body pride and shame on dietary restraint and caloric intake. Appetite. 2016;96:375–82.
10. Pila E, et al. Intrapersonal characteristics of body-related guilt, shame, pride, and envy in Canadian adults. Body Image. 2016;16:100–6.
11. Iannaccone M, et al. Self-esteem, body shame and eating disorder risk in obese and normal weight adolescents: a mediation model. Eat Behav. 2016;21:80–3.
12. Higgins MK, et al. Examining impulsivity as a moderator of the relationship between body shame and bulimic symptoms in Black and White young women. Body Image. 2015;14:39–46.
13. Ferreira C, Pinto-Gouveia J, Duarte C. Self-compassion in the face of shame and body image dissatisfaction: implications for eating disorders. Eat Behav. 2013;14(2):207–10.
14. Jankauskiene R, Pajaujiene S. Disordered eating attitudes and body shame among athletes, exercisers and sedentary female college students. J Sports Med Phys Fitness. 2012;52(1):92–101.
15. Claudat K, Warren CS, Durette RT. The relationships between body surveillance, body shame, and contextual body concern during sexual activities in ethnically diverse female college students. Body Image. 2012;9(4):443–54.
16. Jambekar SA, Masheb RM, Grilo CM. Gender differences in shame in patients with binge-eating disorder. Obes Res. 2003;11(4):571–7.
17. Forman EM, et al. Acceptance-based behavioral treatment for weight control: a review and future directions. Curr Opin Psychol. 2015;2:87–90.
18. Merwin R, Wilson K. Understanding and treating eating disorders. An ACT perspective. In: Blackledge J, Ciarrochi J, Deane P, editors. Acceptance and commitment therapy. Contemporary theory, research, and practice. Australia: Australian Academic Press; 2009. p. 87–117.
19. Thompson T, Dinnel DL. Construction and initial validation of the self-worth protection scale. Br J Educ Psychol. 2003;73(Pt 1):89–107.
20. Tangney JP, Wagner PE, Gramzow R. The test of self-conscious affect (TOSCA). Fairfax, VA: George Mason University; 1989.
21. Troop NA, Redshaw C. General shame and bodily shame in eating disorders: a 2.5-year longitudinal study. Eur Eat Disord Rev. 2012;20(5):373–8.
22. Cavalera C, et al. A short version of the state shame and guilt scale (SSGS-8). TPM Test Psychom Methodol Appl Psychol. 2017;24(1):99–106.
23. Troop NA, et al. Establishing a useful distinction between current and anticipated bodily shame in eating disorders. Eat Weight Disord. 2006;11(2):83–90.
24. Gilbert P. What is shame? Some core issues and controversies. In: Gilbert P, Andrews B, editors. Shame: interpersonal behaviour, psychopathology and culture. New York: Oxford University Press; 1998. p. 3–38.
25. Castilho P, et al. Recall of threat and submissiveness in childhood and psychopathology: the mediator effect of self-criticism. Clin Psychol Psychother. 2014;21(1):73–81.
26. Gilbert P. Body shame: a biopsychosocial conceptualisation and overview with treatment implications. In: Gilbert P, Miles J, editors. Body shame: conceptualisation, research and treatment. New York: Brunner Routledge; 2002. p. 3–54.
27. Goss K, Gilbert P. Eating disorders, shame and pride: a cognitive–behavioural functional analysis. In: Gilbert P, Miles J, editors. Body shame: conceptualisation, research and treatment. New York: Brunner Routledge; 2002. p. 219–55.
28. Arnow B, Kenardy J, Agras WS. The Emotional Eating Scale: the development of a measure to assess coping with negative affect by eating. Int J Eat Disord. 1995;18(1):79–90.
29. Goldfield GS, et al. Stress and the relative reinforcing value of food in female binge eaters. Physiol Behav. 2008;93(3):579–87.

30. Heatherton TF, Baumeister RF. Binge eating as escape from self-awareness. Psychol Bull. 1991;110(1):86–108.
31. Leehr EJ, et al. Emotion regulation model in binge eating disorder and obesity—a systematic review. Neurosci Biobehav Rev. 2015;49:125–34.
32. Gillanders DT, et al. The development and initial validation of the cognitive fusion questionnaire. Behav Ther. 2014;45(1):83–101.
33. Luoma J, Hayes SC. Cognitive defusion. In: O'Donohue WT, Fisher JE, Hayes SC, editors. Cognitive behavior therapy: applying empirically supported techniques in your practice. New York: Wiley; 2003. p. 71–8.
34. Barnes-Holmes DCHS, Dymond S. Self and selfdirected rules. In: Hayes S, Barnes-Holmes D, Roche B, editors. Relational frame theory. A post Skinnerian account of human language and cognition. New York: Plenum Press; 2001. p. 119–39.
35. Hayes S. Acceptance and commitment therapy, relational frame theory, and the third wave of behavioral and cognitive therapies. Behav Ther. 2004;35(4):639–65.
36. Hayes SC, et al. Acceptance and commitment therapy: model, processes and outcomes. Behav Res Ther. 2006;44(1):1–25.
37. Forman EM, Butryn ML. A new look at the science of weight control: how acceptance and commitment strategies can address the challenge of self-regulation. Appetite. 2015;84:171–80.
38. Hayes S, Strosahl KD, Wilson K. Acceptance and commitment therapy: an experiential approach to behavior change. New York: Guilford Press; 1999.
39. Ferreira C, et al. Getting entangled with body image: development and validation of a new measure. Psychol Psychother. 2015;88(3):304–16.
40. Trindade IA, Ferreira C. The impact of body image-related cognitive fusion on eating psychopathology. Eat Behav. 2014;15(1):72–5.
41. Miller W. The anatomy of disgust. Cambridge, MA: Harvard University Press; 1997.
42. Weingarden H, et al. Development and validation of the body-focused shame and guilt scale. J Obsessive Compuls Relat Disord. 2016;8:9–20.
43. Andrews B, Qian M, Valentine JD. Predicting depressive symptoms with a new measure of shame: The Experience of Shame Scale. Br J Clin Psychol. 2002;41(Pt 1):29–42.
44. Gilbert P. What is shame? Some core issues and controversies. New York: Oxford University Press; 1998.
45. Matos M, et al. The Other As Shamer Scale-2: development and validation of a short version of a measure of external shame. Pers Individ Dif. 2015;74):6–11.
46. Gilbert P. The evolution of shame as a marker for relationship security: a biopsychosocial approach. In: Tracy J, Robins R, Tangney J, editors. The self-conscious emotions: theory and research. New York: Guilford Press; 2007. p. 283–309.
47. Goss K, Gilbert P, Allan S. An exploration of shame measures-I: the 'Other As Shamer' scale. Pers Individ Dif. 1994;17:713–7.
48. Castelnuovo G, et al. Cognitive behavioral therapy to aid weight loss in obese patients: current perspectives. Psychol Res Behav Manag. 2017;10:165–73.
49. Goss K, Allan S. Compassion focused therapy for eating disorders. Int J Cogn Ther. 2010;3:141–58.
50. Castelnuovo G, et al. Brief strategic therapy vs cognitive behavioral therapy for the inpatient and telephone-based outpatient treatment of binge eating disorder: the STRATOB randomized controlled clinical trial. Clin Pract Epidemiol Ment Health. 2011;7:29–37.
51. Wilson GT, Fairburn CG. Cognitive treatments for eating disorders. J Consult Clin Psychol. 1993;61(2):261–9.
52. Gilbert P, Irons C. A pilot exploration of the use of compassionate images in a group of self-critical people. Memory. 2004;12(4):507–16.
53. Neff KD. The development and validation of a scale to measure selfcompassion. Self Identity. 2003;2(3):223–50.
54. Hayaki J, Friedman MA, Brownell KD. Shame and severity of bulimic symptoms. Eat Behav. 2002;3(1):73–83.

55. Gale C, et al. An evaluation of the impact of introducing compassion focused therapy to a standard treatment programme for people with eating disorders. Clin Psychol Psychother. 2012;21:1–12.
56. Calogero RM. Objectification theory, self-objectification, and body image. In: Cash TF, editor. Encyclopedia of body image and human appearance. San Diego: Academic Press; 2012. p. 574–80.
57. Fredrickson BL, Roberts T-A. Objectification theory. Psychol Women Q. 1997;21(2):173–206.
58. Tiggemann M, Slater A. NetGirls: the Internet, Facebook, and body image concern in adolescent girls. Int J Eat Disord. 2013;46(6):630–3.
59. Bair CE, et al. Does the Internet function like magazines? An exploration of image-focused media, eating pathology, and body dissatisfaction. Eat Behav. 2012;13(4):398–401.
60. Beuf A. Beauty is a beast. New York: University of Pennsylvania Press; 1990.
61. Cohen R, Blaszczynski A. Comparative effects of Facebook and conventional media on body image dissatisfaction. J Eat Disord. 2015;3:23.
62. Fardouly J, et al. The mediating role of appearance comparisons in the relationship between media usage and self-objectification in young women. Psychol Women Q. 2015;39(4):447–57.
63. Fardouly J, et al. Social comparisons on social media: the impact of Facebook on young women's body image concerns and mood. Body Image. 2015;13:38–45.
64. Tufekci Z. Grooming, Gossip, Facebook and Myspace. Inform Commun Soc. 2008;11(4):544–64.
65. Utz S, Tanis M, Vermeulen I. It is all about being popular: the effects of need for popularity on social network site use. Cyberpsychol Behav Soc Netw. 2012;15(1):37–42.
66. Blease C. Too many 'friends,'too few 'likes'? Evolutionary psychology and 'Facebook depression'. Rev Gen Psychol. 2015;19(1):1.
67. Feinstein B. Negative social comparison on Facebook and depressive symptoms: Rumination as a mechanism. 2013.
68. Meier EP, Gray J. Facebook photo activity associated with body image disturbance in adolescent girls. Cyberpsychol Behav Soc Netw. 2014;17(4):199–206.
69. Cruz C. Facebook users don't always have a poor body image or a risky diet. 2015. http://www.medicaldaily.com/social-networking-facebook-users-dont-always-have-poor-body-image-or-risky-diet-344048. Accessed 21 July 2015.
70. Preidt R. Does Facebook lead young women to dangerous diets? 2015. http://health.usnews.com/health-news/articles/2015/07/27/does-facebook-lead-young-women-to-dangerous-diets. Accessed 27 July 2015.
71. Nadkarni A, Hofmann SG. Why do people use Facebook? Pers Individ Dif. 2012;52(3):243–9.
72. Toma CL, Hancock JT. Self-affirmation underlies Facebook use. Pers Soc Psychol Bull. 2013;39(3):321–31.
73. Kwan GCE, Skoric MM. Facebook bullying: an extension of battles in school. Comput Hum Behav. 2013;29(1):16–25.
74. Hinduja S, Patchin JW. Bullying, cyberbullying, and suicide. Arch Suicide Res. 2010;14(3):206–21.
75. Puhl R, Peterson JL, Luedicke J. Motivating or stigmatizing? Public perceptions of weight-related language used by health providers. Int J Obes (Lond). 2013;37(4):612–9.
76. Eisenberg ME, Neumark-Sztainer D, Perry CL. Peer harassment, school connectedness, and academic achievement. J Sch Health. 2003;73(8):311–6.
77. Haines J, et al. V.I.K. (Very Important Kids): a school-based program designed to reduce teasing and unhealthy weight-control behaviors. Health Educ Res. 2006;21(6):884–95.
78. Menzel JE, et al. Appearance-related teasing, body dissatisfaction, and disordered eating: a meta-analysis. Body Image. 2010;7(4):261–70.
79. Stice E, Shaw HE. Role of body dissatisfaction in the onset and maintenance of eating pathology: a synthesis of research findings. J Psychosom Res. 2002;53(5):985–93.

Studies on Weight Stigma and Body Image in Higher-Weight Individuals

28

Angela Meadows and Rachel M. Calogero

28.1 Introduction

Weight stigma can be broadly defined as negative attitudes and behaviors toward higher-weight individuals because of their weight or size. Negative attitudes include endorsement of stereotypes of higher-weight people, for example, that they are greedy, lazy, or unintelligent. Stigmatizing behaviors can range from social exclusion to rude or presumptuous comments, from staring or pointing to overt discrimination, or even verbal and physical attacks.

Understanding the causes and consequences of weight stigma is essential for scholars and practitioners in want of a more complete understanding of negative body image and eating disorders. Fear of fat, negative evaluations of weight and body shape, and overvaluations of body size and shape for self-worth constitute core features of eating disorders—features that have not emerged in a vacuum but rather emerge in the context of experienced and internalized forms of weight stigma in fat-phobic societies.

This chapter provides a summary of the scientific evidence for the relationship between weight stigma and negative body image in higher-weight individuals.[1] Due to space restraints, an exhaustive review of the literature on weight stigma and body image is beyond the scope of this chapter. Our aim is to highlight select studies that

[1] In this chapter, we use the phrase "higher-weight" to describe individuals with a body mass index in the "overweight" or "obese" categories, and avoid "person-first language." For the rationale behind this usage and a discussion on best practice for avoiding stigmatizing terminology when describing larger bodies, see [95].

A. Meadows (✉)
School of Psychology, University of Exeter, Exeter, UK

R. M. Calogero
Department of Psychology, Western University, London, ON, Canada
e-mail: rcaloger@uwo.ca

M. Cuzzolaro, S. Fassino (eds.), *Body Image, Eating, and Weight*,
https://doi.org/10.1007/978-3-319-90817-5_28

provide a good representation of the research in this area. Where existing reviews are available, we will direct your attention to these resources. We will also focus on two forms of target-directed weight stigma—experiencing stigma from others and stigmatizing oneself. We will not here consider the impact of outwardly directed anti-fat attitudes, i.e., dislike of fat others.

28.2 Experienced Weight Stigma

Experienced weight stigma refers to public and private encounters of being stigmatized by others because of your weight. Higher-weight individuals report experiencing weight stigma in practically every domain of daily living, including at work, in education, healthcare, and interpersonal relationships (for a review, see [1]), and weight stigma appears to be on the increase [2, 3]. The frequency of stigma experiences increases markedly with increasing body weight, but most forms of weight stigma also occur more frequently in women, and are prevalent at lower body weights than in men [2, 4]. Weight-related stigma and bullying are also prevalent among children and adolescents. Weight is now one of the most common targets for bullying in schools, with 92% of adolescents reported observing weight-related bullying in one large US study [5].

One difficulty when attempting to explore the impact of experienced weight stigma is that, when considered retrospectively, it may be difficult to remember specific instances that have occurred, sometimes many years previously. Additionally, without example of what might constitute "stigma," many instances of weight-related bias might not be recognized as such by the victim, being written off as deserved, well meaning, simple truths, or just innocent statements, especially when originating from children [6, 7]. This is likely to be particularly true of the more subtle forms of stigma and discrimination—most people are likely to remember being physically attacked, for example, but people making assumptions about your lifestyle based solely on your weight might not stand out. Yet, for most people, their lifetime exposure to stigma will consist primarily of these "lesser" but more pervasive incidents. Additionally, micro-aggressions—sometimes-ambiguous verbal, behavioral, or environmental "messages" that confer some form of negative valuation or hostility toward higher-weight individuals, whether intentional or not—are commonplace and act as a cumulative stressor [8]. In a qualitative study of "obese" Australian adults drawn from diverse community sources, half of the participants reported experiencing environmental forms of stigma, two-thirds had experienced direct stigma, and three-quarters discussed indirect forms of stigma [6]. These latter included experiences such as feeling ignored by customer service staff, friends, or family members ridiculing other higher-weight individuals in front of them, and strangers peering inquisitively into their supermarket trolleys. The participants found these subtle occurrences more difficult to respond to, and felt that subtle forms of stigma had the most negative impact on their health and well-being [6].

To partially address issues of recall and attribution, Myers and Rosen developed one of the first complex measures of experienced weight stigma, the Stigmatizing Situations Inventory (SSI) [9]. The SSI prompts respondents using a list of 50 specific situations, across eleven different domains (family, strangers, employment, doctors, etc.), and participants indicate how often they have ever experienced each type of stigma. Studies using the SSI find that, overall, most people indicate having experienced some form of stigma at least once in their lifetimes, with some studies reporting certain types of stigma occurring as often as weekly. Even so, retrospective studies that rely on recall over a lifetime likely underestimate the prevalence of weight stigma. In confirmation, a US study in which 50 higher-weight women completed a daily diary each day for seven days, indicating whether any of the 50 items of the SSI had occurred to them that day, resulted in over 1000 incidents being recorded, or approximately 3 incidents per person over the seven days [10]. Additionally, none of the currently used measures of experienced weight stigma include the media as a possible source of stigma. Representations of higher-weight bodies in both news and entertainment media are most often stigmatizing in nature [11, 12], and the media is frequently mentioned as a source of weight stigma in qualitative studies [6, 13] and studies that capture stigma experiences in real time [14]. Thus, in addition to issues with the reliability of recall, it is likely that existing quantitative studies of experienced weight stigma may further underestimate the extent of exposure to such negative messages. In an Australian study of 46 higher-weight Australian adults, in which the media was included as a potential source of stigma in the instructions to participants, participants completed the SSI at the start of the study and reported, on average, having experienced weight stigma "several times in [their] life." By comparison, using a personal digital assistant to record stigmatizing events as they occurred, these same participants recorded an average of 11.1 episodes of weight stigma over the subsequent 2-week study period, or approximately 0.8 episodes per day [15].

28.3 Internalized Weight Stigma

When higher-weight individuals endorse negative stereotypes and ascribe those negative attributes to themselves, they are said to express internalized weight stigma, or weight-related self-stigma. Internalized weight stigma is most commonly defined as not just awareness, or even endorsement, of negative stereotypes, but also as applying those negative attributes to yourself *and* subsequently devaluing yourself because of it. This last step is important. As a fat person, I may be aware that many people consider fat people to be lazy; I may or may not agree that this is usually true (I don't), and I may even happily admit that I, myself, am indeed both fat and lazy. But if I do not judge myself morally for this purported deficit, if my self-worth is unaffected by this admission, then I cannot be said to have internalized weight stigma.

Unlike experienced weight stigma, internalized weight stigma appears to affect men and women fairly equally, although a few studies have found slightly higher internalized weight stigma scores in women (e.g., [16, 17]). Internalized weight stigma is related to the construct of body image, involving, as it does, negative appearance evaluation, but differs in key aspects. First, the negative judgments are specific to facets of body image related to weight. Second, there is a strong element of self-blame involved. For example, while one might have poor body image related to a specific body part, such as height, or a disliked facial feature, this is unlikely to be tainted by a belief that one is to blame for that aspect of one's appearance.

Most studies of IWS have been conducted in adults. To date, only one study has examined internalized weight stigma in children. In a German study of 1000 children aged 7–11 years, girls reported higher internalized weight stigma than boys, and "overweight," but not "non-overweight," children tended to agree with self-stigmatizing statements [18].

28.4 Correlates of Experienced and Internalized Weight Stigma

Both experienced and internalized weight stigma have been linked with a range of physical, psychological, and behavioral outcomes, even after controlling for body mass index (BMI)[2] and other potential confounding factors, including disordered eating patterns, reduced motivation to exercise, avoidant coping strategies, substance dependence, and social and behavioral problems in adolescents, including substance use, self-harm, and suicidality. Weight stigma is also strongly associated with healthcare avoidance among higher-weight individuals, including reduced engagement with preventive screening programs [19, 96]. Perceived weight discrimination is associated with higher risk of chronic morbidity [21] and mortality [22], and with poorer self-reported physical and psychological health and health-related quality of life [23]. Indeed, both actual experience of stigma and simply fear of being stigmatized by others appear to mediate the relationship between higher BMI and poorer self-reported health [24]. In another study, the association between higher BMI and poorer physical health-related quality of life was only observed in those individuals who also had high levels of internalized weight stigma [25].

Importantly, internalized weight stigma appears to mediate the relationship between experienced weight stigma and health and well-being outcomes in higher-weight individuals, including depression and anxiety [26], low self-esteem, emotional and externally cued eating, as opposed to responding to internal hunger signals [27], binge eating [28], and exercise behavior [27, 29]. That is, being stigmatized by others can lead to more self-stigmatization, and it is this internalized weight stigma that then influences health and behavioral outcomes, suggesting that targeting internalized weight stigma may be a useful approach in health interventions.

[2] All outcomes in included studies are controlled for BMI unless otherwise specified.

28.5 Experienced Weight Stigma and Body Image

28.5.1 Cross-Sectional Studies

Despite the difficulties of reliably measuring experienced weight stigma, even studies using relatively crude measures consistently indicate associations between stigma history and body image, as well as other psychological outcomes. In a sample of 174 higher-weight adults considering weight-loss surgery, a single-item question asking whether they had been teased about their weight when they were a child identified significantly greater weight and shape concern and body dissatisfaction among those with a history of childhood weight teasing compared with those who had only minimal or no experience of childhood weight-related teasing [30].

Most studies using the SSI use a composite score across all sources of stigma. Such studies have found that frequency of stigmatizing experiences is strongly correlated with body image distress in weight-loss treatment-seeking populations [9, 31], and the effect is exacerbated when the targets also hold stronger anti-fat attitudes themselves [32]. In a community sample of higher-weight individuals, 97% of the 111 participants reported having ever experienced weight stigma, with half having such experiences at least once per week. Scores were strongly correlated with body dissatisfaction, although the relationship was attenuated a little when controlling for BMI [33]. An adapted version of the SSI that examined experienced weight stigma at different life points found formative experiences of weight stigma during childhood, in particular, have lingering effects on adult body image problems [34].

A small number of studies have reported outcomes independently for the different domains of the SSI, allowing for a more nuanced understanding of the impact of experiencing different forms of weight stigma. In an international sample of higher-weight adults, social exclusion had the strongest impact on appearance evaluation, but poorer body image was also linked with receiving rude comments from one's family, from children, or other people; embarrassment about your weight from loved ones; people making negative assumptions about you; and experiencing work-based discrimination. Inappropriate comments from doctors, experiencing physical barriers in daily life—for example seats too narrow, not being able to fit through turnstiles, being stared at in public, and even being physically attacked were not significantly associated with body image in this sample [27]. While it is to be expected that interpersonal forms of weight stigma have a strong impact on body image, it is a little surprising that some of the more systemic forms of stigma did not have an effect.

One of the most common forms of experienced weight stigma, particularly among younger people, is that of weight-related teasing. By its nature, teasing is most likely to come from an individual's immediate circle, such as family or friends, and thus can often be a pervasive occurrence in daily life. In an extensive review and meta-analysis of the literature between January 1991 and December 2009, Menzel and colleagues [35] examined the evidence for a relationship between weight-related teasing and body image in adults and children, and reported a medium-large effect overall, with the effects being somewhat stronger in children than in adults, and in female than male samples. Studies that used more comprehensive measures of teasing, rather than a single question about teasing experience, reported higher effects still, suggesting that methodological limitations of some studies may underestimate the true relationship between weight-related teasing and body dissatisfaction. One limitation of these findings is that all but four of the studies were conducted in all, or predominantly, "normal-weight" samples, making it unfeasible to explore, or control for, the role of BMI in this relationship. Studies that independently assess the effects of weight-based teasing across different weight groups have produced conflicting results: while studies report significantly higher levels of weight-related teasing in heavier students, one study that compared response to teasing by weight status found no difference in affective responses to victimization, including body-related distress, between weight groups [36], whereas in another study, heavier individuals reported greater distress as a result of weight-based victimization than did slimmer individuals [37].

28.5.2 Longitudinal Studies

To our knowledge, there are no longitudinal studies that prospectively assess the impact of experienced weight stigma on body image in adults. However, a number of studies have prospectively explored the impact of weight-related teasing in children and adolescents over time. Cattarin and Thompson conducted the first such study, exploring the impact of weight-related teasing in adolescence on subsequent body image and eating disturbances [38]. The study took baseline measures from 210 adolescent girls, aged 10–15, although only approximately 40% of this sample was available at 3-year follow-up. Higher-weight girls experienced significantly more weight-related teasing, which in turn predicted subsequent global appearance dissatisfaction, although not dissatisfaction with specific body sites, after controlling for age, weight, and maturational status. However, only body-site dissatisfaction subsequently predicted restrictive and bulimic eating disturbances when controlling for all other factors.

One of the longest-established cohorts in this field is the Eating and Activity in Teens and Young Adults cohort (Project EAT), with the first wave of data collected from 4746 adolescent boys and girls at 31 middle and high schools in a Midwest US city in 1999 [39]. Second-wave data collection in 2003–2004 indicated that weight-related teasing at baseline had a small but significant correlation with body dissatisfaction at 5-year follow-up, but was not a significant independent predictor of body image after controlling for baseline body dissatisfaction and BMI [40]. Thus, the detrimental impact of weight-related teasing may be most profound during earlier adolescent body image development. However, just published fourth-wave data collected in 2015 from 1830 participants, now in young adulthood, indicated that women who had experienced weight-based teasing from family or peers as adolescents reported poorer body image, as well as more binge eating behavior, eating to cope, and unhealthy weight control practices 15 year later, even after controlling for baseline BMI and other potential confounding factors, than did women who had not experienced such teasing. Men who had experienced weight-related teasing from peers also experienced more body dissatisfaction, although the long-term impact on dysfunctional eating behaviors was not pronounced in males. Weight-related teasing from family members did not appear to have the same effect in men as it did in women [41].

More recently, a prospective longitudinal study of intrapersonal development risk factors in childhood assessed the impact of weight-related teasing and social exclusion in 1486 children (mean age 8.4 years) from 33 German primary schools on their body dissatisfaction and disordered eating behaviors 1 year later [42]. The sample was predominantly "normal weight," with only 13.6% classified as "overweight" or "obese" by BMI z-scores. Experiences of weight stigma were reported in over half of "obese" children, compared with just over one in four "overweight" children, and one in twelve "normal-weight" participants; higher-weight girls reported more stigma than higher-weight boys and also reported greater body dissatisfaction and disordered eating at follow-up. Although baseline weight status significantly predicted body dissatisfaction 1 year later in both genders, the significant relationship between experienced weight stigma and body dissatisfaction at follow-up was present only in girls. Similarly, in girls, but not boys, body dissatisfaction mediated the relationship between baseline weight stigma experience and disordered eating behavior 1 year later [42].

28.5.3 Experimental Studies

The field of weight stigma research has been largely dominated by cross-sectional studies, which preclude drawing reliable inferences regarding causality. Recently, a number of well-designed experimental manipulation studies have been published, which attempt to elucidate the processes by which the harms associated with weight stigma are transmitted. Such studies randomize participants to either a stigma condition or a control condition, thus isolating exposure to the stigmatizing experience as the driver of any resultant differences in outcome between the groups. However, to date, only one study has included a measure of body image as an outcome of interest [43]. As this study explores the impact of both experienced and internalized weight stigma, it will be discussed in detail in the section on internalized weight stigma, below Sect. 28.6.3.

28.5.4 Intervention Studies

A number of weight-stigma reduction interventions have been tested, with generally unimpressive results [44]; however, few consider the body image of the intervention participants as an outcome measure. Interventions aimed at increasing acceptance of size diversity among higher-weight individuals themselves sometimes include content targeting general anti-fat attitudes; however, most of these interventions involve multiple components, including content directed at changing self-directed attitudes. While these complex approaches are likely to be more effective at producing changes in psychological outcomes and well-being from a clinical point of view than are interventions targeting a single construct or risk factor, it is then difficult to identify the effect of targeting weight stigma *per se* on changing body image. School-based interventions aimed at reducing weight-related bullying and harassment are another potential source of information. Most school-based interventions also take a multivariate approach, targeting multiple risk factors for body dissatisfaction and disordered eating, and some of these have successfully improved student body image but failed to impact on weight-related teasing ([45]; for a review, see [46]). To our knowledge, only one school-based intervention has *specifically* targeted weight-related teasing as its primary outcome. The V.I.K. (Very Important Kids) program is an extensive, multi-component intervention aiming to reduce weight-related teasing in elementary schools, although the ultimate goal was prevention of unhealthy weight-control behaviors. In a small pilot study, V.I.K. was trialed in 63 4th–6th graders at an ethnically diverse, primarily low-income US Midwest school and their families. Approximately half of the students were "overweight" or "obese" by BMI *z*-score. Eight months after the intervention, weight-related teasing was significantly reduced at the school, whereas a matched control school saw an increase in teasing over the same period. Students in the intervention school also felt more confident in their ability to address weight-related teasing if it occurred. However, the intervention did not have any effect on body satisfaction, dieting behavior, or unhealthy weight control practices [47].

28.6 Internalized Weight Stigma and Body Image

28.6.1 Cross-Sectional Studies

The majority of studies that have assessed internalized weight stigma have been cross-sectional, which makes it impossible to elucidate the relationship between internalized weight stigma and body image beyond saying they are strongly associated with each other. In contrast, the relationship between both self-reported and objectively measured BMI tends to only weakly correlate with measures of body image [17, 48]. That is, poor body image is less related to *actual* body weight and shape, but is, rather, dependent upon negative self-evaluation due to weight. In fact, in two separate studies conducted in higher-weight community samples, BMI and general dislike of fat individuals accounted for only a small amount of the variance in body image concerns, whereas internalized weight stigma explained between a third and half of the variation in scores [49, 50].

The robust negative relationship between internalized weight stigma and body image has been consistently replicated across studies using numerous different measures of body image, including general appearance evaluation [27], weight-related body self-consciousness [50], body satisfaction [51], weight dissatisfaction [52], weight and shape concerns [53], body-related pride [54], and body shame and body image flexibility [55]—a form of distress tolerance defined as the ability to accept sometimes negative body-related thoughts and feelings. The relationship is also consistent in clinical [50, 56] as well as community samples, and in adolescents [57, 58] and children [59] as well as in adults.

Internalized weight stigma has also been shown to mediate the relationship between experienced weight stigma and appearance evaluation [27] and weight dissatisfaction [28, 57]. That is, being stigmatized by others because of one's weight is associated with higher levels of internalized weight stigma, which in turn is linked with poorer body image. Many of the measures of body image used in these studies were assessed as part of an evaluation of eating-disordered cognitions and behaviors, and, unsurprisingly, internalized weight stigma also mediates the relationship between experienced weight stigma and problem eating, in slimmer as well as in higher-weight samples [60, 61].

It is worth noting that the majority of these studies have used the Weight Bias Internalization Scale (WBIS), which comprises 11 items relating to negative global self-judgments due to weight status, appearance of the higher-weight body, and how the individual thinks they appear to others [49], and therefore this strong relationship is not unexpected. Nevertheless, an alternative, and increasingly popular measure of internalized weight stigma, the Weight Self-Stigma Questionnaire (WSSQ) [16], distinguishes between self-devaluation and fear of being stigmatized by others, and doesn't focus on the appearance of the body. A recent comparative study of internalized weight stigma measures found no association between the WSSQ Self-Devaluation subscale and body image in a weight-loss surgery sample, but did find a moderate association between the WSSQ Fear of Stigma subscale and appearance evaluation; in contrast, the WBIS was significantly correlated with appearance evaluation and with appearance orientation—how focused the individual is on their appearance [56]. However, a psychometric evaluation of the WSSQ in a sample of higher-weight French-Canadian adolescents reported high correlation between physical appearance evaluation and both subscales of the WSSQ [58]. Further studies are needed to more clearly elucidate the relationship between internalized weight stigma and body image, and to clarify whether alternative conceptualizations of weight-related self-stigma differentially predict body image in clinical and non-clinical populations.

28.6.2 Longitudinal Studies

Prospective longitudinal studies in community samples of adults rarely consider body image as an outcome measure, although body image may be an outcome of interest in studies conducted in eating disorder or weight-loss treatment-seeking populations. However, specific measures of internalized weight stigma have only recently been developed and have therefore not been included in existing long-term prospective or cohort studies.

To our knowledge, only one study has so far tracked both internalized weight stigma and body image over time. In a pre-post design, 14-week behavioral weight-loss intervention, change in internalized weight stigma between baseline and the end of the intervention was significantly associated with improvements in general appearance evaluation [62]. It is worth noting that changes in BMI were small, and the reductions in internalized weight stigma and body image were not due to changes in actual body size.

28.6.3 Experimental Studies

Few studies have utilized experimental designs to identify any causative role of internalized weight stigma in psychological outcomes, although a few have explored its role in eating behavior. To our knowledge, only one study has included a measure of body image as an outcome variable. In an online study, 260 higher-weight participants read about a female employee denied a promotion to a sales position because of her weight [43]. They were then randomized to either an "Experienced" stigma condition, where they read about the employee's outrage and were asked to write about a similar experience of their own when they had been treated unfairly because of their weight, or to an "Internalized" stigma condition, where they read how the employee blamed herself and felt worthless, and again asked to write about a similar experience of their own. Compared with the Experienced stigma condition, those in the Internalized stigma condition reported more negative affect, less positive affect, and lower self-esteem following the intervention. In the Experienced stigma condition, women reported significantly more body dissatisfaction than did men. They also reported slightly more body dissatisfaction than men in the Internalized stigma condition, but this was not statistically significant. Surprisingly, while men reported greater body dissatisfaction in the Internalized condition than in Experienced stigma condition, there were no differences in the effect on body dissatisfaction between Experienced and Internalized stigma for women. The authors hypothesized that internalized weight stigma may be so ingrained in most higher-weight women that it may have been less responsive to the manipulation than was the case in the male participants [43]. While findings from several cross-sectional studies have suggested that internalized weight stigma may be a more important driver of negative health outcomes than experienced weight stigma, this study provided the first confirmatory experimental evidence. Further research is needed to replicate and clarify these findings.

28.6.4 Intervention Studies

A small number of studies that specifically target internalized weight stigma have now been conducted, and have demonstrated significant improvements in quality of life, psychological outcomes, and problematic eating behaviors in the experimental group compared with a control [63–65]. However, only one of these included body image as an outcome measure [65]. In a small pilot trial of "Accept Yourself!"—an 11-week manualized self-acceptance program created using a Health At Every Size® and Acceptance Commitment Therapy framework [66], 21 higher-weight women with major depressive disorder saw marked improvements in internalized weight stigma and body image flexibility, as well as in depressive symptoms and quality of life, at the end of the program, and these were maintained at 3-month follow-up; no changes in weight occurred among the participants [65].

Other studies have targeted internalized weight stigma as part of a broader intervention. For example, one randomized controlled trial of two different behavioral weight-loss approaches compared a typical program with one that included psycho-education around weight stigma, both experienced and internalized, media literacy, and body acceptance [67]. Both programs included information about nutrition and exercise, and weight-loss maintenance. The extent to which weight stigma can be successfully targeted within a weight-loss treatment context is debatable, and indeed both programs produced similar reductions in internalized weight stigma and small improvements in body satisfaction. It is reasonable to assume that individuals who stigmatize themselves because of their weight will report lower self-stigma on achieving weight loss; however, it is likely that subsequent increases in internalized weight stigma will be observed when weight is regained, unless underlying negative attitudes toward weight are also altered. Interestingly, the participants in the traditional weight-loss group continued to assign negative stereotypes to both themselves and to higher-weight others after the intervention, whereas those receiving the program with the stigma-reduction component saw large reductions in negative stereotypes, both toward themselves and to higher-weight individuals in general [67], suggesting that the program may have been effective in changing attitudes, despite the weight-loss setting. Nevertheless, it would be interesting to see whether these changes would be maintained in the face of weight regain.

Similar findings were reported from another comparative trial of two "healthy living" programs—a traditional weight-loss intervention and a weight-neutral program [68, 69]. The weight-neutral program promoted health behaviors for intrinsic reasons, such as personal enjoyment and well-being, with no focus on weight loss as a goal. Although the weight-neutral program emphasized size acceptance and an appreciation of natural body size diversity, the program did not specifically target internalized weight stigma. Nevertheless, while the weight-loss program resulted in significant weight-loss after the 6-month trial period and no weight loss was observed in the weight-neutral group, both programs produced a similar reduction in internalized weight stigma post-study. Reductions in weight and shape concerns also decreased in both groups, although the effect was larger in the weight-neutral group. However, at 24-month follow-up, weight regain was apparent in the weight-loss group, as was a rebound in internalized weight stigma scores, whereas improvements were maintained in the weight-neutral group. Likewise, a significant interaction effect of internalized weight stigma and time on weight concerns was observed in the weight-neutral but not the weight-loss group, and a marginal effect was observed for shape concerns [68, 69]. Thus, it seems likely that improvements in internalized weight stigma and body image that occur as a result of weight loss are due, at least in part, to changes in weight rather than changes in views about weight, and benefits may be contingent upon weight-loss maintenance, and therefore somewhat tenuous. Interventions are clearly needed that result in reduced internalized weight stigma independent of weight loss. Earlier studies of weight-neutral interventions, while not measuring internalized weight stigma *per se*, do suggest that improvements in body image measures (or other psychosocial, eating-related, or physical activity outcomes) resulting from such programs are not generally matched or maintained in weight-loss comparison groups [70–73].

28.7 Ethnic and Cultural Differences

Although early cross-cultural studies suggested differences in anti-fat attitudes between countries [74], negative attitudes toward higher-weight bodies are becoming the norm worldwide, even in countries where fat was previously admired [75], and experienced weight stigma is now prevalent in both developed and developing countries [76, 77] (see also Chap. 31 of this book). The majority of studies of internalized weight stigma have been conducted in the USA, although a small but growing number of studies have recently emerged from countries in Europe [26, 78–80] and the Middle East [81–83].

In a recent study of 379 higher-weight adults from 16 different countries, frequency of experienced weight stigma did not differ by geographical region after controlling for BMI; however, the relationship between experienced weight stigma and appearance evaluation, controlling for BMI, was much stronger among participants from Oceania, than among those from the UK, North America, and Europe [27]. The reasons for this difference are unclear, and future cross-cultural studies are needed to identify other sociocultural factors that moderate these relationships. Some differences in levels of internalized weight stigma were also apparent. Approximately two-thirds of participants from the UK and Oceania reported at least some degree of internalized weight stigma, compared with only around 40% of participants from the USA and Europe. Interestingly, regional averages were inversely proportional to regional mean BMI, such that participants with the highest mean BMI by region had the lowest levels of internalized weight stigma, and vice versa, possibly due to a norming effect whereby higher-weight bodies are less obviously deviant from regional norms. However, the relationship between internalized weight stigma and body image was the same across all regions [27].

Looking at patterns of experienced weight stigma by ethnicity and race, baseline data from the Project EAT cohort indicated similar rates of weight-related teasing experiences among higher-weight adolescents, independent of race or ethnicity, although there was some variation in source of teasing, i.e., family or peers, and White girls tended to express more distress as a result of weight-related teasing than did girls from other racial or ethnic groups [84]. Cross-sectional data from a subsequent wave of Project EAT, comprising a racially and socioeconomically diverse sample of nearly 3000 middle- and high-school students, found that ever having been harassed or teased because of weight was independently associated with significantly lower body dissatisfaction in both boys and girls, as well as self-esteem, and, in girls only, depressive symptoms [85]. After controlling for weight-based harassment, no effects on body image were observed for having experienced sexual harassment or harassment due to race or socioeconomic status, underscoring the distinctive negative impact of this form of weight stigma for young people.

Most studies of internalized weight stigma that have explored race/ethnicity as a potential covariate have reported no difference between groups [27, 86, 87]. There is some evidence from US samples that internalized weight stigma may be lower in African-American participants than in non-Hispanic White and Latino/Latina participants, but again, the relationship between internalized weight stigma and body image appears to be the same across ethnicities and racial groups, with African-American participants also tending to report less body dissatisfaction than other racial/ethnic groups [88, 89].

Little is known about the processes by which weight-related teasing is associated with body image issues and distal health outcomes across ethnic or cultural groups. A study in 100 Australian Caucasian females and 48 Hong Kong Chinese females, aged 17–28, found different associations between weight-related teasing, body dissatisfaction, and eating disturbance between the two groups [90]. Models were constructed including BMI, ever having Dieted, internalization and pressure to conform to the thin ideal, self-esteem, and experience of weight-based teasing as predictors of body dissatisfaction, and body dissatisfaction as a mediator between these predictors and a measure of eating disturbance (bulimia and drive for thinness). In the full model, self-esteem was the only significant predictor of body dissatisfaction, and body dissatisfaction and ever having dieted predicted eating disturbance in the Australian sample. In the Hong Kong sample, body dissatisfaction did not significantly predict eating disturbance, whereas self-esteem and weight-related teasing experience directly predicted problematic eating [90]. However, this sample had only a single participant with a BMI over 25, and it has yet to be established that weight-related teasing impacts on outcomes in the same way in higher-weight individuals.

28.8 Future Research

Although researchers have been cataloguing the prevalence and correlates of weight stigma for over 50 years, there are still many gaps in our knowledge. Longitudinal cohort studies are now providing evidence of the serious long-term, cumulative harms associated with experienced weight stigma, but little is known about the long-term impacts of internalized weight stigma. Additionally, while some studies have explored mechanisms between weight stigma and health and behavioral outcomes, most have utilized cross-sectional designs that preclude determination of causal pathways.

Another area that requires attention is that much of the research in the field of weight stigma continues to be conducted in predominantly White populations. Exploring cultural and ethnic differences in weight stigma serves not only to document the extent of the problem within the wider social context, but also enables consideration of intersectional effects, more accurately mirroring the lived experience of individuals in marginalized groups. Most people do not fit neatly into a single box, based solely on their size, gender, ethnicity, age, socioeconomic status, sexuality, or other singular identity. In reality, there is a non-additive effect of the multiple identities that we all possess, which may overlap in complex ways in terms of exposure to oppression and inequality [91, 92].

Additionally, much research on weight stigma is still conducted in student samples or other predominantly "normal-weight" populations. From an ethical standpoint, this situation serves to obliterate the voices of the marginalized group. However, there are also scientific reasons why this practice may result in findings of uncertain validity. While anti-fat attitudes, fear of fat, weight-related teasing, and body dissatisfaction are present across the weight range, the *experience* of experienced stigma is almost certainly different in an individual whose body weight is considered to fall outside the normative range. These experiences occur within a pervasively hostile environment in which higher-weight people additionally carry the burden of their recognized subordinate status in society, in a way unlikely to be experienced by members of the privileged, i.e., normative, group [93], and are likely to be complicated by aspects of blame and shame, again, not experienced by slimmer individuals. Thus, the generalizability of research conducted in lower-weight populations to higher-weight individuals is far from proven, and any distal effects on affective, cognitive, or behavioral outcomes may well be transmitted via different mechanisms [94]. Research that aims to elucidate the pathways via which weight-related discrimination impacts on such outcomes should be conducted in populations that are the primary target of such discrimination and prejudice, or in mixed-weight populations that allow for any moderating effects of weight status to be explored. Nevertheless, it is critical that the roles of both experienced and internalized weight stigma as causal and complicit forces in negative body image and eating pathology across eating disorder diagnoses not be minimized or missed altogether among lower- and average-weight clients in eating disorders prevention and treatment efforts.

28.9 Concluding Remarks

The multiple injurious effects of weight stigma on higher-weight individuals are incontrovertible. One mechanism by which these harms are effectuated is via the impact of weight stigma on body image. While in the short term, interventions that reduce internalized weight stigma may increase individual resilience and help to offset some of the psychological harms associated with weight stigma, a focus on internalized weight stigma will only get us so far. It is essential to target intrapersonal-level factors that operate in ways to keep people vulnerable to stigma. However, these efforts, too, are ultimately futile if socio-structural factors that contribute to systemic weight stigma are not directly and effectively addressed. Although the scientific literature has clearly linked weight stigma to poorer body image and its corresponding downstream effects, the same literature essentially ignores why higher-weight bodies are stigmatized in the first place and how weight-based oppression operates in the lives of higher-weight people [95].

In closing, weight is central to body image and eating-related pathology in myriad ways, and body image and eating disorders scholars and practitioners are on the front lines when it comes to modeling and communicating attitudes and behaviors around weight with vulnerable individuals. We cannot address weight stigma or its downstream consequences on body image and eating pathology until we become informed advocates for those clients and communities who suffer most acutely from experienced and internalized forms of weight stigma. It is long past time to heed the call for cultivating size diversity as a means of challenging weight bias in community and clinical populations.

References

1. Puhl RM, Heuer CA. The stigma of obesity: A review and update. Obesity. 2009;17:941–64. https://doi.org/10.1038/oby.2008.636.
2. Andreyeva T, Puhl RM, Brownell KD. Changes in perceived weight discrimination among Americans, 1995-1996 through 2004-2006. Obesity. 2008;16:1129–34. https://doi.org/10.1038/oby.2008.35.
3. Kyle TK, Thomas DM, Ivanescu AE, et al. Indications of increasing social rejection related to weight bias. Obes. Week. 2015.
4. Hatzenbuehler ML, Keyes KM, Hasin DS. Associations between perceived weight discrimination and the prevalence of psychiatric disorders in the general population. Obesity. 2009;17:2033–9. https://doi.org/10.1038/oby.2009.131.
5. Puhl RM, Luedicke J, Heuer C. Weight-based victimization toward overweight adolescents: observations and reactions of peers. J Sch Health. 2011;81:696–703. https://doi.org/10.1111/j.1746-1561.2011.00645.x.
6. Lewis S, Thomas SL, Blood RW, et al. How do obese individuals perceive and respond to the different types of obesity stigma that they encounter in their daily lives? A qualitative study. Soc Sci Med. 2011;73:1349–56 https://doi.org/10.1016/j.socscimed.2011.08.021.
7. Lozano-Sufrategui L, Carless D, Pringle A, et al. "Sorry mate, you're probably a bit too fat to be able to do any of these": Men's experiences of weight stigma. Int J Men's Heal. 2016. https://doi.org/10.3149/jmh.1501.4.
8. Munro L. Everyday indignities: using the microaggressions framework to understand weight stigma. J Law Med Ethics. 2017;45:502–9. https://doi.org/10.1177/1073110517750584.
9. Myers A, Rosen JC. Obesity stigmatization and coping: relation to mental health symptoms, body image, and self-esteem. Int J Obes. 1999;23:221–30. https://doi.org/10.1038/sj.ijo.0800765.
10. Seacat JD, Dougal SC, Roy D. A daily diary assessment of female weight stigmatization. J Health Psychol. 2016;21:228–40. https://doi.org/10.1177/1359105314525067.
11. Ata RN, Thompson JK. Weight bias in the media: a review of recent research. Obes Facts. 2010;3:41–6. https://doi.org/10.1159/000276547.
12. Heuer CA, McClure KJ, Puhl RM. Obesity stigma in online news: a visual content analysis. J Health Commun. 2011;16:976–87. https://doi.org/10.1080/10810730.2011.561915.
13. Couch D, Thomas SL, Lewis S, et al. Obese adults' perceptions of news reporting on obesity SAGE Open. 2015;5:215824401561252. https://doi.org/10.1177/2158244015612522.
14. Vartanian LR, Pinkus R, Smyth JM. The phenomenology of weight stigma in everyday life. J Context Behav Sci. 2014;3:196–202. https://doi.org/10.1016/j.jcbs.2014.01.003.
15. Vartanian LR, Pinkus RT, Smyth JM. Experiences of weight stigma in everyday life: implications for health motivation. Stigma Heal. 2016. https://doi.org/10.1037/sah0000077.
16. Lillis J, Luoma JB, Levin ME, Hayes SC. Measuring weight self-stigma: the Weight Self-Stigma Questionnaire. Obesity. 2010;18:971–6. https://doi.org/10.1038/oby.2009.353.

17. Schvey NA, Roberto CA, White MA. Clinical correlates of the Weight Bias Internalization Scale in overweight adults with binge and purge behaviours. Adv Eat Disord Theory Res Pract. 2013;1:213–23. https://doi.org/10.1080/21662630.2013.794523.
18. Zuba A, Warschburger P. The role of weight teasing and weight bias internalization in psychological functioning: a prospective study among school-aged children. Eur Child Adolesc Psychiatry. 2017;26(10):1245–55. https://doi.org/10.1007/s00787-017-0982-2.
19. Puhl RM, King KM. Weight discrimination and bullying. Best Pract Res Clin Endocrinol Metab. 2013;27:117–27. https://doi.org/10.1016/j.beem.2012.12.002.
20. Janell L. Mensinger, Tracy L. Tylka, Margaret E. Calamari, (2018) Mechanisms underlying weight status and healthcare avoidance in women: A study of weight stigma, body-related shame and guilt, and healthcare stress. Body Image 25:139–147.
21. Udo T, Purcell K, Grilo CM. Perceived weight discrimination and chronic medical conditions in adults with overweight and obesity. Int J Clin Pract. 2016;70:1003–11. https://doi.org/10.1111/ijcp.12902.
22. Sutin AR, Stephan Y, Terracciano A. Weight discrimination and risk of mortality. Psychol Sci doi. 2015;26(11):1803–11. https://doi.org/10.1177/0956797615601103.
23. Rosenthal L, Earnshaw VA, Carroll-Scott A, et al. Weight- and race-based bullying: health associations among urban adolescents. J Health Psychol. 2015;20:401–12. https://doi.org/10.1177/1359105313502567.
24. Hunger JM, Major B. Weight stigma mediates the association between BMI and self-reported health. Heal Psychol. 2015;34:172–5. https://doi.org/10.1037/hea0000106.
25. Latner JD, Barile JP, Durso LE, O'Brien KS. Weight and health-related quality of life: the moderating role of weight discrimination and internalized weight bias. Eat Behav. 2014;15:586–90. https://doi.org/10.1016/j.eatbeh.2014.08.014.
26. Magallares A, Bolanos-Rios P, Ruiz-Prieto I, et al. The mediational effect of weight self-stigma in the relationship between blatant and subtle discrimination and depression and anxiety. Span J Psychol. 2017;20:1–7. https://doi.org/10.1017/sjp.2017.1.
27. Meadows A, Higgs S. Impact of experienced and internalised weight stigma on eating behaviour and psychological outcomes—an international study. In: 142nd Annu. Meet. Am. Public Heal. Assoc; 2014.
28. Durso LE, Latner JD, Hayashi K. Perceived discrimination is associated with binge eating in a community sample of non-overweight, overweight, and obese adults. Obes Facts. 2012;5:869–80. https://doi.org/10.1159/000345931.
29. Pearl RL, Puhl RM, Dovidio JF. Differential effects of weight bias experiences and internalization on exercise among women with overweight and obesity. J Health Psychol. 2015;20:1626–32. https://doi.org/10.1177/1359105313520338.
30. Rosenberger PH, Henderson KE, Bell RL, Grilo CM. Associations of weight-based teasing history and current eating disorder features and psychological functioning in bariatric surgery patients. Obes Surg. 2007;17:470–7. https://doi.org/10.1007/s11695-007-9082-6.
31. Friedman KE, Ashmore JA, Applegate KL. Recent experiences of weight-based stigmatization in a weight loss surgery population: psychological and behavioral correlates. Obesity. 2008;16:S69–74. https://doi.org/10.1038/oby.2008.457.
32. Friedman KE, Reichmann SK, Costanzo PR, et al. Weight stigmatization and ideological beliefs: relation to psychological functioning in obese adults. Obes Res. 2005;13:907–16. https://doi.org/10.1038/oby.2005.105.
33. Vartanian LR, Novak SA. Internalized societal attitudes moderate the impact of weight stigma on avoidance of exercise. Obesity. 2011;19:757–62. https://doi.org/10.1038/oby.2010.234.
34. Annis NM, Cash TF, Hrabosky JI. Body image and psychosocial differences among stable average weight, currently overweight, and formerly overweight women: the role of stigmatizing experiences. Body Image. 2004;1:155–67. https://doi.org/10.1016/j.bodyim.2003.12.001.
35. Menzel JE, Schaefer LM, Burke NL, et al. Appearance-related teasing, body dissatisfaction, and disordered eating: a meta-analysis. Body Image. 2010;7:261–70. https://doi.org/10.1016/j.bodyim.2010.05.004.

36. Puhl RM, Luedicke J. Weight-based victimization among adolescents in the school setting: emotional reactions and coping behaviors. J Youth Adolesc. 2012;41:27–40. https://doi.org/10.1007/s10964-011-9713-z.
37. Quick VM, McWilliams R, Byrd-Bredbenner C. Fatty, fatty, two-by-four: weight-teasing history and disturbed eating in young adult women. Am J Public Heal. 2013;103:508–15. https://doi.org/10.2105/AJPH.2012.300898.
38. Cattarin JA, Thompson K. A three-year longitudinal study of body image, eating disturbance, and general psychological functioning in adolescent females. Eat Disord. 1994;2:114–25. https://doi.org/10.1080/10640269408249107.
39. Neumark-Sztainer D, Falkner N, Story M, et al. Weight-teasing among adolescents: correlations with weight status and disordered eating behaviors. Int J Obes Relat Metab Disord. 2002;26:123–31. https://doi.org/10.1038/sj.ijo.0801853.
40. Paxton SJ, Eisenberg ME, Neumark-Sztainer D. Prospective predictors of body dissatisfaction in adolescent girls and boys: a five-year longitudinal study. Dev Psychol. 2006;42:888–99. https://doi.org/10.1037/0012-1649.42.5.888.
41. Puhl RM, Wall MM, Chen C, et al. Experiences of weight teasing in adolescence and weight-related outcomes in adulthood: a 15-year longitudinal study. Prev Med. 2017;100:173–9. https://doi.org/10.1016/j.ypmed.2017.04.023.
42. Jendrzyca A, Warschburger P. Weight stigma and eating behaviours in elementary school children: a prospective population-based study. Appetite. 2016;102:51–9. https://doi.org/10.1016/j.appet.2016.02.005.
43. Pearl RL, Puhl RM. The distinct effects of internalizing weight bias: an experimental study. Body Image. 2016;17:38–42. https://doi.org/10.1016/j.bodyim.2016.02.002.
44. Daníelsdóttir S, O'Brien KS, Ciao A. Anti-fat prejudice reduction: a review of published studies. Obes Facts. 2010;3:47–58. https://doi.org/10.1159/000277067.
45. Richardson SM, Paxton SJ. An evaluation of a body image intervention based on risk factors for body dissatisfaction: a controlled study with adolescent girls. Int J Eat Disord. 2010;43:112–22. https://doi.org/10.1002/eat.20682.
46. Yager Z, Diedrichs PC, Ricciardelli LA, Halliwell E. What works in secondary schools? A systematic review of classroom-based body image programs. Body Image. 2013;10:271–81. https://doi.org/10.1016/j.bodyim.2013.04.001.
47. Haines J, Neumark-Sztainer D, Perry CL, et al. V.I.K. (Very Important Kids): a school-based program designed to reduce teasing and unhealthy weight-control behaviors. Health Educ Res. 2006;21:884–95. https://doi.org/10.1093/her/cyl123.
48. Boswell RG, White MA. Gender differences in weight bias internalisation and eating pathology in overweight individuals. Adv Eat Disord Theory Res Pract. 2015;3:259–68. https://doi.org/10.1080/21662630.2015.1047881.
49. Durso LE, Latner JD. Understanding self-directed stigma: development of the weight bias internalization scale. Obesity. 2008:16(Suppl 2):S80–6. https://doi.org/10.1038/oby.2008.448.
50. Durso LE, Latner JD, Ciao AC. Weight bias internalization in treatment-seeking overweight adults: psychometric validation and associations with self-esteem, body image, and mood symptoms. Eat Behav. 2016;21:104–8. https://doi.org/10.1016/j.eatbeh.2016.01.011.
51. Carels RA, Burmeister J, Oehlhof MW, et al. Internalized weight bias: ratings of the self, normal weight, and obese individuals and psychological maladjustment. J Behav Med. 2013;36:86–94. https://doi.org/10.1007/s10865-012-9402-8.
52. Pearl RL, Dovidio JF. Experiencing weight bias in an unjust world: impact on exercise and internalization. Heal Psychol. 2015;34:741–9. https://doi.org/10.1037/hea0000178.
53. Pearl RL, White MA, Grilo CM. Overvaluation of shape and weight as a mediator between self-esteem and weight bias internalization among patients with binge eating disorder. Eat Behav. 2014;15:259–61. https://doi.org/10.1016/j.eatbeh.2014.03.005.
54. Pila E, Brunet J, Crocker PRE, et al. Intrapersonal characteristics of body-related guilt, shame, pride, and envy in Canadian adults. Body Image. 2016;16:100–6. https://doi.org/10.1016/j.bodyim.2016.01.001.

55. Webb JB, Hardin AS. An integrative affect regulation process model of internalized weight bias and intuitive eating in college women. Appetite. 2016;102:60–9. https://doi.org/10.1016/j.appet.2016.02.024.
56. Hübner C, Schmidt R, Selle J, et al. Comparing self-report measures of internalized weight stigma: the Weight Self-Stigma Questionnaire versus the Weight Bias Internalization Scale. PLoS One. 2016;11:e0165566. https://doi.org/10.1371/journal.pone.0165566.
57. Roberto CA, Sysko R, Bush J, et al. Clinical correlates of the weight bias internalization scale in a sample of obese adolescents seeking bariatric surgery. Obesity. 2012;20:533–9. https://doi.org/10.1038/oby.2011.123.
58. Maïano C, Aimé A, Lepage G, Morin AJS. Psychometric properties of the Weight Self-Stigma Questionnaire (WSSQ) among a sample of overweight/obese French-speaking adolescents. Eat Weight Disord. 2017. https://doi.org/10.1007/s40519-017-0382-0.
59. Zuba A, Warschburger P. Weight bias internalization across weight categories in childhood. In: 5th Annu. Int. Weight Stigma Conf. 2017.
60. Sienko RM, Saules KK, Carr MM. Internalized weight bias mediates the relationship between depressive symptoms and disordered eating behavior among women who think they are overweight. Eat Behav. 2016;22:141–4. https://doi.org/10.1016/j.eatbeh.2016.06.002.
61. O'Brien KS, Puhl RM, Vartanian LR, et al. The relationship between weight stigma and eating behavior is explained by weight bias internalization and psychological distress. Appetite. 2016;102:70–6. https://doi.org/10.1016/j.appet.2016.02.032.
62. Carels RA, Wott CB, Young KM, et al. Implicit, explicit, and internalized weight bias and psychosocial maladjustment among treatment-seeking adults. Eat Behav. 2010;11:180–5. https://doi.org/10.1016/j.eatbeh.2010.03.002.
63. Pearl RL, Hopkins CH, Berkowitz RI, Wadden TA. Group cognitive-behavioral treatment for internalized weight stigma: a pilot study. Eat Weight Disord. 2018;23(3):357–62. https://doi.org/10.1007/s40519-016-0336-y.
64. Palmeira L, Pinto-Gouveia J, Cunha M. Exploring the efficacy of an acceptance, mindfulness & compassionate-based group intervention for women struggling with their weight (Kg-Free): a randomized controlled trial. Appetite. 2017;112:107–16. https://doi.org/10.1016/j.appet.2017.01.027.
65. Berman MI, Morton SN, Hegel MT. Uncontrolled pilot study of an acceptance and commitment therapy and health at every size intervention for obese, depressed women: accept yourself! Psychotherapy. 2016;53:462–7. https://doi.org/10.1037/pst0000083.
66. Berman MI, Morton SN, Hegel MT. Health at every size and acceptance and commitment therapy for obese, depressed women: treatment development and clinical application. Clin Soc Work J. 2016;44:265–78. https://doi.org/10.1007/s10615-015-0565-y.
67. Carels RA, Burmeister JM, Koball AM, et al. A randomized trial comparing two approaches to weight loss: differences in weight loss maintenance. J Health Psychol. 2014;19:296–311. https://doi.org/10.1177/1359105312470156.
68. Mensinger JL, Calogero RM, Stranges S, Tylka TL. A weight-neutral versus weight-loss approach for health promotion in women with high BMI: a randomized-controlled trial. Appetite. 2016;105:364–74. https://doi.org/10.1016/j.appet.2016.06.006.
69. Mensinger JL, Calogero RM, Tylka TL. Internalized weight stigma moderates eating behavior outcomes in women with high BMI participating in a healthy living program. Appetite. 2016;102:32–43. https://doi.org/10.1016/j.appet.2016.01.033.
70. Tanco S, Linden W, Earle T. Well-being and morbid obesity in women: a controlled therapy evaluation. Int J Eat Disord. 1998;23:325–39. https://doi.org/10.1002/(SICI)1098-108X(199804)23:3<325::AID-EAT10>3.0.CO;2-X.
71. Gagnon-Girouard MP, Begin C, Provencher V, et al. Psychological impact of a "health-at-every-size" intervention on weight-preoccupied overweight/obese women. J Obes. 2010. https://doi.org/10.1155/2010/928097.
72. Bacon L, Stern JS, Van Loan MD, Keim NL. Size acceptance and intuitive eating improve health for obese, female chronic dieters. J Am Diet Assoc. 2005;105:929–36. https://doi.org/10.1016/j.jada.2005.03.011.

73. Borkoles E, Carroll S, Clough P, Polman RCJ. Effect of a non-dieting lifestyle randomised control trial on psychological well-being and weight management in morbidly obese pre-menopausal women. Maturitas. 2016;83:51–8. https://doi.org/10.1016/j.maturitas.2015.09.010.
74. Crandall CS, D'Anello S, Sakalli N, et al. An attribution-value model of prejudice: anti-fat attitudes in six nations. Personal Soc Psychol Bull. 2001;27:30–7. https://doi.org/10.1177/0146167201271003.
75. Brewis AA, Wutich A, Falletta-Cowden A, Rodriguez-Soto I. Body norms and fat stigma in global perspective. Curr Anthropol. 2011;52:269–76. https://doi.org/10.1086/659309.
76. Puhl R, Suh Y. Health consequences of weight stigma: implications for obesity prevention and treatment. Curr Obes Rep. 2015;4:182–90. https://doi.org/10.1007/s13679-015-0153-z.
77. Hackman J, Maupin J, Brewis AA. Weight-related stigma is a significant psychosocial stressor in developing countries: evidence from Guatemala. Soc Sci Med. 2016;161:55–60. https://doi.org/10.1016/j.socscimed.2016.05.032.
78. Hübner C, Baldofski S, Zenger M, et al. Influences of general self-efficacy and weight bias internalization on physical activity in bariatric surgery candidates. Surg Obes Relat Dis. 2015;11:1371–6. https://doi.org/10.1016/j.soard.2014.11.013.
79. Conradt M, Dierk J-M, Schlumberger P, et al. Development of the Weight- and Body-Related Shame and Guilt Scale (WEB–SG) in a nonclinical sample of obese individuals. J Pers Assess. 2007;88:317–27. https://doi.org/10.1080/00223890701331856.
80. Duarte C, Stubbs J, Pinto-Gouveia J, et al. The impact of self-criticism and self-reassurance on weight-related affect and well-being in participants of a commercial weight management programme. Obes Facts. 2017;10:65–75. https://doi.org/10.1159/000454834.
81. O'Hara L, Tahboub-Schulte S, Thomas J. Weight-related teasing and internalized weight stigma predict abnormal eating attitudes and behaviours in Emirati female university students. Appetite. 2016;102:44–50. https://doi.org/10.1016/j.appet.2016.01.019.
82. Schulte SJ. Predictors of binge eating in male and female youths in the United Arab Emirates. Appetite. 2016;105:312–9. https://doi.org/10.1016/j.appet.2016.06.004.
83. Farhangi MA, Emam-Alizadeh M, Hamedi F, Jahangiry L. Weight self-stigma and its association with quality of life and psychological distress among overweight and obese women. Eat Weight Disord. 2017;22(3):451–6. https://doi.org/10.1007/s40519-016-0288-2.
84. van den Berg P, Neumark-Sztainer D, Eisenberg ME, Haines J. Racial/ethnic differences in weight-related teasing in adolescents. Obesity. 2008;16:S3–S10. https://doi.org/10.1038/oby.2008.445.
85. Bucchianeri MM, Eisenberg ME, Wall MM, et al. Multiple types of harassment: associations with emotional well-being and unhealthy behaviors in adolescents. J Adolesc Heal. 2014;54:724–9. https://doi.org/10.1016/j.jadohealth.2013.10.205.
86. Meadows A, Nolan LJ, Higgs S. Self-perceived food addiction: prevalence, predictors, and prognosis. Appetite. 2017;114:282–98. https://doi.org/10.1016/j.appet.2017.03.051.
87. Schvey NA, Sbrocco T, Bakalar JL, et al. The experience of weight stigma among gym members with overweight and obesity. Stigma Heal. 2017;2(4):292–306. https://doi.org/10.1037/sah0000062.
88. Evans PC, McConnell AR. Do racial minorities respond in the same way to mainstream beauty standards? Social comparison processes in Asian, Black, and White women. Self Identity. 2003;2:153–67. https://doi.org/10.1080/15298860309030.
89. Eisenberg MH, Street RL, Persky S. "It runs in my family …": the association of perceived family history with body dissatisfaction and weight bias internalization among overweight women. Women Health. 2017;57:478–93. https://doi.org/10.1080/03630242.2016.1170095.
90. Sheffield JK, Tse KH, Sofronoff K. A comparison of body-image dissatisfaction and eating disturbance among Australian and Hong Kong women. Eur Eat Disord Rev. 2005;13:112–24. https://doi.org/10.1002/erv.641.
91. Crenshaw K. Demarginalizing the intersection of race and sex: a Black feminist critique of antidiscrimination doctrine, feminist theory and antiracist policies. Univ Chic Leg Forum. 1989;140:139–67.

92. Bauer GR. Incorporating intersectionality theory into population health research methodology: challenges and the potential to advance health equity. Soc Sci Med. 2014;110:10–7. https://doi.org/10.1016/j.socscimed.2014.03.022.
93. Fiske ST, Fiske TS. Interpersonal stratification: status, power, and subordination. In: Fiske ST, Gilbert DT, Lindzey G, editors. Handb. Soc. Psychol. 5th ed. Hoboken, NJ: Wiley; 2010. p. 941–82.
94. Meadows A, Daníelsdóttir S, Calogero R, O'Reilly C. Why fat suits do not advance the scientific study of weight stigma. Obesity. 2017;25(2):275. https://doi.org/10.1002/oby.21742.
95. Calogero RM, Tylka TL, Mensinger JL. Scientific weightism: a view of mainstream weight stigma research through a feminist lens. In: Roberts T-A, Curtin N, Duncan LE, Cortina LM, editors. Feminist perspectives on building a better psychological science of gender. New York: Springer; 2016. p. 9–28.
96. Mensinger JL, Tylka TL, Calamari ME. Mechanisms underlying weight status and healthcare avoidance in women: a study of weight stigma, body-related shame and guilt, and healthcare stress. Body Image. 2018;25:139–47.

Studies on Body Image, Eating, and Weight in Models, Dancers, and Aesthetic Athletes

29

Rita Francisco

29.1 Introduction

In aesthetic activities—which include fashion, dance, and aesthetic sports (e.g., gymnastics, synchronized swimming, or figure skating)—physical appearance is considered fundamental and lean bodies are required. For these reasons, they are considered high-risk contexts for the development of body image concerns and eating disorders (ED), as several studies of populations around the world have shown since the 1980s. Garner and Garfinkel [1] were the first to examine a population of female professional dance students and fashion models. The authors found that excessive dieting concerns and ED were overrepresented in the dance and modeling students compared to music students and normal controls. Especially at the elite level, in addition to the aesthetic and artistic components of these activities, the competitive aspects become essential in the pursuit of perfection and success and in overcoming the limits of the body [2–4]. However, it is important to keep in mind the multifactorial conception of body image concerns and ED, since the individual, family, and sociocultural variables all contribute to their development. Some contributory factors appear to be necessary for the appearance of these kinds of problems, but no single factor is sufficient to explain them [5]. Therefore, the contexts of fashion, dance, or aesthetic sports can be considered subcultures in which social pressures to be thin are reinforced; thus, their practitioners are frequently encouraged to adopt unhealthy eating and weight control behaviors [6–10] in the incessant search for perfection. The perfection of movement is the perfection of the body; in this sense, the body is often worked to exhaustion in an attempt to achieve the ideal form, which is also the leanest possible [11]. However, the requirements in each of these specific contexts are different, particularly in terms of body image. For

R. Francisco
Católica Research Centre for Psychological, Family and Social Wellbeing (CRC-W), School of Human Sciences, Universidade Católica Portuguesa, Lisboa, Portugal
e-mail: ritafrancisco@ucp.pt

M. Cuzzolaro, S. Fassino (eds.), *Body Image, Eating, and Weight*,
https://doi.org/10.1007/978-3-319-90817-5_29

Table 29.1 Summary of the reviewed studies on fashion models

Author(s)	Year	Type of study[a]	Sample
Garner and Garfinkel [1]	1980	Quant, Cr	Female modeling students and other groups (ballet students, patients with AN, music students, and controls)
Brenner and Cunningham [20]	1992	Quant, Cr	Male and female professional fashion models and controls
Santonastaso, Mondini, and Favaro [19]	2002	Quant, Cr	Female professional fashion models and controls
Preti, Usai, Miotto, Petretto, and Masala [18]	2008	Quant, Cr	Female professional fashion models and controls
Swami and Szmigielska [10]	2013	Quant, Cr	Female professional fashion models and controls

[a]*Cr* cross-sectional, *Quant* Quantitative

example, gymnasts are required, above all, to be short, lean, and muscular, while dancers are expected to be thin, light, and delicate. In turn, fashion models should be tall and slender. Thus, it is important to understand better how fashion models, dancers, and aesthetic athletes address their eating and body image, the protective and risk factors for the development of body image concerns and ED, and the incidence of these problems in these contexts. Tables 29.1, 29.2, and 29.3 summarize the empirical studies reviewed in this chapter on fashion models, dancers, and aesthetic athletes, respectively.

29.2 Models

Despite some important initiatives—for example, a Madrid Fashion Week ban of models with an excessively low body mass index (BMI) [12] or the recent law passed by the French parliament that models must have a medical certificate to prove that they are a healthy weight [13]—and a flood of media coverage of the debates subsequent to the deaths of young models as a result of complications of ED [14], fashion models continue to be "so unrepresentative of the everyday woman that they are offensive" [15]. Most of them are far too slender and have a hazardously low BMI, especially as a consequence of pressure from agencies to lose weight, as recently revealed by Erin Heatherton, a famous former Victoria's Secret model [16].

As noted in a recent systematic review of the literature, there are few studies on body image and ED among fashion models. In addition, relatively small samples and frequently low response rates of fashion models limit the generalization of any conclusions [17]. However, the existing studies may help us to understand this population better. Compared to non-models, female fashion models often report more disordered eating [1, 18, 19], and this is especially true for partial-syndromes ED since full syndromes are often not statistically more prevalent [18, 19]. However, fashion models are on average slightly underweight with significantly lower BMI than controls, report more dysfunctional investment in their appearance, and even

Table 29.2 Summary of the reviewed studies on dancers

Author(s)	Year	Type of study[a]	Sample
Garner and Garfinkel [1]	1980	Quant, Cr	Female professional ballet students and other groups (modeling students, patients with AN, music students, and controls)
Bettle, Bettle, Neumärker and Neumärker [25]	1998	Quant, Cr	Male and female adolescent ballet dancers and controls
Neumärker, Bettle, Bettle, Dudeck and Neumärker [64]	1998	Quant, Cr	Male and female adolescent ballet dancers, patients with AN and controls
Neumärker, Bettle, Neumärker and Bettle [29]	2000	Quant, Cr	Male and female adolescent ballet dancers and controls
Anshel [26]	2004	Quant, Cr	Female adolescent ballet dancers and controls
Doumenc, Sudres and Sztulman [33]	2005	Quant, Cr	Female professional ballet students and amateurs
Ravaldi, Vannacci, Bolognesi, Mancini, Faravelli and Ricca [28]	2006	Quant, Cr	Female non-elite ballet dancers, female gymnasium users, male non-competitive body builders, female and male controls
Ringham, Klump, Kaye, Stone, Libman, Stowe et al. [30]	2006	Quant, Cr	Female ballet dancers, patients with AN and BN, and controls
Aalten [11]	2007	Qual, Cr	Female professional ballet dancers and dance students
Gvion [7]	2008	Qual, Cr	Female professional ballet students
de Bruin, Bakker and Oudejans [36]	2009	Quant, Cr	Female artistic gymnasts and modern dancers
Toro, Guerrero, Sentis, Castro and Puértolas [34]	2009	Quant, Cr	Female adolescent dance students and controls
Langdon and Petracca [24]	2010	Quant, Cr	Female modern dancers (and controls from previous studies)
Pollatou, Bakali, Theodorakis and Goudas [32]	2010	Quant, Cr	Female professional and amateur dancers
Schluger [23]	2010	Quant, Cr	Female modern and ballet dancers
Nordin-Bates, Walker and Redding [63]	2011	Quant, Cr	Male and female professional dance students
Francisco, Alarcão and Narciso [9]	2012	Qual, Cr	Male and female professional ballet students and elite gymnasts
Francisco, Narciso and Alarcão [2]	2012	Quant, Cr	Male and female ballet dancers and gymnasts
Swami and Harris [31]	2012	Quant, Cr	Female ballet and contemporary dancers
Goodwin, Arcelus, Marshall, Wicks and Meyer [35]	2014	Quant, Cr	Female dance students
Kong and Harris [3]	2015	Quant, Cr	Female athletes from leanness-focused (including dance) and nonleanness-focused sports
Nerini [27]	2015	Quant, Cr	Female preadolescent ballet dancers and controls
Nordin-Bates, Schwarz, Quested, Cumming, Aujla and Redding [37]	2015	Quant, Cr	Male and female professional dance students

[a] *Cr* cross-sectional, *L* longitudinal, *Quant* Quantitative, *Qual* Qualitative

Table 29.3 Summary of the reviewed studies on aesthetic athletes

Author(s)	Year	Type of study[a]	Sample
Byrne and McLean [6]	2002	Quant, Cr	Male and female elite athletes from leanness-focused and nonleanness-focused sports and controls
Sundgot-Borgen and Torstveit [38]	2004	Quant, Cr	Male and female elite athletes (from aesthetic and other sports) and controls
Torstveit and Sundgot-Borgen [43]	2005	Quant, Cr	Female elite athletes (from aesthetic and other sports) and controls
Torstveit and Sundgot-Borgen [44]	2005	Quant, Cr	Female elite athletes (from aesthetic and other sports) and controls
Bachner-Melman, Zohar, Ebstein, Elizur and Constantini [54]	2006	Quant, Cr	Female aesthetic and nonaesthetic athletes, patients with AN, and controls
Kerr, Berman and De Souza [8]	2006	Quant+Qual, Cr	Female current and retired artistic gymnasts, parents, coaches, and judges
Milligan and Pritchard [45]	2006	Quant, Cr	Male and female lean and nonlean sport athletes
de Bruin, Oudejans and Bakker [59]	2007	Quant, Cr	Female elite and non-elite and gymnasts, and controls
Muscat and Long [58]	2008	Quant, Cr	Female athletes and sport participants
de Bruin, Bakker and Oudejans [36]	2009	Quant, Cr	Female artistic gymnasts and modern dancers
de Bruin, Oudejans, Bakker and Woertman [53]	2011	Quant, Cr	Female aesthetic or endurance athletes and other sport participants
Krentz and Warschburger [51]	2011	Quant, Cr	Male and female elite athletes from aesthetic sports
Francisco, Alarcão and Narciso [9]	2012	Qual, Cr	Male and female elite gymnasts and professional ballet students
Francisco, Narciso and Alarcão [2]	2012	Quant, Cr	Male and female elite and non-elite gymnasts and ballet dancers
Francisco, Narciso and Alarcão [46]	2013	Quant, Cr	Male and female elite and non-elite gymnasts and ballet dancers, and controls
Krentz and Warschburger [49]	2013	Quant, L	Male and female elite athletes from aesthetic sports
Kong and Harris [3]	2015	Quant, Cr	Female athletes from leanness- and nonleanness-focused sports
Thiemann, Legenbauer, Vocks, Platen, Auyeung and Herpertz [47]	2015	Quant, Cr	Female elite aesthetic and ball game sports athletes, and controls
Galli, Petrie and Chatterton [57]	2017	Quant, Cr	Male collegiate athletes from different sports

[a]*Cr* cross-sectional, *L* longitudinal, *Quant* Quantitative, *Qual* Qualitative

desire to become thinner. These worrisome indicators are considered to be associated with the intense competitiveness of the fashion world and with the widespread methods used to control weight, which are thought to be too prevalent in the world of top models [18].

Nevertheless, compared to controls, models seem to report higher levels of body satisfaction [18, 20] or no differences [10]. For female (but not for male) models, body satisfaction was associated to self-esteem [20], which can derive from conforming to societal and industry ideals. Self-esteem can buffer against the development of body image disturbances [10] or ED [19], considering the great pressure to maintain a thin shape to continue to work [17].

29.3 Dancers

Ballet is considered an art by those who practice it but is also the most physical of the performing arts [21], which is why dancers are also considered special athletes. Contemporary dance is rarely included in studies on body image and ED, because of the lesser demands made on these dancers to be thin and the greater acceptance of diversity in terms of body shape and weight. Thus, the lower incidence of constraints and restrictions, both physical and artistic [22], seems to place contemporary dancers at lower risk of developing ED. For example, Schluger [23] found twice the prevalence of disturbed eating behaviors in ballet dancers than in modern dancers (24.4% vs. 12.2%), and Langdon and Petracca [24] identified more positive body image in modern dancers, when compared with previous samples of ballet dancers.

Even though they have lower BMI than control groups, female ballet dancers and dance students at professional ballet schools frequently present a higher desire to lose weight and greater body image dissatisfaction than female non-dancers [25–27]. Consistently, most studies also have found a higher prevalence of ED among ballet dancers than non-dancers [28, 29], including the finding that female dancers and individuals with ED are similar in measures of eating pathology [26, 30].[1] However, recent research has suggested that the effects of dance participation on body image and disordered eating could also be related to the dancer identity, considering that modern dancers with lower dancer identity had more positive general and dance specific body image [24], or to the dance performance level. When adolescent elite ballet dancers and non-elite dancers were compared, elite dancers appeared more dissatisfied with their bodies [31–33] and had significantly higher levels of disordered eating [2].

[1] Studies that include male dancers are scarce; thus, results for gender differences are less congruent. For example, equal proportions of disordered eating were found among female and male talented young dancers from the UK centers for advanced training [63], but other studies have found significantly lower levels among male than female dancers [2, 64]. These results suggest that further research is warranted.

The differences reported above seem to be especially related to the perception of the pressure to be thin and to the competitive nature of these contexts. A ballet dancer's extra-thin body is looked upon as a sign of ultimate control and professional achievement [7], and the culture of "thinness = success" is widespread. Dancers are motivated by a drive to achieve perfection, and some researchers have found that the higher levels of perfectionism found among them than among non-dancers seem to be encouraged [26, 29]. A qualitative study of young elite ballet dancers found that this pressure to be thin is viewed as an implicit and an explicit rule among ballet schools and the ballet subculture [9]. Diverse studies have confirmed that the pressure to be thin is especially transmitted through critical comments by teachers and peers about eating, weight, and shape [34], and that more severe critical comments are associated with higher eating psychopathology through reduced self-esteem [35]. In general, the pressure to be thin influences dancers' disordered eating both directly and indirectly through reduced self-esteem and reduced body satisfaction [2].

Another important contextual variable that influences body dissatisfaction and disordered eating among dancers is the perspective towards the success. Those who are actively ego-oriented (with an emphasis on social comparison and outcome) tend to display more disordered eating correlates. By contrast, perceptions of task-involving motivational climates (focused on learning and personal development) are associated with higher self-esteem and lower weight-related pressure from peers and teachers [36]. However, a more recent study indicates that an ego-involving climate in the dance environment could be more salient for male than for female dancers [37]. Future research should further explore these context characteristics, which seem very important for the development of preventive interventions that include teachers and peers, in order to create and improve a climate of mastery [36].

29.4 Aesthetic Athletes

One of the methodologically more robust prevalence studies was conducted in two phases with all Norwegian elite athletes, between 15 and 39 years of age ($n = 1620$), and a representative sample from the general Norwegian population. This research revealed a higher prevalence of ED (AN, BN, or EDNOS, based on clinical interviews) among athletes (both female and male) than in the general population. The prevalence was notably higher among athletes competing in sports that focus on leanness and weight (e.g., aesthetic sports) than athletes competing in other sports and controls [38].

When disordered eating or ED (also related to low energy availability) are associated with amenorrhea and osteoporosis, they represent the presence of a syndrome very common in female athletes—the Female Athlete Triad—with potentially irreversible consequences. This triad is often triggered by extreme diets in response to pressures to achieve an unrealistic body weight or shape, resulting in a deficit of energy, menstrual irregularities, and a decrease in bone density that increases the risk of injury [39, 40].

Recently, the International Olympic Committee (IOC) updated and replaced its Consensus Statement, since studies have shown that the clinical phenomenon is a "syndrome resulting from relative energy deficiency that affects many aspects of physiological function including metabolic rate, menstrual function, bone health, immunity, protein synthesis, cardiovascular and psychological health" [41]. Thus, and because the relative energy deficiency also affects men, IOC began to use a new terminology for the overall syndrome—Relative Energy Deficiency in Sport (RED-S), instead of the former "Female Athlete Triad". ED have consistently been found to be more prevalent among both male and female athletes who compete in leanness sports than athletes from other sports and non-athletes [6, 42–47].

Gymnasts (competing in rhythmic, artistic, or acrobatic gymnastics) are the most studied group of aesthetic athletes regarding body image and ED [48]. Nevertheless, despite some slight differences among some disciplines, studies that also include athletes who practice, for example, figure skating, synchronized swimming and cheerleading show, in general, similar results. The desire to be leaner to improve sports performance is predictive of disordered eating, and it seems to mediate the relationship between social pressure from the sports environment and disordered eating [49]. Although previous studies have indicated an equal or slightly more positive body image among athletes than controls [50], more recent studies have focused on sports-related body dissatisfaction (instead of general body dissatisfaction) and identified it as a better predictor of disordered eating among aesthetic athletes [2, 51].

The difference between the ideal body image conveyed by society and the one for the practice of a particular sport leads many athletes, especially females, to experience a paradox in relation to their body image [52]. As suggested by de Bruin et al. [53], an athlete may be satisfied with his/her body shape and figure in the social environment but not with his/her "sporting" body. In this sense, the fact that male athletes perceive a higher similarity between these two images and are less subject to this paradox may be the reason that they frequently present better body image satisfaction than their female counterparts, even when the sporting body image is evaluated [2, 45].

For many athletes, sports participation is their life, which potentiates some individual traits that make them vulnerable to the development of ED. Some of these characteristics, manifested by "good athletes," are often encouraged and reinforced in elite sporting environments [54–56]. These features are, to some extent, similar to those of AN patients [56]: (a) perfectionism; (b) persistence that leads athletes to train and compete to exhaustion (sometimes to please coaches); (c) determination to be the best; (d) placing the interests, priorities, and needs of the team before their own; (e) tolerance of physical suffering.

In addition to these individual traits, some other contextual factors have been identified in the literature as contributing significantly to the development of body image dissatisfaction and ED. Regular weigh-ins (sometimes in front of the whole team and/or public posting of weights) are frequently used by coaches to monitor athletes' physical progress, which may lead both male and female athletes to engage in unhealthy behaviors [8, 9, 57]. At the same time, as we noted previously with dancers, several studies have found that critical comments about eating, weight, and shape from coaches are important risk factors for disordered eating [2, 3, 8, 51, 58]. These two elements are important and visible signs of the pressure to be thin frequently found in these contexts, which was found to be a better predictor of disordered eating among aesthetic athletes than the elite (vs. non-elite) level of competition [2, 59]. It is possible that high levels of pressure to be thin perceived by aesthetic athletes in their clubs or teams explains the absence of differences in body image dissatisfaction or disordered eating between elite and non-elite athletes, as found in many studies [48].

Conclusion

Fashion models, dancers, and aesthetic athletes are indeed high-risk groups for the development of body image problems and eating disorders, and different individual, relational, and contextual factors contribute to that risk. It seems inevitable that thinness will continue to be a "rule" in these three studied contexts since any attempt to bring about change would conflict with the history, values, and culture of these pursuits. The problem emerges when thinness is taken to the extreme and places at risk models', dancers', and athletes' health. It is often difficult to find the balance between aesthetic/artistic leanness and the extreme thinness that is in conflict with healthy human limits, and even coaches may have difficulty recognizing the symptoms [60].

Systemic preventive actions—targeting not only models, dancers, and athletes, but also coaches, teachers, support personnel, and parents—are necessary for these contexts, similar to Piran's work in a highly competitive professional ballet school for 15 years, with positive long-term effects [61, 62]. For example, it is essential the promotion of task-involving and caring climates in which critical comments about eating, weight, and shape are avoided. Such actions should equip fashion models, dancers, and athletes with tools to develop a more positive and healthy experience of their body, as well as higher well-being, self-esteem, and activity-specific body image satisfaction. See also Chaps. 12, 24 and 30 of this book.

References

1. Garner D, Garfinkel P. Socio-cultural factors in the development of anorexia nervosa. Psychol Med. 1980;10:647–56.
2. Francisco R, Narciso I, Alarcão M. Specific predictors of disordered eating among elite and non-elite gymnasts and ballet dancers. Int J Sport Psychol. 2012;43:479–502.
3. Kong P, Harris LM. The sporting body: body image and eating disorder symptomatology among female athletes from leanness focused and nonleanness focused sports. J Psychol. 2015;149:141–60.
4. Scoffier S, Corrion K, D'Arripe-Longueville F. Effects of achievement goals on female aesthetic athletes' disordered eating attitudes. Sci Sport. 2013;28:e151–7.
5. Polivy J, Herman CP. Causes of eating disorders. Annu Rev Psychol. 2002;53:187–213.
6. Byrne SM, McLean N. Elite athletes: effects of the pressure to be thin. J Sci Med Sport. 2002;5:80–94.
7. Gvion L. Dancing bodies, decaying bodies: the interpretation of anorexia among Israeli dancers. Young. 2008;16(1):67–87.

8. Kerr G, Berman E, De Souza MJ. Disordered eating in women's gymnastics: perspectives of athletes, coaches, parents, and judges. J Appl Sport Psychol. 2006;18:28–43.
9. Francisco R, Alarcão M, Narciso I. Aesthetic sport as high-risk context for eating disorders: young elite dancers and gymnasts perspectives. Span J Psychol. 2012;15:265–74.
10. Swami V, Szmigielska E. Body image concerns in professional fashion models: are they really an at-risk group? Psychiatry Res. 2013;207:113–7.
11. Aalten A. Listening to the dancer's body. Sociol Rev. 2007;55:109–25.
12. CNN. Skinny models banned from catwalk. 2006. http://edition.cnn.com/2006/WORLD/europe/09/13/spain.models/.
13. Willsher K. Models in France must provide doctor's note to work. The Guardian [Internet]. 2015. https://www.theguardian.com/world/2015/dec/18/models-doctors-note-prove-not-too-thin-france.
14. Soltis CA. Dying to be a supermodel: can requiring a healthy BMI be fashionable? J Contemp Health Law Policy. 2013;26(1):49–71.
15. Mears A. Size zero high-end ethnic: cultural production and the reproduction of culture in fashion modeling. Poetics. 2010;38:21–46.
16. Oppenheim M. Former Victoria's Secret model Erin Heatherton says she left the company after being told to lose weight. The Independent [Internet]. 2016. http://www.independent.co.uk/news/people/victorias-secret-erin-heatherton-weight-loss-body-image-lingerie-img-a6970671.html.
17. Zancu SA, Enea V. Eating disorders among fashion models: a systematic review of the literature. Eat Weight Disord. 2017;22:395–405.
18. Preti A, Usai A, Miotto P, Petretto DR, Masala C. Eating disorders among professional fashion models. Psychiatry Res. 2008;159:86–94.
19. Santonastaso P, Mondini S, Favaro A. Are fashion models a group at risk for eating disorders and substance abuse? Psychother Psychosom. 2002;71:168–72.
20. Brenner JB, Cunningham JG. Gender differences in eating attitudes, body concept and self-esteem among models. Sex Roles. 1992;27:413–37.
21. Aalten A. "The moment when it all comes together": embodied experiences in ballet. Eur J Women's Stud. 2004;11:263–76.
22. Clabaugh A, Morling B. Stereotype accuracy of ballet and modern dancers. J Soc Psychol. 2004;144:31–48.
23. Schluger AE. Disordered eating attitudes and behaviors in female college dance students: comparison of modern dance and ballet dance majors. N Am J Psychol. 2010;12:117–28.
24. Langdon SW, Petracca G. Tiny dancer: body image and dancer identity in female modern dancers. Body Image. 2010;7(4):360–3. https://doi.org/10.1016/j.bodyim.2010.06.005.
25. Bettle N, Bettle O, Neumärker U, Neumärker K-J. Adolescent ballet school students: their quest for body weight change. Psychopathology. 1998;31:153–9.
26. Anshel MH. Sources of disordered eating patterns between ballet dancers and non-dancers. J Sport Behav. 2004;27(2):115–33.
27. Nerini A. Media influence and body dissatisfaction in preadolescent ballet dancers and non-physically active girls. Psychol Sport Exerc. 2015;20:76–83.
28. Ravaldi C, Vannacci A, Bolognesi E, Mancini S, Faravelli C, Ricca V. Gender role, eating disorder symptoms, and body image concern in ballet dancers. J Psychosom Res. 2006;61:529–35.
29. Neumärker K-J, Bettle N, Neumärker U, Bettle O. Age- and gender-related psychological characteristics of adolescent ballet dancers. Psychopathology. 2000;33:137–42.
30. Ringham R, Klump K, Kaye W, Stone D, Libman S, Stowe S, et al. Eating disorder symptomatology among ballet dancers. Int J Eat Disord. 2006;39:503–8.
31. Swami V, Harris AS. Dancing toward positive body image? Examining body-related constructs with ballet and contemporary dancers at different levels. Am J Danc Ther. 2012;34:39–52.
32. Pollatou E, Bakali N, Theodorakis Y, Goudas M. Body image in female professional and amateur dancers. Res Danc Educ. 2010;11:131–7.
33. Doumenc A, Sudres JL, Sztulman H. Approche des dimensions pondérales et corporelles de jeunes danseuses classiques amatrices vs professionnelles [Approach to the weight and body

dimensions of young amateur vs. professional dancers]. Neuropsychiatr Enfance Adolesc. 2005;53:299–308.
34. Toro J, Guerrero M, Sentis J, Castro J, Puértolas C. Eating disorders in ballet dancing students: problems and risk factors. Eur Eat Disord Rev. 2009;17:40–9.
35. Goodwin H, Arcelus J, Marshall S, Wicks S, Meyer C. Critical comments concerning shape and weight: associations with eating psychopathology among full-time dance students. Eat Weight Disord. 2014;19:115–8.
36. de Bruin AP, Bakker F, Oudejans R. Achievement goal theory and disordered eating: relationships of disordered eating with goal orientations and motivational climate in female gymnasts and dancers. Psychol Sport Exerc. 2009;10:72–9.
37. Nordin-Bates SM, Schwarz JFA, Quested E, Cumming J, Aujla IJ, Redding E. Within- and between-person predictors of disordered eating attitudes among male and female dancers: findings from the UK Centres for Advanced Training. Psychol Sport Exerc. 2016;27:101–11.
38. Sundgot-Borgen J, Torstveit M. Prevalence of eating disorders in elite athletes is higher than in the general population. Clin J Sport Med. 2004;14:25–32.
39. Yeager KK, Agostini R, Nattiv A, Drinkwater B. The female athlete triad: disordered eating, amenorrhea, osteoporosis. Med Sci Sports Exerc. 1993;25(7):775.
40. Nattiv A, Loucks AB, Manore MM, Sanborn CF, Sundgot-Borgen J, Warren MP. The female athlete triad. Med Sci Sports Exerc. 2007;39:1867–82.
41. Mountjoy M, Sundgot-Borgen J, Burke L, Carter S, Constantini N, Lebrun C, et al. The IOC consensus statement: beyond the Female Athlete Triad-Relative Energy Deficiency in Sport (RED-S). Br J Sports Med. 2014;48(7):491.
42. Melin A, Torstveit M, Burke L, Marks S, Sundgot-Borgen J. Disordered eating and eating disorders in aquatic sports. Int J Sport Nutr Exerc Metab. 2014;24:450–9.
43. Torstveit M, Sundgot-Borgen J. Participation in leanness sports but not training volume is associated with menstrual dysfunction: a national survey of 1276 elite athletes and controls. Br J Sports Med. 2005;39:141–7.
44. Torstveit M, Sundgot-Borgen J. The female athlete triad: are elite athletes at increased risk? Med Sci Sports Exerc. 2005;37(2):184–93.
45. Milligan B, Pritchard M. The relationship between gender, type of sport, body dissatisfaction, self esteem and disordered eating behaviors in Division I athletes. Athl Insight. 2006;8:1–15.
46. Francisco R, Narciso I, Alarcão M. Individual and relational risk factors for the development of eating disorders in adolescent aesthetic athletes and general adolescents. Eat Weight Disord. 2013;18:403–11.
47. Thiemann P, Legenbauer T, Vocks S, Platen P, Auyeung B, Herpertz S. Eating disorders and their putative risk factors among female German professional athletes. Eur Eat Disord Rev. 2015;23(4):269–76.
48. Smolak L, Murnen SK, Ruble AE. Female athletes and eating problems: a meta-analysis. Int J Eat Disord. 2000;27:371–80.
49. Krentz EM, Warschburger P. A longitudinal investigation of sports-related risk factors for disordered eating in aesthetic sports. Scand J Med Sci Sport. 2013;23:303–10.
50. Hausenblas HA, Downs DS. Comparison of body image between athletes and nonathletes: a meta-analytic review. J Appl Sport Psychol. 2001;13:323–39.
51. Krentz EM, Warschburger P. Sports-related correlates of disordered eating in aesthetic sports. Psychol Sport Exerc. 2011;12:375–82.
52. Russell K. On versus off the pitch: the transiency of body satisfaction among female rugby players, cricketers, and netballers. Sex Roles. 2004;51:561–74.
53. de Bruin AP, Oudejans R, Bakker F, Woertman L. Contextual body image and athletes' disordered eating: the contribution of athletic body image to disordered eating in high performance women athletes. Eur Eat Disord Rev. 2011;19:201–15.
54. Bachner-Melman R, Zohar AH, Ebstein RP, Elizur Y, Constantini N. How anorexic-like are the symptom and personality profiles of aesthetic athletes? Med Sci Sports Exerc. 2006;38:628–36.
55. Leung F, Geller J, Katzman M. Issues and concerns associated with different risk models for eating disorders. Int J Eat Disord. 1996;19(3):249–56.

56. Thompson RA, Sherman RT. "Good athlete" traits and characteristics of anorexia nervosa: are they similar? Eat Disord. 1999;7:181–90.
57. Galli N, Petrie T, Chatterton J. Team weigh-ins and self-weighing: relations to body-related perceptions and disordered eating in collegiate male athletes. Psychol Sport Exerc. 2017;29:51–5.
58. Muscat AC, Long BC. Critical comments about body shape and weight: disordered eating of female athletes and sport participants. J Appl Sport Psychol. 2008;20:1–24.
59. de Bruin AP, Oudejans R, Bakker F. Dieting and body image in aesthetic sports: a comparison of Dutch female gymnasts and non-aesthetic sport participants. Psychol Sport Exerc. 2007;8(4):507–20.
60. Nowicka P, Eli K, Ng J, Apitzsch E, Sundgot-Borgen J. Moving from knowledge to action: a qualitative study of elite coaches' capacity for early intervention in cases of eating disorders. Int J Sport Sci Coach. 2013;8:343–56.
61. Piran N. Eating disorders: a trial of prevention in a high risk school setting. J Prim Prev. 1999;20:75–90. http://search.ebscohost.com/login.aspx?direct=true&db=eoah&AN=4276601&site=ehost-live&scope=site.
62. Bar RJ, Cassin SE, Dionne MM. The long-term impact of an eating disorder prevention program for professional ballet school students: a 15-year follow-up study. Eat Disord. 2017;25(5):375–87. https://www.tandfonline.com/doi/full/10.1080/10640266.2017.1308731.
63. Nordin-Bates SM, Walker IJ, Redding E. Correlates of disordered eating attitudes among male and female young talented dancers: findings from the UK centres for advanced training. Eat Disord. 2011;19:211–33.
64. Neumärker K-J, Bettle N, Bettle O, Dudeck U, Neumärker U. The eating attitudes test: comparative analysis of female and male students at the Public Ballet School of Berlin. Eur Child Adolesc Psychiatry. 1998;7:19–23.

Body Image in the Integrated Prevention of Eating and Weight Disorders

30

Ottavio Bosello, Angiola Vanzo, and Massimo Cuzzolaro

30.1 The Concept of Integrated Prevention

To *integrate* means to coordinate, or blend into a functioning or unified whole. The expression *integrated care* is commonly used to describe a multidimensional (e.g., bio-psycho-social) and multi-professional approach to the treatment of a disease. Conversely, *integrated prevention* is used to indicate interventions designed to prevent two or more diseases altogether. A short historical note may introduce and elucidate this concept.

In the 1970s, Toma Strasser, Chief Officer of the World Health Organization (WHO), was very concerned about the prospect of cardiovascular disease (CVD) pandemic. He formulated a basic preventive strategy: "there is only a single motto for the future: Prevention" [1] (p. 225). Strasser coined the terms *protoprophylaxis* or *primordial prevention* to indicate actions aimed to promote healthy lifestyles (e.g., smoking cessation, proper nutrition, appropriate physical activity) and healthy environments and to hinder the factors that increase the risk of CVD.

In the 1980s, the WHO recognized the need for *integrated prevention* of chronic, non-communicable diseases (NCDs) and developed the *Inter-Health Programme* aimed to demonstrate how such integrated programs could be implemented in several different countries. Programs for action were organized on the basis of two main beliefs: (a) most major NCDs share common risk factors; (b) "those that are

O. Bosello
Department of Medicine, University of Verona, Verona, Italy
e-mail: ottavio.bosello@univr.it

A. Vanzo
Department of Food Hygiene and Nutrition, ULSS 8 Berica, Vicenza, Italy
e-mail: angiola.vanzo@aulss8.veneto.it

M. Cuzzolaro (✉)
Formerly Medical Pathophysiology Department, Eating Disorders and Obesity Unit, Sapienza University of Rome, Rome, Italy

M. Cuzzolaro, S. Fassino (eds.), *Body Image, Eating, and Weight*,
https://doi.org/10.1007/978-3-319-90817-5_30

lifestyle related are modifiable through efficient interventions using multifactorial strategies, involving community participation and behavior changes, carried out at the primary health care level" [2] (p. 99).

So, to get back to the initial issue, an integrated prevention program is designed "to provide in 'one package' a coordinated set of health measures that hopefully will serve to prevent a series of chronic disorders simultaneously" [3] (p. 135).

Few years before the obesity pandemic of the last four decades, Strasser wrote that the outbreak of risk factors in the consumer societies had not reached the majority of the developing world [1]. But now obesity, body image concerns, disordered eating, and harmful weight-control behaviors are altogether a growing global health problem [4–8]. Campaigns against obesity and actions that in some way stigmatize fat people are likely to increase shape and weight concerns, especially among children and adolescents, and the incidence of eating disorders (ED).

Interventions explicitly aimed at preventing risk factors for both obesity and ED emerged in the early 2000s when it appeared manifest that taking care of a small number of individuals at high risk for obesity or ED may give temporary results that cannot reduce the incidence of these conditions significantly.

For example, in 2000, a systematic review of 20 empirical intervention studies on ED prevention found that, in the final two decades of the twentieth century, most studies had been designed to measure change on the individual level. The author concluded with a recommendation "for new attention to a model of proactive primary prevention targeted at environmental change and cross-disciplinary collaboration to achieve a reduction in the incidence of eating disorders" [9] (p. 1249).

30.2 Integrated Prevention of Obesity and Eating Disorders

In the literature on integrated prevention, the spectrum of eating- and weight-related problems usually include anorexia nervosa (AN), bulimia nervosa (BN), binge-eating disorder (BED), subthreshold eating disorders, unhealthy dieting and weight-control practices, overweight, and obesity [10].

In this section of the chapter, the salient findings from the literature are divided into four sections: theoretical pros, potential and practical obstacles, strategies, and efficacy evidence.

30.2.1 Theoretical Pros

The integrated prevention model for both obesity and ED in adolescence seems reasonable for four main reasons [11–13].

Firstly, on the scientific level, the integrated approach can be "the strategy of choice" only if different chronic diseases share several common causes and risk factors [3]. ED and obesity present similarities in a number of risk factors (shared susceptibility genes, low self-esteem, body weight and shape concerns, weight-related teasing, dieting, external locus of control, media exposure, etc.) [14–16] (Table 30.1).

Table 30.1 An alphabetical list of some shared risk factors for obesity and ED

Body weight and shape concerns
Childhood overweight/obesity
External locus of control
Family negative weight-related messages
Family unhealthy eating patterns
Family unhealthy physical activity habits
Low self-esteem
Media uncritical exposure and use
Parental overweight/obesity
Susceptibility genes possibly shared
Unhealthy dieting
Weight-related talk
Weight-related teasing

Furthermore, disordered eating behaviors are a risk factor for excessive weight gain and, conversely, being overweight is a significant risk factor for the development of unhealthy weight-control behaviors, above all in adolescence and youth.

Secondly, ED and obesity present phenotypic similarities (e.g., loss of control over eating, binge eating, unhealthy restriction, body weight and shape concerns, etc.).

Thirdly, ED and obesity may co-occur or occur sequentially.

Fourthly, on the logistic level, the integration of preventive plans makes better use of available resources both in terms of human resources and funds [3].

Consequently, a growing number of clinicians and researchers have considered appropriate and well-grounded to address the broad spectrum of eating and weight disorders through integrated prevention programs, particularly in adolescence, taking into account both shared and distinct risk factors [17].

The theoretical reasons for integrated prevention start from the knowledge that several risk factors are involved in the natural history of both obesity and ED and interact additively and perhaps multiplicatively when they are present at the same time.

Common behavioral and physiological risk factors related to ED and obesity are already present at young ages. According to a recent study of 5-year-old girls, unhealthy dieting tendencies appear very early in life [18].

A prospective study on 2516 female and male adolescents (*Project EAT*, Eating among Teens) found that weight-teasing by family, personal weight concerns, and unhealthy dieting and weight-control behaviors strongly and consistently predicted overweight status, binge eating, and extreme weight-control behaviors after 5 years [19].

The *Project EAT-II* found a longitudinal association between dieting and BMI increase that was partially mediated via the long-term adoption of the following behavioral patterns: increased binge eating, decreased breakfast consumption, and decreased physical activity [20].

The *Growing Up Today Study*, a prospective cohort study of 6022 girls and 4518 boys, showed that concern for weight, parental weight-related teasing, dieting, and family meals frequency had a shared effect on the eating- and weight-related problems [21].

A cross-cultural comparison between North American (2793, 53% girls) and Spanish (1501, 48% girls) adolescents detected in both population-based samples the intersection between risk factors for ED and obesity. The report of dieting and unhealthy weight-control behaviors was high in both groups, especially among girls and overweight and obese youth [22].

In a sample of women, the so-called *normal-weight obesity syndrome* significantly overlapped with ED in terms of eating attitudes and behaviors [23].

Another argument in favor of the integrated prevention model is that, from a transdiagnostic point of view, eating and weight disorders frequently co-occur and a person can move from one condition to another [24–26].

Binge eating is a symptom that crosses the entire field of ED and the whole spectrum of body weights [27, 28]. Increasing numbers of individuals with BN are also obese [29–33]. The *Project EAT* found that about 20% of overweight boys and 40% of overweight girls engaged in disordered eating and unhealthy weight-control behaviors [19]. Adolescents with a history of overweight/obesity represent a significant portion of patients with restrictive ED [34]. Childhood or parental obesity has been shown to be a specific risk factor for the development of BN [35]. On the other hand, dieting is a behavior that reinforces shape and weight concerns [36].

By the way, the concept of *weight suppression* is defined as a person's highest past weight minus the current weight. Recent studies on AN, BN, and BED suggest the importance of weight suppression as an outcome predictor. In particular, it predicts weight gain and disordered eating symptoms in bulimia-spectrum disorders [37], and a faster rate of weight gain with bulimic symptoms during intensive treatment of AN [38]. On the other hand, in obesity, weight cycling and binge eating are strongly associated [39]. Lastly, severe ED are frequent among bariatric surgery candidates, also adolescents [40, 41], and may persist or appear as new symptoms after surgery [42]. It is likely that such postoperative symptoms are underreported [43, 44].

30.2.2 Potential and Practical Obstacles

Connections and overlaps between ED and obesity are essential and it seems appropriate to use wide-ranging expressions like *non-homeostatic eating disorders* or *weight-related disorders* to indicate the broad spectrum of the conditions from anorexia nervosa to obesity [45]. Common environmental risk factors should inspire integrated prevention programs while more specific factors should be tackled by selective interventions for high-risk individuals [16].

However, thus far, a significant obstacle has been that obesity is traditionally regarded as a medical illness [46] and a domain of the biological sciences, while ED are classified as mental disorders [47] and a domain of psychiatry and psychology. As a consequence, very few health professionals have experience and expertise in both clinical fields [48].

Besides, cognitive/caloric restriction is a key component of obesity treatment but is a risk factor, a defining symptom, and a perpetuating cause of ED. Brownell and

Rodin chose the expression "the dieting maelstrom" to indicate the unsolved debate over the virtues and dangers of dieting [49] (p. 781).

The BODY (*Beyond Obesity and Disordered eating in Youth*) study was a qualitative research aimed to highlight the different meanings that individuals attribute to the spectrum of weight-related problems. Findings from the BODY study shed light on some possible causes of the tension between the two fields: e.g., ideology, power, knowledge, gender [50].

Finally, public and media attitudes to obesity and ED are often different: "indifference or blame in the case of obesity, and sympathy and awe in the case of eating disorders" [48] (p. 151).

It remains a challenging and ongoing problem to bridge the two areas [13, 50].

30.2.3 The Role of Body Shape and Weight Concerns in Integrated Prevention Programs for Adolescents

In spite of the global obesity pandemic, the westernized context of visual and social media enhances the ideal of thinness, perpetuates stigma and prejudice about fat, and reinforces the misconception that shape and size of one's body can be easily controlled and manipulated.

There is limited agreement on the ways to package or combine interventions to achieve integrated prevention-oriented goals. Approaches aimed only to raise awareness of healthy eating and physical activity are insufficient. The delivery of body image education is considered essential [51].

In addition to broader community interventions, most programs for adolescents are school- or family-based. Interventions aimed at minority ethnic groups, vulnerable groups, and vulnerable life stages are implemented as well.

Strategies include [52–55]:

- *Ecological* approaches, that aim at aspects of the sociocultural context (e.g., body-based teasing; thin ideal disseminated by the fashion industry).
- *Activism* approaches, that are created by community members who work together through voluntary participation (e.g., campaigns to protest advertisements which disseminate weight bias and promote unhealthy thinness).
- *Public policy* approaches, that are the actions of governments concerning the prevention of body image disturbances and related eating and weight disorders (e.g., legislation, codes of conduct, community-based initiatives, digitally delivered universal interventions).
- *School-based* approaches, that were first employed in the 1980s and remain the most common. The early studies increased nutrition knowledge, provided information about the harmful effects of unhealthy dieting, and tried to improve body image through the analysis of the cultural roots of female body ideals. The primary target was preventing ED in female students. These interventions improved knowledge but had little effects on attitudes, body image concerns, and behaviors. Later, many more interventions were interactive and, in some cases, peer-

led [56]. Different models were implemented such as *Healthy Schools-Healthy Kids* [57], *New Moves* [58–60], *Very Important Kids* [61], *Media-Smart Youth* [62], and *Everybody's Different* [63]. Several programs are aimed to prevent body image concerns among both female and male students. However, it is still uncertain whether boys should have gender-specific programs or be included in mixed-gender interventions with girls.

There are different types of school-based approaches:

- The early school programs were *psychoeducational interventions*. They used didactic instruments and counseling techniques focused on the way students (usually girls) perceived their own bodies. In general, they did not produce significant results.
- In the 1990s were designed interventions aimed at body image improvement via *self-esteem* protection and enhancement. Low self-esteem is very common in adolescents and more common among those with weight problems. It is considered a major risk factor for eating and weight disorders. A notable result was the improvement of body image worries in adolescence, in both boys and girls even if with higher weight [64]. Conversely, the *Everybody's Different* program did not result effective among fifth-grade school children [65].
- The *media literacy approaches* aim to teach students how to assess critically the media messages and the bombardment of clichéd body images that contribute to continuous comparisons and body dissatisfaction. Programs such as *Media-Smart Youth* seem to be able to reduce the internalization of the media stereotypical ideal of muscularity among boys and thinness among girls [62].

In the last two decades, a *cognitive dissonance* (CD) approach has been used in some prevention studies, mainly for young women at high risk for eating and weight disorders. The expression CD refers to an uncomfortable state of tension that occurs in a person when a choice has to be made between equally attractive or repulsive alternatives or when she/he holds mutually contradictory beliefs, attitudes, behaviors, and knowledge. It is supposed that CD can motivate to change some of the conflicting cognitions to mitigate the confused mental state and the anxiety.

30.2.4 Evidence of Efficacy

The integrated prevention of both obesity and ED is of a very complex nature. It is hard to quantify the results of the ecological, activism and public policy approaches to the prevention of body image problems. For *universal* prevention, more research-to-policy translation efforts are required targeting macro-environmental change (e.g., dietary supplements for weight loss and muscle building) [66].

Empirical research in this field is still poor and inhomogeneous, and many studies did not use a randomized design.

Table 30.2 Some RCT studies on integrated prevention of eating and weight disorders

First author, year (reference)	Study design	Participants	Follow-up (months)
Atkinson, MJ 2015 [67]	RCT	Adolescent girls	6
Atkinson, MJ 2016 [68]	RCT	Young adult women	6
Austin, SB 2005 [69]	RCT	Early adolescent girls	21
Doyle, AC 2008 [70]	RCT	Overweight adolescent girls and boys	4
Neumark-Sztainer, D 2010 [60]	RCT	Adolescent girls	9
Rohde, P 2014 [71]	RCT	Early adolescent girls	3
Rohde, P 2017 [72]	RCT	Women	6
Stice, E 2001 [73]	RCT	Young women	1
Stice, E 2006 [74]	RCT	Adolescent girls	6–12
Stice, E 2013 [75]	RCT	Female college students	12–24
Wade, TD 2017 [62]	RCT	Early adolescent girls and boys	12
Wilksch S 2015 [76]	RCT	Early adolescent girls and boys	12

Table 30.2 synoptically summarizes twelve randomized controlled trials (RCT) that showed some promising effects on body dissatisfaction, disordered eating, and weight-related problems. Follow-up was usually short. Most interventions concerned girls and young women.

A systematic review of randomized controlled trials (RCT) on prevention of ED found that media literacy, dissonance-based, and cognitive-behavior therapy were empirically supported approaches [77].

Another systematic review and meta-analysis confirmed that promising preventive interventions for ED risk factors and behaviors included cognitive dissonance, cognitive-behavior therapy, and media literacy. In particular, regarding *universal* programs, media literacy reduced body weight and shape worries for both males and females. As to *selective* prevention, cognitive dissonance interventions decreased ED symptoms in late adolescent and young adult females. Conversely, some *indicated* prevention programs were not effective in reducing ED risk factors [78].

As to cognitive dissonance (CD), a first randomized controlled trial was performed in a sample of 87 young women with severe body image concerns [73]. Participants in the CD-intervention reported decreased thin-ideal internalization, body dissatisfaction, dieting, negative affect, and bulimic symptoms, at termination and 4-week follow-up.

The *Body Project* is a *selective* prevention program for young women with body dissatisfaction. It is a CD-based prevention program that targets body image, unhealthy weight-control behaviors, decreased physical activity, smoking, and negative affect. In 2017, it was being implemented in 125 countries [79].

A recent fMRI (functional magnetic resonance imaging) study found that the *Body Project* reduces reward regions (caudate) response to images of thin models in high-risk young women with body dissatisfaction [80].

The *Body Project* has three variants: clinician-led groups, undergraduate peer educator-led groups, and an Internet-delivered version (*eBody Project*). A recent study compared the three versions and found that age moderated intervention results. The *eBody Project* produced superior effects with older women (≥25) regarding both BMI and ED symptoms reductions. Conversely, girls up to 20 benefitted more from the group-based versions [72].

A randomized controlled trial found that a mindfulness-based approach improved weight and shape concerns, thin-ideal internalization, and eating disordered behaviors in a sample of young adult women with body image concerns. However, most intervention gains were lost at 6-month follow-up [68].

Sanchez-Carracedo et al. demonstrated efficacy and effectiveness of an integrated approach to the prevention of ED and weight-related problems. Beauty ideal internalization significantly decreased in the girls of the intervention group [81, 82].

A media literacy (*Media Smart*) program showed also benefit on disordered eating behaviors, obesity risk factors, and weight and shape concerns [62, 76].

30.3 Conclusive Remarks

The advantages of prevention can be assessed only in the long run [83]. The benefits of chronic disease prevention are recognized, even though some studies have shown that prevention usually adds to medical costs instead of reducing them [84].

Programs designed for integrated prevention of ED and obesity are still in the beginning stages but are here to stay all over the world. An Australian study found that, from 1995 to 2015, there were statewide significant increases in the independent and comorbid prevalence of obesity, binge eating, and very strict dieting/fasting [85]. The authors concluded that "These findings support the need for more integrated approaches to both the prevention and treatment of obesity and eating disorder behaviors" (p. 1148). In Malaysia, the *EPal* is an integrated health education intervention aimed to prevent overweight and disordered eating among secondary school adolescents (13–14 years old). The acronym stands for *Eat right, be Positive about your body and live actively* [86].

Adolescents and young adults with higher body weight represent a subset of the population particularly at risk for disordered eating behaviors. Body dissatisfaction and depressive symptoms appear as the main predictors [87]. Integrated primary prevention programs should seek to simultaneously improve these risk factors and those that lead to excessive weight gain. Alternatively, environments that promote and skill young people in healthy eating can be of mutual benefit to obesity and ED.

Follow-up analysis of the *US Planet Health obesity prevention intervention*, aimed at early high-school years, showed that the interdisciplinary program produced combined and cost-effective benefits for both obesity prevention and prevention of disordered eating and weight-control behaviors. There was a significant reduction in the number of girls using extreme weight-loss practices compared with those in control schools [88, 89].

Although some positive results have been identified, the long-term efficacy of combined obesity and ED prevention programs has not yet been demonstrated, and the value of preventive programs is still uncertain.

We have much to learn about optimizing the use of integrated prevention for ED and obesity, in particular how intensive to make the intervention. A 2017 review article concluded that "combined ED and obesity prevention interventions require further research" (p. 46). Many questions that are essential to advise practice and policymaking remain unanswered, such as:

- Is integrated prevention a truly effective way to reduce the incidence of both obesity and eating disorders?
- How intensive should be the intervention?
- Which strategies are cost-effective?
- Could similar integrated programs be implemented in different countries and cultures?
- What is the best role in integrated prevention programs of the crucial but elusive concept of *body image*? (see Chap. 1 of this volume)
- Which gender-specific risk and protective factors play a role in the development of body shape and weight experiences in children and adolescents?
- Which are the variations by age, ethnicity, religious practices, and social groups?

References

1. Strasser T. Reflections on cardiovascular diseases. Interdiscip Sci Rev. 1978;3(3):225–30.
2. Berrios X, Koponen T, Huiguang T, Khaltaev N, Puska P, Nissinen A. Distribution and prevalence of major risk factors of noncommunicable diseases in selected countries: the WHO Inter-Health Programme. Bull World Health Organ. 1997;75(2):99–108.
3. Epstein FH, Holland WW. Prevention of chronic diseases in the community—one-disease versus multiple-disease strategies. Int J Epidemiol. 1983;12(2):135–7.
4. Finucane MM, Stevens GA, Cowan MJ, Danaei G, Lin JK, Paciorek CJ, et al. National, regional, and global trends in body-mass index since 1980: systematic analysis of health examination surveys and epidemiological studies with 960 country-years and 9.1 million participants. Lancet. 2011;377(9765):557–67.
5. N.C.D. Risk Factor Collaboration. Trends in adult body-mass index in 200 countries from 1975 to 2014: a pooled analysis of 1698 population-based measurement studies with 19.2 million participants. Lancet. 2016;387(10026):1377–96.
6. Makino M, Tsuboi K, Dennerstein L. Prevalence of eating disorders: a comparison of Western and non-Western countries. MedGenMed. 2004;6(3):49–56.
7. Pike KM, Dunne PE. The rise of eating disorders in Asia: a review. J Eat Disord. 2015;3:33–46.
8. Chisuwa N, O'Dea JA. Body image and eating disorders amongst Japanese adolescents. A review of the literature. Appetite. 2010;54(1):5–15.
9. Austin SB. Prevention research in eating disorders: theory and new directions. Psychol Med. 2000;30(6):1249–62.
10. Sanchez-Carracedo D, Neumark-Sztainer D, Lopez-Guimera G. Integrated prevention of obesity and eating disorders: barriers, developments and opportunities. Public Health Nutr 2012;15(12):2295–309.
11. Cuzzolaro M. Eating disorders. In: Sbraccia P, Finer N, editors. Obesity: pathogenesis, diagnosis, and treatment. Cham: Springer; 2017. p. 1–24.
12. Neumark-Sztainer D. Obesity and eating disorder prevention: an integrated approach? Adolesc Med. 2003;14(1):159–73.
13. Neumark-Sztainer D. The interface between the eating disorders and obesity fields: moving toward a model of shared knowledge and collaboration. Eat Weight Disord. 2009;14(1):51–8.

14. Haines J, Neumark-Sztainer D. Prevention of obesity and eating disorders: a consideration of shared risk factors. Health Educ Res. 2006;21(6):770–82.
15. Day J, Ternouth A, Collier DA. Eating disorders and obesity: two sides of the same coin? Epidemiol Psichiatr Soc. 2009;18(2):96–100.
16. Krug I, Villarejo C, Jimenez-Murcia S, Perpina C, Vilarrasa N, Granero R, et al. Eating-related environmental factors in underweight eating disorders and obesity: are there common vulnerabilities during childhood and early adolescence? Eur Eat Disord Rev. 2013;21(3):202–8.
17. Golden NH, Schneider M, Wood C, Committee on Nutrition, Committee on Adolescence, Section on Obesity. Preventing obesity and eating disorders in adolescents. Pediatrics. 2016;138(3):1–10.
18. Damiano SR, Paxton SJ, Wertheim EH, McLean SA, Gregg KJ. Dietary restraint of 5-year-old girls: associations with internalization of the thin ideal and maternal, media, and peer influences. Int J Eat Disord. 2015;48(8):1166–9.
19. Neumark-Sztainer DR, Wall MM, Haines JI, Story MT, Sherwood NE, van den Berg PA. Shared risk and protective factors for overweight and disordered eating in adolescents. Am J Prev Med. 2007;33(5):359–69.
20. Neumark-Sztainer D, Wall M, Haines J, Story M, Eisenberg ME. Why does dieting predict weight gain in adolescents? Findings from project EAT-II: a 5-year longitudinal study. J Am Diet Assoc. 2007;107(3):448–55.
21. Haines J, Kleinman KP, Rifas-Shiman SL, Field AE, Austin SB. Examination of shared risk and protective factors for overweight and disordered eating among adolescents. Arch Pediatr Adolesc Med. 2010;164(4):336–43.
22. Lopez-Guimera G, Neumark-Sztainer D, Hannan P, Fauquet J, Loth K, Sanchez-Carracedo D. Unhealthy weight-control behaviours, dieting and weight status: a cross-cultural comparison between North American and Spanish adolescents. Eur Eat Disord Rev. 2013;21(4):276–83.
23. Di Renzo L, Tyndall E, Gualtieri P, Carboni C, Valente R, Ciani AS, et al. Association of body composition and eating behavior in the normal weight obese syndrome. Eat Weight Disord. 2016;21(1):99–106.
24. Sim LA, Lebow J, Billings M. Eating disorders in adolescents with a history of obesity. Pediatrics. 2013.
25. Darby A, Hay P, Mond J, Quirk F, Buttner P, Kennedy L. The rising prevalence of comorbid obesity and eating disorder behaviors from 1995 to 2005. Int J Eat Disord. 2009;42(2):104–8.
26. Neumark-Sztainer D, Story M, Hannan PJ, Perry CL, Irving LM. Weight-related concerns and behaviors among overweight and nonoverweight adolescents: implications for preventing weight-related disorders. Arch Pediatr Adolesc Med. 2002;156(2):171–8.
27. Stunkard A. Eating patterns and obesity. Psychiatry Q. 1959;33:284–95.
28. Fairburn CG, Wilson GT. Binge eating: definition and classification. In: Fairburn CG, Wilson GT, editors. Binge eating nature assessment and treatment. New York: The Guilford Press; 1993. p. 3–14.
29. Hudson J, Pope H, Wutman J. Bulimia in obese individuals. J Nerv Ment Dis. 1988;176:144–52.
30. Mitchell JE, Pyle RL, Eckert ED, Hatsukami D, Soll E. Bulimia nervosa in overweight individuals. J Nerv Ment Dis. 1990;178(5):324–7.
31. Rotella F, Castellini G, Montanelli L, Rotella CM, Faravelli C, Ricca V. Comparison between normal-weight and overweight bulimic patients. Eat Weight Disord. 2013;18(4):389–93.
32. Bulik CM, Marcus MD, Zerwas S, Levine MD, La Via M. The changing "weightscape" of bulimia nervosa. Am J Psychiatry. 2012;169(10):1031–6.
33. Hay P, Chinn D, Forbes D, Madden S, Newton R, Sugenor L, et al. Royal Australian and New Zealand College of Psychiatrists clinical practice guidelines for the treatment of eating disorders. Aust N Z J Psychiatry. 2014;48(11):977–1008.
34. Lebow J, Sim LA, Kransdorf LN. Prevalence of a history of overweight and obesity in adolescents with restrictive eating disorders. J Adolesc Health. 2015;56(1):19–24.
35. Fairburn CG, Welch SL, Doll HA, Davies BA, O'Connor ME. Risk factors for bulimia nervosa: a community-based case-control study. Arch Gen Psychiatry. 1997;54(6):509–17.
36. Fairburn CG, Harrison PJ. Eating disorders. Lancet. 2003;361(9355):407–16.

37. Herzog DB, Thomas JG, Kass AE, Eddy KT, Franko DL, Lowe MR. Weight suppression predicts weight change over 5 years in bulimia nervosa. Psychiatry Res. 2010;177(3):330–4.
38. Wildes JE, Marcus MD. Weight suppression as a predictor of weight gain and response to intensive behavioral treatment in patients with anorexia nervosa. Behav Res Ther. 2012;50(4):266–74.
39. Venditti EM, Wing RR, Jakicic JM, Butler BA, Marcus MD. Weight cycling, psychological health, and binge eating in obese women. J Consult Clin Psychol. 1996;64(2):400–5.
40. Utzinger LM, Gowey MA, Zeller M. Jenkins TM, Engel SG, Rofey DL, et al. Loss of control eating and eating disorders in adolescents before bariatric surgery. Int J Eat Disord. 2016;49(10):947–52.
41. Herget S, Rudolph A, Hilbert A, Bluher S. Psychosocial status and mental health in adolescents before and after bariatric surgery: a systematic literature review. Obes Facts. 2014;7(4):233–45.
42. Sondike SB, Pisetsky EM, Luzier JL. Development of significant disordered eating in an adolescent following gastric bypass surgery. Eat Weight Disord. 2016;21(1):133–6.
43. Segal A, Kinoshita Kussunoki D, Larino MA. Post-surgical refusal to eat: anorexia nervosa, bulimia nervosa or a new eating disorder? A case series. Obes Surg. 2004;14(3):353–60.
44. Marino JM, Ertelt TW, Lancaster K, Steffen K, Peterson L, de Zwaan M, et al. The emergence of eating pathology after bariatric surgery: a rare outcome with important clinical implications. Int J Eat Disord. 2012;45(2):179–84.
45. Cuzzolaro M. Eating and weight disorders: studies on anorexia, bulimia, and obesity turns 19. Eat Weight Disord. 2014;19(1):1–2.
46. American Medical Association House of Delegates. Report of the Council on Science and Public Health (CSAPH). Recognition of obesity as a disease. Resolution. 420 (A-13). 2013. http://www.ama-assn.org/assets/meeting/2013a/a13-addendum-refcomm-d.pdf#page=19. Accessed 11 Nov 2014, 25 June 2013.
47. American Psychiatric Association. Diagnostic and statistical manual of mental disorders, DSM-5. 5th ed. Arlington, VA: American Psychiatric Publishing; 2013.
48. Hill AJ. Obesity and eating disorders. Obes Rev. 2007;8(Suppl 1):151–5.
49. Brownell KD, Rodin J. The dieting maelstrom. Is it possible and advisable to lose weight? Am Psychol. 1994;49(9):781–91.
50. Ferrari M. Understanding the feasibility of integrating the eating disorders and obesity fields: the beyond obesity and disordered eating in youth (BODY) study. Eat Weight Disord. 2015.
51. Piran N. New possibilities in the prevention of eating disorders: the introduction of positive body image measures. Body Image. 2015;14:146–57.
52. Piran N, Mafrici N. Preventing body image problems: ecological and activism approaches. In: Cash TF, editor. Encyclopedia of body image and human appearance. 2nd ed. Amsterdam: Elsevier Academic Press; 2012 p. 674–9.
53. Paxton S. Preventing body image problems: public policy approaches. In: Cash TF, editor. Encyclopedia of body image and human appearance. 2nd ed. Amsterdam: Elsevier Academic Press; 2012. p. 680–5.
54. O'Dea J. Preventing body image problems: school-based approaches. In: Cash TF, editor. Encyclopedia of body image and human appearance. 2nd ed. Amsterdam: Elsevier Academic Press; 2012. p. 686–92.
55. Piran N. Prevention of eating disorders: a review of outcome evaluation research. Isr J Psychiatry Relat Sci. 2005;42(3):172–7.
56. Becker CB, Bull S, Schaumberg K, Cauble A, Franco A. Effectiveness of peer-led eating disorders prevention: a replication trial. J Consult Clin Psychol. 2008;76(2):347–54.
57. McVey G, Tweed S, Blackmore E. Healthy Schools-Healthy Kids: a controlled evaluation of a comprehensive universal eating disorder prevention program. Body Image. 2007;4(2):115–36.
58. Neumark-Sztainer D, Flattum CF, Story M, Feldman S, Petrich CA. Dietary approaches to healthy weight management for adolescents: the New Moves model. Adolesc Med State Art Rev. 2008;19(3):421–30, viii.
59. Neumark-Sztainer D, Story M, Hannan PJ, Rex J. New Moves: a school-based obesity prevention program for adolescent girls. Prev Med. 2003;37(1):41–51.

60. Neumark-Sztainer DR, Friend SE, Flattum CF, Hannan PJ, Story MT, Bauer KW, et al. New moves-preventing weight-related problems in adolescent girls. A group-randomized study. Am J Prev Med. 2010;39(5):421–32.
61. Haines J, Neumark-Sztainer D, Perry CL, Hannan PJ, Levine MP. V.I.K. (Very Important Kids): a school-based program designed to reduce teasing and unhealthy weight-control behaviors. Health Educ Res. 2006;21(6):884–95.
62. Wade TD, Wilksch SM, Paxton SJ, Byrne SM, Austin SB. Do universal media literacy programs have an effect on weight and shape concern by influencing media internalization? Int J Eat Disord. 2017;50(7):731–8.
63. O'Dea JA. Prevention of child obesity: "First, do no harm". Health Educ Res. 2005;20(2):259–65.
64. O'Dea J. Body image and self-esteem. In: Cash TF, editor. Encyclopedia of body image and human appearance. 1st ed. Amsterdam: Elsevier Academic Press; 2012. p. 141–7.
65. Ghaderi A, Martensson M, Schwan H. "Everybody's different": a primary prevention program among fifth grade school children. Eat Disord. 2005;13(3):245–59.
66. Austin SB, Yu K, Tran A, Mayer B. Research-to-policy translation for prevention of disordered weight and shape control behaviors: a case example targeting dietary supplements sold for weight loss and muscle building. Eat Behav. 2017;25:9–14.
67. Atkinson MJ, Wade TD. Mindfulness-based prevention for eating disorders: a school-based cluster randomized controlled study. Int J Eat Disord. 2015;48(7):1024–37.
68. Atkinson MJ, Wade TD. Does mindfulness have potential in eating disorders prevention? A preliminary controlled trial with young adult women. Early Interv Psychiatry. 2016;10(3):234–45.
69. Austin SB, Field AE, Wiecha J, Peterson KE, Gortmaker SL. The impact of a school-based obesity prevention trial on disordered weight-control behaviors in early adolescent girls. Arch Pediatr Adolesc Med. 2005;159(3):225–30.
70. Doyle AC, Goldschmidt A, Huang C, Winzelberg AJ, Taylor CB, Wilfley DE. Reduction of overweight and eating disorder symptoms via the Internet in adolescents: a randomized controlled trial. J Adolesc Health. 2008;43(2):172–9.
71. Rohde P, Auslander BA, Shaw H, Raineri KM, Gau JM, Stice E. Dissonance-based prevention of eating disorder risk factors in middle school girls: results from two pilot trials. Int J Eat Disord. 2014;47(5):483–94.
72. Rohde P, Stice E, Shaw H, Gau JM, Ohls OC. Age effects in eating disorder baseline risk factors and prevention intervention effects. Int J Eat Disord. 2017;50(11):1273–80.
73. Stice E, Chase A, Stormer S, Appel A. A randomized trial of a dissonance-based eating disorder prevention program. Int J Eat Disord. 2001;29(3):247–62.
74. Stice E, Shaw H, Burton E, Wade E. Dissonance and healthy weight eating disorder prevention programs: a randomized efficacy trial. J Consult Clin Psychol. 2006;74(2):263–75.
75. Stice E, Rohde P, Shaw H, Marti CN. Efficacy trial of a selective prevention program targeting both eating disorders and obesity among female college students: 1- and 2-year follow-up effects. J Consult Clin Psychol. 2013;81(1):183–9.
76. Wilksch SM, Paxton SJ, Byrne SM, Austin SB, McLean SA, Thompson KM, et al. Prevention across the spectrum: a randomized controlled trial of three programs to reduce risk factors for both eating disorders and obesity. Psychol Med. 2015;45(9):1811–23.
77. Watson HJ, Joyce T, French E, Willan V, Kane RT, Tanner-Smith EE, et al. Prevention of eating disorders: a systematic review of randomized, controlled trials. Int J Eat Disord. 2016;49(9):833–62.
78. Le LK, Barendregt JJ, Hay P, Mihalopoulos C. Prevention of eating disorders: a systematic review and meta-analysis. Clin Psychol Rev. 2017;53:46–58.
79. Becker CB. From efficacy to global impact: lessons learned about what not to do in translating our research to reach. Behav Ther. 2017;48(5):718–30.
80. Stice E, Yokum S, Waters A. Dissonance-based eating disorder prevention program reduces reward region response to thin models; how actions shape valuation. PLoS One. 2015;10(12):e0144530.
81. Sánchez-Carracedo D, López-Guimerà G, Fauquet J, Barrada JR, Pàmias M, Puntí J, et al. A school-based program implemented by community providers previously trained for the pre-

vention of eating and weight-related problems in secondary-school adolescents: the MABIC study protocol. BMC Public Health. 2013;13:955.
82. Sanchez-Carracedo D, Fauquet J, Lopez-Guimera G, Leiva D, Punti J, Trepat E, et al. The MABIC project: an effectiveness trial for reducing risk factors for eating disorders. Behav Res Ther. 2016;77:23–33.
83. Wilson JF. Can disease prevention save health reform? Ann Intern Med. 2009;151(2):145–8.
84. Russell LB. Preventing chronic disease: an important investment, but don't count on cost savings. Health Aff. 2009;28(1):42–5.
85. da Luz FQ, Sainsbury A, Mannan H, Touyz S, Mitchison D, Hay P. Prevalence of obesity and comorbid eating disorder behaviors in South Australia from 1995 to 2015. Int J Obes. 2017;41(7):1148–53.
86. Sharif Ishak SI, Chin YS, Mohd Taib MN, Mohd SZ. School-based intervention to prevent overweight and disordered eating in secondary school Malaysian adolescents: a study protocol. BMC Public Health. 2016;16(1):1101.
87. Goldschmidt AB, Wall MM, Loth KA, Neumark-Sztainer D. Risk factors for disordered eating in overweight adolescents and young adults. J Pediatr Psychol. 2015;40(10):1048–55.
88. Wang LY, Nichols LP, Austin SB. The economic effect of Planet Health on preventing bulimia nervosa. Arch Pediatr Adolesc Med. 2011;165(8):756–62.
89. Austin SB, Kim J, Wiecha J, Troped PJ, Feldman HA, Peterson KE. School-based overweight preventive intervention lowers incidence of disordered weight-control behaviors in early adolescent girls. Arch Pediatr Adolesc Med. 2007;161(9):865–9.

31 Body Image, Eating, and Weight. Some Cultural Differences

Carla Gramaglia, Claudia Delicato, and Patrizia Zeppegno

31.1 Introduction

Body image is not a "neutral" construct, but depends on sociocultural models which may change from one cultural context to another. Research within the body image literature has consistently shown weight importance (defined as the self-reported emphasis or importance one places on weight and body shape in determining self-views) to be a strong predictor of disordered eating and persistent dieting [1]. Moreover, weight importance predicts the continuity of these behaviors between adolescence and adulthood. Reviews of the literature on body image concerns and disordered eating in women have revealed significant ethnic differences, at least historically [2–4]. Actually, some authors in the nineties considered eating disorders (EDs) themselves as culture-bound syndromes, which are more prevalent in industrialized countries and Western cultures, and far more common among females than males, mirroring cross-cultural differences in the importance of thinness for women [3, 5]. Culture-bound syndromes are described as "a collection of signs and symptoms (excluding notions of cause) which is restricted to a limited number of cultures primarily by reason of certain of their psychosocial features" [5]. Nonetheless, evidence of anorexia nervosa (AN) in non-Western cultures would not decrease the extent to which it represents a culture-bound syndrome because AN cannot be understood separated from its cultural context [6], as well as from the historical one. Body image, as well as eating and weight-related

C. Gramaglia · P. Zeppegno (✉)
Department of Translational Medicine, Psychiatry Institute,
Università del Piemonte Orientale, Novara, Italy

SC Psichiatria—AOU Maggiore della Carità di Novara, Novara, Italy
e-mail: patrizia.zeppegno@med.uniupo.it

C. Delicato
Department of Translational Medicine, Psychiatry Institute,
Università del Piemonte Orientale, Novara, Italy

M. Cuzzolaro, S. Fassino (eds.), *Body Image, Eating, and Weight*,
https://doi.org/10.1007/978-3-319-90817-5_31

behaviors, changes in different historical periods and should be interpreted within both the social and historical frame. It is clear from the art of different eras that representations of female bodies have shifted from symbols of fertility (e.g., the Venus of Willendorf) to mathematically calculated proportions. These dramatic changes in what is considered a beautiful body follow the transformation of women's role in society: from mother and mistress to a career-oriented individual [7]. Hence, identical symptoms now may mean different things from what they meant in the late nineteenth century, when the disorder was first documented as it is currently recognized. Nonetheless, divergent patterns emerged from the examination of epidemiological, cross-historical, and cross-cultural evidence of EDs as culture-bound syndromes by Keel and Klump, who concluded that while bulimia nervosa is culture bound, AN is not [8].

Interestingly, and offering a more thorough perspective on the notion of culture-bound syndrome, recently the DSM-5 [9] replaced it with the following concepts which may offer a frame for the interpretation of body image and related EDs: (1) cultural syndromes: "clusters of symptoms and attributions that tend to co-occur among individuals in specific cultural groups, communities, or contexts [...] that are recognized locally as coherent patterns of experience"; (2) cultural idioms of distress: "ways of expressing distress that may not involve specific symptoms or syndromes, but that provide collective, shared ways of experiencing and talking about personal or social concerns"; and (3) cultural explanations of distress or perceived causes: "labels, attributions, or features of an explanatory model that indicate culturally recognized meaning or etiology for symptoms, illness, or distress" [8].

One early review concluded that "Whites experience greater eating disturbance and body dissatisfaction than their non-White counterparts" [4]; ethnic minority women may have more flexible beauty ideals [10] or be less willing to internalize mainstream Euro-American norms of beauty, particularly the thin ideal [11–13]. Reports about this last issue are mixed, and increasing levels of body dissatisfaction among ethnic minority women in post-industrial societies may reflect increasing idealization of thinness in media aimed at a greater internalization of the thin ideal [14, 15], which eventually contributes to increased body dissatisfaction, drive for thinness, body change behaviors, and disordered eating [12, 16–20].

Research consistently supports the negative impact of thinness pressures on body image, and socio-cultural theories may provide a useful framework for understanding the unique experiences of individuals of differing ethnicities [21]. Two well-supported socio-cultural theories implicating appearance-related pressure have been proposed: the Tripartite Influence Model [16] and the Dual Pathway Model [17]. The Tripartite Influence Model posits that thinness pressures from family, peers, and media may lead to internalization of the thin ideal and appearance comparisons, resulting in body dissatisfaction and disordered eating. The Dual Pathway Model posits that thinness pressures and thin-ideal internalization likely combine to produce negative effects on body image and eating patterns.

Side by side with the "thin ideal," in the last years and likely due to the emphasis on the "healthy" concept in all fields of everyday life, in Western countries the "healthy ideal" has emerged. While the ideal of maintaining one's body weight within the boundaries of a "healthy" range does not totally overlap with the thin ideal, it may impact on body image as well and be somewhat involved in the development of weight concerns. This may happen through the internalization of anti-fat attitudes, and a strong focus on the possibility and need to control one's weight by dieting and exercising [22]. A wide body of research has described the relationships between health and weight status, and between weight status and body self-perception in different populations and environmental contexts [23–26]. The increasing incidence of overweight and obesity worldwide is now reaching alarming proportions. As an effect of the nutritional transition, these diseases concern both developed and developing countries. Hence the latter are facing a dual burden of malnutrition, with a high prevalence of both underweight and overweight/obesity [27–29]. Previous studies in Western countries have reported lower accurate perceptions of overweight in low socioeconomic status groups and this misperception contributes to the persistence of unhealthy lifestyles [30, 31]. This aspect is particularly burdensome in immigrants from low-to-medium-income countries who have migrated to high-income countries; they seem to be more susceptible to overweight and obesity than their local counterparts [32]. Furthermore, since they misperceive their overweight/obesity, they do not attempt to lose weight, leading to an increase of these nutritional disorders.

Nevertheless, it is not so clear if the recent preference for slimmer body size is only due to the Westernization process. It is also probably related to the idea that "plumpness" is revered only when it is a rare condition in a context of food scarcity, while it loses desirability when overweight and obesity become more prevalent [33].

Anti-fat attitudes are influenced by actual and perceived weight, weight importance, and ethnicity. Some studies found that overweight and obese individuals appear to endorse anti-fat attitudes at rates similar to normal-weight individuals, such that all weight groups demonstrate anti-fat bias [34, 35], whereas others found stronger anti-fat bias in thinner individuals than in heavier ones [36]. As a function of ethnicity, anti-fat attitudes are expressed by Black women to a lesser extent than by White women [37]. Hispanic women may respond in a similar manner to Black women and demonstrate lower anti-fat attitudes than White ones, whereas Asian women may respond in a similar manner to White women and endorse high levels of anti-fat attitudes [38, 39]. Nevertheless, it is important to consider that rates of overweight and obesity have been increasing in Asia with wide variability among different geographic regions which may impact weight stigma [40]. Global trend towards increased weight stigma even in cultures previously characterized as "fat positive" (e.g., Mexico and American Samoa) suggests it is important to continue to examine ethnicity as fluctuations in obesity rates and global acceptance of weight stigma occur [41] (see also Chap. 28 of this book).

Regarding individual differences in psychological vulnerability to socio-cultural messages concerning body image and weight, these may be influenced by the cultural value placed on the concept of self-esteem. In Western societies, where greater emphasis is placed on individual performance rather than on the maintenance of group cohesiveness, individuals are encouraged to assert themselves and to develop a robust self-esteem [42]. In contrast, in more collectivist societies like Japan, the focus is less on the individual developing a robust self-esteem but more on defining a sense of self in terms of interpersonal relationships with significant others [42, 43]. Within these societies, individual abilities, feelings, and views may need to be controlled or downplayed to maintain group cohesiveness, and the ability to adjust, restrain the self, and maintain group harmony is viewed as desirable and encouraged. The concepts of individualism and collectivism may provide a further framework for exploring the association between cultural values and psychological processes [44]; for instance, there are suggestions that women in collectivistic societies which are in a changing cultural environment, such as modern exposure and experimentation with individualistic models, might develop an ED as a reaction to socio-cultural disconnection and transition [45]. Nonetheless, currently it is lacking the literature about the possible role of the individualism and collectivism concepts in the clinical manifestations of EDs, especially AN.

Last, a brief note about the meaning attributed to some terms in different cultural contexts; for instance, the term overweight designates a culturally acceptable body size (i.e., overweight bodies are not too fat) in African American populations. Therefore the same word (e.g., overweight or obese) may be used with different meanings by different people; this may represent an obstacle also in the effective communication between clinician and patient about the health risks of large body size and have an impact on help-seeking for weight loss [46, 47].

31.2 Ethnic Differences in Body Satisfaction and Appearance Evaluation

31.2.1 Black and Hispanic Women

Research reports from the United States are mixed, with some studies suggesting higher thinness pressures in White women compared to Black [48], and Hispanic women [49], and other studies suggesting comparable thinness pressures among these ethnic groups [12]. Lower levels of media appearance pressure in Black women compared to White and Hispanic women [50] have been described. Regarding parental messages, their influence on women's body image could operate in different ways in Black and White young women [51]. In White samples, parental communication (such as the encouragement to lose weight) has more consistent and stronger effects on daughters' body image than parental modeling [52, 53]; nonetheless, communication constructs and perceived parental modeling seem to have a similar impact on body image after controlling for body mass index [51]. Greater maternal than paternal influence has been suggested [52, 54], and high perceived levels of maternal criticism about childhood appearance are associated with increased weight concern in both Black and White adult women [55, 56].

African Americans are more satisfied with their body size than are Whites, independent of BMI and socio-economic status [57–61], being one potential explanation for the lower prevalence of EDs and the higher prevalence of obesity among African Americans compared to Whites [57, 58, 60, 62–65]. The prevalence of obesity is significantly higher among non-Hispanic African American women than White women [66, 67]; specifically, they and their female children have the highest obesity prevalence of any demographic group [67]. African American women are more likely to underestimate their body weight [57, 68–73], and underestimation of weight is associated with poor weight management behavior [74], greater weight gain over time [62], and an underestimation of health risk [73]. Overweight and obese African American women are almost twice as likely as overweight and obese White women to respond that they are "about the right weight," or "underweight" [68–71]. Because Black women are more likely to be overweight than White women, they may disengage from the thin ideal; hence Black parents may be less likely to pressure their daughters to lose weight or to criticize their weight, which may protect them from developing a negative body image [48, 75]. On the other hand, given concerns about obesity and related health risks in the Black population [76], parents may exert pressure on their daughters to lose weight which may have implications for their body image [51].

31.2.2 Japanese Women

Recent cross-cultural research findings have suggested that individuals from non-Western countries are equally susceptible than those from Western-industrialized countries to beauty ideals and thinness pressures [77, 78]. Several studies have reported high levels of body dissatisfaction, drive for thinness, dieting, and disordered eating in the Japanese population [79, 80]. The Japanese women's "ideal" BMI is lower than that of American women, who usually have a higher average BMI [81], and their ideal female body shape is significantly thinner [82]. Etiological explanations, also for the increased prevalence of EDs in Japan, include the crucial role of socio-cultural influences such as the popular media in promoting the "thinness ideal" and the internalization of Western beauty ideals [83, 84]. The strong ideal for thinness of modern Japanese society likely combines Japanese traditions (that encourage thinness) with the Western thin ideal of beauty [85]. On the other hand, the rise of EDs in Japan may partly be due to the rapid westernization and industrialization that has occurred in that country, which brings along rapid changes in the social system, an enhanced vulnerability of the family structure, and insufficient social support systems [86]. This conceptualization is echoed in Nishizono-Maher's description of ED as a "culture change syndrome." She argued that young women in Japan are faced with trying to build a personal identity inside and outside the family context and are caught between the conflicting pressures of traditional rules of the family and an increasingly individualistic society focused on personal freedoms [87].

31.2.3 Indian Women

In India the number of EDs appears to be on the rise [88, 89], but research on this topic is still scant [90]. In India females with an ED may not present with signs typical of EDs reported in western clinical samples, particularly as regards body image disturbances, fear of fatness and of weight gain [91]. The exception is in cases of premorbid overweight or obesity that subsequently lose a significant, unhealthy amount of weight and report a fear of fatness and body image disturbance [92]. Moreover, along with a thinner body image ideal of Indian women, fear of fatness and body image disturbance is growing in females that are more exposed to western beauty ideals [93]. A lack of "fat phobia" could suggest that South Asians do not have a strong association of "fat" as being undesirable. It should be noted that Indians in India and those in the UK would most likely experience different pressures from their family, stressors, and levels of exposure to western ideals [94]. Evidence to date is inconsistent regarding body dissatisfaction, with reports of Indians having greater [95], similar [96, 97] and lower levels of dissatisfaction [98] than Caucasians.

31.2.4 Immigrants

As described above, socio-cultural factors influence the standards of desirable body weight within cultures, and body image perception and body shape preferences are culturally determined [23]. Furthermore, the ideals of beauty may change as a result of immigration, leading immigrant people, especially women, to pursue ideals of thinness. Thus, in immigrants in which the beauty ideals determine an increased level of body and weight dissatisfaction, the risk for the development of nutritional disorders increases. As is the case of immigrants, the comparison of body image perception and body shape preference across populations living in developing countries is complicated by the variety of environmental and cultural conditions, including "modernization," media influence, and recent rapid transitions of the economy and urbanization [33, 99, 100].

Body size and body image perception have mainly been investigated among immigrant groups in the USA [32] and there are few data regarding immigrants from Africa to Europe. In many non-Western and low-income countries, body fat is seen as an indicator of health and prosperity since only high-status individuals have the possibility to put on body weight because of the scarcity of food. Conversely, in many industrialized countries with food abundance, fatness is associated with poverty and poor health [33] while slimness is a sign of high economic status [101]. During the complex immigration process, everything that surrounds the person changes, including diet, social and family relationships, climate and culture [102]. Factors such as acculturation, enculturation, and socioeconomic status have a strong effect on many parameters, including weight status and perception of body size. For instance, African residents generally show a preference for heavier body size than their immigrant peers [103]. When more aligned with Western values, South African overweight/obese women wished to be thinner, whereas those who were still more aligned with the African values and with the idea that higher body weight is a positive factor were more satisfied with their body size [104].

31.2.5 Ethnic Differences in Drive for Muscularity

Little is known about ethnic differences in men's body image. Studies consistently show that men have significantly higher scores on measures of drive for muscularity compared to women [105] and higher drive for muscularity among men has been associated with a host of adverse outcomes, including lower self-esteem and life satisfaction, higher rates of anabolic steroid and supplement use, and greater symptoms of depression and body dysmorphic disorder [106]. Most research on drive for muscularity has focused on men in Western cultures [107], but emerging work has examined cross-cultural differences as well [108, 109].

In a socio-political context wherein muscularity symbolizes dominance and power [110], drive for muscularity may be a means of negotiating masculine ideals and countering a perceived lower status through the development of muscle mass [110, 111]. Studies that have specifically examined ethnic differences in drive for muscularity within singular national contexts have produced mixed results. The majority of research about body image among ethnic minority men has been performed in North America, and findings from North America may not be exactly mirrored in other national settings [11]. A study in men from the community in Greater London (White, Black British, and South Asian) found ethnic minority groups—specifically Black British and South Asian British men—showing greater drive for muscularity compared with White ones [15]. Asian-American identity was a significant predictor of muscle dissatisfaction [112] and higher drive for muscularity [113]. It might not be ethnic minority status per se that contributes to higher risk of drive for muscularity, but rather the specific experience of Asian ancestry [107, 114, 115]: Asian men typically have smaller body frames and may be perceived as less masculine compared to African American and White men. Asian men may also experience competing pressures to conform to masculine and muscular ideals, on the one hand, and traditional Asian values that run counter to the highly muscular and "macho" concept of Western masculinity [116].

31.3 Future Perspectives

Interventions to improve body image through reductions in thin-ideal internalization typically focus on changing patient's attitudes regarding their own body shape and weight, embracing positive body image approaches [117–119]. Positive body image is multi-faceted, including body appreciation, body acceptance, adaptive appearance investment, and filtering information in a manner that is protective to the self [120]. The availability of local data on body image perception is essential to plan health strategies and to support noncommunicable disease management. Besides, future research should examine how personality dimensions and social relationships may contribute to weight stigma. As evidence suggests that culturally adapted interventions may lead to improved treatment outcomes [121], understanding these differences may aid in the continued evolution of culturally sensitive interventions. One option such as assessing and targeting family pressure may prove particularly beneficial for Black women, while an emphasis on both family and media pressures may particularly benefit Hispanic women. White women may benefit from an approach addressing all three sources of pressure. Interventions should be culturally adapted to more readily respond to the unique characteristics of women from diverse cultural backgrounds [21].

References

1. Loth KA, MacLehose R, Bucchianeri M, Crow S, Neumark-Sztainer D. Predictors of dieting and disordered eating behaviors from adolescence to young adulthood. J Adolesc Health. 2014;55(5):705–12.
2. Crago M, Shisslak CM, Estes LS. Eating disturbances among American minority groups: a review. Int J Eat Disord. 1996;19(3):239–48.
3. Pate JE, Pumariega AJ, Hester C, Garner DM. Cross-cultural patterns in eating disorders: a review. J Am Acad Child Adolesc Psychiatry. 1992;31(5):802–9.
4. Wildes JE, Emery RE, Simons AD. The roles of ethnicity and culture in the development of eating disturbance and body dissatisfaction: a meta-analytic review. Clin Psychol Rev. 2001;21(4):521–51.
5. Miller MN, Pumariega AJ. Culture and eating disorders: a historical and cross-cultural review. Psychiatry. 2001;64(2):93–110.
6. Swartz L. Anorexia nervosa as a culture-bound syndrome. Soc Sci Med. 1985;20(7):725–30.
7. Bonafini BA, Pozzilli P. Body weight and beauty: the changing face of the ideal female body weight. Obes Rev. 2011;12(1):62–5.
8. Keel PK, Klump KL. Are eating disorders culture-bound syndromes? Implications for conceptualizing their etiology. Psychol Bull. 2003;129(5):747–69.
9. American Psychiatric Association. Diagnostic and statistical manual of mental disorders. 5th ed. Arlington: American Psychiatric Association; 2013.
10. Webb JB, Warren-Findlow J, Chou YY, Adams L. Do you see what I see? An exploration of inter-ethnic ideal body size comparisons among college women. Body Image. 2013;10(3):369–79.
11. Swami V, Airs N, Chouhan B, Padilla Leon MA, Towell T. Are there ethnic differences in positive body image among female British undergraduates? Eur Psychol. 2009;14:288–96.
12. Shaw H, Ramirez L, Trost A, Randall P, Stice E. Body image and eating disturbances across ethnic groups: more similarities than differences. Psychol Addict Behav. 2004;18(1):12–8.
13. White EK, Warren CS. Body checking and avoidance in ethnically diverse female college students. Body Image. 2013;10(4):583–90.
14. Snapp S. Internalization of the thin ideal among low-income ethnic minority adolescent girls. Body Image. 2009;6(4):311–4.
15. Swami V. Masculinities and ethnicities: Ethnic differences in drive for muscularity in British men and the negotiation of masculinity hierarchies. Br J Psychol. 2016;107(3):577–92.
16. Thompson JK, Heinberg LJ, Altabe M, Tantleff-Dunn S. Exacting beauty: theory, assessment, and treatment of body image. Washington, DC: American Psychological Association; 1999.
17. Stice E, Nemeroff C, Shaw HE. Test of the dual pathway model of bulimia nervosa: evidence for dietary restraint and affect regulation mechanisms. J Soc Clin Psychol. 1996;15(3):340–63.
18. Culbert KM, Racine SE, Klump KL. Research review: what have we learned about the causes of eating disorders—a synthesis of sociocultural, psychological, and biological research. J Child Psychol Psychiatry. 2015;56(11):1141–64.
19. Rogers Wood NA, Petrie TA. Body dissatisfaction, ethnic identity, and disordered eating among African American women. J Couns Psychol. 2010;57(2):141–53.

20. Stice E, Shaw HE. Role of body dissatisfaction in the onset and maintenance of eating pathology: a synthesis of research findings. J Psychosom Res. 2002;53(5):985–93.
21. Ordaz DL, Schaefer LM, Choquette E, Schueler J, Wallace L, Thompson JK. Thinness pressures in ethnically diverse college women in the United States. Body Image. 2017;24:1–4.
22. Rodgers RF. The role of the "Healthy Weight" discourse in body image and eating concerns: an extension of sociocultural theory. Eat Behav. 2016;22:194–8.
23. Paeratakul S, White MA, Williamson DA, Ryan DH, Bray GA. Sex, race/ethnicity, socioeconomic status, and BMI in relation to self-perception of overweight. Obes Res. 2002;10(5):345–50.
24. Mama SK, Quill BE, Fernandez-Esquer ME, Reese-Smith JY, Lee RE. Body image and physical activity among Latina and African American women. Ethn Dis. 2011;21(3): 281–7.
25. Gillen MM, Lefkowitz ES. Gender and racial/ethnic differences in body image development among college students. Body Image. 2012;9(1):126–30.
26. Brown SR, Hossain MB, Bronner Y. African American male and female student perceptions of pulvers body images: implications for obesity, health care, and prevention. J Health Care Poor Underserved. 2014;25(3):1328–40.
27. Ng M, Fleming T, Robinson M, Thomson B, Graetz N, Margono C, Mullany EC, Biryukov S, Abbafati C, Abera SF, Abraham JP, Abu-Rmeileh NM, et al. Global, regional, and national prevalence of overweight and obesity in children and adults during 1980–2013: a systematic analysis for the Global Burden of Disease Study 2013. Lancet. 2014;384(9945):766–81.
28. Swami V, Frederock DA, Aavik T, Alcalay L, Allik J, Anderson D, Andrianto S, Arora A, Brännström A, Cunningham J, Danel D, Doroszewicz K, et al. The attractive female body weight and female body dissatisfaction in 26 countries across 10 world regions: results of the international body project I. Pers Soc Psychol Bull. 2010;36(3):309–25.
29. Gualdi-Russo E, Zaccagni L, Manzon VS, Masotti S, Rinaldo N, Khyatti M. Obesity and physical activity in children of immigrants. Eur J Pub Health. 2014;24(Suppl 1):40–6.
30. Pampel FC, Krueger PM, Denney JT. Socioeconomic disparities in health behaviors. Annu Rev Sociol. 2010;36:349–70.
31. Joh HK, Oh J, Lee HJ, Kawachi I. Gender and socioeconomic status in relation to weight perception and weight control behavior in Korean adults. Obes Facts. 2013;6:17–27.
32. Delavari M, Sønderlund AL, Swinburn B, Mellor D, Renzaho A. Acculturation and obesity among migrant populations in high income countries—a systematic review. BMC Public Health. 2013;13:458.
33. Tlili F, Mahjoub A, Lefevre P, Bellaj T, Romdhane HB, Eymard-Durvernay S, et al. Tunisian women's perception of desicerable body size and chronic disease risk. Ecol Food Nutr. 2008;47(4):399–414.
34. Crandall CS. Prejudice against fat people: ideology and self-interest. J Pers Soc Psychol. 1994;66:882–94.
35. Wang SS, Brownell KD, Wadden TA. The influence of the stigma of obesity on overweight individuals. Int J Obes. 2004;28:1333–7.
36. Schwartz MB, Vartanian LR, Nosek BA, Brownell KD. The influence of one's own body weight on implicit and explicit anti-fat beliefs. Obesity. 2006;14:440–7.
37. Hebl M, King EB, Perkins A. Ethnic differences in the stigma of obesity: identification and engagement with a thin ideal. J Exp Soc Psychol. 2009;45:1165–72.
38. Pepper AC, Ruiz SY. Acculturation's influence on antifat attitudes, body image, and eating behaviors. Eat Disord. 2007;15:427–47.
39. Neumark-Sztainer D, Croll J, Story M, Hannan PJ, French SA, Perry C. Ethnic/racial differences in weight-related concerns and behaviors among adolescent girls and boys: findings from Project EAT. J Psychosom Res. 2002;53(5):963–74.
40. Asia Pacific Cohort Study Collaboration. Cholesterol, diabetes and major cardiovascular diseases in Asia Pacific region. Diabetologia. 2007;50(11):2289–97.
41. Brewis AA, Wutich A, Falletta-Cowden A, Rodriguez-Soto I. Body norms and fat stigma in global perspective. Curr Anthropol. 2011;52(2):269–76.

42. Markus HR, Kitayama S. Culture and the self: implications for cognition, emotion and motivation. Psychol Rev. 1991;98(2):224–53.
43. Dryer R, Uesaka Y, Manalo E, Tyson G. Cross-cultural examination of beliefs about the causes of bulimia nervosa among Australian and Japanese females. Int J Eat Disord. 2015;48(2):176–86.
44. Triandis HC. Individualism-collectivism and personality. J Pers. 2001;69(6):907–24.
45. Katzman MA, Lee S. Beyond body image: the integration of feminist and transcultural theories in the understanding of self starvation. Int J Eat Disord. 1997;22(4):385–94.
46. Annunziato RA, Lee JN, Lowe MR. A comparison of weight-control behaviors in African American and Caucasian women. Ethn Dis. 2007;17(2):262–7.
47. Tovée MJ, Swami V, Furnham A, Mangalparsad R. Changing perceptions of attractiveness as observers are exposed to a different culture. Evol Hu Behav. 2006;27:443–56.
48. Striegel-Moore RH, Wilfley DE, Caldwell MB, Needham ML, Brownell KD. Weight-related attitudes and behaviors of women who diet to lose weight: a comparison of Black dieters and White dieters. Obes Res. 1996;4(2):109–16.
49. McKnight Risk Factor Study. Ethnic group differences in disordered eating attitudes and behaviors and related risk factors. In: Paper presented at the Ninth International Conference on Eating Disorders; 2000.
50. Quick VM, Byrd-Bredbenner C. Disordered eating, socio-cultural media influencers, body image, and psychological factors among a racially/ethnically diverse population of college women. Eat Behav. 2014;15(1):37–41.
51. Bardone-Cone AM, Harney MB, Sayen L. Perceptions of parental attitudes toward body and eating: associations with body image among Black and White college women. Body Image. 2011;8(2):186–9.
52. Baker CW, Whisman MA, Brownell KD. Studying intergenerational transmission of eating attitudes and behaviors: methodological and conceptual questions. Health Psychol. 2000;19(4):376–81.
53. Rodgers R, Chabrol H. Parental attitudes, body image disturbance and disordered eating amongst adolescents and young adults: a review. Eur Eat Disord Rev. 2009;17(2):137–51.
54. Wertheim EH, Martin G, Prior M, Sanson A, Smart D. Parent influences in the transmission of eating and weight related values and behaviors. Eat Disord. 2002;10(4):321–34.
55. Thompson SH, Sargent RG. Black and white women's weight-related attitudes and parental criticism of their childhood appearance. Women Health. 2000;30(3):77–92.
56. Brown KM, Schreiber GB, McMahon RP, Crawford P, Ghee KL. Maternal influences on body satisfaction in black and white girls aged 9 and 10: the NHLBI Growth and Health Study (NGHS). Ann Behav Med. 1995;17(3):213–20.
57. Lynch E, Liu K, Spring B, Hankinson A, Wei GS, Greenland P. Association of ethnicity and socioeconomic status with judgments of body size: the Coronary Artery Risk Development in Young Adults (CARDIA) Study. Am J Epidemiol. 2007;165(9):1055–62.
58. Altabe M. Ethnicity and body image: quantitative and qualitative analysis. Int J Eat Disord. 1998;23(2):153–9.
59. Smith DE, Thompson JK, Raczynski JM, Hilner JE. Body image among men and women in a biracial cohort: the CARDIA study. Int J Eat Disord. 1999;25(1):71–82.
60. Schuler PB, Vinci D, Isosaari RM, Philipp SF, Todorovich J, Roy JL, Evans RR. Body-shape perceptions and body mass index of older African American and European American women. J Cross Cult Gerontol. 2008;23(3):255–64.
61. Wilfley DE, Schreiber GB, Pike KM, Striegel-Moore RH, Wright DJ, Rodin J. Eating disturbance and body image: a comparison of a community sample of adult black andwhite women. Int J Eat Disord. 1996;20(4):377–87.
62. Lynch E, Liu K, Wei GS, Spring B, Kiefe C, Greenland P. The relation between body size perception and change in body mass index over 13 years. Am J Epidemiol. 2009;169(7):857–66.
63. Swanson SA, Crow SJ, Le Grange D, Swendsen J, Merikangas KR. Prevalence and correlates of eating disorders in adolescents: results from the national comorbidity survey replication adolescent supplement. Arch Gen Psychiatry. 2011;68(7):714–23.

64. Striegel-Moore RH, Dohm FA, Kraemer HC, Taylor CB, Daniels S, Crawford PB, Schreiber GB. Eating disorders in white and black women. Am J Psychiatry. 2003;160(7):1326–31.
65. Rucker CE, Cash TF. Body images, body-size perceptions, and eating behaviors among African-American and white college women. Int J Eat Disord. 1992;12:291–9.
66. Flegal KM, Carroll MD, Ogden CL, Curtin LR. Prevalence and trends in obesity among US adults, 1999-2008. JAMA. 2010;303:235–41.
67. Ogden CL, Lamb MM, Carroll MD, Flegal KM. Obesity and socioeconomic status in adults: United States 1988–1994 and 2005–2008. NCHS Data Brief. 2010;50:1–8.
68. Chang VW, Christakis NA. Extent and determinants of discrepancy between self-evaluations of weight status and clinical standards. J Gen Intern Med. 2001;16(8):538–43.
69. Chang VW, Christakis NA. Selfperception of weight appropriateness in the United States. Am J Prev Med. 2003;24(4):332–9.
70. Bennett GG, Wolin KY. Satisfied or unaware? Racial differences in perceived weight status. Int J Behav Nutr Phys Act. 2006;3:40.
71. Dorsey RR, Eberhardt MS, Ogden CL. Racial/ethnic differences in weight perception. Obesity. 2009;17(4):790–5.
72. Hendley Y, Zhao L, Coverson DL, Din-Dzietham R, Morris A, Quyyumi AA, Gibbons GH, Vaccarino V. Differences in weight perception among blacks and whites. J Womens Health. 2011;20(12):1805–11.
73. Powell TM, De Lemos JA, Banks K, Ayers CR, Rohatgi A, Khera A, McGuire DK, Berry JD, Albert MA, Vega GL, Grundy SM, Das SR. Body size misperception: a novel determinant in the obesity epidemic. Arch Intern Med. 2010;170(18):1695–7.
74. Dorsey RR, Eberhardt MS, Ogden CL. Racial and ethnic differences in weight management behavior by weight perception status. Ethn Dis. 2010;20(3):244–50.
75. Parker S, Nichter M, Nichter M, Vuckovic N, Sims C, Ritenbaugh C. Body image and weight concerns among African American and White adolescent females: differences that make a difference. Hum Organ. 1995;54(2):103–14.
76. Hedley AA, Ogden CL, Johnson CL, Carroll MD, Curtin LR, Flegal KM. Prevalence of overweight and obesity among US children, adolescents, and adults, 1999–2002. JAMA. 2004;291(23):2847–50.
77. Lee S, Lee AM. Disordered eating in three communities of China: a comparative study of female high school students in Hong Kong, Shenzhen, and rural Hunan. Int J Eat Disord. 2000;27(3):317–27.
78. Pike KM, Borovoy A. The rise of eating disorders in Japan: issues of culture and limitations of the model of 'Westernization'. Cult Med Psychiatry. 2004;28(4):493–531.
79. Kowner R. When ideals are too "far off": physical self-ideal discrepancy and body dissatisfaction in Japan. Genet Psychol Monogr. 2004;130(4):333–61.
80. Nishizawa Y, Kida K, Nishizawa K, Hasiba S, Saito K, Mita R. Perception of self-physique and eating behaviour of high school students in Japan. Psychiat Clin Neurosci. 2003;57(2):189–96.
81. Mukai T, Kambara A, Sasaki Y. Body dissatisfaction, need for social approval, and eating disturbances among Japanese and American college women. Sex Roles. 1998;39(9–10):751–63.
82. Smith AR, Joiner TE. Examining body image discrepancies and perceived weight status in adult Japanese women. Eat Behav. 2008;9(4):513–5.
83. Stark-Wroblewski K, Yanico BJ, Lupe S. Acculturation, internalization of Western appearance norms, and eating pathology among Japanese and Chinese international student women. Psychol Women Q. 2005;29(1):38–46.
84. Yamamiya Y, Shroff H, Thompson JK. The tripartite influence model of body image and eating disturbance: a replication with a Japanese sample. Int J Eat Disord. 2008;41(1):88–91.
85. Chisuwa N, O'Dea JA. Body image and eating disorders amongst Japanese adolescents: a review of the literature. Appetite. 2010;54(1):5–15.
86. Yasuhara D, Homan N, Nagai N, Naruo T, Komaki G, Nakao K, Nozoe S. A significant nationwide increase in the prevalence of eating disorders in Japan: 1998-year survey. Int Congr Ser. 2002;1241:297–301.

87. Nishizono-Maher A. Eating disorders in Japan: finding the right context. Psychiat Clin Neurosci. 1998;52:S320–3.
88. Malik SC. Eating disorders. In: Vyas JN, Ahuja N, editors. Postgraduate society. New Delhi: B. I. Churchill Livingstone; 1992. p. 260–79.
89. Makino M, Tsuboi K, Dennerstein L. Prevalence of eating disorders: a comparison of Western and non-Western countries. MedGenMed. 2004;6(3):49.
90. Mammen P, Russell S, Russell PS. Prevalence of eating disorders and psychiatric comorbidity among children and adolescents. Indian Pediatr. 2007;44(5):357–9.
91. Mendhekar DN, Mehta R, Srivastav PK. Bulimia nervosa. Indian J Pediatr. 2004;71(9):861–2.
92. Khandelwal SK, Sharan P, Saxena S. Eating disorders: an Indian perspective. Int J Soc Psychiatry. 1995;41(2):132–46.
93. Mendhekar DN, Arora K, Lohia D, Aggarwal A, Jiloha RC. Anorexia nervosa: an Indian perspective. Natl Med J India. 2009;22(4):181–2.
94. Tareen A, Hodes M, Rangel L. Non-fat-phobic anorexia nervosa in British South Asian adolescents. Int J Eat Disord. 2005;37(2):161–5.
95. Mumford DB, Whitehouse AM, Platts M. Sociocultural correlates of eating disorders among Asian schoolgirls in Bradford. Br J Psychiatry. 1991;158:222–8.
96. Gupta MA, Chaturvedi SK, Chandarana PC, Johnson AM. Weight-related body image concerns among 18-24-year-old women in Canada and India: an empirical comparative study. J Psychosom Res. 2001;50(4):193–8.
97. Rubin B, Gluck ME, Knoll CM, Lorence M, Geliebter A. Comparison of eating disorders and body image disturbances between Eastern and Western countries. Eat Weight Disord. 2008;13(2):73–80.
98. Walker AR, Walker BF, Locke MM, Cassim FA, Molefe O. Body image and eating behaviour in interethnic adolescent girls. J R Soc Health. 1991;111(1):12–6.
99. Nicolau M, Benjelloun S, Stronks K, van Dam RM, Seidell JC, Doak CM. Influences on body weight of female Moroccan migrants in the Netherlands: a qualitative study. Health Place. 2012;18(4):883–91.
100. Swami V, Tovée MJ. Female physical attractiveness in Britain and Malaysia: a cross-cultural study. Body Image. 2005;2(2):115–28.
101. Bush HM, Williams RG, Lean ME, Anderson AS. Body image and weight consciousness among South Asian, Italian and general population women in Britain. Appetite. 2001;37(3):207–15.
102. Toselli S, Gualdi Russo E, Marzouk D, Sundquist J, Sundquist K. Psychosocial health among immigrants in Central and Southern Europe. Eur J Pub Health. 2014;24(Suppl 1):26–30.
103. Toselli S, Rinaldo N, Gualdi-Russo E. Body image perception of African immigrants in Europe. Global Health. 2016;12(1):48.
104. Soh NL-W, Walter G. Publications on cross-cultural aspects of eating disorders. J Eat Disord. 2013;1:4.
105. McCreary DR, Saucier DM. Drive for muscularity, body comparison, and social physique anxiety in men and women. Body Image. 2009;6(1):24–30.
106. McCreary DR. Muscularity and body image. In: Cash TF, editor. Encyclopedia of body image and human appearance, vol. 2. San Diego, CA: Academic Press; 2012. p. 561–7.
107. Ricciardelli LA, McCabe MP, Williams RJ, Thompson JK. The role of ethnicity and culture in body image and disordered eating among males. Clin Psychol Rev. 2007;27(5):582–606.
108. Jung J, Forbes GB, Chan P. Global body and muscle satisfaction among college men in the United States and Hong Kong-China. Sex Roles. 2010;63(1-2):104–17.
109. Campana ANNB, Tavares MCGCF, Swami V, da Silva D. An examination of the psychometric properties of Brazilian Portuguese translations of the Drive for Muscularity Scale, the Swansea Muscularity Attitudes Questionnaire, and the Masculine Body Ideal Distress Scale. Psychol Men Masc. 2013;14(4):376–88.
110. Swami V, Neofytou R-V, Jablonska J, Thirlwell H, Taylor D, McCreary DR. Social dominance orientation predicts drive for muscularity among British men. Body Image. 2013;10(4):653–6.

111. Swami V, Voracek M. Associations among men's sexist attitudes, objectification of women and their own drive for muscularity. Psychol Men Masc. 2013;14(2):168–74.
112. Grammas DL, Schwartz JP. Internalization of messages from society and perfectionism as predictors of male body image. Body Image. 2009;6(1):31–6.
113. Kelly NR, Cotter EE, Tanofsky-Kraff M, Mazzeo SE. Racial variations in binge eating, body image concerns, and compulsive exercise among men. Psychol Men Masc. 2015;16(3):326–36.
114. Yang CF, Gray P, Pope HG Jr. Male body image in Taiwan versus the West: Yanggang Zhiqi meets the Adonis complex. Am J Psychiatry. 2005;162(2):263–9.
115. Wilkins CL, Chan JF, Kaiser CR. Racial stereotypes and interracial attraction: phenotypic prototypicality and perceived attractiveness of Asians. Cultur Divers Ethnic Minor Psychol. 2011;17(4):427–31.
116. Pompper D. Masculinities, the metrosexual, and media images: across dimensions of age and ethnicity. Sex Roles. 2010;63(9–10):682–96.
117. Becker CB, Hill K, Greif R, Han H, Stewart T. Reducing self-objectification: are dissonance-based methods a possible approach? J Eat Disord. 2013;1:10.
118. Becker C, Smith LM, Ciao AC. Peer-facilitated eating disorder prevention: a randomized effectiveness trial of cognitive dissonance and media advocacy. J Counsel Psychol. 2006;53(4):550–5.
119. Stice E, Mazotti L, Weibel D, Agras WS. Dissonance prevention program decreases thin-ideal internalization, body dissatisfaction, dieting, negative affect, and bulimic symptoms: a preliminary experiment. Int J Eat Disord. 2000;27(2):206–17.
120. Tylka TL, Wood-Barcalow NL. What is and what is not positive body image? Conceptual foundations and construct definition. Body Image. 2015;14:118–29.
121. Hall GC, Ibaraki AY, Huang ER, Marti CN, Stice E. A meta-analysis of cultural adaptations of psychological interventions. Behav Ther. 2016;47(6):993–1014.

Printed by Printforce, the Netherlands